Policy and Politics in Nursing and Health Care
Third Edition

Diana J. Mason, PhD, RN, FAAN

Professor
Department of Graduate Studies
Lienhard School of Nursing
Pace University
Pleasantville and New York, New York

Partner
Transformations
New York, New York, and Brandon, Mississippi

Producer and Moderator
Healthstyles
WBAI-FM, Pacifica Radio
New York, New York

Judith K. Leavitt, MEd, RN, FAAN

Associate Professor
School of Nursing
University of Mississippi Medical Center
Jackson, Mississippi

Partner
Transformations
New York, New York, and Brandon, Mississippi

W.B. SAUNDERS COMPANY
A Division of Harcourt Brace & Company
Philadelphia London Toronto Montreal Sydney Tokyo

W.B. SAUNDERS COMPANY

A Division of Harcourt Brace & Company

The Curtis Center
Independence Square West
Philadelphia, Pennsylvania 19106

Library of Congress Cataloging-in-Publication Data

Policy and politics in nursing and health care / [edited by] Diana J.
    Mason, Judith K. Leavitt. — 3rd ed.
        p.   cm.
        Rev. ed. of: Policy and politics for nurses. 2nd. ed. c1993.
        Includes bibliographical references and index.
        ISBN 0-7216-7038-5
        1. Nurses—United States—Political activity.   2. Nursing—
Political aspects—United States.   3. Medical policy—United
States.   4. Medical care—Political aspects—United States.
I. Mason, Diana J.   II. Leavitt, Judith K. (Judith Kline)
III. Policy and politics for nurses.
        [DNLM: 1. Nursing.   2. Public Policy—United States.   3. Politics—
United States.   4. Delivery of Health Care—United States.   WY 16
P7662 1998]
RT86.5.P58   1998
362.1'73—dc21
DNLM/DLC
                                                                            98-21520

POLICY AND POLITICS IN NURSING AND HEALTH CARE   ISBN 0-7216-7038-5

Last digit is the print number: 9   8   7   6   5   4   3   2   1

ABOUT THE EDITORS

Diana J. Mason, PhD, RN, FAAN, is professor at the Lienhard School of Nursing, Pace University in New York City and Pleasantville, New York. She is co-founder and partner in Transformations, a consulting service to assist nurses and health care organizations in preparing for, designing, implementing, and evaluating strategies for change. She is a noted speaker and writer on policy and politics in nursing and health care. She has been a leader in professional nursing organizations on local, state, and national levels. She is co-producer and moderator of *Healthstyles,* a weekly, award-winning radio program on health matters that airs in the New York City metropolitan area. She is also a researcher, most recently focusing on health policy and health services research. She has received numerous awards, including the Lavinia Dock Award from the New York Counties Registered Nurses Association, the Legislative Award from the New York State Nurses Association, the Media Award from the National Association of Childbirthing Centers and from the Public Health Association of New York City, and fellowship in the American Academy of Nursing. She serves on the editorial board of the *American Journal of Nursing* and is a reviewer for several research journals in nursing and health care. She earned the BSN at West Virginia University, an MSN from St. Louis University, and the PhD from New York University.

Judith Kline Leavitt, MEd, RN, FAAN, is associate professor at the University of Mississippi Medical Center, School of Nursing. She is co-founder and partner in Transformations. She was formerly the Executive Director of Generations United, a national organization dedicated to intergenerational public policies and programs. She served on the National Advisory Council on Education and Practice for the Division of Nursing, U.S. Public Health Service. She was selected by President Clinton to serve on the Health Professional Advisory Group to the White House Task Force on Health Care Reform. She was also the upstate coordinator for Geraldine Ferraro's 1992 campaign for the U.S. Senate, chairperson of the American Nurses Association's Political Action Committee, chairperson of New York State Nurses for Political Action, and instrumental in the founding of the New York State Nurses Association's Political Action Committee. She is a noted speaker and author. Her many awards include the Chancellor's Award for Teaching Excellence from the State University of New York, the Health Policy Award from the Division of Nursing at New York University, the Legislative Award from the New York State Nurses Association, and fellowship in the American Academy of Nursing. She earned a BSN from the University of Pennsylvania and an MEd from Teacher's College, Columbia University.

Dedicated To

The Contributors to This Book
and All Nurses Who Make a Difference

CONTRIBUTORS

Sheila Abood, MS, RN

Associate Director, Federal Government Relations, American Nurses Association, Washington, District of Columbia
Legislative and Regulatory Processes

Jeanne Anselmo, BSN, RN

CoDirector, Holistic Nursing Associates; Consultant; Private Practice, New York, New York
Dancing with the Chaos: A Grassroots Approach to Transformation and Healing in Nursing

Mila Ann Aroskar, EdD, RN, FAAN

Associate Professor, School of Public Health, and Faculty Associate, Center for Bioethics, University of Minnesota, Minneapolis, Minnesota
Ethical Issues: Politics, Power, and Policy

Rosemary L. Auth, JD, MSN

Research Associate, Center for Health Services and Policy Research, University of Pennsylvania, Philadelphia, Pennsylvania
Dynamics of Public Policy: Community-based Practice Meets Managed Care

Barbara A. Backer, DSW, RN

Professor of Nursing, Lehman College, Bronx, New York
Feminist Perspectives on Policy and Politics

Susan Scoville Baker, PhD, RN, CS

Director and Associate Professor, Dr. F. M. Canseco School of Nursing, Texas A&M International University, Laredo, Texas
Contemporary Issues in the Community

Karen A. Ballard, MA, RN

Director, Nursing Practice and Services Program, New York State Nurses Association, Latham, New York
Nurses, Consumers, Activists, and the Politics of AIDS

Theresa L. Beck, MPA, RN, OCN

Vice President of Strategic Services, Visiting Nurse Association of Central Jersey, Red Bank, New Jersey
Working with the Community for Change

Geraldine Polly Bednash, PhD, RN, FAAN

Adjunct Professor, George Mason University, Fairfax, Virginia; Executive Director, American Association of Colleges of Nursing, Washington, District of Columbia
Federal Government

Andrea Berne, MPH, CPNP

Adjunct Faculty Member, Pace University and Hunter College, City University of New York; Nurse Practitioner, Private Practice, LaGuardia Place Pediatrics, New York, New York
Ensuring the Future of Nurse Practitioners in Clinical Practice

Virginia Trotter Betts, JD, MSN, RN, FAAN

Senior Advisor on Nursing Policy to the Secretary and Assistant Secretary for Health, United States Department of Health and Human Services, Washington, District of Columbia
Nursing and the Courts

Katherine McDermott Blackburn, MPA, RN, OCN

Senior Consultant, Ernst & Young, LLP, New York, New York
Oncology Nursing Society

Linda Burnes Bolton, DrPH, RN, FAAN

Vice President and Chief Nursing Officer, Cedars-Sinai Medical Center, Los Angeles, California
Transforming a Nursing Organization to Influence Public Policy: National Black Nurses Association

Elizabeth Bonham, MSN, CS, RN

Clinical Adjunct Professor, Indiana University; Family Support Services Program Director, Indiana Juvenile Justice Task Force, Indianapolis, Indiana; Past President, Association of Child and Adolescent Psychiatric Nurses (ACAPN), Philadelphia, Pennsylvania
Association of Child and Adolescent Psychiatric Nurses

Dorothy Brooten, PhD, RN, FAAN

Associate Dean for Research and Graduate Studies and John Burry Jr. Professor of Nursing, Case Western Reserve University, Cleveland, Ohio
The Politics of Nursing Research

Linda P. Brown, PhD, RN, FAAN

Miriam L. Stirl Professor in Nutrition, School of Nursing, University of Pennsylvania, Philadelphia, Pennsylvania
The Politics of Nursing Research

Virginia Burggraf, DNS, RN, C

Adjunct Faculty, George Mason University, Fairfax, Virginia; Grants Development Associate, American Nurses Foundation, Washington, District of Columbia
Affordable Long-term Care: Nursing Models of Care Delivery

Anna Marie Butrie, MSN, MPH

Senior Manager, Ernst & Young, New York, New York
Communicating and Collaborating for Change in the Workplace

Debra M. Campbell, MSN, RN

Political Director for the Psychiatrists' Political Action Committee, Washington, District of Columbia
Nursing Organizations in Action

Cecelia Capuzzi, PhD, RN

Professor in Community Health Care Systems Division and Chair of Population-based Nursing Department, Oregon Health Sciences University, Portland, Oregon
Rationing Health Care: The Oregon Story

Toni G. Cesta, PhD, RN

Director of Case Management Programs and Adjunct Professor, Pace University, Pleasantville, New York; Director of Case Management, St. Vincents Hospital and Medical Center, New York, New York
The Politics of Case Management

Mary Chaffee, BSN, BS, RN, CNA, CCRN, CEN

Commander, Nurse Corps, United States Navy
Political Activity and Government-employed Nurses

Theresa Chalich, MPH, RN

Health Care Director, Rainbow Health Center, Homestead, Pennsylvania
The Rainbow Kitchen: Developing a Neighborhood Health Center

Mary Ann Christopher, MSN, RNCS, FAAN

Executive Vice President and Chief Operating Officer, Visiting Nurse Association of Central Jersey, Red Bank, New Jersey
Working with the Community for Change

Sally S. Cohen, PhD, RN, FAAN

Assistant Professor and Director, Center for Health Policy, Yale University School of Nursing, New Haven, Connecticut
Political Analysis and Stategy; Lobbying Policymakers: Individual and Collective Strategies

Mary Beth Conroy, MPH

Program Research Specialist II—Health Systems, New York State Department of Health, Office of Managed Care, Albany, New York
The Economics of Health Care

Donna M. Costello-Nickitas, PhD, RN

Associate Professor, Hunter-Bellevue School of Nursing, Hunter College, City University of New York, New York, New York
Feminist Perspectives on Policy and Politics

Barbara Thoman Curtis, RN

Legislative Political Consultant, Washington, District of Columbia
Political Action Committees

Candy Dato, MS, RN

Assistant Professor, School of Nursing, Long Island University, Brooklyn, New York; Clinical Specialist, Lenox Hill Hospital, New York, New York
The American Voter: Political Campaigns and Nursing's Leadership

Judith S. Dempster, DNSc, NP-C, FNP

Chair, National Alliance of Nurse Practitioners, Washington, District of Columbia
National Alliance of Nurse Practitioners

Christine M. deVries, MA

Deputy Executive Director for Programs, American Nurses Association, Washington, District of Columbia
You and Your Professional Organization

Betty R. Dickson, BS

Executive Director and Lobbyist, Mississippi Nurses Association, Madison, Mississippi
Political Appointments

Donna Diers, MSN, RN, FAAN

Annie W. Goodrich Professor, School of Nursing; Lecturer, Department of Epidemiology and Public Health, School of Medicine, Yale University; Project Director, Nursing/Resource Information Management Systems (RIMS) Office, Yale New Haven Hospital, New Haven, Connecticut
Research as Policy/Political Tool

Joanne M. Disch, PhD, RN, FAAN

Adjunct Associate Professor, University of Minnesota School of Nursing; Vice President, Patient/Family Services, Fairview—University Medical Center, Minneapolis, Minnesota
The Healthy Work Environment as Core to an Organization's Success

Alma Yearwood Dixon, EdD, MPH, RN

Assistant Professor, Bethune-Cookman College, Daytona Beach, Florida
Conflict Management

Catherine J. Dodd, MS, RN

Lecturer, San Francisco State University, San Francisco, California; Executive Director, American Nurses Association—California
The Role of the Media in Influencing Policy: Getting the Message Across; Free Media Coverage: Using Letters (Messages) to the Editor; Political Parties

Diane Carlson Evans, RN

Chair and Founder, Vietnam Women's Memorial Project, Inc., Washington, District of Columbia
Moving a Vision: The Vietnam Women's Memorial

Suzanne Feetham, PhD, RN, FAAN

Professor and Harriet Werley Research Chair, College of Nursing, University of Illinois at Chicago, Chicago, Illinois; Chair, Policy Committee, Society of Pediatric Nurses
Society of Pediatric Nurses

Karen S. Fennell, MS, RN

Senior Policy Analyst, American College of Nurse-Midwives, Washington, District of Columbia
American College of Nurse-Midwives

Linda M. Finke, PhD, RN

Professor and Associate Dean for Graduate Programs, Indiana University, Indianapolis, Indiana; President, Association of Child and Adolescent Psychiatric Nurses (ACAPN), Philadelphia, Pennsylvania
Association of Child and Adolescent Psychiatric Nurses

Mary E. Foley, MS, RN

Director of Nursing/Chief Nurse Executive, Saint Francis Memorial Hospital, San Francisco, California
Collective Action in the Workplace

Patricia Ford-Roegner, MSW, RN, FAAN

Advisory Committee and Field Practicum Faculty, University of Georgia, Athens, Georgia; Faculty Advisor, Georgia State University; Regional Administrator, United States Department of Health and Human Services, Atlanta, Georgia
The American Voter: Political Campaigns and Nursing's Leadership

Eve Franklin, MSN, RN

Assistant Professor of Nursing, College of Nursing, Montana State University—Bozeman, Great Falls Campus, Great Falls, Montana; State Senator, Montana State Senate
Pilgrim in Politics

Terri Gaffney, MPA, RN

Director, State Government Relations, American Nurses Association, Washington, District of Columbia
State Government

Deborah B. Gardner, PhD, RN, CS

Adjunct faculty, Department of Nursing, George Mason University, Fairfax, Virginia; Health Care Consultant, Learningworks, Falls Church, Virginia
Contemporary Issues in Government

Elaine Gelman, BS, CPNP

Executive Director, New York State Coalition of Nurse Practitioners, Inc., Albany, New York
Ensuring the Future of Nurse Practitioners in Clinical Practice

C. Alicia Georges, MA, RN, FAAN

Lecturer, Lehman College of The City University of New York, Bronx, New York

Transforming a Nursing Organization to Influence Public Policy: National Black Nurses Association

Shirley Girouard, PhD, RN, FAAN

Vice President, Child Health and Financing, National Association of Children's Hospitals and Related Institutions, Alexandria, Virginia

Policy, Politics, and Foundations

Barbara Glickstein, MPH, MS, RN

Associate Director, The Program for Humanistic Health Care, Beth Israel Medical Center; Producer and Moderator, *Healthstyles*, WBAI-FM Pacifica Radio, New York, New York

The Role of the Media in Influencing Policy: Getting the Message Across

Jody Glittenberg, PhD, RN, HNC, FAAN

Professor of Nursing and Research Professor of Psychiatry and Anthropology, College of Nursing, The University of Arizona, Tucson, Arizona

The Power of Literacy

Suzanne Gordon, BA

Journalist and Author, Arly, Massachusetts; Cofounder, Nurses Network for a National Health Program

Afterword

Janet Gottschalk, DrPH, RN, FAAN

Visiting Professor, Canseco School of Nursing, Texas A&M International University, Laredo, Texas

Contemporary Issues in the Community

Hurdis M. Griffith, PhD, RN, FAAN

Dean and Professor, Rutgers College of Nursing, Newark, New Jersey

Developing and Implementing a Health Promotion Initiative

Sharron Guillett, PhD, RN

Associate Director, Child Health and Finance, National Association of Children's Hospitals and Related Institutions, Alexandria, Virginia

Contemporary Issues in Government

Mary R. Haack, PhD, RN, FAAN

Senior Research Staff Scientist, The George Washington University Center for Health Policy Research, Washington, District of Columbia

Impact of the New Welfare Law on Child Health

Barbara E. Hanley, PhD, RN

Assistant Professor, Nursing–Health Policy Program, University of Maryland School of Nursing, Baltimore, Maryland

Policy Development and Analysis

Mary Ellen Hatfield, MN, RN

Adjunct Faculty, College of Nursing, University of South Carolina; State School Health Nurse Consultant, South Carolina Department of Health and Environmental Control, Columbia, South Carolina

National Association of State School Nurse Consultants

Terri Havill, RN, RPN

Vancouver Pretrial Services Center, Vancouver, British Columbia

Blowing the Whistle

Pamela J. Haylock, MA, RN

President, Oncology Nursing Society (1997–1998), and Cancer Care Consultant, Kerrville, Texas

Oncology Nursing Society

Janet Heinrich, DrPH, RN, FAAN

Director, American Academy of Nursing, Washington, District of Columbia

Organization and Delivery of Health Care in the United States: The Health Care System That Isn't

G. Brockwel Heylin, JD, LLM

Director of Government Affairs, American Association of Colleges of Nursing, Washington, District of Columbia

Federal Government

Melinda Jenkins, PhD, RN, CS

Assistant Professor of Primary Care and Director, Family Nurse Practitioner Program, School of Nursing, University of Pennsylvania; Family Nurse Practitioner, Abbottsford Community Health Center, Philadelphia, Pennsylvania

Dynamics of Public Policy: Community-based Practice Meets Managed Care

Anie Kalayjian, EdD, DDL, RN, C

Adjunct Professor, Fordham University, New York, New York, and College of New Rochelle, New Rochelle, New York; Treasurer, United Nations Non-Governmental Organization, Human Rights Committee; President, International Society for Traumatic Stress Studies, New York Chapter; Co-chair, World Federation for Mental Health, Human Rights Committee

The Fourth World Conference on Women: The Road to Beijing and Beyond

David Keepnews, JD, MPH, RN

Consultant in health policy and law, Boston, Massachusetts

Ensuring the Future of Nurses in Clinical Practice: Issues and Strategies for Staff Nurses and Advanced Practice Nurses; Nursing and the Courts

Karren Kowalski, PhD, RN, FAAN

Associate Professor, and Chairperson, Department of Maternal Child Nursing, Rush College of Nursing; Assistant Vice President and Administrator, Women's and Children's Hospital, Rush–Presbyterian–St. Luke's Medical Center, Chicago, Illinois

Strategies for Change in the Workplace

Franklin N. Laufer, PhD

Research Assistant Professor, Center for Policy Research, Rockefeller College of Public Affairs and Policy, State University of New York at Albany; Program Manager, Bureau of Health Economics, New York State Department of Health, Albany, New York

The Economics of Health Care

Judith K. Leavitt, MEd, RN, FAAN

Associate Professor, School of Nursing, University of Mississippi Medical Center, Jackson, Mississippi

Policy and Politics: A Framework for Action; Political Analysis and Strategy; Coalitions for Action; Rising to the Top: An Interview with Sheila Burke

Margaret A. Leonard, MS, RN, C, FNP, Cm

Adjunct Faculty, College of New Rochelle, New Rochelle, New York; Vice President of Clinical Services, Westchester Prepaid Health Service Plan, Inc., Tarrytown, New York; Producer and Host, *Community Nurse On-Call*, WBAU, 90.3 FM, New York, New York

One Nurse's Perspective on Managed Care

Mary Alice Leonhardt, JD, BSN

Member, Brown, Rudnick, Freed & Gesmer, P.C., Hartford, Connecticut; Lobbyist, Connecticut Nurses' Association, Meriden, Connecticut

Political Analysis and Strategy

Sandra Beth Lewenson, EdD, RN

Associate Professor and Associate Dean of the Graduate Program, Lienhard School of Nursing, Pace University, Pleasantville, New York

Historical Overview: Policy, Politics, and Nursing

Phyllis J. Lewis, MSN, RN

Coordinator of Health Programs, Indiana Department of Education, Indianapolis, Indiana

National Association of State School Nurse Consultants

Kae Livsey, MPH, RN

Associate, American College of Healthcare Executives; Member, American Society of Association Executives, Atlanta, Georgia

American Association of Occupational Health Nurses

Ruth Watson Lubic, EdD, RN, CNM, FAAN

Adjunct Professor, School of Nursing, Georgetown University, Washington, District of Columbia, and Division of Nursing, School of Education, New York University, New York, New York; Project Director, Project NACC Foundation, Washington, District of Columbia

The Community and Childbearing Centers

Barbara Lumpkin, BS, RN

Associate Executive Director, Florida Nurses Association, Orlando, Florida

Political Action Committees

Bonnie Mackey, MSN, ARNP, CMT, CHN

Adjunct Professor, School of Nursing—Graduate Level, Florida International University, North Miami, Florida; Owner, Director, Mackey Health Institute, Inc.; Clinical Advanced Registered Nurse Director, Complementary HealthCare Center, North Shore Hospital, Miami, Florida; Vice President, National Association of Nurse Massage Therapists, Durham, North Carolina

National Association of Nurse Massage Therapists

Diane Mahoney, PhD, RN, CS

Director of Nursing Research, Research and Training Institute, Hebrew Rehabilitation Center for the Aged, Boston, Massachusetts
Health Care Financing

Judith A. Maire, MN, RN

Health Services Supervisor, Office of the Superintendent of Public Instruction, Olympia, Washington
National Association of State School Nurse Consultants

Juanita V. Majewski, BSN, RN

School Nurse, Eden Central School District, Eden, New York; Board of Trustees, New York State Nurses Association Political Action Committee, Latham, New York
Local Government

Beverly L. Malone, PhD, RN, FAAN

Professor, School of Nursing, North Carolina A&T State University, Greensboro, North Carolina; President, American Nurses Association, Washington, District of Columbia
Ensuring the Future of Nurses in Clinical Practice: Issues and Strategies for Staff Nurses and Advanced Practice Nurses

Diana J. Mason, PhD, RN, FAAN

Professor, Department of Graduate Studies, Lienhard School of Nursing, Pace University, Pleasantville and New York, New York; Producer and Moderator, *Healthstyles*, WBAI-FM, Pacifica Radio, New York, New York
Policy and Politics: A Framework for Action; Feminist Perspectives on Policy and Politics; Political Analysis and Strategy; The Role of the Media in Influencing Policy: Getting the Message Across

Angela Barron McBride, PhD, RN, FAAN

Distinguished Professor and Dean, Indiana University School of Nursing, Indianapolis, Indiana
Feminist Perspectives on Policy and Politics

Judith L. Miller, MS, RN

Director of Primary Care and Public Health, Visiting Nurse Association of Central Jersey, Red Bank, New Jersey
Working with the Community for Change

Susan M. Miovech, PhD, RNC

Assistant Professor of Nursing, Rutgers, The State University of New Jersey, College of Nursing, Newark, New Jersey; Staff nurse, Temple University–Lower Bucks Hospital, Bristol, Pennsylvania
The Politics of Nursing Research

Pamela Mittelstadt, MPH, RN

Associate Vice President of Quality Management, PHP Healthcare Corporation, Reston, Virginia
Legislative and Regulatory Processes

Lillian H. Mood, MPH, RN, FAAN

Adjunct Faculty, College of Nursing, School of Public Health, University of South Carolina, Columbia; Director of Risk Communication and Community Liaison, South Carolina Department of Health and Environment Control, Columbia, South Carolina
Environmental Health Policy: Environmental Justice

Nancy E. Mooney, MA, RN, ONC

Director of Patient Care Services, Beth Israel Medical Center, North Division, New York, New York; Past President, National Association of Orthopedic Nurses, Pitman, New Jersey
National Association of Orthopaedic Nurses

Suzanne Moore, PhD, RN

Associate Adjunct Professor, Columbia University School of Nursing, New York, New York; Director, Bureau of Health Economics, New York State Department of Health, Albany, New York
The Economics of Health Care

Hank Nowoholnik, MBA

Principal, The Huntington Group, IDX Systems, Inc., Boston, Massachusetts
Communicating and Collaborating for Change in the Workplace

Marjory C. O'Brien, MS, RN

Legislative Analyst, New York State Assembly, Albany, New York
Local Government

Jeffrey P. O'Donnell, MS, RN, FNP

Adjunct Instructor and Systems Analyst, Center for Nursing Research, Clinical Practice, and International Affairs, Lienhard School of Nursing, Pace University, Pleasantville, New York
Internships in Policy and Politics

Jane B. Pinsky, BA

Political and Legislative Consultant, Raleigh, North Carolina
Coalitions for Action

Sallie Porter, MS, RN

Director, Society of Pediatric Nurses Policy Committee; Hudson Cradle, A Home for Infants, Jersey City, New Jersey
Society of Pediatric Nurses

Tim Porter-O'Grady, EdD, PhD, FAAN

Assistant Professor, Emory University; Senior Partner, Tim Porter-O'Grady Associates Inc.; Senior Consultant, Affiliated Dynamics Inc., Atlanta, Georgia
Contemporary Issues in the Workplace: A Glimpse Over the Horizon into the New Age of Health Care

Belinda E. Puetz, PhD, RN

Puetz and Associates, Inc., Pensacola, Florida
Networking

Joyce Pulcini, PhD, RN, CS

Associate Professor, Hunter-Bellevue School of Nursing, City University of New York, New York, New York
Health Care Financing

Joanne W. Rains, DNS, RN

Dean of Nursing and Associate Professor, Indiana University East, Richmond, Indiana
Managing a Campaign

Susan C. Reinhard, PhD, RN, FAAN

Assistant Professor, Rutgers University College of Nursing, Newark, New Jersey; Deputy Commissioner, New Jersey Department of Health and Senior Services, Trenton, New Jersey
Lobbying Policymakers: Individual and Collective Strategies

Anne M. Rhome, MPH, RN

Director, Member Education, American Association of Colleges of Nursing
Federal Government; American Association of Colleges of Nursing

Judy Biros Robson, MSN, RN

State Representative, Wisconsin Legislature, State Assembly, 45th Assembly District
One Nurse's Journey to Becoming a Policymaker

Candace L. Romig, MA, RN

Legislative Program Coordinator, Association of Operating Room Nurses, Denver, Colorado
Association of Operating Room Nurses

Pauline M. Seitz, MS, MPA, RN

National Program Director, Robert Wood Johnson Foundations Local Initiatives Funding Partners Program and New Jersey Health Initiatives, Health Research and Educational Trust of New Jersey, Princeton, New Jersey
Policy, Politics, and Foundations

Judy Sheridan-Gonzalez, BS, RN, CEN

Staff Nurse, Emergency Department, Montefiore Medical Center, Bronx, New York; Chairperson, Council of Nursing Practitioners (Montefiore), and Member, Delegate Assembly, New York State Nurses Association
Every Patient Deserves a Nurse

Linda J. Shinn, MBA, RN, CAE

Principal, Consensus Management Group, Fairfax Station, Virginia
Networking; Contemporary Issues in Professional Organizations

Betty J. Skaggs, PhD, RN

Assistant Professor of Clinical Nursing and Director, Learning Center, The University of Texas at Austin School of Nursing, Austin, Texas
You and Your Professional Organization

Gloria Smith, PhD, RN, FAAN

Vice President—Programs, W. K. Kellogg Foundation, Battle Creek, Michigan
Introduction

Kathleen T. Smith, BS, RN, CNN

Director of Legislative Services, *Nursing Economic$*, Washington, District of Columbia
American Nephrology Nurses Association; National Federation for Specialty Nursing Organizations: Nurse in Washington Internship

Sandra R. Smoley, BSN

Secretary, California Health and Welfare Agency, Sacramento, California
Political Parties

Julie Sochalski, PhD, RN, FAAN

Assistant Professor of Health Services Research and Nursing and Associate Director, Center for Health Services and Policy Research, University of Pennsylvania, Philadelphia, Pennsylvania
Dynamics of Public Policy: Community-based Practice Meets Managed Care

David O. Sprouse, EdD, RN

President-Elect, American Assembly for Men in Nursing, Brooklyn, New York
American Assembly for Men in Nursing

Lisa Summers, MSN, CNM

Senior Technical Advisor, Professional Services, American College of Nurse-Midwives, Washington, District of Columbia
The Community and Childbearing Centers

Linda Tarr-Whelan, MS, RN

United States Ambassador to United Nations Commission on the Status of Women; President, Center for Policy Alternatives, Washington, District of Columbia
From Bedside to Beijing

Betsy Todd, MPH, RN

Adjunct Lecturer, Hunter-Bellevue School of Nursing, City University of New York; School Nurse, Trevor Day School, New York, New York
The Ad Hoc Committee to Defend Health Care: A Collaborative Nurse-Physician Effort

Sue M. Towey, MS, RN, CS, LP

Lecturer, Psychiatric–Mental Health Nursing, University of Minnesota School of Nursing; Community Associate, Center for Spirituality and Healing, University of Minnesota Academic Health Center; Minneapolis, Minnesota; Project Coordinator, Nursing Administration, Methodist Hospital, St. Louis Park, Minnesota
The Healthy Work Environment as Core to an Organization's Success

Peter J. Ungvarski, MS, RN, ACRN, FAAN

Clinical Nurse Specialist, HIV Infection; Clinical Director, AIDS Services, Visiting Nurse Service of New York, New York, New York
Nurses, Consumers, Activists, and the Politics of AIDS

Connie Vance, EdD, RN, FAAN

Dean and Professor, College of New Rochelle, New Rochelle, New York
Feminist Perspectives on Policy and Politics

Irene Van Slyke, MN, MS

Family Nurse Practitioner, Fashion Institute of Technology, New York, New York
Bicycling, Public Policy, and Health: The Nurse as Community Activist

Barbara Velsor-Friedrich, PhD, RN

Associate Professor, Department of Maternal Child Health Nursing, Niehoff School of Nursing, Loyola University Chicago, Chicago, Illinois; Vice Chair, Council of Nurse Researchers, Illinois Nurses Association; Policy Committee, Society of Pediatric Nurses
Society of Pediatric Nurses

Mary B. Wachter, MSN, RN

Director of Legislative Affairs, New Jersey State Nurses Association, Trenton, New Jersey; Staff Nurse, Cooper Health Systems, Camden, New Jersey
Nurses as Appointed Leaders in State Government

Marva Wade, AAS, RN

Clinical Staff Nurse, Operating Room, Mount Sinai Medical Center, New York, New York; Past President, Chairperson, Council of Nursing Practitioners (Mount Sinai), and Member, Delegate Assembly, New York State Nurses Association
Every Patient Deserves a Nurse

Mary Wakefield, PhD, RN, FAAN

Professor, Department of Nursing, and Director, Center for Health Policy, George Mason University, Fairfax, Virginia
Contemporary Issues in Government

Christine M. Wallin, MA

Research Associate, Center for Health Policy Research, The George Washington University Medical Center, Washington, District of Columbia
Impact of the New Welfare Law on Child Health

Virginia A. Walter, MSA, RN

Manager, Medical Procedures Unit, The University of Michigan Health System, Ann Arbor, Michigan
Society of Gastroenterology Nurses and Associates

Jane Weaver, JD, MN, RN, FNP

Assistant Professor and Director of International Programs, University of Maryland School of Nursing, Baltimore, Maryland; Colonel, United States Air Force Reserve Nurse Corps; Chair, International Task Force, The American Association (Ellicott City, Maryland) of Nurse Attorneys; Former Director, International Nursing Center, American Nurses Association/Foundation

Nursing, Health, and Health Care in the International Community

Joyce Penrose White, DrPH, FNP

Associate Professor of Nursing, Slippery Rock University; Coordinator, Clarion University–Slippery Rock University, Family Nurse Practitioner Graduate Program, Slippery Rock, Pennsylvania

The Rainbow Kitchen: Developing a Neighborhood Health Center

Jerry Williamson, MN, RN, CAE

Director of Public Affairs, American Association of Occupational Health Nurses, Atlanta, Georgia

American Association of Occupational Health Nurses

Rita Wray, MBA, BSN, RN, CNA

Chief Executive Officer, Choices, Inc., Jackson, Mississippi

Lobbying Policymakers: Individual and Collective Strategies

CONTENTS

Unit *V*
CONTEMPORARY ISSUES IN PROFESSIONAL ORGANIZATIONS

Unit *VI*
POLICY AND POLITICS IN THE COMMUNITY

FOREWORD

At no other time in our nation's history has our country so needed the expertise of nurses in the development of health policy. As our nation struggles to reverse the tide of rising numbers of uninsured children and adults, to increase consumer involvement in health choices, and to care for our expanding aging population, we must turn to the expertise of our nations nurses. These are complex issues that do not lead to simple answers.

You are the profession that can put a face to health. Your touch expertise is essential as we struggle to create caring health care systems, redefine the role of government in providing care, and help consumers become knowledgeable about maintaining and improving their own health. Your voice is needed to move policy debates out of the realm of theory and into the everyday lives of real people with real health needs. You are closest to the patients and consumers of health care, and you have devoted your lives to empowering your patients. Now you must empower yourselves to help this country by taking an active role in the political and policy process.

Policy and Politics in Nursing and Health Care provides the information, the personal stories, and the how-to's to find creative policy solutions and to influence the policy process. It provides a context in which to analyze the complex questions that emerge from and lead to health policy options. And it reinforces, through the stories of nurses themselves, why you need to be part of the solution. Can politics and policy, whether in the workplace, government, organizations, or our community, be different if more nurses are involved? How can you as nurses provide the leadership to transform our health care system?

I have spent many years with nurses. In Congress I worked closely with the American Nurses Association on issues of pay equity and equal rights. In 1984, ANA was the first group to endorse my candidacy for Vice President. In my 1992 race for the U.S. Senate I reached out to a nurse, Judy Leavitt, to work on health policy and be a leader in my campaign. And again in 1998 I turned to the nurses for their expertise in my U.S. Senate campaign.

I don't know one politician who would not welcome your support and your knowledge about health care. Policymakers need you, politicians need you, and the American public needs you to help us create affordable access to health care for every American.

Geraldine A. Ferraro

PREFACE

As we began work on this third edition of *Policy and Politics in Nursing and Health Care*, we were struck by the evolution of nursing's political development since the first edition was published in 1985. At that time, nurses were still struggling with whether being professional included being political. The present edition of *Policy and Politics in Nursing and Health Care* represents the profession's coming of age in the world of policy and politics. Indeed, we have changed the title of this edition to emphasize the role and responsibility of the profession in leading policy-related initiatives in the broader health care arena. Although we have omitted the subtitle that accompanied the prior two editions—Action and Change in the Workplace, Government, Organizations and Community—this edition continues to use a framework that reflects the interaction among these four spheres.

Cohen et al. (1996) have described nursing's stages of political development, noting that we are beginning to show signs of moving into the highest stage, in which nurses are leading health policy initiatives. Certainly, nurses hold an unprecedented number of policymaking positions in local, state, and federal governments. It is now the expectation that nurses be represented on major health-related commissions and task forces. And nurses are moving into executive positions in the private sector, shaping health policies within health care organizations.

The question is no longer, Can nurses be political and professional at the same time? Today, the questions are, How do we become more sophisticated in our political strategy without embracing behaviors that are in conflict with nurs-

ing's values? How do we change the face of politics and policy to reflect a valuing of health as a human right and a community—a global—responsibility? We have been embracing the concept that influencing policymaking is the responsibility of all nurses. Even nurse researchers are being more attentive to the policy implications of their work. The challenge to nursing is in preparing nurses to expect a seat at the table, hold their own, and lead interdisciplinary initiatives in policy development. We must build upon nursing's traditional holistic approach, recognizing that it actually positions us to lead efforts that connect health to the broader economic and social issues of our times.

Although many nursing schools have integrated politics and policy discussions into their curricula, many faculties continue to struggle with how to move beyond teaching simply the basics of the legislative process and how to make the connections between public policy and the health of individuals and communities. The third edition of this book was designed to help faculties, students, clinicians, administrators, researchers, and even politically experienced nurses expand their understanding, knowledge, and skills in participating and leading policy development in various arenas.

One of the premises that we have used in framing this book is that nurses must value and use mentoring so that we can count on the next generation to lead the profession in ways that we never thought possible. Policymaking and political processes are best learned by jumping into the fray with those who know the ropes. For some, it is a family member, a friend, or colleague. Other nurses have sought out a political leader. Faculty and professional organizations can be instrumental in helping students and practicing nurses to become involved.

In keeping with the belief of encouraging other nurses to learn about policy and politics, we and the publisher, W.B. Saunders, have sponsored a scholarship for a nurse to attend the Nurse in Washington Internship (NIWI), a description of which is included in this edition. This donation is made on behalf of all of the books' contributors, who have demonstrated their commitment to the next generation of nurses by donating their time and expertise to the development of this book. We have enormous faith and hope in that next generation and hope that readers will embrace our commitment.

This edition of the book also reflects changing times. We are in the midst of a global shift to market-driven economies. The nursing and health care communities have struggled with this shift in the United States, as health care has become viewed as a privilege and a commodity, rather than a right. As a result, there is less support for the government's role in providing health care and even in oversight of the private sector's role. And yet, the public is demanding government oversight of managed care to protect patients' rights and is increasingly supporting regulation of what was heretofore seen as a private matter—smoking. Furthermore, in 1997, Congress passed legislation authorizing the Child Health Insurance Program (CHIP), the largest federal health program since Medicare and Medicaid in the mid-1960s. CHIP and other federal initiatives are providing evidence of a shift in locus of control to the states. This opens up opportunities for nurses to be closer to where decisions are made; after all, all politics is still local.

The interplay between the private and public sectors, the individual and the community, human rights and economic realities will continue to require careful, value-driven policy deliberations that nurses can and should not only participate in but also lead. This edition has been developed to raise nurses' awareness and understanding of these issues, to enable them to analyze policy issues, to enhance their political knowledge and skills, and to prepare them for leadership roles in shaping policies that determine the public's health.

It builds on the prior edition in the following ways:

1. The policy focus and content of the book have been increased. Whereas prior editions have emphasized the political process, this edition emphasizes the policy process and provides in-depth analysis of current policy issues, such as Social Security, Medicare, and Medicaid reform. These issues may change from year to year, but their analysis can inform nurses' understanding of the historical context of current debates. We have enlarged the focus on policymaking in the private sphere, as this sector has proven to be just as influential (if not more so) than the government in determining who will receive what kind of health care, where, and how.

2. Health care financing is driving policy decisions. Nurses must be more knowledgeable about how health care is financed, as well as about how to frame policy matters in economic terms. The chapter on health care financing has been expanded substantially, and we have added a chapter on health care economics. In Chapter 2 a vignette on the Fourth International Women's Congress in Beijing points out the connections between economics and women's health and welfare across the globe.

3. We received both support and questioning about our overtly stated feminist perspective in the first two editions. We have carefully examined the issues that the language of feminism raises and decided that there continues to be a need to frame a perspective that incorporates what we have defined as feminist principles. As more women are in policymaking positions, the gender differences have become evident but are also showing signs of be-

coming integrated into mainstream be-liefs, rather than being seen as marginal. What we and others have referred to as feminist process is now being seen as a preferred approach to decision making, leading, and managing. We support this integration and hope that in the next edi-tion we will be referring to it as a human perspective.

4. We have continued to include nursing or-ganizations as an important sphere for nurses' political activism. As in prior edi-tions, we invited national nursing organi-zations to submit examples of their in-volvement in policy and politics for inclusion in the case study in Unit V. We were unable to include all that were sub-mitted but were impressed with the broad range of issues, the use of collective strate-gies, and the leadership that many have taken in shaping public policies. A special thanks to Debra Campbell for doing such a fine job of putting this section together.

5. This edition has continued the format of using vignettes and case studies to bring content alive, with a particular emphasis on the stories of individual nurses who were successful in shaping policy issues. The saying "the personal is political" is re-flected in vignettes and case studies that include one nurse's courageous story of establishing the Vietnam Women's Memo-rial, an interview with a nurse who was one of the most powerful persons in the country during the past two decades, and the story of the nurse who is the U.S. am-bassador for women at the United Na-tions. We believe that these stories are powerful examples of nurses' leadership in policy and politics.

USING THE BOOK

As with the previous two editions, this book is designed for nurses at all levels of political devel-opment, from novice to expert. We did not ask the contributors to write with one level in mind.

We wanted to continue to provide a resource that students and nurses would enjoy reading while learning the basics of policymaking and political action. We also wanted to include critical analy-ses that would be of interest to those with more expertise. We knew it would be difficult to speak to so many levels at once, but we believe the book continues to succeed in doing so.

The book is organized to provide the reader with a context for exploring policy and politics, generic strategies for policy development and political action, and the application of these strategies in the four spheres of workplace, gov-ernment, organizations, and community. Unit I provides the context. The introductory chapter gives an organizing framework, followed by feminist and historical perspectives and the or-ganization of health care in the United States.

Unit II explores generic concepts beginning with policy analysis and the dynamics of the policy process. Political analysis and strategy, conflict management, collective strategies, the use of media, research as a political tool, the economics of health care, and ethical dimen-sions of policy and politics are explored in this unit's chapters.

Unit III begins with the application of these generic concepts to the specific spheres of nurses' political action. The workplace is the first sphere discussed to emphasize the impor-tance of nurses' recognizing the political nature of their everyday work. Unit IV explores the sphere of government; Unit V, professional orga-nizations; and Unit VI, the community. Every unit contains a case study illustrating the con-cepts presented. Two End Case Studies describe the starting of a nurse-run health center in an underserved community and the interplay be-tween policy and politics in relation to HIV/AIDS.

The reader should note that although these units are separated according to sphere, the four spheres overlap. Indeed, for nurses to be effec-tive in one sphere, this interplay must be recog-nized and developed.

The book concludes with three appendixes: an updated listing of internships and fellowships available for nurses who are interested in learning more about particular dimensions of policy or politics, an important review of the Hatch Act for nurses who are employees of federal organizations and institutions and the military, and an executive summary of nursing's agenda for health care reform.

ACKNOWLEDGMENTS

As with the previous editions, one of the remarkable features of this book is the large number of contributors who donated their time, energy, and expertise to further nurses' political development. Over 100 nurses participated in writing this edition. They are all extraordinarily busy people yet graciously responded to our pressures for meeting tight deadlines and collaborating with us to shape the book into a progressive contribution to the nursing literature. We are indebted to them for their commitment to this project and have dedicated the book to them. We are acknowledging their commitment through sponsoring the NIWI scholarship on their behalf.

This book is reflective of the work of contributors in the previous edition who helped establish the book's preeminence in the field. We continue to be grateful for their contributions as well.

Susan Talbott was one of the original editors of this book. Her vision, activism, and energy were instrumental in shaping the direction and substance of both the first and second editions. Although she was unable to continue as an editor on the current edition, we are grateful for her continued support of this endeavor and of furthering nurses' political development.

Sabrina Shange Sutherland dropped into our lives as a young "wise woman." She was a thoroughly professional and competent project coordinator. She lent not only her expertise to the project but also her support, encouragement, sense of humor, and collaborative spirit, which were crucial to completing the book. Her true dedication to this book became evident when she continued her responsibilities while coping

with being a new mother. No amount of thanks can truly express our gratitude.

Books require a full team of people who never appear in the table of contents but who are crucial to the production of a quality publication. We continue to be indebted to the W.B. Saunders Company and Thomas Eoyang, our editor, for their support of nurses' political development, not only through the publication of this book but also through co-sponsorship of the NIWI scholarship. Our thanks to W.B. Saunders' Joan Sinclair, who coordinated the production process. Mary Espenschied of Book Production, Inc., was masterful in producing such a complex book in a short period of time. It is always a pleasure to work with such a competent nonnurse who understands nursing's unique perspective and appreciates it.

We called upon three important women to write the introduction, foreword, and endnote. Geraldine Ferraro continues to be a tireless advocate for nursing, women, and health care. As the Vice President for Programs at the W.K. Kellogg Foundation, Gloria Smith is a wonderful role model of nursing's leadership in policy arenas. Her vision of resource sharing and community partnerships is shaping the next generation of policy priorities and political strategy. And Suzanne Gordon, who has become one of nursing's foremost champions through her writing and speaking, at the same time continues to challenge us to reach new heights in policy arenas. We are honored to have these three women lend their support to this book.

This book has provided us with a unique opportunity to hear nurses' stories of struggle, success, and challenges in political matters. Nurses such as Terri Havill, who writes about blowing the whistle on injustices in a Canadian workplace, or Diane Carlson Evans, who struggled against unbelievable odds to create a tribute to women's caring during wartime, have inspired and sustained us during these turbulent times in health care. We are grateful to nurses such as these who are our unsung heroines and heroes.

Our families continue to sustain us. A heartfelt acknowledgment goes to James Ware for his encouragement and support of Diana. She is sustained by his love, his support of her work, and his understanding of the special perspectives that nurses and women have on life and living. Judy's sons, Noah and David, though continuing to believe that she is super-mom, have never failed to recognize their role in providing the support and love she needs to carry on. One of the individuals who was a major support for the second edition was Richard Leavitt. He fed us, supported us, and nurtured us. We are sorry that he was not able to see this edition become a reality but know that his spirit was with us.

This book was produced amidst multiple changes in our personal and professional lives. We are grateful to those who understood our many demands and struggles, and who, in spite of it all, were patient and forgiving. And we are thankful for our own friendship, which has been strengthened over these past years. This book is a tribute to the creative and energizing context that can be created when friends and colleagues work together to meet tomorrow's challenges.

Diana J. Mason
Judith K. Leavitt

REFERENCE

Cohen, S. S., Mason, D.J., Kovner, C., Leavitt, J.K., Pulcini, J., Sochalski, J. (1997). Stages of nursing's political development: Where we've been and where we ought to go. *Nursing Outlook, 44*(6), 259–266.

INTRODUCTION

This book teaches skills for *influencing policy*. To influence policy, nurses must learn a new way of thinking. The heart of making policy is resource allocation. New thinking about controlling and allocating resources can frame the profession's work to influence policy. In the new thinking the paradigm shifts from the resource-scarcity model to the power-sharing model.

Greater awareness of the resource allocation that occurs in policy making, which is sometimes plain and sometimes obscure, will be helpful in applying this new thinking. Through this book you may test your skills in policy analysis with questions concerning who wins and who loses in terms of cost and control, who gains resources, from whom and to whom are resources being transferred, whose dollars are being spent to serve whose interests, and how could those dollars otherwise be spent. Some advocates maintained, for example, that close analysis of prominent national tax and expenditure policies adopted in the 1980s disclosed that the policies' effect was to shift resources from the have-nots to the haves. As you study, you may find it useful to ask, "In what way does a policy manifest the relative power of those with interests in it?"

The scarcity model holds that there are only so many resources to go around and that, if you give up some, you have less of the total available than you had before. You seek to make *your piece* of the pie bigger. The power-sharing model posits that, through sharing, total resources can be increased. It says that the *whole* pie can get bigger, the enterprise richer, and the infrastructure stronger. But for that to happen, it is necessary to give up some power. This defies how we have been taught to think about the world.

The scarcity model justifies grabbing resources and denying them to others. An illustration may suggest how **the scarcity model itself contributes to scarcity of resources for health.** Awash in high technology the world envies, the United States is unable to attain the goal of Health for All enunciated in the 1978 Alma-Ata Declaration, which responded, primarily, to the plight of the Third World. In the United States the following could happen: A single young male without any health insurance and no regular primary care provider could yet receive miraculous life-saving treatment using spectacular procedures for trauma the likes of which could only be dreamed of in most of the globe. In this example, he is likely to be black or Hispanic, poor and poorly educated, and living in an inner city. He is treated for a gunshot wound in the emergency room of what may well be a teaching hospital.

The gunshot wound occurs during criminal activity in which he is either participant or victim. This activity diverts attention from the real crime, which occurs throughout the years of his young life as he, his family, and his community are systematically denied resources *for* life. This young man only gains access to the unjustly allocated wealth as perpetrator or victim of street crime.

Several futurists can educate us about the power-sharing paradigm. For example, Alvin and Heidi Toffler report that, to speed decision making in order to stay competitive, today's corporations and the military push decisional authority to the lowest level possible. Through training and information technology, workers and soldiers have a share of their organizations' assets—namely knowledge. They exercise a share of their organizations' power to make decisions.

Practical experience is growing in the use of power sharing to increase resources. In community-engagement strategies such as asset-based community development, communities—no matter how disadvantaged—are recognized as having assets and expertise to bring to decision making, problem solving, and resource allocation. Although the physician still dominates the health care delivery model, more recognition is being given to alternative providers, such as acupuncturists, who bring new resources and perspectives to the healing process. Chief among alternative providers is the advanced practice nurse, without whom health care would be inaccessible to many people. Practice models that incorporate community health workers employ one of the most important approaches to linking community expertise with professional expertise. The Kellogg Foundation has funded community-institution partnerships for health professionals in training to work in multidisciplinary teams, but true *multidisciplinary* team practice is in its infancy in America, and its capacity to expand resources for cost-effective delivery remains to be fully developed.

Can power sharing correct cumulative inequity? Should not nurses pursue power sharing on the side while focusing on the main battle, where the scarcity model still prevails? Yes, nurses must employ two contradictory models at once. While the scarcity model is still strong, we live in an age of sweeping transformations. Nurses must be aware and ready and recognize the potential value of concentrated work in the power-sharing model for the future of health care. Daniel Yankelovich, a public-opinion expert, believes that unformed public opinion moves to public judgment over a ten-year period. He concluded that in 1993–94, when the Clinton Health Plan failed, public opinion was still in the first stage of change. Today, in 1998, more than 41 million Americans are uninsured while national health spending exceeds that of any other country. Where will public opinion be in five years, when Yankelovich's ten years are up? It may be important then to demonstrate to the public and policy makers that, through a new paradigm for managing resources, it is possible to improve health status and provide primary care and prevention cost-effectively. Such a demonstration would open a new policy option for affordable coverage for the uninsured (and all people). This is the possibility to which nurses—above all other providers—as thinkers, leaders, educators, practitioners, and policy activists, can contribute and must aspire!

Gloria Smith, PhD, RN, FAAN

Unit *I*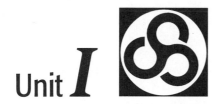

POLICY AND POLITICS:
A Nursing Perspective

Unit I

provides the context for the discussions of policy and politics throughout the rest of this book. In Chapter 1, policy and politics are defined and discussed within a values framework that is relevant to the four spheres of nurses' political activism: the workplace, government, professional organizations, and community. Throughout the book, readers are challenged to explore how their own professional values will influence their attitudes and actions toward policy and politics.

The interaction between feminist and nursing values is explored in depth in Chapter 2 and provides a context for examining how policies and political behavior might look different if women and nurses had more influence over policymaking. Two vignettes illustrate this interaction. The first is one nurse's experience from being a nurse at the bedside to being a major player in setting an international agenda for women. The second vignette, on "dancing with the chaos" of the turbulent changes in health care, is an example of how these values can lead to supportive approaches for helping nurses not only to survive but to grow and to shape tomorrow's health care system.

Chapter 3 is a historical overview of policy and politics as experienced by women and nurses in the United States. The chapter interweaves two women's movements in this century with the nursing profession's development and involvement in political and policy matters.

Chapter 4 explores the evolution of the health care system in the United States and illustrates how limited our progress has been in confronting issues of access and continuity of care. A vignette on long-term care describes nursing models of care delivery that need to be expanded. Another vignette, on a national health promotion initiative, challenges nursing to become a major player in developing, implementing, and evaluating primary care standards and policy.

In Chapter 5, health care financing is explored in considerable detail and scope because it is so critical to understanding the present state of our health care system. The vignette that follows this chapter presents one nurse's involvement with influencing the regulation of managed care organizations.

This unit ends with the extraordinary story of one nurse's reaction to a national memorial that ignored the contributions of women and nurses in Vietnam. It illustrates how one nurse learned to use political strategy and determination to move the nation to recognize and honor these women.

Chapter 1

POLICY AND POLITICS:
A Framework for Action

JUDITH K. LEAVITT AND DIANA J. MASON

What is difficult can be done at once. What is impossible takes a little longer. — Priscilla Sears (1996, p. 179)

The tumultuous changes in health care in the 1990s provide multiple lessons in the political forces that shape health care policy in the public and private sectors. They also illustrate how nursing itself is one of these forces. Whether it will be a force in the future depends on how well nurses understand the policy process and its political dynamics, and how engaged they are in the process.

This chapter provides a framework for nurses to view policy and politics. It does so within the context of the so-called "health care reform" movement in the 1990s and discusses the values that underpin the political and policy processes. The chapter concludes with an examination of policy and politics in each of the four spheres of a nurse's influence: the government, workplace, organizations, and community. It proceeds with the assumption that change is continuous—it's the pace and direction that can be shaped by nurses' deliberate efforts.

THE CONTEXT FOR HEALTH CARE IN THE 1990s

The approach of the twenty-first century has been associated with profound shifts in societal values, actions, and advances in technology, particularly in relation to health care in the 1990s. It provides an opportunity to take stock of where we've been and where we need to go to ensure that nursing values are reflected in a changing health care system. Because national efforts to create a "new" health care system involved so many sectors in society—government, health care industry, providers, businesses, foundations, communities, and individual citizens—an analysis of the process is a useful context for understanding the policy process.

Nursing and the Health Security Act

In 1991 the American Nurses Association's Political Action Committee (ANA-PAC) was the first health professional organization to endorse William Jefferson Clinton for President of the United States (Trotter-Betts, 1996). His health platform was consistent with Nursing's Agenda for Health Care Reform (1991; see Appendix C), thus reflecting the centrality of a nursing perspective to quality health care. Both Clinton and nursing embraced a belief that government had a responsibility to guarantee access to quality health care for all. They also shared the belief that nurses had a significant role in providing that care. The term *nurses* appeared in his campaign speeches, organized rallies, interviews with the press, and policy statements. Nurses across the country campaigned energetically and extensively for his election. Nurses such as Pat Ford-Roegner, a long-time political activist and former Political Director for the ANA and the Service Employees International Union, held leadership positions in the campaign. In November of 1991, Clinton was elected president. He was the first presidential candidate endorsed by organized nursing to win.

Nurses were infused with excitement and hope in the potential for their influence with national health policy. There was also a great sense of accomplishment and collaboration within organized nursing. More than 70 national nursing organizations had signed on to Nursing's Agenda for Health Care Reform. Developed in 1989, this document defines the principles that nursing believed should undergird the U.S. health care system. It was timely and reflected the values of many progressive health groups, such as the American Public Health Association, in relation to promoting access to care, ensuring universality of coverage through public and private financing, shifting resources to primary care, involving consumers in health care decision making, and emphasizing quality (Joel, 1993; Richardson, 1993). So when health care reform took center stage in the 1990 and 1991 elections, nursing was ready.

It was ready because there was a growing sophistication about the worlds of policy and politics (Cohen et al., 1996). Nurses understood that they had to be players in shaping public and private policies that determined the nature of health care in this country and in their workplaces. They knew that mobilizing community support for their issues was paramount. And they knew that their efforts would in turn influence the level of health in the community. Nurses no longer questioned whether being professional included being political. It did.

Health care reform was one of Clinton's primary domestic policy agendas during his election campaign. Once in office, he involved nurses in the process of developing and reviewing his plan for health care reform, eventually the Health Security Act (HSA). Nurses were appointed to the many task forces that worked on defining the elements of the HSA and also participated in major coalitions organized around health care reform that included consumers, the business community, and other health care provider groups. Nursing was visible and influential. For the first time, nurses were included as providers in a major health policy initiative. From 1992 to 1993, media coverage of nursing increased by 300%, and 95% of the coverage was positive (Trotter-Betts, 1996). Advanced practice nurses were mentioned on the front pages of major newspapers and in more than 700 electronic and print news reports.

The HSA never passed in Congress. The many analyses of its demise suggest the following factors (Blumenthal, 1995; Fallows, 1996; Hacker, 1996; Yankelovich, 1995):

- The legislation was too complex and Americans never fully understood it.
- The media covered the politics of health care reform more than the substantive content issues.
- Major opponents to the plan developed effective counter strategies, including the Health Insurance Association of America's *Harry and Louise* commercials.
- The public was comfortable with existing health care and became overwhelmed with a sense of fear that current health assurances would be lost. The majority were not willing to risk change, in the name of extending health care benefits to the uninsured. People will always resist change, and radical policy changes are enormously difficult to achieve in a society that is more comfortable with incremental reform.
- The process of the development and movement of the HSA took so long that the opposition was able to grow and solidify. Clinton brought a different set of values to the politics of policymaking. He embraced consensus building, a style that was new to Washington. While consensus was building among 500 people in multiple groups addressing various aspects of health care reform, the opposition attacked the process as being closed and secretive (even though it was the most inclusive, democratic process used to

develop a major public policy in this country) (Fallows, 1996).

With the demise of the HSA, the implicit policy governing the health care system became one in which market forces, which had already begun to reshape health care because of cost concerns, were left to control the system with minimal government oversight. Subsequently, efforts have been launched at the state and federal levels to redefine the role of government in ensuring access to quality health care.

The Effects of the Demise of the Health Security Act

Was nursing's effort in the Clinton campaign wasted? What were some of the outcomes of the rise and fall of the HSA? How have workplaces, communities, and nursing organizations responded?

• Nurses demonstrated that they understand the importance of political action by contributing an unprecedented amount of money to the ANA-PAC, making it the third largest national health PAC in the United States in 1994.

• Employers' concerns over rising health care costs fueled a shift from acute care in hospitals to prevention and long-term care in the home and community. This shift was envisioned by the nursing organizations in Nursing's Agenda for Health Care Reform and has provided many entrepreneurial opportunities for nurses in their own communities. Other nurses have been challenged to move into roles such as case management, where they are the linchpin in a health care team's determination of clinical policies and practices (Cohen & Cesta, 1997).

• Initially, nursing tried to use its influence to gain support for long-standing goals, including reimbursement for advanced practice nurses (APNs) in all settings, for all groups, and at full levels of compensation. Although these issues continue to need the profession's attention, a major breakthrough occurred in 1997, when Congress included in its budget bill an extension of Medicare reimbursement to all APNs regard-

less of geographic location. Policymakers are now much more familiar with APN roles and outcomes. In states such as Oregon, nurses have used the media and other strategies to garner public support for a more progressive state practice act, as well as other policy initiatives to remove barriers to practice (Bifano, 1996).

• The locus of control has shifted from the federal to state and local governments in a movement termed *devolution*. Fox-Piven and Cloward's (1971) classic work *Regulating the Poor: The Functions of Public Welfare* suggests that throughout the history of the Western World, devolution has occurred in relation to economic prosperity and is accompanied by cutbacks in social welfare programs. It further demonstrates that when the economy again slides, social upheaval will increase and the cycle of increased federal control will return as local communities are unable to support the growing needs of their people. For nurses, devolution has meant that efforts long targeted at the federal level must shift to the state and local levels. It has created opportunities for experimentation with new ideas for delivering health and social services. Nurses have been rising to this challenge through innovative practices in local communities (Lamb, 1995). Nevertheless, nurses must be mindful of the societal trends that may indicate a shift back to central control.

• The preeminence of market forces has made cost containment the primary driving force and has moved health care organizations (e.g., hospitals and home care agencies) to reorganize, reengineer, and otherwise change their own policies around employees and patient care. For-profit corporations have proliferated amid rising concern that they are dedicating fewer resources to the actual delivery of care (Woolhandler & Himmelstein, 1997). As the largest and most visible part of the hospital budget, nurses have come to be seen as a financial liability and have sometimes been replaced by unlicensed assistive personnel (UAPs). Unions have begun to compete with state nursing organizations, doing collective bargaining on the basis of who could better protect nurses from layoffs. This threatens the viability of some state nurses associations while failing to alleviate the increasing anxiety of many staff nurses over their job security and the delivery of safe patient care. In the late 1990s, state and federal proposals and bills to mandate staffing ratios, supervision of UAPs, layoff protections, and other protections surfaced but were seldom approved (Moore, 1997).

• With the mounting threats to nursing practice, some have criticized nurses for turning inward toward self-protection at the expense of the broader health issues. Staff nurses have felt demoralized as their values of caring have been discounted by business values that focused on the bottom line. On the other hand, nurses in Oregon, Mississippi, Texas, and New York have been proactive in defining the preferred future for nursing and health care, developing strategies to move toward that future, and capitalizing on opportunities to develop innovative practice partnerships. In New York and other states, media campaigns promoted "Every Patient Deserves a *Real Nurse*"—and mobilized public concern. Soon after, hospitals began to advertise that patients coming to them would be guaranteed to see a registered nurse (RN) (see advertisement on p. 199).

• Communities across the country have been left without adequate health services as for-profit corporations have bought and then closed community hospitals. Mounting public concern over these and individual assaults on people's rights to quality care may be creating a public constituency that will increase pressure on the government to return "health care for people, not for profits" (Blumenthal, 1995). The number of uninsured has been increasing at the rate of more than one million people a year since the demise of the HSA (U.S. Bureau of the Census, 1996). A radical change in the nation's welfare policies threatened to increase these numbers, as eligibility for Medicaid and Supplemental Security Insurance (SSI) was disconnected from welfare entitlements (see Chapter 21 and the subsequent vignette). The question for communities at the end of the decade was whether they could provide for their members' health and welfare needs.

• Nurses have responded to a growing community need for health care through innovations and risk taking. In academia, financial pressures have led faculty to develop practices that have received national recognition as models for promoting health through community partnerships and the use of a health framework that embraces other community sectors such as education and social welfare (U.S. Department of Health and Human Services, 1996). In fact, nursing has been in the forefront of the community empowerment movement (Reinhard et al., 1996).

• Although many physicians made a quick turnaround by not only embracing managed care but also learning how to control it and benefit from it, in 1997 there continued to be few practice networks composed of and initiated by nurses, leaving nurses to be the invisible provider in group medical practices (Cohen, Mason, Arsenie, Sargese, & Needham, 1998; Mason, Cohen, O'Donnell, Baxter, & Chase, 1997). Early on, comparatively few nurses were positioned to be inside players in managed care systems. Many of the managed care organizations have therefore developed policies reflecting medical and corporate models that, for example, failed to see the importance of credentialling and listing APNs as primary care providers. A highly publicized demonstration project between Columbia University and the Oxford Health Plan increased the visibility and inclusion of APNs in provider panels but also served to mobilize physician opposition (Grandinetti, 1997).

• Nurses continue to be mentioned in the media and appointed to important policymaking bodies (three were appointed to Clinton's Quality Commission in 1997), and they are now moving into leadership positions within managed care organizations, where they are shaping corporate policies and influencing the kind and quality of care that people receive.

• The attention received by APNs in the media caused a rift between APNs and staff nurses, with the latter claiming that they had been ignored and neglected in the health care reform debate, even by their own nursing organizations. And the collaborative work done around Nursing's Agenda for Health Care Reform seems to have been lost. With no common goal, nursing organizations seem to be turning inward or focusing on their own singular agendas. Nevertheless, there remains hope that these organizations will have another common goal. The Ad Hoc Committee to Defend Health Care (1997), a grassroots collaborative effort by physicians and nurses, began in 1997 to return the country from a focus on profits to one of quality, accessible care.

• Although questions have arisen about the cost-effectiveness of prevention, society has begun to embrace prevention as a value. For example, communities have taken action to address exposure to smoke, especially in young people. This marked a shift in societal attitudes toward prevention, with the paradoxical expectation that the government do more to limit tobacco production and use during a time when deregulation is the dominant value.

This cursory review of the outcomes of the rise and fall of the HSA and the nursing community's involvement illustrates the complex interactive and cyclical nature of policy and politics. It reflects the different values that drove the debate and public actions. Instead of a belief that health care is a right, the values that emerged to undermine the HSA reflected a belief in profits and market forces as the solution to developing efficient, cost-effective health care. Government was viewed as an inflated bureaucracy that overregulates and interferes with people's lives. The primacy of health care for all was a value that lost out to the fear of big government.

This example also demonstrates the impact that public and private policies have on nursing practice, as well as the potential for nursing's power and influence. In addition, it serves as a lens through which to view the connections among the government, organizations, work-

places, and communities in shaping public and private policies.

NURSING, POLICY, AND POLITICS

Cohen et al. (1996) have developed a conceptualization of nursing's political development. From stages one through three, the profession has moved from marginal participation in political and policy matters, to leading collective efforts to act on behalf of nursing's self-interest, and to participating in coalitions on broader health care issues. The fourth stage of nursing's development is characterized as one in which nursing takes the lead in mobilizing health and public constituencies to act on these broader health issues. The profession has begun to move into this latter stage but continues to be well grounded in the earlier ones.

As recently as the 1980s, recurrent shortages of nurses prompted several blue ribbon panels to identify factors that were influencing who came into and stayed in nursing. One of the consistent conclusions of these studies was that nurses must participate more fully in policymaking within and outside their workplaces (National Commission on Nursing, 1981; Secretary's Commission on Nursing, 1988). The multidisciplinary National Commission on Nursing (1981), sponsored by the American Hospital Association, Hospital Research and Education Trust, and American Hospital Supply Corporation, recommended that

> nursing participates in policy development and in management decisions at every level of the [health care] organization. . . . Nurses should participate in community activities and in public policy forums about health care on a local, state, and national basis. Such efforts should be encouraged by educators and supported by employers. [pp. 15, 28]

During that decade and the next, nurses did become more involved in governmental politics, as evidenced by increases in the numbers of nurses writing on politics, candidates for political offices who sought endorsement and contributions from nurses' political action committees, nurses running for elective office, and nurses receiving political appointments. Nursing's influence in the public arena grew and continues to be evident in the passage of legislation and involvement in electoral politics. However, many are less certain about the gains made in the private sector, which is now driving health care. In a study of the readership of the *American Journal of Nursing* (Shindul-Rothschild & Berry, 1997), 60% of the more than 7500 nurses who responded reported that their institutions had reduced the number of RN positions; 42% reported that UAPs were being substituted for RNs, and more than one third noted that their nurse executive had been eliminated without a replacement. The workplace was seen as limiting nurses' numbers and influence as providers and leaders.

For too many nurses, politics and policy continue to be remote, ethereal topics. Policy needs to be related to nurses' everyday practice in ways that will frame their personal and professional experiences as political ones; policy and politics, that is, need to be explicitly related to bedside nursing. For example, the nurse who is caring for a patient who has had bypass surgery needs to understand that this nurse-patient interaction is occurring within the context of a health care system that is still a disease-oriented system. Health care financing policies ensure that the bypass surgery will be funded but won't ensure that the nurse's time to teach the patient and family about posthospital care and to provide emotional support are valued. Some public and private health policies should raise concerns in the minds of nurses who are concerned with quality care. For example, when health care financing policies emphasize reducing hospital lengths of stay, the following behaviors are reinforced:

- It is much quicker to feed the elderly patient by a nasogastric tube than to feed the patient slowly by mouth.

- It is quicker to catheterize the incontinent patient than to teach bladder control after a stroke.

Outside the hospital, public policies suggest the following:

- It is ostensibly cheaper for a local community to lay off the school health nurse than to ensure that children receive the primary and urgent care that school nurses can provide.
- As home care nurses become pressured to see more patients per day, they often leave the patient and family with the impression that it's the home health aide whom they can really count on.
- In one state, a nurse practitioner can administer controlled substances but in an adjoining state be unable to do so.

All these scenarios are driven by public and private policies. Politics shapes these policies at every point along their development and execution, from which policies are considered to how an implemented policy is evaluated. Knowing the process enables nurses to know where to focus their efforts to influence policies that support their vision for health and health care.

POLICY DEFINED

Policy has been defined as "the principles that govern action directed towards given ends" (Titmus, 1974, p. 23) and "a consciously chosen course of action (or inaction) directed toward some end" (Kalisch & Kalisch, 1982, p. 61). It is a plan, direction, or goal for action. It is "authoritative decision making" (Stimpson & Hanley, 1991, p. 12). Policy encompasses the choices that a society, segment of society, or organization makes regarding its goals and priorities and the ways it will allocate its resources. It reflects the values of those setting the policy.

Consider the example of policies related to tobacco. Earlier in this century, the federal government began to subsidize tobacco farming and the nation watched the Marlboro man riding across television screens with the implicit message that smoking was manly (later womanly, as in "You've come a long way, baby"), "cool," good for social interaction, and sexy. By the 1990s, the Marlboro man had died of lung cancer, tobacco ads were banned from television and radio, the attorneys general of states were developing an agreement for cigarette companies to pay for the health bills that resulted from lifetimes of smoking, and tobacco companies began shifting their marketing plans to Third World countries (Annas, 1997).

Public policy is policy formed by governmental bodies—for example, legislation passed by Congress and the regulations written from that legislation. Public policy related to tobacco use includes a law that bans the selling of cigarettes within a specified radius of a school, or one that requires health warning labels on cigarette packaging.

Social policy pertains to the directives that promote the welfare of the public. For example, a local ordinance might set an age limit on the purchase of tobacco products. This policy would promote the welfare of children.

Health policy includes the directives for promoting the health of citizens. For example, the federal government could decide to pay for smoking-prevention programs for all people in the military and their families. The state government might require such coverage by companies providing Medicaid managed care.

Institutional policies are those governing workplaces, what the institution's goals will be and how it will operate, how the institution will treat its employees, and how employees will work. For example, a hospital can institute a no-smoking policy that prohibits both patients and staff from smoking anywhere in the building.

Organizational policies are the rules governing and positions taken by organizations, such as state nurses association or specialty nursing organizations. For example, a state nurses association can develop a policy banning smoking at its meetings, or a member might put forth a resolution calling on the association to offer free or at-cost continuing education programs to nurses on how to help themselves and their patients quit smoking.

All these policies are shaped by politics and reflect societal values, beliefs, and attitudes.

POLITICS DEFINED

Politics is often associated with negative images—smoke-filled rooms, with deals made by power brokers, bribes, unethical compromises, pork barreling, bureaucracies, payoffs, and vote buying, to name only a few. These images arise from newspaper headlines of scandals in local, state, and federal government, political parties, and campaigns. The negative associations are highly visible and prevalent enough to leave the impression that all politics is tainted, if not dirty and unethical.

Yet *politics* is a neutral term. It means "influencing"—specifically, influencing the allocation of scarce resources. Politics is a process by which one influences the decisions of others and exerts control over situations and events. It is a means to an end.

The statement "She plays politics" is often viewed negatively by nurses when it describes a peer. However, ask the same nurses if they want a chief nurse officer who is politically astute, and they will usually say yes.

Politics is thus a term associated with conflicting values. Politics is a necessary part of operating where multiple interest groups are competing for scarce resources of money, time, supplies, personnel, or access to information. Whether the perception of politics is negative or positive depends largely on these factors:

- An individual's own biases, experiences, and knowledge of politics
- How the game of politics is played—that is, the system in which politics is operating and the rules that have been established as acceptable within that system
- Whether the goals or ends are important

• Whether one has a vision for different ways of influencing and is in a position to change the rules of the system

The last factor is one that nurses, as members of a profession that continues to be predominantly female, must address. Do nurses want to be accomplices in political processes that are too often corrupt and oppressive, or should nurses play a leadership role in transforming political systems?

POLITICS, POLICY, AND VALUES

The development of policy is a value-laden process, beginning with which problems become policy issues and including who will decide how a policy will be evaluated. Figure 1–1 illustrates the interconnections among values, politics, and policy.

Policymaking is a complex, multidimensional, dynamic process that reflects the values of those who are setting the policy agenda,

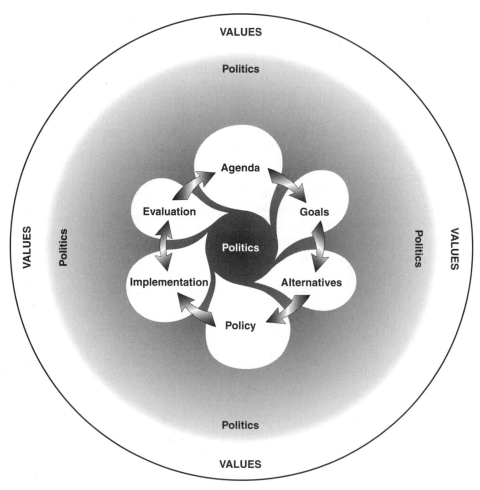

Figure 1–1   A values framework for politics and the policy process. The figure illustrates the steps in the policy process. Politics can influence the process at any step. Both the politics of policy development and the policy itself are grounded in and influenced by values.

determining policy goals and alternatives, formulating policy, and implementing and evaluating policy. When values are in conflict, as they often are in policy arenas with diverse constituencies, politics necessarily comes into play.

The values underlying the politics and policies related to tobacco and smoking illustrate this conflict. Should the focus be on the economy of tobacco-growing areas or on the health of the public? Should the federal government support tobacco growers as businesses, or should it discourage smoking through laws and regulations that limit the age for purchasing tobacco products and that restrict where one can smoke? Should state or federal governments, or both, engage in legal action against tobacco companies to recover the costs of health care of smokers who have Medicare or Medicaid, even if it means that the tobacco company's viability is threatened? Should public monies be used to help people to stop smoking, or is this a private issue?

Nursing's values of caring, collaboration, collectivity, and high-touch care are often in conflict with the dominant values of society: competition, individuality, and high-tech care (MacPherson, 1987). When women and nurses are not at policy tables in sufficient numbers, the policies that result often do not support the health and development of individuals, families, and communities. Several examples illustrate this point:

• A coalition of women's organizations, scientists, and legislators brought to the public's attention that most of the federally funded research in this country excluded women. The body of biomedical knowledge that was being used to treat both men and women may not be accurate when applied to women. The coalition worked to develop a policy to require all federally funded research to address the issue of women as subjects. Similar policies were developed to promote the inclusion of ethnic minorities who had also been excluded from most studies.

• While giving lip service to valuing the family, the United States is the only industrialized country without policies that support workers' taking paid leaves of absence from their jobs to care for an infirm child or elder, and the only one that does not guarantee the availability of child care for working families.

• Because prenatal care is not guaranteed in this country, some women receive no or too little prenatal care and therefore deliver very low birth weight infants who require immediate and prolonged care in a neonatal intensive care unit. Yet prenatal care in this country costs relatively little compared with the high cost of neonatal intensive care that is most often provided regardless of the family's wishes and financial situation. The infant will be sent home without a guarantee that the mother will receive the support she needs to provide for the infant, or that the infant will receive the developmental support and special education that may be needed.

• In a thorough review of research and demonstration projects aimed at improving the odds for high-risk children and families, Schorr (1989) noted that the successful programs have repeatedly shown that this risk can be reduced through comprehensive, intensive, and responsive services with "staffs with the time and skill to establish relationships based upon mutual respect and trust" (p. xxii). Since Schorr's review, Olds et al. (1997) have reported that home visits by nurses to low-income families reduced the risk of child abuse and neglect 15 years later. A replication of this study found that nurses' home visits to low-income African American women during pregnancy and the 2-year postpartum period resulted in a reduced rate of additional pregnancies and fewer childhood injuries, as well as other positive maternal-child health outcomes (Kitzman et al., 1997). Such humanistic approaches to health and social problems are too seldom embraced by policymakers. What predominates in the public policy arena is a disease-oriented value system, rather than a holistic wellness model.

Although much is being said about limited resources in society, Smith (1997) has argued that we could embrace a resource-sharing framework instead of a resource-limited one. A resource-sharing framework requires embracing values of empowerment, community collaboration, and partnerships. It assumes that such partnerships can discover previously unknown resources and develop new ones to meet the needs of individuals, families, and communities.

Such a framework also embraces the need for a global perspective on policymaking. Although most citizen action occurs on a local level, the decisions made there increasingly have a global impact. Promoting the health of local communities requires a focus on what is good for the world community and vice versa. As a global perspective proliferates, the potential conflict in culture-bound values will need to be addressed. Nurses can be a leading voice in advocating for the values clarification that will be needed to integrate global perspectives on public policies and political action.

Public and private policies are a matter of choices. These choices are based on values that come into play in the political dynamics of policymaking. When individuals and groups with disparate values enter into the policymaking process, consensus around policies can be difficult unless values are clarified and agreement is reached on how to work within any differences. Although groups with markedly different values sometimes agree to the same solution, they may do so because the solution manages to reflect these value sets. In addition, values around appropriate political behavior and strategies to move an issue should be clarified.

FOUR SPHERES OF POLITICAL ACTION

Although politics and policy are usually associated with government, there are three other spheres for nurses' political action: the workplace, professional organizations, and community. Figure 1–2 illustrates the spheres of the government, workplace, and organizations contained in the broader sphere of the community. These four spheres are interconnected and overlapping. The political effectiveness of nurses

Figure 1–2 The four spheres of political influence where nurses can effect change: workplace, government, organizations, and community (the encompassing sphere).

in one sphere will be influenced by nurses' involvement in the other spheres. Although this book is structured to address each of these spheres separately, their interaction and interdependence are evident throughout. The reader is encouraged to look for this interaction and integrate it into his or her own plan for political activism.

Workplace

Most nurses are familiar with "policies and procedures" manuals, and these certainly are workplace policies, as are policies that determine what kind of care is provided by whom—whether written or unwritten. Following are other policies that can be found in many workplaces:

- Designation of no-smoking areas, or a ban on smoking in the entire facility.
- Whether nurses have input into the governing structure of the organization.
- Working conditions, including whether sexual harassment is dealt with aggressively.
- Parental leave policies.
- Whether home care patients can be seen without an initial referral and, if so, for how many visits.
- Whether coordinated services are provided to persons infected with human immunodeficiency virus (HIV).
- Whether unlicensed personnel are substituted for RNs in care delivery in hospital or home.

The workplace can be public or private. It can be a for-profit or a nonprofit organization. The type of organization can influence who sets what policies and even the values that underlie the policies. For example, a for-profit home care agency is more likely to terminate care for a chronically ill patient whose insurance has run out than is a charitable health care organization whose mission is to serve the poor.

Because so much of a nurse's time is spent at work, the policies and political nuances of the workplace can have a profound impact on the quality of the nurse's professional life. Therefore it is important to examine what influence nurses have over their organizations' policies, recognizing that these policies may be influenced by the policies of government, nursing organizations, and the community. For example, occupational and health standards established by the federal government may drive a nurse's workplace to develop policies on the handling of hazardous wastes. In addition, a nurses' association may keep this issue visible and, through a resolution of its own, decide to pressure nurses' workplaces to use particular protective equipment in high-risk areas. And communities can pressure workplaces to keep operating services that the agency may prefer to eliminate during a time of fiscal constraints.

At the end of the 1990s, there was a growing concern within the nursing community regarding whether a nursing presence would continue at policy tables in many health care organizations. The elimination of nurse managers and chief nurse officers portended a lack of a nursing voice in the policies of the workplace. It is up to all nurses to ensure that a nursing perspective on workplace policies is available, listened to, and incorporated into final decisions.

Government

We live in a very collective, very organized society in which we are all connected, in which the welfare and safety of each one of us is dependent upon the health and welfare of a cooperative and collective enterprise. Government has become bigger and more centralized, not because we have become careless of our freedoms or morally lazy in our commitment to individual values, but because the important tasks that need to be done in our nation today are beyond the reach of single men and women. Making our society work—the flourishing of civilization—is everyone's business. It's what *we* do. Our individual freedom depends upon our participating membership in democracy. [Moyers, 1991, p. 14]

In spite of societal attitudes that government has overstepped its boundaries in a free society, government plays an enormously important role for nursing and health care. The sphere of government provides society with a legal definition of nursing. It influences reimbursement systems for health care and nursing services, and to a great extent it determines who will get what kind of health care. It determines whether society's children will have a healthy and educated start in life, and whether we will use military approaches to managing world conflicts.

Throughout the last part of the twentieth century, federal, state, and local governments decided:

- Whether women could receive full information about reproductive rights and who could provide that information.
- Where smoking may take place, and where alcohol and smoking may be advertised.
- What health services are available in schools and whether schools should distribute condoms to prevent the spread of acquired immunodeficiency syndrome (AIDS).
- Whether public funds will be used to distribute clean needles to intravenous-drug users as a harm-reduction strategy to reduce the spread of HIV/AIDS.
- What resources are available to communities for low-income housing development and maintenance.
- Whether violence is treated solely as a crime rather than as a public health issue, and whether the use of handguns is controlled.

The sphere of government is far-reaching. The interplay between the public and private sectors can result in public policies' becoming policy for the private sector as well. It often drives the policies and programs in health care organizations. The Institute of Medicine (1988) argues that although not all efforts to improve and promote the health of the public must be made by government, the government does have the responsibility for providing guidance in the policy process:

> Policy formulation takes place as the result of interactions among a wide range of public and private organizations and individuals. . . . Although it joins with the private sector to arrive at decisions, government has a special obligation to ensure that the public interest is served by whatever measures are adopted. [p. 44]

The government's actions are, in turn, shaped by private individuals and organizations, including nursing.

Professional Organizations

Professional organizations are instrumental in shaping the practice of nursing—for example, in developing standards of practice, lobbying for progressive changes in the scope of nurses' practice, and playing a role in collective action in the workplace. They are increasingly a significant force in the development of health policy.

Although a powerful force, these organizations could increase their power if more nurses supported them. The American Nurses Association represents only 10% of the nurses in this country. Some specialty organizations include a greater percentage of potential members but rarely exceed 30%. Yet these organizations are essential for advocating for nurses and for values of caring and health promotion. A strong professional organization should be a visible force within its community: a national organization should have a national presence, and a local organization should be known in the local community. These organizations can and should identify issues of concern to nursing and health care, bring them to the attention of the public, and take a leadership role in calling for the development of policies that can improve the health of communities and ensure the provision of quality nursing care.

To achieve this mandate, these organizations need the collective participation and support of nurses who will develop and use their political savvy to promote progressive policies for and by the organizations.

Community

In years past, leaders such as Lillian Wald viewed the community as more than a practice site. It is a social unit with a variety of special interest groups, community activities, health and social problems, and numerous resources for solving those problems. The community can be one's neighborhood, or it can be the international connections that will be needed for moving the world into the twenty-first century. The other three spheres of influence are an integral part of the community. As members of a community, we have a responsibility to promote the welfare of the community and its members. In turn, the community's resources can be invaluable assets to health promotion and health care delivery. Government officials, hospital administrators, patients, corporate managers, presidents of private and public organizations—all players who can effect change in health policy—are affiliated with at least one community, the one in which they live. When nurses become visible in the affairs of their communities, they represent an entire profession. Community networks can be called upon to support nursing agendas.

Likewise, nursing should be called upon to support the agendas of communities that are trying to develop a better place in which to live. Nurses can be and are involved in parent-teacher associations, senior citizens councils, community planning boards, advocacy and civic organizations, and business groups. They can be instrumental in organizing and mobilizing communities on issues such as recycling, environmental cleanup, and safety. Although such activism may arise out of the private concerns of nurses for their own well-being and that of their families, it can also affect nurses' professional lives as, for example, they care for the victims of toxic waste disposal, pollution, or crime.

The interrelationship among these four spheres becomes more obvious as the nurse develops and uses political skills. Ignoring one sphere can endanger one's effectiveness as a change agent. Developing one's influence in all four spheres, however, takes time and effort. While a nurse is striving to develop such influence, networking and collaborating with colleagues who have already achieved significant influence in any one arena should be sought.

NURSING'S HISTORIC MANDATE

Today's nurses were given a mandate for political activism in these four spheres by nurse heroines throughout the profession's history. Although numerous, a few exemplary nurse heroines illustrate this point.

Florence Nightingale was a consummate politician. She transformed the British and Indian health care systems, and military health care as well. She knew the value of data in influencing policy and came to be recognized as the first statistician. Reflecting on her first administrative position in nursing, Nightingale wrote:

> When I entered into service here, I determined that, happen what would, I never would intrigue among the Committee. Now I perceive that I do all my business by intrigue. I propose in private to A, B, or C the resolution I think A, B, or C most capable of carrying in Committee, and then leave it to them, and I always win. [Huxley, 1975, p. 53]

Nightingale oversaw the development of British health policy from her bed; she became frail after the Crimean War and took to her bed for much of the remainder of her life. Policymakers came to her. She sent flowers to her new student graduates, invited them to tea, and then sent

them on difficult assignments that they rarely protested. She was a leader who knew how to garner the support of her followers, colleagues, and policymakers.

Sojourner Truth was born into slavery and later provided nursing care to Union soldiers and civilians during the Civil War. She became an ardent and eloquent advocate for abolishing slavery and supporting women's rights. As a great orator, her words helped to transform the racist and sexist policies that limited the health and well-being of African Americans and all women. As an activist, she worked to free slaves through the underground railroad, fought for human rights, and lobbied for federal funds to train nurses and physicians (Carnegie, 1986).

Lillian Wald's political activism and vision reflected feminist values. At the turn of the century, she recognized the connections between health and social conditions as she established the Henry Street Settlement House on the Lower East Side of New York City. The settlement house was a "safe place" where Wald and a group of nurse and nonnurse colleagues used consensus building to establish programs for the largely poor immigrant population living—and dying—in squalid conditions. She was a driving force behind the federal government's development of the Children's Bureau, arguing that it was shameful for a nation to have policies and departments protecting animals but not children. An ardent peace activist, she was called on by the White House on frequent occasions to participate in the development of national and international policy. A suffragette, she campaigned for presidents even when she herself could not vote (Coss, 1989; Daniels, 1989).

Finally, Margaret Sanger transformed a nation's attitudes and approaches to family planning, risking jail and her own life to do so. She knew the power of information and civil disobedience as she distributed literature on birth control when it was illegal (Chesler, 1992).

These nurse heroines all had a vision that reflected an understanding of the connections between health and the broader social issues of their times. This vision was grounded in values that reflected a caring for the well-being of individuals, families, and communities. They did not silence their voices when they realized that their values were not shared by policymakers. Instead, they developed and used their political skills to transform neighborhoods, cities, states, nations, and the world. Today's nurses must follow in this tradition.

REFERENCES

Ad Hoc Committee to Defend Health Care. (1997). A call to action. *Journal of the American Medical Association, 28*(21), 1733–1738.

Annas, G. J. (1997). Tobacco litigation as cancer prevention: Dealing with the devil. *New England Journal of Medicine, 336*(4), 304–308.

Bifano, L. (1996). Advanced practice politics and the Oregon nurses' trail. *Nursing Administration Quarterly, 20*(3), 54–62.

Blumenthal, D. (1995). Health care reform—past and future. *New England Journal of Medicine, 332*(7), 465–468.

Carnegie, E. M. (1986). *The path we tread: Blacks in nursing, 1854–1984.* Philadelphia: Lippincott.

Chesler, E. (1992). *Woman of valor: Margaret Sanger and the birth control movement in America.* New York: Simon & Schuster.

Cohen, E., & Cesta, T. (1997). *Nursing case management: From concept to evaluation* (2nd ed.). St. Louis: Mosby.

Cohen, S., Mason, D., Kovner, C., Leavitt, J., Pulcini, J., & Sochalski, J. (1996). Stages of nursing's political development: Where we've been and where we ought to go. *Nursing Outlook, 44*(6), 259–266.

Cohen, S., Mason, D. J., Arsenie, L., Sargese, S., & Needham, D. (1998). Nurse practitioners' experiences with managed care organizations. *Nurse Practitioner, 23*(6).

Coss, C. (Ed.). (1989). *Lillian Wald: Progressive activist.* New York: The Feminist Press.

Daniels, D. G. (1989). *Always a sister: The feminism of Lillian Wald.* New York: The Feminist Press.

Fallows, J. (1996). *Breaking the news: How the media undermine American democracy.* New York: Vintage Books.

Fox-Piven, F., & Cloward, R. (1971). *Regulating the poor: The functions of public welfare.* New York: Pantheon.

Grandinetti, D. A. (1997). Will patients choose NPs over doctors? *Medical Economics, 74*(14), 134–142.

Hacker, J. (1996). National health care reform: An idea whose time came and went. *Journal of Health Politics, Policy and Law, 21*(4), 647–696.

Huxley, E. (1975). *Florence Nightingale.* New York: Putnam's Sons.

Institute of Medicine. (1988). *The future of public health.* Washington, DC: National Academy Press.

Joel, L. (1993). Contemporary issues in nursing organizations. In D. J. Mason, S. W. Talbott, & J. K. Leavitt (Eds.), *Policy and politics for nurses: Action and change in the workplace, government, organizations and community* (2nd ed., pp. 539–559). Philadelphia: Saunders.

Kalisch, B. J., & Kalisch, P. A. (1982). *Politics of nursing.* Philadelphia: Lippincott.

Kitzman, H., Olds, D., Henderson, C. R., Hanks, C., Cole, R., Tatelbaum, R., McConnochie, K. M., Sidora, K., Luckey, D. W., Shaver, D., Engelhardt, K., James, D., & Barnard, K. (1997). Effect of prenatal and infancy home visitation by nurses on pregnancy outcomes, childhood injuries and repeated childbearing: A randomized controlled trial. *Journal of the American Medical Association, 278*(8), 644–653.

Lamb, G. (1995). Early lessons from a capitated community-based nursing model. *Nursing Administration Quarterly, 19*(3), 18–26.

MacPherson, K. (1987). Health care policy, values and nursing. *Advances in Nursing Science, 9,* 1–11.

Mason, D. J., Cohen, S. S., O'Donnell, J., Baxter, K., & Chase, A. (1997). Managed care organizations' arrangements with nurse practitioners. *Nursing Economics, 15*(6), 306–314.

Moore, J. D. (1997, May 26). Mass. nurses push staffing bill. *Modern Healthcare, 6.*

Moyers, B. (1991). Yearning for democracy. *In Context, 30,* 14–17.

National Commission on Nursing. (1981). *Initial report and preliminary recommendations.* Chicago: Hospital Research and Educational Trust.

Nursing's Agenda for Health Care Reform. (1992). Washington, DC: American Nurses Publishing.

Olds, D., Eckenrode, J., Henderson, C. R., Kitzman, H., Powers, J., Cole, R., Sidora, K., Morris, P., Pettitt, L. M., & Luckey, D. (1997). Long-term effects of home visitation on maternal life course and child abuse and neglect: Fifteen-year follow-up of a randomized trial. *Journal of the American Medical Association, 278*(8), 637–844.

Reinhard, S., Christopher, M. A., Mason, D. J., McConnell, K., Rusca, P., & Toughill, E. (1996). Promoting healthy communities through neighborhood nursing. *Nursing Outlook, 44*(5), 223–228.

Richardson, D. (1993). Federal government. In D. J. Mason, S. W. Talbott, & J. K. Leavitt (Eds.), *Policy and politics for nurses: Action and change in the workplace, government, organizations and community* (2nd ed., pp. 451–466). Philadelphia: Saunders.

Rogers, B. (1989). Exploring health policy as a concept. *Western Journal of Nursing Research, 11*(6), 694–702.

Schorr, L. (1989). *Within our reach: Breaking the cycle of disadvantage.* Garden City, NY: Doubleday.

Sears, P. (1996). What is difficult can be done at once. What is impossible takes a little longer: The Beijing Conference. *National Women's Studies Association Journal, 8*(1), 179–185.

Secretary's Commission on Nursing (1988). *Final Report* (Vol. 1). Washington, DC: U.S. Department of Health and Human Services.

Shindul-Rothschild, J., & Berry, D. (1997). Ten keys to quality care. *American Journal of Nursing, 97*(11), 35–43.

Smith, G. (1997, June 18). Shaping the future health system through community-based approaches. Keynote address, International Council of Nurses' Congress, Vancouver, British Columbia, Canada.

Stimpson, M., & Hanley, B. (1991). Nurse policy analysts. *Nursing and Health Care, 12*(1), 10–15.

Titmus, R. M. (1974). *Social policy: An introduction.* New York: Pantheon Books.

Trotter-Betts, V. (1996). Nursing's agenda for health care reform: Policy, politics and power through professional leadership. *Nursing Administration Quarterly, 20*(3), 1–9.

U.S. Bureau of the Census. (1996). *Current population survey, March 1996 Supplement.* Washington, DC: Author.

U.S. Department of Health and Human Services. (1996). *Models that work.* Washington, DC: U.S. Government Printing Office.

Woolhandler, S., & Himmelstein, D. U. (1997). Costs of care and administration at for-profit and other hospitals in the United States. *New England Journal of Medicine, 336*(11), 769–774.

Yankelovich, D. (1995). The debate that wasn't: The public and the Clinton plan. *Health Affairs, Spring,* 7–23.

Chapter 2

FEMINIST PERSPECTIVES ON POLICY AND POLITICS

BARBARA A. BACKER, DONNA M. COSTELLO-NICKITAS, DIANA J. MASON, ANGELA BARRON MCBRIDE, AND CONNIE VANCE

There's an old Chinese proverb: Women Hold Up Half the Sky. *It means that half the work and half the thinking in the world is done by women. For the sky to be complete, both halves must work together; nothing can be truly human that excludes one half of humanity. Until recently, the half of the sky assigned to women has been the private half; the public half has been ceded to men. But as women assume positions of leadership in the public realm, they are bringing their values with them, and the ancient dichotomies—between male and female, between public and private—are dissolving.*

— Sally Helgesen (1990, p. xxi)

Throughout the world, considerable progress is being made in women's calls for equity in the public sphere—in the world outside the private sphere of the home where societal and institutional decisions are made and actions taken. Combining work and family is increasingly seen as the norm for both sexes, and playing multiple roles is no longer assumed to be inherently problematic for women (Crosby & Jaskar, 1993). In spite of signs of progress, barriers to women's full participation in the public sphere persist, as evidenced in the following statistics:

- In 1994, 58.8% of women in the United States were in the full-time labor force; however, women still earned approximately 75% of what men earned (Institute for Women's Policy Research, 1996; Lewin, 1997).
- Only 5% of senior managers at Fortune 2000 industrial and service companies are women (Women Figures, 1997).

- Women are represented by pictures and quotes in the news media only 8% to 15% of the time; they are more likely to be shown in television programs, films, commercials, and magazines as preoccupied with romance rather than having jobs or going to school (Friedan, 1990; Smith, D., 1997).
- Although American women are struggling to increase their number and clout in the United States Congress, in 1997 they held only about 10% of the 535 seats in the House and Senate (Ayres, 1997).
- Women hold only 11.7% of all the seats in the world's parliaments, even though they make up 50% of the world's population (Lewis, 1997).

If the challenges of the twenty-first century are to be met and equality in the policy process established, it is essential to understand the inequities of women's real life experiences as they struggle with removing the barriers to full participation in the public sphere, rather than being limited to the private sphere. Binion (1995) suggests that the consequences for women over the public-private dichotomy are fundamental and profound. "A separate spheres approach has relegated women to the home (private sphere), away from the political institutions that make policy and away from a substantial role as well in the other public institutions that determine the nature and quality of life in a community" (p. 515). According to the report of the Fourth World Conference on Women, held in Beijing, China, in 1995, women's equal participation in political life and policymaking is pivotal in ensuring the advancement of women. "Without the active participation of women and the incorporation of women's perspectives at all levels of decision-making, the goals of equality, development and peace cannot be achieved" (Fourth World Conference on Women, 1996, p. 109).

Feminist scholars have consistently called on women to recognize and respect their own voices and to use them to transform and change their local communities, their workplaces, and government and public policy (Friedan, 1981, 1990; Tobias, 1997). Nurses and women have an urgent and historic mission to change societal systems that lack caring and foster violence and abuse of power, which, in turn, destroy and violate people's wholeness. In fact, women policymakers are showing that this is possible. Regardless of their political affiliation, they are promoting agendas that their male counterparts have previously not prioritized, including issues such as maternity leave, divorce law, and domestic violence (Ayres, 1997; Brenner, 1997). An analysis of voting patterns in recent elections demonstrated that women are more supportive than men of the social safety net and a governmental role in solving society's problems, as well as being concerned about the human impact of public policies and budget cuts (Dodson, 1997).

More than 25 years ago, a nurse and president of the National Organization for Women, Wilma Scott Heide (1973), called on nurses to become leaders in bringing about a humanistic society, as well as to humanize health care. A noted feminist theorist and psychiatrist, Jean Baker Miller (1982, 1988), has suggested that true social advancement can emerge when women put forth feminist concerns and perspectives. A feminist reformulation of work, leadership, and relationships is essential. This will occur if we listen to, value, and articulate our voices and bring them to the public worlds of politics and policymaking.

This chapter will explore feminist perspectives on power, politics, and policy, with an aim to provide visions for new models and directions for "holding up the sky." In this new vision, people will have confidence in their voices in the public sphere and will participate fully in shaping institutional and societal policy and the methods for developing such policy. As Chinn (1989) has stated:

> [F]eminist thinking brings another dimension to the possibilities that we can envision for the future, a dimension that enables us to think about how to move towards that reality. This dimension is best expressed by a foundational premise of feminism: the personal is political. . . . This premise of feminism is much more than a slogan. It is a profound insight about the world that creates a tremendous shift in how we think, what we identify as the most important problems in our world today, and what solutions we envision for these problems. This insight brings us face to face with issues of power and freedom . . . what it means to be powerful, and what it means to exercise power in the world. [p. 73]

A FEMINIST MODEL OF CARING

Caring is a concept that is central to feminist and nurses' values (Benner & Wrubel, 1989). Contrary to what is often popularly believed, feminist thinking and values are not limited to women but include all people who are concerned with equality, human rights, connectedness, and humanism. Feminist researchers and theorists have focused their work on understanding gender differences in life experiences, values, and perspectives, even though they are often quick to point out that these differences are not strictly gender based. Women do not "own" nurturance, compassion, or caring. These are human traits (Pinch, 1996). Caring is not gender specific, nor is it mere sentiment. To view it in this way trivializes it and precludes it from being basic to the public world. Caring is a value that must become central to the foundations, operations, and priorities of the workplace, government, organizations, and community.

The feminist value of caring has been devalued in the past. It has typified the private sphere but has not been the dominant value in the public sphere, where policy is made and where nurses work (MacPherson, 1987). As Reverby (1987) notes, nurses have been ordered to care by a society that does not value caring. This conflict of engaging in work that a society does not value has taken its toll on the profession. It has led to the replacement of nurses with less skilled or in some cases unskilled personnel, the absence of whistle-blower protection for nurses reporting unsafe conditions in health care institutions, opposition to reimbursement of nurse practitioners and clinical nurse specialists, and attempts to control nurses and nursing.

Caring is the basis of any spirit of community among people (Farson, 1996). Pinch (1996) points out that creating a caring community belongs to everyone, each of whom is charged with protecting, rather than exploiting, the community. "We can no longer afford to restrict feminine values to the private domestic sphere. They must be integral in group functioning, community building, and world peace" (p. 87). To build meaningful communities of caring in which people can live and grow, Blickman (1996) suggests that the following elements be present: trust, unity, interdependence, and stability. "Nurses and the patient relationships they forge create that kind of community. They not only help us heal, they embody the more powerful and enduring victory of care" (Gordon, 1997, p. 308). To remain victorious in promoting care and compassion while simultaneously facing historic changes in the health care delivery system (hospital restructuring, layoffs, replacement of nurses by unlicensed personnel, and managed care and other private sector forces), nurses must be clear about their values and bring them forth in the new world order.

A feminist model of caring fits this new world order. A caring model encompasses the values of wholeness, interconnectedness, equality, process, support, diversity, and collaboration. These values are tied to women's ways of knowing, interacting, and decision making. They contrast with the dominant societal values in the United States of individualism, competition, and inequality (MacPherson, 1987). Although the feminist model does not necessarily exclude individualism and competition, it puts these concepts into balance with collectivity and cooperation. The feminist emphasis on caring and community is based on the concept of the "web of inclusion" (Helgesen, 1990). This web is a way to portray a model of living and working in which relationships are affirmed, collaboration is encouraged, and diversity and equality are highly valued. It emphasizes collectivity and connectedness, in contrast to individualism and isolation; working together in a blend of collaboration and competition; and attending to many voices, in contrast to one authority. Working collectively requires that process be valued as much as product; in fact, the valuing of process can lead to a better product.

Caring involves a belief system that encourages empowerment and emancipation of both nurses and patients. It is the power to act according to one's own values instead of being acted on by other people and events. Caring also encompasses fostering a health care system that comprises enabling and supportive activities. Caring in nursing includes the following:

> a) a way of being for people which is responsive rather than judgmental or hierarchial—what might be termed a care ethic; b) a health care system which encourages health care and not just disease management; and c) a range of nurturing and protective acts devoted to assessing and responding to patient conditions. To be concerned about care is to be involved at the macro level (e.g., social values and policies), as well as the micro level (e.g., interpersonal processes and caring acts). [McBride, 1989, p. 6]

Caring within a feminist model goes beyond bottom-line performance and clinical outcomes. Gordon (1997) explains that although it is essential to analyze scientifically the results of nursing care, measures must be sensitive enough to capture what caring means to and does for patients as individuals and the health care system as a whole.

The concepts of the caring community and web of inclusion have tremendous relevance for a shifting health care system. There is a far greater role for inclusion, community partnerships, cooperation, and caring if we are to survive and to address the multiple human problems that confront us daily. The U.S. health care system suffers from a lack of caring; it is devoid of enabling and supportive activities, including attending to patients' emotional and social needs as well as their physical pain and suffering (Gordon, 1997). There is a critical need to build the power of caring through a feminist perspective. This will be difficult, because current power holders will struggle against anything that challenges the status quo and their control of power. Nevertheless, this new model is not about taking power away; rather, it seeks a redistribution of power that confers respect for each person's voice.

EMPOWERMENT: FEMINIST PERSPECTIVES ON POWER

The feminist values identified above suggest that there may be ways of understanding, getting, and using power that differ from those of the traditional model that has dominated society and, in its extreme Machiavellian form, has led to continuing, blatant abuses of power. In a classic work, *Towards a New Psychology for Women,* Miller (1976) noted that women and men often view power very differently. The traditional male model is one of power grabbing—hoarding information and control, taking power from others, and wielding authority. Rowan (1984) suggests that those who seek to wield power over others want to enhance their own power at the expense of others. On the other hand, those who prefer to share power want to share influence, information, and control. They seek power "with" rather than power "over." This notion of sharing is central to feminist values of equality and connectedness. It is dynamic and reflects an understanding of the strength that occurs when resources and abilities are pooled and developed in collaboration with others.

Power sharing is increasingly being embraced as a model for operating in various spheres. Contemporary models of leadership and management reflect the significance of shared decision making in organizations and of leaders' providing employees with both the freedom and support needed to perform their jobs (Belasco & Gorham, 1996; Keller & Dansereau, 1995). New paradigms for health care delivery promote collaborative teamwork that encompasses the possibility of nonhierarchical distribution of power and decision making. Nurses' awareness of, and skills in, implementing these new paradigms and policies are vital if we are to maintain our voices in this new ideology of partnerships. Power sharing enhances respect for others and self, and it leads to empowerment. It is a process aimed at changing the nature and distribution of power in a particular cultural context. "Empowerment requires a commitment to connection between self and others, enabling individuals or groups to recognize their own strengths, resources, and abilities to make changes in their personal and professional lives. It is a process of confirming one's self and/or one's group" (Mason, Backer, & Georges, 1991, p. 73).

For empowerment of nurses to participate in the policy process, three overlapping dimensions must be addressed (Mason et al., 1991):

1. **Consciousness raising** about the sociopolitical realities of a nurse's life and work within society. This includes an understanding of gender, racial, cultural, and class biases that impede equal participation by nurses in making policy decisions in their places of work and in government.
2. **A sense of self-efficacy or self-esteem** regarding nurses' ability to participate in the policymaking process. Nurses must value their voices and speak at policy tables, in clinical settings, their communities, and in academe.
3. **Development of skills** to influence the policymaking process—knowing how to use

traditional methods of power and politics in policymaking, as well as how to use new methods of relating to power and politics. In recognition of the importance of skill development, participants at the Fourth World Conference on Women, in Beijing, China, in 1995, included in their action plan a strategic objective to increase women's capacity to participate in decision making and leadership through providing leadership and self-esteem training (Fourth World Conference on Women, 1996).

Chinn (1995) and others (Mason et al., 1991; Fourth World Conference on Women, 1996) have identified some of the methods for actualizing these three dimensions to empower nurses:

- Involving those affected by a decision in the decision-making process but making certain that they are educated on techniques of effective communication and problem solving
- Flattening organizational charts to decentralize decision making
- Using consensus building when possible
- Using brainstorming techniques to devise approaches for managing conflict and problem solving
- Being attentive to the dynamics of the process of work, giving attention to ground rules such as encouraging dissenting voices, and respecting disagreement
- Encouraging deliberative mentoring
- Developing peer review approaches to evaluation
- Using self-governance models in health care institutions
- Valuing the connections that people develop with each other in the process of daily work and deliberations

Diverse mechanisms for sharing power must be developed and tested in a variety of settings. Studies reported in the nursing literature support the relationship between staff nurses' empowerment and the degree of authority and autonomy they possess (Backer, Costello-Nickitas, & Mason-Adler, 1994; Blanchfield & Biordi, 1996). Rodwell (1996) noted in her concept analysis of empowerment that "practitioners appear to value the interpersonal process element of empowerment, whereas managers see empowerment as returning power and control to the practitioners" (p. 307).

Traditional methods of power acquisition need to be carefully examined in terms of their consistency with or violation of the value of caring. For example, to the extent that positional power requires unequal, hierarchical relationships, it violates equality as an essential part of caring; however, development and use of expert power does not, unless expertise is narrowly defined (e.g., only those with "credentials" have expert knowledge, or only the professional nurse has expertise—the nurse's aide has none). Developing an empowered, collective nursing voice in partnership relationships includes the valuing of all caregivers' contributions to patient care, including family, technicians, and community healers.

Power sharing has been embraced by other groups that are shaping health policy and health care. Dr. Gloria Smith, RN, vice president of programs for the W. K. Kellogg Foundation, has extended the power-sharing model as a challenge to the "limited resource model" that is driving health care. In her keynote address before the 1997 International Council of Nurses' Quadrennial Congress, she noted that resources to promote the health of communities are limited only if people fight over who will get and control which resources, rather than embracing the power-sharing approach of community partnerships. With this approach, the strengths of public and private community entities are shared to expand rather than constrict resources. Nurses have long understood and demonstrated this model with communities (Reinhard et al., 1996). We now need to articulate it, integrate it into our politics, and support policies that will enable it.

FEMINIST PERSPECTIVES ON POLITICS

The world of politics has historically presented obstacles and challenges to women and nurses. Politics has been perceived by many women as a corrupt, masculine, and coercive arena best left to the machinations of male politicians. Although Lewenson (1996) has documented that nursing's early leaders were political activists around public policy and nursing issues, nurses have often viewed the political world as unprofessional, unfeminine, and unrelated to their care of patients. Further, nurses and women have been characterized as oppressed victims who lack the self-esteem, cohesiveness, and political savvy to improve their situation. Until politics was understood as the mechanism that influences practically every sphere of professional and personal life, many women and nurses preferred distancing themselves from the political realm and did not attempt to gain political know-how. The prevalent societal view perpetuated by political philosophers has been that men by nature are rational and politically adept and that women are emotional and therefore incapable of being effective in politics (Lloyd, 1984). Socialization and internalization of values, attitudes, and behaviors have produced structures and norms with a built-in power and political balance toward men.

A worldwide movement toward democratization has opened up the political process in many nations, but the participation of women in politics and governance, as full and equal partners with men, has yet to be achieved. As supported by the data at the beginning of this chapter on women's political representation in policymaking bodies worldwide, women are still dramatically underrepresented in the centers of political power. American women are still struggling to increase their number and clout in the United States Congress. In state legislatures, about 21.5% (or 1,593) of the 7,424 legislative seats are held by women (Ayres, 1997). In 1997, two nurses held Congressional seats and approximately 80 nurses held positions in state legislatures. Although the numbers present a dismal picture as we move toward the twenty-first century, there are growing pockets of remarkable political involvement by women and nurses. For example, in the State of Washington, there are almost as many female legislators in

the Senate as male—22 of 49. "Nowhere else in American politics is there a sight quite like it" (Ayres, 1997). In 1997, three nurses were appointed by President Bill Clinton to the 32-member Advisory Commission on Consumer Protection and Quality in the Health Care Industry.

As women and nurses are inventing new paradigms of teaching and learning (Belenky, Clinchy, Goldberger, & Tarule, 1986), of leadership (Helgesen, 1990; Jamieson, 1995; Rogers, 1988; Rosener, 1990), and of mentoring (Vance & Olson, 1998), they are developing new methods of political involvement. Friss (1994) argues that nursing is politically alive and that its struggles are symptomatic of societal conflicts over issues of education, work, and the private and public lives of women. A new political paradigm and substantive changes will be required for women and nurses to realize their full and equal participation in economic, sociocultural, educational, and political life. In *Megatrends for Women,* Aburdene and Naisbitt (1992) state that women are finding new routes to political power. It is their contention that women dominate the electorate and support their own; that they get higher marks in dealing with crucial social and domestic issues such as day care, education and health, and helping the poor, and that they have uncovered new routes to political clout, as lobbyists, as appointed commissioners and policymakers, and in elected offices of mayor, state treasurer, and governor.

Women's ways of political activity have the capacity to transform politics so that a plurality of voices and perspectives can be heard and acted on. This plurality is essential in a complex global society that will require new ways of living and working. At the first Women's Economic Leadership Summit, cosponsored by the Center for Policy Alternatives and the White House Office for Women's Initiatives and Outreach, held in April 1997 in Washington, D.C., it was stated that "women do not yet have the power to insure outcomes that can transform their lives and the broader society," nor do they have a "critical mass in economic or political decision-making" (American Council on Education, 1997). This critical mass of women activists in politics will be required in order to move social, health, educational, and economic agendas that will ultimately benefit the entire society. The Leadership Summit is prepared to launch a series of roundtable events to determine how women in various realms of influence can join together to move society's mandates. These deliberate initiatives will be required in order to solidify women's political influence.

Nurses and nursing students in the new millennium will need to be political activists and to work together to ensure that their voices are heard and that policy decisions are collectively determined. Several political writers in the profession have suggested that nursing's move to a more sophisticated stage of political development must be deliberately planned if the perspective and values of the profession are to be mobilized to reshape the health care system (Cohen et al., 1996). They suggest that the essential strategies in this stage include the building of coalitions and constituencies, leadership development, campaign involvement, integration of health policy into educational curricula, and the development of public media expertise and of sophistication in policy analysis and research. Nurses have several notable strengths in the political arena: their numbers (more than 2.5 million), their values and concerns for people, and their positive public image (Hadley, 1996). Nurses represent a substantial group of educated, professional citizens who can be a collective lobbying voice and a powerful voting bloc. By converting their considerable power into political action, nurses can be a strong force for transforming health care systems and societal values.

FEMINIST PERSPECTIVES ON POLICY

Public policy is a matter of choices. These choices are driven by the values of those who determine what the policies will be. If women's and nurses' voices are not represented at the policy table, as historically has been the case,

the policies that result will be driven by the dominant values of the public sphere, which have left many of our communities struggling for survival. When policy is developed with a focus limited to "bottom line" issues at the expense of concern for the growth and development of communities, then choices become limited. Caring becomes a lost value.

Nurses know well the emphasis that society has placed on both curing and the use of high technology, often at the expense of models of care that require a great deal of human interaction, connectedness, and intuitive knowing. Schorr (1989) pointed out that research and demonstration projects have repeatedly documented the successful strategies for improving maternal and infant outcomes in high-risk teen pregnancies, such as reduction of repeated teenage pregnancies, return of the mother to education or employment, and reduction of infant and maternal morbidity and mortality rates. These strategies involve intense, well-coordinated human interaction over time—characteristics that doom these strategies to be considered "too costly," even though society unquestioningly pays for the expensive high-tech care of a very low birth weight infant. Since Schorr's review, Olds et al. (1997) have reported on the long-term outcomes of postpartum home visits by nurses to high-risk mothers and infants, concluding that the $7000 spent per mother on the follow-up care was cost-effective. Nevertheless, such nursing care is seldom supported by the private or public sector.

How different would public policies look if women's and nurses' voices were more influential in shaping them? In 1977, 20,000 women from the United States and its territories were elected to participate in the first National Women's Conference to draft a comprehensive feminist agenda for public policy (Fund for the Feminist Majority, 1990). Following are some of the major concepts and examples of policies consistent with these concepts:

- **Equality:** Support for ratification of and compliance with human rights treaties and international conventions on women's rights.

- **Reproductive freedom:** Support for funding international family planning.
- **Peace and disarmament:** Support for reduction in military spending, disarmament treaties, the development of peace initiatives, and the promotion of peace education.
- **Civil rights:** Support of measures to eliminate racial and ethnic discrimination of all kinds.
- **Economic justice:** Support for the right of workers to collective bargaining, fair labor standards, a livable minimum wage, decent occupational health and safety standards, and adequate and secure pension rights, and support for pay equity.
- **Elimination of poverty:** Support for equality for women in education and employment, as well as support programs to provide adequate food and health levels to people in poverty.
- **Elimination of discrimination on the basis of disabilities:** Support for barrier-free access to public accommodations.
- **Increase in quality human services:** Support for a comprehensive nationwide system of quality child care with adequate public and private funding; support for national health insurance; and increase in spending for education, health care, and medical and scientific research for human services.
- **Elimination of violence:** Support for laws and programs to decrease the incidence of violence.

Although progress has been made on some of these issues, women are continuing to define policy agendas that reflect their priorities and values (Brenner, 1997). By 1997, women leaders were recognizing the preeminence of the economic context of their concerns. At the first Women's Economic Leadership Summit, 80 women leaders developed a national economic plan that identifies the needs of families and communities, highlights critical economic issues, and incorporates women's ideas, solutions, and priorities. The plan included the following:

- Expanding **access to education and training** as a key step toward economic efficiency.

- Expanding the **Family and Medical Leave Act** to guarantee paid leave, broader eligibility, and mandatory posting of and education about the act in the workplace.
- Ensuring a **critical mass of women** in economic and political decision making.
- Making **fair pay** for all workers a top priority.
- Passing **comprehensive domestic violence legislation** in all states.
- **Improving the welfare reform law** passed in 1996 by emphasizing education and training (American Council on Education, 1997).

Add nurses' voices to this agenda, and the result is Nursing's Agenda for Health Care Reform (*see* Appendix D), which emphasizes primary care and public health. Additional specific policies might include the following:

- **An emphasis on the development of provider-client relationships,** the "knowing" of the client, and health counseling based on this understanding, rather than the "seven-minute visit" promoted in some managed care systems.
- **Prevention and treatment of addictions** to legal (e.g., nicotine and alcohol) and illegal drugs would be free and readily available.
- **Decision making about priorities for health initiatives and resource allocation** would be made via true partnerships with communities in a power-sharing model.
- **Behavioral, high-touch interventions** would be embraced and reimbursed for their long-term cost-effectiveness and emphasis on self-care. For example, behavioral approaches to incontinence that are currently being used by clinical nurse specialists would be reimbursed just as surgical interventions are.
- **Treatment plans for pregnant women with substance abuse problems** would include day care centers, with the recognition that the **care of the women's children** is an integral part of the care of the women.
- A variety of **approaches to sustain and support the family** would be endorsed. For example, respite care would be available for women and men who are providing care for ill family members at home.

- **Education would be a priority** for society and would be recognized as essential to the health and well-being of individuals and communities. Education would be adequately funded to permit effective teacher-student ratios and on-site health care services. The importance of human interaction and connectedness to the growth and development of our children would be recognized and supported—documented as successful and cost-effective in the Head Start programs.
- **Resources and plans would be devoted to community development,** including community organizing and decision making, development of youth organizations, control of environmental issues (traffic, pollution, noise), community education on nonviolent approaches to conflict management, and community-based health programs that include outreach efforts.

Nurses' voices can be particularly effective at advocating a policy agenda based on an ethic of care because they consider both the instrumental (i.e., objective, rational) and the expressive (i.e., affective values and beliefs) components of issues. Women have lived the expressive component, but they have had to learn the instrumental component to be effective in the public world. The integration of both components has the potential to blend both feminist and traditional voices in policymaking. However, because the expressive component has not been valued in the public world, the full integration of this component into nurses' professional work needs further development and exploration.

SUMMARY

As women increasingly move into policymaking roles and other positions that can influence the policy agendas of the public and private sectors, they have the opportunity to transform their professions, their workplaces, their professional organizations, and health care in general. The political skills necessary for nurses to transform the health care and social systems will include traditional ones such as lobbying, know-

ing parliamentary procedure, and negotiating tradeoffs; however, nurses—both men and women—with feminist values will bring new skills to policy formulation and implementation. These skills will include listening to all voices until consensus is reached, recognizing multiculturalism in the expansion of frontiers of knowledge and practice, and sharing power. We as nurses must acknowledge our selves: "But primarily for us all, it is necessary to teach by living and speaking those truths which we believe and know beyond understanding. Because in this way alone we can survive, by taking part in a process of life that is creative and continuing, that is growth" (Lorde, 1984, p. 43).

REFERENCES

Aburdene, P., & Naisbitt, J. (1992). *Megatrends for women*. New York: Villard Books.

Allen, D. (1984). Division of labor by gender, professionalism and the control of nursing practice. In S. Geiger (Ed.), *Sex/gender division of labor: Feminist perspectives* (pp. 93–103). Minneapolis: University of Minnesota Press.

American Council on Education. (1997). Women leaders express need for expanding access to education. *Higher Education & National Affairs, 46*(8), 1, 4.

Ashley, J. (1980). Power in structural misogyny: Implications for the politics of care. *Advances in Nursing Science, 2*(2), 3–22.

Ayres, B. D. (1997, April 14). Women in Washington statehouse lead U.S. tide. *The New York Times*, A1.

Backer, B. A., Costello-Nickitas, D., & Mason-Adler, M. (1994). Nurses' experiences of empowerment in the workplace: A qualitative study. *The Journal of the New York State Nurses Association, 25*(2), 4–7.

Belasco, J. A., & Gorham, G. (1996). Why empowerment does not empower: The bankruptcy of current paradigms. *Seminar for Nurse Managers, 4*(1), 20–27.

Belenky, M. F., Clinchy, B. M., Goldberger, N. R., & Tarule, J. N. (1986). *Women's ways of knowing: The development of self, voice, and mind*. New York: Basic Books.

Benner, P., & Wrubel, J. (1989). *The primacy of caring: Stress and coping in health and illness*. Menlo Park, CA: Addison-Wesley.

Binion, G. (1995). Human rights: A feminist perspective. *Human Rights Quarterly, 3*(8), 509–526.

Blanchfield, K. C., & Biordi, D. L. (1996). Power in practice: A study of nurse authority and autonomy. *Nursing Administration Quarterly, 20*(3), 42–49.

Blickman, L. (1996). A continuum of care: More is not always better. *American Psychology, 51*(7), 689–701.

Brenner, E. (1997, January 19). The power women share as lobbyists. *The New York Times,* Section 13, p. 1.

Care, N. S. (1984). Career choice. *Ethics, 94,* 283–302.

Chinn, P. (1989). Nursing patterns of knowing and feminist thought. *Nursing and Health Care, 10*(2), 70–75.

Chinn, P. (1995). *Peace and power: Building communities for the future* (4th ed.). New York: National League for Nursing.

Cohen, S. S., Mason, D. J., Kovner, C., Leavitt, J., Pulcini, J., & Sochalski, J. (1996). Stages of nursing's political development: Where we've been and where we ought to go. *Nursing Outlook, 44,* 259–266.

Cole, J. (1991, May 26). Commencement speech, College of New Rochelle, New Rochelle, NY.

Costello-Nickitas, D. (1989). *The lived experience of choosing among life goals: A qualitative study.* Unpublished doctoral dissertation. Garden City, NY: Adelphi University.

Crosby, F. J., & Jaskar, K. L. (1993). Women and men at home and at work: Realities and illusions. In S. Oskamp & M. Costanzo (Eds.), *Gender issues in contemporary society* (pp. 143–172). Newbury Park, CA: Sage Publications.

Dalton, G. W., Thompson, P. H., & Price, R. L. (1977). The four stages of professional careers: A new look at performance by professionals. *Organizational Dynamics, 6*(1), 19–42.

Dodson, D. L. (1997). Women voters and the gender gap. In W. Crotty & J. Mileur (Eds.), *America's choice: The election of 1996.* New York: McGraw-Hill.

Fact sheet on women's political progress. (1991). Washington, DC: National Women's Political Caucus and American Council of Life Insurance.

Farson, R. (1996). *Management of the absurd: Paradoxes in leadership.* New York: Simon & Schuster.

Fourth World Conference on Women (1996). *Platform for action and the Beijing Declaration.* New York: United Nations.

Fox Keller, E. (1985). *Reflections on gender and science.* New Haven, CT: Yale University Press.

Fox Keller, E. (1986). Making gender visible in the pursuit of nature's secrets. In T. de Laurentis (Ed.), *Feminist studies: Critical studies* (pp. 67–77). Bloomington: Indiana University Press.

Friedan, B. (1981). *The second stage.* New York: Dell.

Friedan, B. (1990, November 3). The new feminine mystique. Paper presented at the American Academy of Psychoanalysis, New York, NY.

Friss, L. (1994). Nursing studies laid end to end form a circle. *Journal of Health Politics, Policy and Law, 19*(3), 597–631.

Fund for the Feminist Majority. (1990). *The feminization of power in government.* Arlington, VA: The Fund.

Gilligan, C. (1982). *In a different voice: Psychological theory and women's development.* Boston: Harvard University Press.

Gordon, S. (1997). *Life support: Three nurses on the front lines.* Boston: Little, Brown.

Hadley, E. H. (1996). Nursing in the political and economic marketplace: Challenges for the 21st century. *Nursing Outlook, 44,* 6–10.

Heide, W. S. (1973). Nursing and women's liberation: A parallel. *American Journal of Nursing, 73,* 824–826.

Helgesen, S. (1990). *The female advantage: Women's ways of leadership.* New York: Doubleday.

Howe, M. (1991, June 16). Sex discrimination persists, U.N. says. *New York Times,* p. 7.

Institute for Women's Policy Research. (1996). *The status of women in the states.* Washington, DC: Author.

Jamieson, K. H. (1995). *Beyond the double bind: Women and leadership.* New York: Oxford University Press.

Keller, T., & Dansereau, F. (1995). Leadership and empowerment: A social exchange perspective. *Human Relations, 48*(2), 127–145.

Lewenson, S. (1996). *Taking charge: Nursing, suffrage and feminism in America, 1873–1920.* New York: National League for Nursing Press.

Lewin, T. (1997, September 5). Equal pay for equal work is No. 1 goal of women. *The New York Times,* p. A20.

Lewis, P. (1997, March 16). In the world's parliaments, women are still a small minority. *The New York Times,* p. A10.

Lloyd, G. (1984). *The man of reason: "Male" and "female" in Western philosophy.* Minneapolis: University of Minnesota.

Lorde, A. (1984). *Sister outsider.* Freedom, CA: The Crossing Press.

MacPherson, K. (1987). Health care values, policy, and nursing. *Advances in Nursing Science, 9*(3), 1–11.

Mason, D. J., Backer, B., & Georges, A. (1991). Towards a feminist model for the political empowerment of nurses. *Image: Journal of Nursing Scholarship, 23*(2), 72–77.

Mason, D. J., & Costello-Nickitas, D. (1990). Empowering nurses for politically astute change in the workplace. *The Journal of Continuing Education in Nursing, 22*(1), 5–10.

McBride, A. B. (1989). Knowledge about care and caring: State of the art and future development. *Sigma Theta Tau International Reflections, 15*(2), 5–7.

Miller, J. B. (1976). *Towards a new psychology for women.* Boston: Beacon.

Miller, J. B. (1982). *Women and power: A work in progress.* Wellesley, MA: Stone Center, Wellesley College.

Miller, J. B. (1988). *Connection, disconnections, and violations: A work in progress.* Wellesley, MA: Stone Center, Wellesley College.

National Center for Children in Poverty. (1991). Number of poor children growing. *News and Issues, Fall Issue,* 1.

Olds, D. L., Eckenrode, J., Henderson, C. R., Kitzman, H., Powers, J., Cole, R., Sidora, K., Morris, P., Pettitt, L. M., & Luckey, D. (1997). Long-term effects of home visitation on maternal life course and child abuse and neglect: Fifteen-year follow-up of a randomized trial. *Journal of the American Medical Association, 278,* 637–643.

Pinch, W. J. (1996). Is caring a moral trap? *Nursing Outlook, 44*(2), 84–88.

Public Health Service Task Force on Women's Health Issues. (1985). *Women's health: Report of the public health service task force on women's health issues,* Vols. 1 & 2. Washington, DC: U.S. Department of Health and Human Services.

Reinhard, S., Christopher, M. A., Mason, D. H., McConnell, K., Rusca, P., & Toughill, E. (1996). Neighborhood nursing. *Nursing Outlook, 44*(5), 223–228.

Reverby, S. (1987). *Ordered to care: The dilemma of American nursing.* New York: Cambridge University Press.

Rodwell, C. M. (1996). An analysis of the concept of empowerment. *Journal of Advanced Nursing, 23,* 305–313.

Rogers, J. L. (1988). New paradigm leadership: Integrating the female ethos. *Initiatives, 51*(4), 1–8.

Rosener, J. B. (1990). Ways women lead. *Harvard Business Review,* November–December, 119–134.

Rowan, G. R. (1984, Spring). Looking for a new model of power. *Women of Power, 1,* 67–68.

Schorr, L. (1989). *Within our reach: Breaking the cycle of disadvantage.* New York: Doubleday.

Smith, D. (1997, May 1). Media more likely to show women talking about romance than at a job, study says. *The New York Times,* p. B15.

Smith, G. (1997, June). Shaping the future health system through community-based approaches. Keynote address, International Council of Nurses' Quadrennial Congress, Vancouver, BC.

Tobias, S. (1997). *Faces of feminism: An activist's reflection on the women's movement.* Boulder, CO: Westview Press.

Vance, C. (1982). The mentor connection. *Journal of Nursing Administration, 12,* 7–13.

Vance, C. (1989–1990). Is there a mentor in your career future? *Imprint, 36,* 41–42.

Vance, C., & Olson, R. (1998). *The mentor connection in nursing.* New York: Springer Publishing.

Watson, J. (1979). *Nursing: The philosophy and science of caring.* Boston: Little, Brown.

Watson, J. (1985). *Human science and human care,* Norwalk, CT: Appleton-Century-Crofts.

Watson, J. (1987). Nursing on the cutting edge: Metaphorical vignette. *Advances in Nursing Science, 10*(1), 10–18.

Watson, J. (1990). The moral failure of the patriarchy. *Nursing Outlook, 38,* 62–66.

Women Figures. (1997, January 15). *The Wall Street Journal,* p. A16.

VIGNETTE
From Bedside to Beijing
Linda Tarr-Whelan

It is not the prerogative of men alone to bring light to the world.   — Aung San Suu Kyi, Nobel Prize winner (1996)

Nurses as Leaders on the Issues Women Share

According to 1996 research results published by the Center for Policy Alternatives in *Women's Voices: Solutions for a New Economy*, there is more that unites women than divides us. Women's common agenda is family economic security. Health is a big worry. Time and money are in short supply; equal pay, retirement, balancing of family and work, and child and elder care top the list of unsolved problems. Respect and dignity for caregiving—at home or in the workplace—are a shared concern for American women.

It is clear from this research that women and men have different views on economic issues close to home. Men largely see family and work as separate and distinct spheres. They are less interested than women in community or employer solutions for benefits, dependent care, or pensions, believing instead that individual families should solve these problems privately. Women, across race, class, party, geography, and age, see the issues differently. Women see family and work as inseparable and intertwined—the *yin* and *yang* of their lives. This difference leads to dramatically different public policy concerns.

Like other women, nurses are working harder and contributing more on the job and at home. Again, our contributions are essential but invisible. Eighty percent of consumer decisions are made by women, and almost that percentage of health decisions are made by women. Yet equal pay is still elusive (*see* Chapter 10, on collective strategies). Pay gaps between women and men still exist in every profession and for every job. Over their lifetimes, male college graduates will average $454,000 more in lifetime earnings than female college graduates.

Economically, women in the United States are now almost half the workforce. More than one in every four American workers is employed in a woman-owned firm. Women are starting businesses two times faster than men and succeeding at a higher rate. Women are the majority of college graduates and graduate school graduates. In an information age with a global economy, the contributions of women are essential to our nation's economic success.

Politically, women's contributions are increasingly important. Women are the majority of voters in our country. In the 1996 elections, the voting pattern of women was very different from that of their husbands, brothers, and fathers. A gender gap of 17% between the votes of women and men resulted in the election of Bill Clinton as president of the United States.

What is true in America is also true for women around the world. There is more that unites us than divides us. In 1995, 50,000 women and men joined together from around the world in Beijing, China, for the United Nations Fourth World Conference on Women.

We came to break the silence—to let the world know that women around the world share problems, aspirations, and solutions and that we have potential economic and political strength in addition to our important family roles. I was one of the 25 delegates representing the United States, and one of two nurses. Virginia Trotter Betts, then president of the American Nurses Association, was the other.

In Beijing, we shared a transforming vision and road map for a new partnership between women and men in all spheres of life. Women's role in the economy, health care, and violence against women were at the center of the discussions. The topics of the conference ranged across the interests of women in their seamless roles of mothers and political leaders, caregivers and financial managers, sisters and daughters, workers and entrepreneurs. The statistics about women in the world are stunning. Women:

- Are 50% of the world's population
- Do 66% of the world's work
- Are, with their children, two thirds of the world's poor and refugees
- Own 10% of the world's land
- Hold 10% of national parliamentary seats
- Have 1% of the world's wealth

The 189 nations of the world agreed in Beijing to a wide-ranging Declaration and Platform for Action to address problems of women and girls throughout the world. The United States was an active participant in this process. President Clinton appointed an inter-agency task force, the White House Council on Women, chaired by Secretary of State Madeline Albright, to provide the leadership for the U.S. Government's implementation of the agreement. Women have come together across the country in nongovernmental organizations to ensure that women's full and equal partnership with men is realized in the public and private spheres of life.

As a nurse I have made the transition from care for individual patients to involvement in national and international issues. The story of my journey is one of increasing awareness of the need to stand up, speak out, and make a difference.

From the Bedside to Beijing and Beyond

Today I lead the Center for Policy Alternatives, a national public policy and leadership center that focuses on action to solve economic and social problems. We work with innovative leaders across the 50 states. My second role is international. I was appointed as U.S. Ambassador by President Bill Clinton to serve as the U.S. Representative to the United Nations Commission on the Status of Women.

I am not a lawyer nor an academic. I'm a nurse—a nurse who believes strongly that our society needs the values, skills, and perspectives that nurses share to be part of public policy development. Anyone watching the dramatic changes in health care in the 1990s knows that decisions are being made and change will continue. Who will be at the policy table is not so clear. Basically we must decide whether nurses are part of policy decisions.

Like most nurses, I have found that the practice of our profession is affected by many issues transcending the nurse-patient relationship. Financial management, economics, politics, and policy are the silent ghosts at every bedside.

So this is the personal story of one nurse and how my concern about patients, nurses, justice, family, and community has brought me into ever-wider circles of public policy and politics. My career has moved me into arenas I never imagined. As the first nurse in the history of our country to serve in the White House and now the first nurse to be a U.S. Ambassador, my journey may help embolden other nurses to expand their horizons.

How and why did a nurse become a negotiator of international documents for women around the world or lead a policy center in Washington, D.C.? Certainly not from personal ambition. This is a tale of awakening and then engagement to leave the world a better place. I have learned to trust my values, beliefs, and instincts. And I stubbornly refuse to sit on the sidelines if I can work with others to change unfair, unjust, or unwise policies.

In 1957, at the age of 17, I began life as a student nurse at the Johns Hopkins Hospital School of Nursing and began wearing our ugly brown "duty booties." The daughter of a suburban middle-class family (my father was a union leader and my mother a librarian), I was the first girl (that's right, "girl") in my family to go on to higher education.

Except for a short flirtation with wanting to be a doctor, an ambition never fostered at home or school, I always wanted to be a nurse. I was a sickly child, and the warm, skillful care of nurses drew me toward nursing. The 1950s preceded the dramatic opening of careers for women fostered by the women's movement. There were relatively few options—secretary, librarian, teacher, nurse, or home "economist." I knew that nursing was what I wanted.

Off I went to the heart of Baltimore and Johns Hopkins. It was and is a bustling world-class medical center. The curriculum was challenging, and our teachers were dedicated professionals. We worked hard, for long hours, and took on awesome responsibility. We grew up fast and learned lessons for life. Hopkins student nurses took responsibility for our actions. We did what needed to be done regardless of the odds. From the beginning, we were taught to respect all our patients and, through public health experiences in the city, to learn about their lives and challenges.

Hopkins gave us the opportunity to care for a variety of patients and families of every race, culture, and class. One of my favorite patients was a Gypsy king dying of stomach cancer amid hundreds of his tribe camped out in the halls. Another was a courageous 3-year-old boy who had been terribly burned in a tenement space-heater fire.

We learned the content and craft of nursing. We were taught that our success was often determined by drawing on the varied perspectives and skills each member of the health team brought to the task of cure and care. Learning was a hands-on experience. Night after night seasoned nurse's aides taught me, supported me, and followed my lead as a skittish 18-year-old student serving as charge nurse on a ward of very sick people.

More a carrier of Florence Nightingale's lamp than a rebel, I liked nursing and did well. Then it seemed the natural order of life that almost all nurses were women and almost all doctors were men. Somewhat uniquely for the time, Hopkins valued the contribution of nurses as professionals. But the lines were still rigid. There was a doctors' dining room and a nurses' dining room. Our nursing notes included circumlocutions such as "the patient appeared blue" to avoid infringing on the prerogative of the doctor to diagnose cyanosis.

The desire to be a change agent evolved slowly over the 10 years that I actively practiced nursing. My nursing career started inauspiciously: I worked as a floor nurse at a small proprietary hospital in the college town where my husband was going to graduate school. Three hours into my first day shift, the director of nursing—and wife of the doctor who owned the hospital—delivered an ultimatum. "Do you want to quit or be fired?" she said. Feeling pretty confident, I asked for the charge against me. I chose to be fired when I heard that the charge was unprofessional conduct. The grounds were that I had not stood up for a doctor when he came on the floor. Not only was this not the hospital for me, but I had learned an important lesson about equality.

Next I took my crisp organdy cupcake cap to a job as the only registered nurse in the office of an ophthalmologist. He was one of very few eye specialists in this midwestern university town. A competent doctor, he saw 75 patients a day. It looked as though I had an ideal full-time job while pursuing my bachelor of science in nursing (BSN) degree full time.

Now my education was of a different sort. The reality of medical economics began to become disturbingly clear. The doctor earned a fortune. I certainly didn't earn enough for tuition and a decent apartment. His time with the patients was minimal and highly technical. This doctor's office was a well-oiled machine aimed at maximizing his earning potential. For most of the patients, the care was impersonal and abrupt even if it was technically superior.

After I moved back east to continue my undergraduate education, two summer experiences really moved me toward changing systems as well as caring for patients. First I was employed to create an in-service education program in a large, underfunded and understaffed city hospital. The next summer was the most difficult in my career. I was hired as an interim head nurse to correct serious problems in a suburban newborn and premature nursery.

Both jobs etched a strong belief in me that it is impossible for real professional nursing practice to exist in a defunct system. No matter how hard one nurse tries, her effort is never enough to make a substantial difference. The core of professionalism must be for nurses to change the institutional policies and practices that stand in the way of good health care.

In 1963, after a total of 6 years in college, I finished my BSN degree at Johns Hopkins and began teaching. A 3-year nursing education was undervalued for college credit. At Johns Hopkins in the early 1960s, women were restricted to the night school; only men could attend the day school. Another lesson in the valuing of women's work and men's work was becoming part of my education.

My first teaching position was in surgical intensive care in an innovative program at a large city hospital. Three instructors and 12 students covered critically ill patients using a 24-hour team coverage approach. There were new learnings here, too. The cost of care for patients was astronomical—and some couldn't pay and were transferred away. Gunshots, knives, and septic abortions took many lives. I began to care more deeply about cause and effect rather than illness and treatment.

After an additional stint of teaching maternal and infant nursing, in 1965 I decided on graduate school with an eye toward using my newfound passion for changing the health care system to be better for patients. Having graduated with honors and with strong work experience, I was naive enough to think that it would be easy to get into a good graduate program in hospital administration. Wrong. "No girls allowed," I was told. By now I knew in my very soul that sex discrimination in education was real. It was time to try to change that reality for the next generation.

Now time moves more quickly. Medicare had just become law. (Although it seems hopelessly naive now, insurance coverage for all elderly citizens was going to be the first step toward universal health care.) There was a building boom in nursing homes. I began to teach at a university school of nursing and developed an instructor's manual to prepare licensed practical nurses for charge responsibilities in nursing homes. The professional nursing organizations worked hard to block the program on the grounds that only registered nurses could perform this role despite a severe shortage at the time.

My dissatisfaction with fighting my own profession led me to become the nurse consultant for a large career ladder program in health care that was funded by the U.S. Department of Labor and the U.S. Department of Health, Education, and Welfare in 1968. The program was a partnership between employers, public employee unions, and colleges in nine states. The most satisfying work I have ever done, my role was to help bridge the aspirations of nonprofessional health workers to become paraprofessionals and professionals through partnerships between unlikely allies.

The American Federation of State, County and Municipal Employees (AFSCME, AFL-CIO) was the sponsor and the fastest-growing union in the country. It was my home for 9 years and the place where I made the transition from nursing to health, from an individual voice to collective strength, from personal ideas and ideals to public policy in Congress and state houses. Shortly after joining AFSCME, I separated from my husband and became a single mother with two young children. And I learned that my insights and experience as a nurse and a mother made a difference in the outcomes of the issues that the union supported.

My work moved me from nurse to union official. I studied the working conditions of nurses in the early 1970s and compared them with international experience. Representing the United States at a joint conference of the World Health Organization and the International Labour Organization in Geneva in 1973 introduced me to the value placed on nurses and nursing in other countries. It had another major effect on my life. My husband of 24 years and I became engaged at this conference. He represented British unions there.

As a union organizer for nurses and health workers, I crisscrossed the country to organize. Most of the members were women. Most of them were supporting families on low wages and skimpy benefits. The members of the union saw immediate improvements in both, and I began to work with other union women to create the Coalition of Labor Union Women to open more opportunities for working women. The platform for action was clear: equality under the Constitution, full partnership in leadership of unions as staff and elected leaders, and pay and working conditions comparable to those of men. That was more than 20 years ago, and none of the goals are yet fully achieved.

My work on issues for health workers led the union to establish a public policy department, which I headed. Now the working experience of public employees across the country was folded into state and national legislation, as well as negotiated as part of collective bargaining agreements. Deinstitutionalization of the state mental hospitals—really more warehouses than hospitals—was under way. We helped write the Community Mental Health Centers Act to enable patients—and workers—to make the transition into the community.

The late 1960s and early 1970s were a dynamic time in our country. The civil rights, antiwar, and women's equality movements were in the headlines, and my job placed me right in the middle of the action. There was no longer a question in my mind. Collective action by people who cared could change the direction of the country politically through policy change.

Tough politics was my next assignment. In 1973, AFSCME decentralized its executive staff and moved my husband and me as a team to lead the union in New York State. It was in many ways an entirely new world. I found myself negotiating statewide contracts for correction

officers after the Attica prison riots, running voter registration and get-out-the-vote campaigns, and lobbying the legislature. One thing hadn't changed. Women working for the State of New York had a tough time. Their career paths were blocked, and few were in management positions. The Center for Women in Government was founded to change that reality. As a statewide union official and nurse, I began to sit on governmental commissions, including New York's groundbreaking health commission, founded to explore the improvement of health care in the state.

In 1976 I moved into state government as the administrative director of the New York State Department of Labor. New York was headed into a recession, and this large agency was responsible for unemployment compensation and worker safety and health. It was early for a woman to hold a high-level management position in government. There was an essential lesson for me. You can make a difference anywhere. We began career ladders, shared jobs, created college classes at the work site, and instituted tuition reimbursement.

My career opened up in unexpected ways. In 1979, the last year that Jimmy Carter was President, I was invited to join the White House staff as deputy assistant to the President for women's concerns. I was amazed to find out that I was the first nurse to hold a position at this level. The job gave me the opportunity to meet with women from all walks of life, work across the country on the passage of the Equal Rights Amendment (ERA), and be involved in the dramatic changes opening up for women in health, education, and employment. As exciting as it was, I would not have been able to hold a White House job without my husband's strong support and his willingness to be the primary caregiver for our children. The position was all encompassing and all consuming.

With the end of the Carter Administration, I moved to the National Education Association, a large union of public-school teachers and employees that had attracted my attention because of its strong support of ERA ratification.

As the director of government relations during the Reagan years, I learned that any public policy advancements are ephemeral. They can disappear with the passage of legislation and the stroke of a pen. Constant vigilance and activity undergird continued public support.

I moved to the Center for Policy Alternatives (CPA), then a small, progressive think tank working across the states. From defending the status quo, we proceeded to a positive, progressive agenda on issues that were stuck in Washington, D.C. As president and chief executive officer, I have been involved in the Center's tenfold growth and have provided leadership on issues of importance to women. CPA is now a 21-year-old policy and leadership development center with a track record of success in creating a horizontal wave of change across the 50 states.

For example, the Family and Medical Leave Act, which provides up to 12 weeks of unpaid leave for care of a newborn infant or emergency health care for oneself, spouse, or family member, was signed into law by President Clinton in January 1993 (*see* Chapter 10). It had languished for 8 years on Capitol Hill and was vetoed twice by President Bush. During that period, with CPA in the lead, family leave legislation passed 30 states in one form or another.

One of the major focal points of CPA's work has been women and the economy. That work was recognized in 1994, when I was tapped to be part of the U.S. delegation preparing for the Beijing Conference. President Bill Clinton named me U.S. representative to the United Nations Commission on the Status of Women. This international body is charged with overseeing implementation of the Beijing Platform to achieve equality for women. Now, with confirmation by the Senate, I am a U.S. Ambassador.

More nurses are needed in the public arena. As I have moved along in my career as an advocate and governmental official, I have credited my nursing roots for much of my success. Nurses have a wider world-view—for us, patients matter as people, family members, and part of the community. Nurses have a "hands on" approach and don't shirk hard work. Nursing today is high touch *and* high tech. Compassion and caring are mixed with professional practice and holistic thinking. That's what our society needs.

It is time that many other nurses join in a journey of self-discovery to understand the value that nurses add to the public dialog and decisions. The nursing profession needs to empower itself to make a difference in wider and wider circles of influence. Nurses must lift their voices for quality health care and access. We must join other women and men to make the contributions of women visible and paid equally. The shared visions and values of nurses are needed to provide solutions for the problems that families and communities face.

VIGNETTE

Dancing with the Chaos: A Grassroots Approach to Transformation and Healing in Nursing

Jeanne Anselmo

Think of the concepts that arise in your mind when the word *chaos* comes to it—random, unpredictable, ever-changing, impermanent, uncertain, disordered. Researchers and physicists tell us that underlying what looks like random, unceasing disorder is the beauty of pattern and organization. From the chaos of downsizing and reengineering, old paradigms are being dismantled, leaving opportunity for our profession to transform itself and the health care system.

Nursing and nurses are learning how to dance with the chaos of these times. Dancing partners learn to respond to each other, to follow the rhythm of the music, and to allow the pattern of the dance steps and the essence of the dance to move through them and guide them. The dance of life is ever changing, as described in ancient wisdom books like the *I Ching*. Nursing, society, health care—all are touched by this constantly changing dance of life. Learning to dance with this chaos allows us to create new opportunities, transform and heal our personal and professional wounds, and learn to be copartners with our colleagues in communities and the world at large. Learning to trust life, to trust that there is a pattern emerging within the

chaos and to understand that by transforming ourselves we may be able to influence larger systems—this is vital to our personal, professional, and collective health, well-being, and wholeness.

Margaret Mead said, "Never doubt that a small group of thoughtful committed citizens can change the world—indeed it is the only thing that ever has." This is not just an inspirational quote by a twentieth-century icon in anthropology. Mead's statement is grounded in physics—the butterfly effect. The beating of a butterfly's wings can create a breeze that, joined by unpredictable forces, culminates in the development of a tornado in another part of the world, according to chaos theorists. Our choices amid chaos can have larger implications and a cumulative impact greater than we can ever imagine. The power of one or a small group is immense.

Friends, Colleagues, and Nursing Circles

In the spring of 1995, the health care system in New York City was beginning to change rapidly. Managed care, downsizing, "right sizing," and reengineering were affecting nurses. Nurses were feeling lost and confused as they grappled with rumors. During this time a number of friends and colleagues who were working together as staff and consultants at a hospital in New York City would gather periodically either by phone or in person. Ideas, information, and possible strategies were shared as these friend-colleagues and I pooled our experiences, knowledge, wisdom, and wit. Being together and working in this way were very special. Each of us had different work roles and

The author acknowledges her friend-colleagues who helped launch the first nursing town meeting and were the seeds starting the Nursing Summit: Barbara Joyce, Barbara Glickstein, and Diana Mason. Special thanks to Susan Luck for her support in opening the door for the summit, and to all the faculty, resource persons, and support persons involved in the creation of this grassroots effort, without whose love, wisdom, and commitment to nursing, these town meetings and the first nursing summit would not have happened.

> **TIPS FOR NURSING CIRCLES**
>
> 1. Begin with creating a safe, nurturing space. Include flowers, music, herbal tea, snacks, and, most important, confidentiality.
> 2. Begin and end with a meditation to center, calm, and relax participants and to practice self-care.
> 3. Leave titles and credentials at the door.
> 4. Invite each person to share from the heart. Remember that everyone needs time to share, so be brief, listen, and be open to what each person is saying.
> 5. Speak from an "I" place, rather than telling people what "they" or "you" should be thinking or doing.
> 6. Learn the principles of conflict resolution and negotiation. (See Chapter 9, on conflict management.) Invite your group to study conflict resolution skills together.
> 7. Use seed questions to begin dialog, or invite issues from the group.
> 8. Don't be afraid to ask for help. If problems arise beyond the scope of skills of the group, call in resource people from human resources, nursing education, social work, or psychology departments. Before a problem arises, make contact with members of other departments and get to know them. Explore whether their philosophy and style match the needs of your group. Build relationships; ask whether they could provide support if necessary.
> 9. If the circle is in the community, call local colleagues in institutions or private practice for support and information. Build relationships.
> 10. Enjoy being together, sharing, supporting each other, building alliances, and creatively solving problems.

positions, making the multifaceted offerings between us nourishing on many levels. The creativity and fun in difficult times was maintained, and we were able to support each other. The unexpected, in-the-moment quality of our informal interactions added an important dimension of spontaneity and demonstrated the authenticity of our connectedness.

During this same time, I was offering self-care and healing circles for nurses at various hospitals and clinics. Some groups consisted of the entire staff, from housekeepers to the medical director, but most focused on self-care for nurses. The multidisciplinary groups offered an opportunity for improving communications, breaking down barriers and stereotypes, and improving conflict resolution and departmental problem solving. Some deep work emerged from these groups, but the deep work around nurses' issues of wounding, experiences of oppression in the system, and hierarchy were unable to be as deeply explored in the interdisciplinary groups as they were in the nursing circles.

The purpose of the nursing circles was to provide a safe place for nurses to share their experiences with and feelings about the changing health care system, as well as to provide mutual support. The nursing-circles format was simple. Chairs were set in a circle in a secluded area of the unit or in a conference room. This was to create an atmosphere of safety and confidentiality. Flowers or a live plant was placed on the floor in the center of the circle as a focus and to bring beauty and centeredness to the group. When possible, herbal tea and healthy snacks (cookies or fresh baked goods from the local green market) were available. The atmosphere of the circle was to offer nurturing support, safety, and care for ourselves and each other.

Each circle began and ended with a centering relaxation, imagery exercise, meditation, or energy practice. This was a way to offer nurses an opportunity to let go of the problems and pressures of the day, to be in touch with their own issues and needs, and to restore and renew themselves. The next step was to go around the circle and "check in." The nurses shared how they were at the moment and what was happening in their work and lives. This was all done voluntarily. The facilitator cultivated an atmosphere of support, encouraging nurses to share ideas, feelings, and needs.

It was amazing how readily nurses accepted a safe forum in which to share their pains, worries, concerns, and interests. For years at Holistic Nursing Associates (HNA), a consulting and practice group formed by a group of holistic nurses, we had been using this format of teaching in a circle. We knew the impact of listening to each other's stories, being able to be heard and be seen by the whole group. This format had a profound impact on the bonding and healing within each of the nurses and within the group and can be used anywhere in nursing practice. HNA's programs differed from unit circles in that the nurses coming to HNA were a self-selected group who were interested in holistic practice and who met outside the hospital. They included nurses from a wide variety of institutions and geographic areas. Rarely were nurses in a class from the same hospital. In the unit- or department-based nursing circles, nurses were sharing their deep concerns with colleagues they worked with each day. The level of need was great, and the fear and the pressures that the nurses were under required a safe, nurturing environment in the nursing circle.

The job of the facilitator is crucial. The role of facilitator is to help each member feel safe, feel vital to the group, and be appreciative of each group member's role and contribution. The group needs to develop an understanding of collaboration and synergy, even while working through problems. In many circumstances, leaderless groups can be extremely nurturing, creative, and effective, though having a facilitator on unit-based groups when the unit or organization is in crisis can be a more effective strategy. I began as the facilitator, but as the group progressed, the facilitator role was taken on by other group members. However, it was often difficult for the charge nurse to be the facilitator. Many times it was hard for the charge nurse to be heard as a fully participating member of the group because she was still in a role of group responsibility. In addition, when difficulties arose between staff members and the charge nurse, issues were less likely to be discussed or resolved. In many cases, charge nurses felt overwhelmed and unprepared to facilitate the group. In these cases, an outside facilitator can help by working with all members of the group, including the charge nurse.

The nursing circles can be initiated by any group of nurses who want to provide a safe place to work through their feelings and con-

---

TIPS FOR TOWN MEETINGS

1. Find a local space or organization interested in copartnering with your group.
2. Begin and end each meeting with a centering meditation, imagery, or relaxation.
3. Keep your meetings simple: invite two to four resource persons to act as catalysts for discussion, information, and support. The resource nurses might be people with experience in professional organizations, innovation, political activism, or community involvement. The purpose of the meeting is to engage the spontaneous sharing of those attending and to learn from each other.
4. If possible, try to offer resource persons an opportunity to meet and socialize before the town meeting, so that they can get to know each other and their areas of interest.
5. Mix various philosophies, ideas, and backgrounds to give depth, variety, and breadth to the meetings. Include all views.

---

cerns while identifying ways to be mutually supportive.

Town Meetings

During the nursing circles, I would try to share some of the insights and information from my friend-colleagues with the unit nurses. I realized that these nurses had missed the excitement, synergy, and fun that my friend-colleagues and I had as we bounced ideas and issues off each other, as well as the deep care we shared as we dealt with the losses going on throughout the system. The unit nurses needed to hear state, national, historical, and holistic perspectives.

The New York Open Center, a holistic institution for education and learning, had been collaborating with HNA to offer an educational series for nurses on holistic practices. The staff of the Open Center are known to be innovators and supporters of growing-edge projects. They offered us a date and space in their catalog to advertise and a room to hold a forum for dialog. We decided that we needed to maintain the circle format, seeing and hearing each other on equal ground. So in the fall of 1995 the first Open Round Table was held at the New York Open Center. Approximately 40 nurses attended, with three nurses and myself serving as resource people or catalysts for the discussions. This and subsequent meetings provided opportunities to expand on the nursing circles by bringing together nurses from different places to network, share their experiences and feelings, and identify other avenues for shifting their own practice and influencing the health care system.

We used a format similar to the one described for the nursing circles. Chairs were placed in a circle in a large room. Music was playing in the background as people came in. Flowers were placed in the center of the circle. We began with a meditation inviting us all to breathe, relax, release the tensions of our day, and be present here and now to what wants to unfold and reveal itself. After the meditation, the four resource people introduced themselves, and we then proceeded around the circle. The 40 nurses introduced themselves and briefly shared why they had come and what interests they wanted to be addressed. The Open Round Table was scheduled for 2 hours, from 8 to 10 P.M. One would expect that after a long day of work in the middle of the week, the nurses would be exhausted. Instead, the energy in the room was enormous. At that first forum, we discussed nurses' being replaced by unlicensed technicians, as well as managed care, political issues in nursing, holistic practices, entrepreneurship, and expanded roles. Nurses in the group participated by voicing their opinions, asking questions, making comments, and listening to each other's ideas.

During the first meeting, nurses asked if we could continue this gathering and suggested that we call future gatherings "nursing town meetings." Each town meeting since has brought together three or four different nursing resource people who shared their vision and experience with approximately 30 to 50 nurses. Mixing together resource nurses of diverse backgrounds, such as nurses from holistic nursing with nurses from state political action commit-

tees, weaves together a variety of ideas and speaks to the wholeness of our profession.

The philosophy of these town meetings and the nursing circles is that each nurse, regardless of position, role, or educational background, has a vital contribution to make. Diversity and inclusiveness of perspectives and ideas are essential to understanding and appreciating nursing's wholeness. Without this we cannot entirely see ourselves, each other, and the truth of our profession. At these forums, we may agree to disagree, but we will always do our best to include all our voices.

A Nursing Summit to Dance with the Chaos

The need to expand on the town meetings became apparent during the summer and fall of 1996, when the downsizing of hospitals began to escalate. Nurses were despairing as they lost jobs, were transferred to clinical areas outside their expertise, saw nursing management wiped out, and tried to cope with financial concerns outweighing the value of caring and quality

---

SEED QUESTIONS FOR USE AT HEALING CIRCLES, TOWN MEETINGS, AND THE NURSING SUMMIT

1. What is your vision for your practice of nursing?
2. How would you like to improve your practice?
3. What skills, personal and professional, would you need to develop? What are your strengths?
4. Why did you become a nurse? Has that reason changed over time?
5. What ways do you stop or undermine your own efforts to move toward your vision? What would help you to change that pattern?
6. What are you learning through personal discussion, reflections, experiences, groups, and workshops that could help you continue to learn and grow?
7. What do you want nursing to become?
8. What do you want nursing practice to be in ten years? Twenty years? Fifty years?
9. Why do you want people to become nurses?
10. What is the true essence of nursing practice? Does your practice today reflect that essence?
11. What do you see nursing's commitment and contribution to society to be? Should be? Could be?

TIPS FOR A NURSING SUMMIT

1. Expect the unexpected. In a volunteer, grassroots group things change and people come and go. Resources may or may not be available. Be flexible! Have a support team. Stay open to what is emerging; it may be better than your original plan.

2. Choose a theme or vision to build the summit. Invite your steering committee to develop a vision, philosophy, and infrastructure for the summit that reflects their shared values and philosophy.

3. Learn about new paradigm leadership. Margaret Wheatley's *Leadership and the New Science* and *A Simpler Way,* David Bohm's *On Dialogue,* and Peter Senges' *The Fifth Discipline* are helpful field books.

4. Leaves titles at the door. Create common ground and an equal playing field for all. Check out your beliefs, expectations, assumptions, and approaches with a variety of nurses from different backgrounds to determine whether you are being inclusive.

5. Diversity brings richness, joy, depth, and deep nurturing. We are all blessed to have a diversity of races, ethnicities, cultures, specializations, education, and ages represented in nursing. Encourage diversity, inclusiveness, and safety. Consciously invite nurses of diverse backgrounds, ethnicities, races, and specializations and education to participate.

6. "Show up for" each other and for ourselves. We will not be able to please everyone; some attendees will want to spring ahead faster, and others will need more time to integrate what is offered. We need to learn to be present for and supportive of each other as nurses. This learning—that nurses were heard, respected, and supported and that they cared about each other—was one of the most highly praised dimensions of the summit.

7. Bring your spirit and deep intention into this work. What touched us all was that, regardless of our tradition, we all wove spirit into our work. Bringing spirit out in ritual, candle-lighting ceremonies, bereavement rituals, dancing, and celebration nourished us deeply, inspired us for the journey ahead, and supported our true intention. Take a risk. Nurses reported that standing together under the stars in a circle, with candles lighted, and being part of a close-knit group in ceremony, has helped to sustain the drive since the summit.

8. Take care of yourself and have fun, and never doubt that a small group of thoughtful, committed nurses can change the world—why not?

patient services. The nursing community was stunned, shocked, and in deep grief. Local nursing groups offered programs on the "threat of the pink slip." Most attendees and presenters seemed to have few answers or ideas, as they grappled with the chaos and the unknown.

Again, we needed to arise out of the chaos to identify ways to transform ourselves, our practices, and the health care system. An opportunity came via the Omega Institute in September 1996. Omega Institute is a campus for holistic education in Rhinebeck, New York. Nestled on a lake amid the beauty of the Hudson River Valley, it offers workshops and retreats. Omega, like the Open Center, has had a long history of offering innovative programs. In 1996 for Omega's twentieth anniversary year, Omega invited an HNA nurse to put together a conference on holistic nursing. Instead of focusing solely on holistic nursing, we joined this opportunity with the issues and momentum building from the town meetings. This was the impetus for the first nursing summit, which a self-formed grassroots steering committee entitled "Dancing With the Chaos."

The beating of the butterfly wings of this grassroots steering committee created a breeze that joined with many unpredictable forces to "shapeshift," form, and re-form the configuration of the summit, leadership group, faculty, and resource persons. Having begun with a plan to gather for 4 days at Omega to strategize and create an action plan for our vision for nursing, we ended up developing a process-oriented healing and visioning summit. The weekend included the following:

- A presummit educational day to help support and develop another generation of nurse facilitators and leaders focusing on diversity, international nursing, environmental nursing, futures visioning, organizational copartnering, creation of a healthy work environment, and self-care.
- Resource faculty sharing their experiences and innovations. More than 30 faculty and resource people, from universities and institu-

tions from Florida to Maine and from Minnesota to Maryland, donated their skills and energy. They continued to share the presummit themes through small group work.

- Time for connecting with others who share a common ground.
- Time for nurses to share their concerns and grief, with rituals to help them acknowledge and then move beyond their losses.
- Small group and large group visioning, offering nurses to think about and write out their vision for nursing and health care, which was then placed in the archives of the New York State Nurses Association to be opened in the year 2020.
- Exploration of new possibilities for nurses and the health care system.
- Time to enjoy each other as nurses and as human beings.

The philosophy of the summit included making this a safe space for all nurses of all backgrounds. Nurses who attended represented nursing's wide range of racial and ethnic diversity, educational backgrounds, and practice settings. There were staff nurses, students, administrators, retired nurses, unemployed nurses, nurse practitioners, researchers, and educators. We were all asked to leave our credentials and roles at the door and sit with each other, nurse to nurse, and person to person. We decided not to have any keynote addresses, though we did have individual presentations and talks. Any language such as "keynote" that would set apart a member from the group, creating a hierarchy, was eliminated.

Those involved in planning the summit discussed how most nurses do not see themselves as leaders and that a leader is "someone with a position of power." They therefore eliminated "leader" and "leadership" from the brochure and reworked the wording to reflect the philosophy that "every nurse is a leader."

We have already planned the date for next year's summit. The National Student Nurses Foundation is providing administrative support and setting up a summit scholarship fund. The Nurses Association of the Counties of Long Island is planning a nursing summit for Long Island; the nurses in Delaware are working on one for Delaware; the Philippines Nurses Association is using the visioning work sheets from the summit as part of their meetings; and various circles and small groups are developing. Individuals and groups are identifying ways that they can continue to shape nursing's future vision. We can't be sure what impact this work will have. We can only be clear about our values and about our intention and commitment to ourselves, each other, our work, nursing, and those we serve. We know that these healing circles, town meetings, and summits are addressing a need in nursing. Two months after the first nursing summit, 80 nurses attended the scheduled nursing town meeting. Two thirds of those nurses had never been to a previous town meeting, summit, or healing circle. As members of the nursing community, we must recognize that this need in nursing is not being acknowledged and addressed in conventional ways. This grassroots movement is filling a gap. I believe this experience invites us to look deeply at the need to reevaluate the current structure of our nursing organizations. We have so much energy and vision yet untapped, waiting and wanting to be developed and supported. Perhaps as many as eight circles, which plan to meet locally, were started that night. They will focus on self-care and self-empowerment to help grassroots nurses create and live their visions. We hope these beginning efforts will be an impetus and inspiration to other nurses.

Chapter 3

HISTORICAL OVERVIEW:
Policy, Politics, and Nursing

SANDRA BETH LEWENSON

The history of the modern nursing movement, which began in 1873, tells the story of a pioneering group of women who responded to the changing role of women in society. They advocated a new profession for women and better health care for the public. In forging the nursing profession in this modern period, nurses had to enter the political arena to gain legitimate authority over their education and practice. However, in the telling of the story, the history has blurred and often obscured from view the rich tapestry of nursing's political past. Nursing's political role and historical activism have been buried in the popular image of the nurse. When remembered at all, nursing has suffered from accusations of conservatism and noninvolvement in the political arena and has been omitted from most women's histories (Lewenson, 1996). This can be explained in part by the way women are perceived by society, which is that women have played a small role in the political arena. Nursing, being closely aligned with women's work, shares with women the many negative, devalued perceptions of the worth of its role (Choon & Skevington, 1984; Heide, 1973; Muff, 1982; Reverby, 1987; Vance, Talbot, McBride, & Mason, 1985). As a result of such a perception, nursing suffers from "nursism," which has been defined as "a form of sexism that specifically maligns the caring role in society" (Lewenson, 1996, p. 226).

Public perception of nursing often depicts nurses as handmaidens to the physicians and subservient members of the health care system.

The old adage that "nurses are born, not made," persists in the 1990s as the purse strings in health care tighten and nursing care is provided by people with less and less professional education. Hospitals cross-train health care workers as a way to cut costs and balance budgets. Like other corporations, hospitals downsize by firing senior nurses with years of experience and advanced professional degrees. This acceptance of less qualified nurses reflects the decreased value society continues to place on professional nursing care. Gordon (1997a, 1997b) writes about the invisibility of nurses' contribution to health care and the lack of recognition for their work. This invisibility and the assumption that women's work is somehow free and expected perpetuate the negative aspects of nursism.

Even more damaging to the profession is the invisibility of nursing's political activism throughout the late nineteenth and the twentieth centuries. Rogge (1987) supports the idea that nursing's use of political power is not new, nor is it confined to this century. Pioneers in nursing honed their political expertise when they persuaded various members of the status quo (e.g., hospital administrators, physicians, community boards of health, state legislators, and politicians) to open nurse-training schools, organize professional associations, and participate in social issues like woman suffrage, birth control, and integration.

The founding and political activities of four national professional nursing groups beginning in the United States in 1893 provide evidence of nursing's political activism. The creation of the American Society of Superintendents of Training Schools for Nurses in 1893 (forerunner of the National League for Nursing), the Nurses' Associated Alumnae of the United States and Canada in 1896 (forerunner of the American Nurses Association), the National Association of Colored Graduate Nurses in 1908, and the National Organization of Public Health Nursing in 1912 provided nursing's political foundation. The history of these organizations illustrates nursing's efforts to control its own education and practice and its strong interest in the *Woman Movement.** They embody nursing's passage through the stages of political development as defined by Cohen et al. (1996). In the early years of each organization, nursing educators and practitioners joined forces to gain control and focus inward on its professional development. Both the self-absorption with professional development and the beginning interest in the larger issues fit the "buy in" stage described by Cohen et al. (1996). Nursing activists educated other nurses on the need for woman suffrage for personal and professional (e.g., to obtain nurse registration laws) reasons. Once established as professional groups, these organizations formed strong coalitions with other nursing organizations (both in this country and abroad) to make their voices heard on social issues like woman suffrage, public health, and women's rights. In this second stage, according to Cohen et al. (1996), nursing moves toward political activism and "develops its own sense of uniqueness" (p. 261). As these organizations matured, they showed interest in issues aside from those that solely affected the profession.

In spite of the historical evidence, accurate memory of political activity in nursing remains scarce. To overcome this dearth of knowledge,

---

Woman Movement is the term used for the late nineteenth and early twentieth centuries' movement to change society's ideas about women; *Women's movement* is the term that describes women's efforts of the 1960s and 1970s.

we must look at cases of political activism from nursing's past. This chapter highlights some historical examples of nursing's political activism such as the influence of Florence Nightingale, the opening of nurse-training schools, the founding of professional nursing organizations, the support of woman suffrage, the work of Lillian Wald in public health and Margaret Sanger in family planning, the efforts of the National Association of Colored Graduate Nurses (NACGN) to integrate African American nurses into the U.S. armed forces, and the formation of the American Nurses Association's Nurses' Coalition for Action in Politics. Because political activism in nursing parallels similar efforts that all women faced throughout the same period, this overview examines the nursing profession's close ties with the Woman Movement of the nineteenth and early twentieth centuries. It also reviews nursing's relationship with the more recent Women's movement of the mid-twentieth century.

BEGINNING WITH THE WOMAN MOVEMENT

The profession of nursing sprang out of the political efforts of women during what is known as the Woman Movement of the middle nineteenth and early twentieth centuries (1848–1920). During this period, women sought political control of their personal lives. They looked to change the laws that regulated their families, their education, and their political freedom. In doing so, women's work came under close scrutiny both by those who wanted to preserve the status quo and by those who wanted reform.

During the nineteenth century, the United States experienced political upheaval, economic changes, and westward expansion. Cities grew out of the rapidly expanding industrial revolution, providing profound economic and political changes in the roles of men and women. Moving away from farms, men found new jobs in the expanding factories and offices in cities. Their labor was no longer dictated by the needs of the farm, which had required them to be available at all hours of the day or night, depending on the season, livestock, or crop. Instead, the time clock now regulated their daily routines. In contrast to the changes in men's lives, women's work continued to be centered around the family's needs. Women worked at home because the family's needs demanded their time, and they had little to do with the world outside. Men's roles dictated that they buffer and protect their wives from the social, political, and economic concerns of the day.

For some women the status quo sufficed, but for many the subordinate role they were expected to play did not, especially for women who did not marry and who did not accept the limitations of women's roles. By the 1830s, schools for women opened and women began to challenge their confined, set role in society. Society conceived women as the "natural born" caretakers for their families, responsible for the moral upbringing of its members. However, some women wanted to branch out of their allotted "separate sphere" and into the more "active sphere" of the world outside the home. For many women (especially middle-class women), this meant obtaining an education, finding a career, and financially supporting themselves. During the nineteenth century, these women sought opportunity for meaningful work, questioned the idea of marriage, and organized to bring about change in the social order (Cott, 1977; Daniels, 1987; Lerner, 1977; Riley, 1986; Rothman, 1978; Zophy, 1978).

POLITICAL AWAKENING AND THE MODERN NURSING MOVEMENT

The modern nursing movement began when Florence Nightingale opened the nurse-training program at St. Thomas Hospital in England in 1860. This landmark event signaled to the world that nurses required schooling for the work they did. It also provided one of the first opportunities for women to work outside the home and be self-supportive. In turn, the rise of modern nursing served as the catalyst for political activities of nurses.

Breaking Ground and the Actions of Florence Nightingale

Nursing was one of the first professions that women sought to control and organize. It is taken for granted that, because nursing is so closely aligned with women's work, women would automatically control the profession. However, historically, this was not the case. Nurses had to maneuver politically to control their professional education, work, and lives. The writings of Florence Nightingale support a feminist stance about who should control the education and work of nurses (Lewenson, 1996). Nightingale believed that nursing should be controlled by nurses. Her "brilliant essence lay in her taking from men's hands a power which did not logically or rightly belong to them, but which they had usurped, and seizing it firmly in her own, from whence she passed it on to her pupils and disciples" (Editorial comment, 1908, pp. 333–334). Like women's education, education for nurses was not considered necessary. The general attitude was that women were natural-born nurses and therefore did not require an education. Yet, after the extraordinary success of Nightingale's ideas about sanitation and nurses' education, an "educated" nurse was sought to reform the deplorable conditions found in hospitals throughout the United States.

Nightingale's letter, sent in 1872 to the founders of the nurse-training school at Bellevue Hospital in New York City, reflected her ideas about separating nursing and medicine. She differentiated between medicine and nursing and clearly saw that nursing's "whole training is to enable them [nurses] to understand how best to carry out medical and surgical orders, including . . . the whole art of cleanliness, ventilation, food, etc., and *the reason* why this is to be done *this* way and not *that* way" (Florence Nightingale's letter of advice to Bellevue, published in the *American Journal of Nursing*, 1911, p. 361). Nightingale further reasoned that "discipline and internal management" of nurses should be "entirely under a woman, a *trained* superintendent, whose whole business is to see that the nursing duties are performed according to this standard" (Florence Nightingale's letter of advice to Bellevue, 1911, p. 362).

Nursing leader and women suffragist Lavinia Dock and her friend Isabel Stewart, professor of nursing education at Teachers College in New York City, commented on how Nightingale's warning to keep control of nursing by nursing was ignored.

> The specially revolutionary feature of Miss Nightingale's plan for nurse-training has been to a singular degree overlooked by commentators and even by nurses. It was, in short, nothing else than the positive mandate that the entire control of a nursing staff, as to discipline and teaching, must be taken out of the hands of men and lodged in those of a woman, who must herself be a trained and competent nurse. [Dock & Stewart, 1931, p. 127]

Nightingale politically advocated health care reforms throughout the world by writing, speaking, and asking for change from people who held powerful positions. Many of her letters illustrate her understanding of the use of power and her ability to articulate clearly what she believed. In a letter written when she had returned from the Crimea to Col. J. H. Lefroy, scientific adviser to the War Office, Nightingale asked for an appointment in the Military Hospitals of the Peace (similar to the appointment she had during the war). She had been invited to meet Queen Victoria of England and sought counsel before meeting her as to how much truth she should share with her at their meeting. Nightingale questioned the integrity and work of the medical men in military hospitals during peacetime and wanted to improve the conditions found there. In her letter, Nightingale stated that the chief reason for her wanting official entrance into the hospital "is the indirect one of having legitimate means of information by which I could suggest reforms not within my power or province to execute" (letter to Col. J. H. Lefroy, in Vicinus & Nergaard, 1989, p. 160). Later in the letter, Nightingale offered that she would be happy to convey her ideas to someone who could accomplish the changes and wrote:

> If I could find a mouth-piece, not obnoxious to the same hostility, which the Army Surgeons

naturally feel towards me, because as a General Officer told me, "they know they have been *found out*," I would gladly give every suggestion which has occurred to me to be worked up & promulgated for the benefit of the Service. [letter to Lefroy, in Vicinus & Nergaard, 1989, p. 162]

After meeting Queen Victoria, Nightingale received a Royal Commission, as she had requested. She wrote of her experiences in the Crimea, as requested, and effected major change in civilian hospitals in England (Vicinus & Nergaard, 1989).

Nightingale the reformer emerges as a complex individual who often achieved her goals "by behind-the-scenes management of the committees and doctors" (Vicinus & Nergaard, 1989, p. 159). It was her letter writing to influential people that helped Nightingale revolutionize health care and nursing education. Moreover, it was the acceptance, around the world, of her ideas about sanitation, education, and separation of nursing and medicine that contributed to her ability to facilitate change.

Professional Education and the Opening of Nurse-training Schools

Political activism of the early nursing pioneers took the form of creating the models for professional education. In the modern nursing movement in the United States, the year 1873 heralded the opening of the Nightingale-influenced nurse-training school. The first three schools credited with this distinction were at Bellevue Hospital in New York City; New Haven Hospital in New Haven, Connecticut; and Massachusetts General Hospital in Boston. Early nursing leaders implemented many of Nightingale's ideas about nursing. They skillfully demonstrated to hospital administrators that using nursing students improved sanitary conditions on wards and led to better patient outcomes. This success created a safer environment for the newly formed medical profession, consequently creating great financial incentives for hospitals to open these schools (Dock & Stewart, 1931). For 20 years (between 1873 and 1893), nurse-training schools proliferated in the United States. In 1880 there were 15 nursing schools, in 1900 432 schools, and by 1910 more than 1,129 schools (Burgess, 1928, p. 35).

The schools opened between 1873 and 1893 were not regulated by any professional group. Hospital administrators recognized the financial advantage of supplying hospitals with students rather than hiring graduate nurses (Kalish & Kalish, 1986; Lewenson, 1996). It was cheaper to use the students than to employ the graduates. Exploitation of the student took on various forms. Education was secondary to work expected. Often the education was limited by the size of the hospital. Many hospitals had too few beds to provide appropriate and sufficient learning opportunities. An early nursing leader and 1885 graduate of the Bellevue Training School for Nurses, Louise Darche (1894), warned the public in a popular magazine of the period, *The Delineator*, of the problems of attending nurse-training programs at small hospitals. Hospitals started those schools to provide the hospital with "a system of cheap nursing" (Darche, 1894, pp. 667–668).

Once nurse training was over, there was no support from the school for the graduate. Graduate nurses found themselves working in the only jobs they could find, such as private duty nursing or public health nursing. Private duty nursing directories, which distributed private duty work, were often controlled by people outside of nursing, such as physicians or pharmacies. This meant that the fee schedule rested outside the nurses' control, which often led to further exploitation of an already exploited group. The exploitation of both the students and the graduate nurses contributed greatly to the strong political stance that early nursing leaders took when they formed professional nursing organizations.

Political Action and the Rise of Professional Organizations

Professional nursing organizations began to form between 1893 and 1912. Their interest first revolved around the issues confronting the profession but later expanded to include social and political reforms affecting society. As each organization formed and matured, political power bases grew and expanded. They moved away from their initial purpose of "the protection and education of one class of women workers" (Palmer, 1909, p. 956) toward interest in more global concerns affecting the health care of the public.

NATIONAL LEAGUE FOR NURSING

The first national nursing organization to form was the American Society of Superintendents for Training Schools, founded in 1893 and renamed the National League of Nursing Education in 1912 and the National League for Nursing in 1952 (hereafter called the NLN). This organization originated at the nurses' congress that convened at the World's Columbian Exposition in Chicago in 1893. Superintendents, chief administrators, and hospital nursing staff sought uniformity in nursing curricula and standards of nursing practice. Alone in their work, they felt isolated and powerless to go before the entrenched powers, such as the hospital boards and medical groups that sought to control the developing profession. By joining together like other women's groups of the day, superintendents created an opportunity to work toward change. Leaders such as Ethel Bedford Fenwick, of England, Isabel Hampton Robb, Lavinia Dock, Louise Darche, Sophia Palmer, and Irene Sutliffe spoke out in favor of collective action. Their early speeches at the first few professional meetings reflected the political tone and progressive nature of the newly founded organization.

Many of the early speeches related the great strides in nursing that had taken place since the opening of nurse-training schools in 1873, while stressing the need to join forces to protect the profession and public from unqualified nurses. They also illustrated the unity and strong sense of political activism that was needed to advance the profession. Lavinia Dock proactively called attention to one of the flagrant problems in nursing practice at the second annual meeting in 1894. Dock (1897) explained how nursing directories exploited private duty nurses by setting fees and paying less to female nurses than male nurses. She demanded that "the woman who nurses ought be paid equally with the man who nurses" (p. 58). Dock urged all private duty nurses to unite and be responsible for setting standards and regulating their work.

AMERICAN NURSES ASSOCIATION

Mindful of the needs of the majority of "trained" or "graduate" nurses, superintendents in the newly formed society urged training schools to form alumnae associations that would provide the basic structure for a second national nursing organization. In doing so, the superintendents spearheaded the founding of the Nurses' Associated Alumnae of the United States and Canada in 1896 (renamed the American Nurses Association in 1911 and hereafter called the ANA). Sophia Palmer, first editor-in-chief of the *American Journal of Nursing* (AJN), called for a grassroots movement that would unite alumnae associations around the country for the purpose of political action and social reform. She urged small and large schools to form alumnae associations that would be able to join together in state associations and form a vital national professional organization. The state societies would form "for the definite and separate purpose of promoting legislation for state registration of nurses" (Palmer, 1909, p. 956). She recognized the inherent power that nurses would wield given organization. Palmer said: "Organization is the power of the day. Without it nothing great is accomplished. All questions having ultimate advancement of the profession are dependent upon united action for success" (1897, p. 55). It was clear to the early pioneer leaders that organizing was the only way to remove the obstacles that nursing experienced on its way to becoming a recognized profession.

Dock (1897) recognized the political importance of a well-organized professional association and laid the groundwork for the organizational structure of the proposed ANA. She did so by studying the structural and political organization of government, labor unions, and other national associations. Dock envisioned a three-tiered organization, with the national organization responsible for developing the ethical, moral, and overriding principles for the graduate nurse; the state organization addressing issues of credentialing and registration; and the alumnae associations supporting the needs of the graduate nurse, such as self-regulating nurse registries and networking opportunities (Dock, 1897; Lewenson, 1996).

The state alumnae associations organized around the highly political issue of state registration. This issue galvanized the nursing membership and forced them to develop their political skills. Up until 1903, anyone could call herself a nurse. It was not until 1903 that the first state nurse registration acts (North Carolina, New York, New Jersey, and Virginia) were passed and the title "nurse" was protected by law. Although the early registration acts varied in their protection of the public from inadequate nursing education, they signified the political efforts of nurses and organized nursing. Nursing leaders in each of these states sought support for this legislation from legislators, politicians, other professionals, and the public through letter-writing campaigns, personal visits to the legislatures, use of the professional journals, and support of the public press (Birnbach, 1985).

Twenty-three nurse alumnae associations joined forces to form the national association and met in New York in April 1898. At their first meeting, they learned at first hand how important it was for them to use their collective strength for political action. Just before the meeting, the United States entered the Spanish-American War. Isabel Hampton Robb, president of the new organization, led the group's effort to serve as gatekeeper for the nurses who served during the war. After a long battle on the home front against Anita Newcomb McGee, a physician and Washington socialite, on who should screen the applicants, organized nursing failed to reach its goal. McGee, as history shows, held on to this pivotal role. Robb believed that this outcome was due to the lack of professional organization. The ANA had organized too late to win this issue (Armeny, 1983; Lewenson, 1996; Robb, 1900). However, nursing learned from this experience. Robb and other nursing leaders recognized their potential political power as an organization and continued to lobby successfully in the years to come.

NATIONAL ASSOCIATION OF COLORED GRADUATE NURSES

Although the first two national organizations addressed the needs of nurses, they primarily focused on those issues confronting the mainstream culture. Discriminatory practices in parts of the United States barred many African American nurses from membership in their state associations. This in turn prevented them from belonging to the ANA. Moreover, segregation and discriminatory practices throughout the country banned black nurses from attending most nurse-training schools and, in some states, prohibited them from sitting for state nurse registration examinations. In keeping with other women's organizations and the need for political activism, black nurses organized the National Association of Colored Graduate Nurses (NACGN) in 1908. It was created to overcome racial hostility and address professional issues. Along with issues of blatant racial discrimination, the NACGN focused on education, standards of practice, and the passage of state nurse registration acts (Hine, 1989, 1990; Johns, 1925; Lewenson, 1996; Staupers, 1937).

To determine the need for such an organization, Martha Franklin, nursing leader and founder of the NACGN, had undertaken a study on black nurses in 1906 and 1907. Franklin sent more than 1,500 surveys to African American graduates of nurse-training schools, most of which had opened in historically black hospital settings (Thoms, 1929). From the survey results, Franklin learned that African American nurses needed an organization to address issues pertaining to their particular needs. Here, too, Franklin recognized that only in the collective would they gain enough power to change conditions in nursing, in health care, and in discriminatory practices (Lewenson, 1996).

At the early meetings, the NACGN members sought to raise professional standards, provide a collegial atmosphere for the graduate nurse, discuss community health nursing, and address issues of racial discrimination. Its members constantly faced the double-edged sword of sexism and racism, which led to the political activism of the NACGN membership. A primary concern for the NACGN was the nurse registration acts that the profession as a whole sought. Not only did the organization support the passage of such acts, but they also fought to ensure that nurses of color could sit for the state examination and that they would be given the same examination as their white counterparts.

Ludie C. Andrews, a 1906 graduate of Spelman College's nurse-training program and superintendent of the Grady Hospital Municipal Training School for Colored Nurses, in Atlanta, vigorously campaigned in Georgia between 1910 and 1920 to ensure the rights of all nurses to sit for state licensure examinations (Hine, 1989). Although Georgia finally, in 1920, ended the discriminatory practice of excluding black nurses from the examinations, the minutes of the NACGN as late as 1917 reflected the concern of its members that "colored nurses were not recognized in the State of Georgia" (letter from Lucy Hale Topley).

Many examples illustrate the political activism of the NACGN in addressing discrimination. Most striking is their effort to fight discriminatory practices in the U.S. armed forces in both World War I and World War II. The American Red Cross barred African American nurses from serving as Red Cross volunteer nurses during World War I. Since membership in the Army Nurse Corps (founded in 1901) required being a Red Cross nurse, black nurses were excluded from serving. Outraged by this affront, Adah Thoms, president of the NACGN, expressed her feelings to Jane Delano, organizer of the American Red Cross Nursing Service and former president of the ANA. In 1918, even while African American nurses were being discriminated against and voicing their anger, they continued to be loyal and patriotic citizens by subscribing to U.S. Liberty Bonds. They believed that the "public should see what we have done and [still] to be ignored professionally" (minutes of the Eleventh Annual Meeting, NACGN, 1918, p. 52).

Delano's response to the Thoms letter was read during the morning session of the NACGN's Eleventh Annual Meeting. Delano said that while she supported the use of NACGN members overseas, the Army had a policy that restricted the number of black nurses selected, and for this reason they were not accepted into the American Red Cross (NACGN, 1918, p. 38). Members of the NACGN continued to argue for the right to serve. However, this policy did not change until 1918, when the ravaging effects of the influenza epidemic in 1917 and 1918 depleted the number of civilian registered nurses and forced the military to accept African American nurses. Eighteen black nurses joined the American Red Cross and were permitted to serve in the Army Nurse Corps in December 1918. Even then, these nurses were denied the right to serve overseas, and integration of the Army Nurse Corps was limited until the end of World War II (Carnegie, 1991; Hine, 1989).

NATIONAL ORGANIZATION FOR PUBLIC HEALTH NURSING

The National Organization for Public Health Nursing (NOPHN) was founded in 1912 by nurses who wanted to ensure the quality and standards of the rapidly growing specialty known as public health nursing. This organization joined with other civic-minded citizens to improve the health of the American public. During the beginning of the twentieth century the need for public health nurses increased as the United States experienced the outcomes of urbanization, industrialization, and immigration. Cities filled with people who wanted to find jobs in these growing industrialized centers. This change in demographics contributed to severely overcrowded housing, unsafe work conditions, inadequate sanitation, spread of epidemics, and poor access to health care, causing progressive reformers to respond. The

public health movement used trained nurses in public health departments and visiting nurse service agencies to bring their ideas about sanitation, immunization, and health care to the public. Between 1895 and 1905, 171 visiting nurse associations opened in more than 110 cities and towns. In 1902 there were only 200 public health nurses; by 1912 there were more than 3,000 (Brieger, 1985; Fitzpatrick, 1975; Gardner, 1933; Lewenson, 1996; Rosenberg & Smith-Rosenberg, 1985; Wald, 1915). With this steady proliferation of visiting nurse associations came unscrupulous home care agencies that offered substandard visiting nurse services. To overcome poor and inferior nursing practices, the ANA and the NLN exerted their political expertise and formed the NOPHN.

In 1911 nursing leaders of the ANA and the NLN developed a plan to organize public health nurses. Letters sent to organizations that employed public health nurses requested that they send a representative to the annual nursing convention of the ANA and the NLN who could vote on the issue of starting a new organization. Most of the agencies responded favorably, and 1 year later, in 1912, the NOPHN organized. The NOPHN objectives were to "stimulate responsibility for the health of the community by the establishment and the extension of public health nursing" and "to develop standards and techniques in public health nursing service" (Gardner, 1933, p. 27). From the outset, the NOPHN recognized the political expediency of forming coalitions with other health professionals and lay people and included them as members. This provided strong affiliations with other groups and a broader political base on which to advocate change.

ORGANIZED NURSING SUPPORTS WOMAN SUFFRAGE

While the ANA, NLN, NACGN, and NOPHN formed, the campaign for suffrage was under way. Suffrage meant personal and political freedom and the means to control the laws that governed women. For nurses, suffrage meant gaining a political voice in the laws that regulated practice, education, and health. Professional nursing organizations provided the medium for nurses to share common experiences and thus find a collective voice. Once these organizations established themselves as viable associations, nurses expanded their horizons to include broader women's issues, such as suffrage, in their political agenda (Lewenson, 1996). This period of political activism in nursing fits the description by Cohen et al. (1996) of the early stages of political development. Nursing, through the four organizations, had developed its identity, formed coalitions, built on its political base, and used the language needed for changing legislation. By advocating for patient rights, nurses began to shape policy. As nursing struggled to come to consensus over the issue of woman suffrage, they published a journal, formed coalitions among themselves and with nonnursing groups, and discussed the political ramifications of both sides of the suffrage question.

In 1900 the ANA and NLN used an important political strategy when they founded the *American Journal of Nursing (AJN)* for the purpose of communicating and sharing ideas. So imperative was the need to find a public forum in which to exchange their views that members funded the journal. The nursing membership raised money to start the journal by buying shares in the journal company. They invested their money, time, and ideas in the professional journal and, in the process, formed a strong coalition from which to carry on their political activities.

The *AJN* provided a public forum for nurses to present ideas about nursing care, nursing interventions, public health, social issues, and other professional issues. Within the pages of the *AJN*, nurses had the opportunity to vent their views on nursing's support of woman suffrage. Although many nurses wanted to maintain the status quo and sought to avoid confrontational political battles, a sufficient number of nurses ardently believed that the survival of the profession rested on gaining suffrage.

Organized nursing's efforts to support the political agenda of the international nursing community led to the formation of the American Federation of Nurses (AFN) between 1901 and 1912. This newly created federation, a coalition forged between the ANA and the NLN, enabled organized nursing in the United States to join the National Council of Women and thus become members of the International Council of Women and later the International Council of Nurses (Lewenson, 1994). It is significant to note that, by 1901, nursing in the United States was ready to form strong coalitions with other nursing groups both here and abroad. They gained a political voice in international health issues affecting women and were specifically interested in supporting suffrage.

Interest in suffrage and connections with women's groups first appeared in the *AJN* in 1906. The *AJN* published letters from the National American Woman Suffrage Association asking nurses to support the sixteenth amendment, giving women the right to vote (Gordon, Myers, & Kelley, 1906). Nursing's staunchest suffragist, Lavinia Dock (1907), argued for nursing's involvement in the suffrage movement and wrote that the national associations would fall short of their mission if they did not get politically involved. She warned against following "the narrow path of purely professional questions" (p. 895). Dock claimed that the modern nursing movement was an outcome of the Woman Movement and that, because nurses were now educated and considered to be "an intelligent army of workers, capable of continuous progress, and fitted to comprehend the idea of social responsibility, it would be a great pity for them to allow one of the most remarkable movements of the day to go on under their eyes without comprehending it" (Dock, 1907, p. 897).

The arguments that nurses used to oppose participation in the political suffrage campaign centered around fear that it would harm political efforts to obtain state nursing registration legislation. In 1908, at the ANA's eleventh annual convention, held in San Francisco, the membership opposed a resolution in favor of the organization's support of woman suffrage. While this event is often used as an example of nursing's conservatism and lack of political activism, this very defeat served as a catalyst for organized nursing to join forces with other women suffragists. Palmer (1908) noted that "the action in San Francisco has brought the matter of suffrage sharply before the nurses of the country" (p. 50). Within four years, nursing responded to the efforts of nursing leaders to support the political franchise. By 1912, nursing organizations voted to support women's right to vote (Ashley, 1976; Chinn, 1985; Christy, 1984; Lewenson, 1996; Wheeler, 1985).

Proponents of nurses' support of woman suffrage linked health issues with the right to vote. Nurses could easily see the relationship between gaining the vote and improving the lives of their patients, families, and communities. Lavinia Dock urged nurses to examine how the franchise would improve social conditions that led to illness. Dock (1908) used tuberculosis as one of the many examples of social issues nurses needed to address and said, in a letter to the AJN, that

> the tuberculosis question is a social question and the causes of tuberculosis (outside of the bacillus) are social causes which need the ballot for their changing, such as bad housing, over-work, underpay, neglect of childhood, etc. . . . Take the present question of the underfed school children in New York. How many of them will have tuberculosis? If mothers and nurses had votes there might be school lunches for all those children. [p. 926]

Progressive-era reform activities and issues such as tuberculosis, Red Cross work, central nursing directories, moral hygiene, state registration, district nursing (public health nursing), school nursing, social work, and nursing the insane were all concerns that members discussed at local alumnae, state, and national organization meetings (Deans, 1910). The NACGN, although not invited to participate in the ANA and NLN resolution to support woman suffrage, did express grave concern for social issues that affected health. The NACGN became

invited members of the international nursing community through its membership in the International Council of Women. This affiliation reflects the NACGN involvement in woman suffrage. The active discussions about woman suffrage, membership in the international women and nursing councils, and the resolution to support suffrage by 1912 indicated strong political activism within the profession.

VISIONARY LEADERS SHAPING HEALTH AND PUBLIC POLICY

Several visionary leaders emerged during this initial period of organization. Some worked with the support of organized nursing, and others did not. Each leader who championed ideas about health care, equal rights, and professional opportunity had to be politically astute to attain the goals. As nursing moved into the stage that Cohen et al. (1996) describes as "self-interest," many of the leaders were paving the way into the next two stages, characterized as "political sophistication" and "leading the way" (p. 260). Women such as Lillian Wald, Margaret Sanger, and Mabel Staupers learned to speak the political language that enabled them to succeed in their respective missions. They spoke to a large audience, served on various national boards and commissions, and built strong coalitions around broad health concerns that went well beyond nursing.

Public Health Nursing

Before the formation of the NOPHN, trained nurses such as Lillian Wald and her friend from training school, Mary Brewster, understood the ramifications of economic, political, social, and cultural factors in regard to health. In 1893, Wald and Brewster opened the Henry Street Nurses' Settlement in New York City, providing nursing care, health education, social services, and cultural experiences to the residents of the Lower East Side (Fitzpatrick, 1975). The nurses at Henry Street lived within the community they served. Wald believed that if nurses educated mothers about health care of the infant, infant mortality would be reduced. Wald (1915) wrote:

> There is a large measure of preventable igno-
> rance, and in the efforts for the reduction of
> infant mortality the intelligent reaction of the
> tenement-house mother has been remarkably
> evidenced. In the last analysis babies of the
> poor are kept alive through the intelligence of
> the mothers. [p. 55]

The work of the nurses at Henry Street reflected their ability to provide care in the home, as well as to lobby for change in the body politic. Backer (1993) noted that Wald "connected her caring with activism by initiating practice and policy changes via administrative and organizational skills, persuasiveness, coalitions, delivering testimony and political power" (p. 128). Wald promoted public health nursing education and the formation of the NOPHN. Moreover, Wald's astute political awareness led to many social changes affecting the health and well-being of the Lower East Side residents.

Children's health and well-being struck a chord with Wald. Concerned for the welfare of children, Wald turned the backyard at Henry Street into a playground. Recognizing that too many children played in the overcrowded streets of the Lower East Side, Wald argued for the opening of city parks and in 1898 successfully formed the Outdoor Recreation League. This group obtained land in New York City and turned it into municipal parks (Siegel, 1983).

Wald's nursing knowledge, social concern, and political savvy joined forces when she maneuvered the board of health into hiring a school nurse in 1902. Wald writes her account in her 1915 book, *The House on Henry Street,* about how she and Brewster recognized a community health problem and kept records on those children excluded from school because of medical problems. After collecting these data, Wald convinced the president of the department of health of the need for nursing services in the public schools. Although the department of health decided to use physicians to inspect the children at schools, when the time was right, Wald encour-

aged the president to hire a public health nurse also. Wald (1915) wrote:

> The time had come when it seemed right to urge
> the addition of the nurse's service to that of the
> doctor. My colleagues and I offered to show that
> with her assistance few children would lose
> their valuable school time and that it would be
> possible to bring under treatment those who
> needed it. Reluctant lest the democracy of the
> school should be invaded by even the most
> socially minded philanthropy, I exacted a prom-
> ise from several of the city officials that if the
> experiment were successful they would use
> their influence to have the nurse, like the
> doctor, paid from public funds. [p. 51]

To Wald's credit, the experiment was successful, and in October 1902 the city of New York paid for the services of a school nurse. The board of estimates had allotted more than $30,000 for the employment of trained nurses who were, in Wald's words, the "first municipalized school nurses in the world" (Wald, 1915, p. 53). New York City's Bureau of Child Hygiene was an outgrowth of this service (Wald, 1915; Siegel, 1983).

The extent to which Wald reached far outside of nursing's boundaries can be seen in the eulogy written by Representative Samuel Dickstein in 1940 for the *Congressional Record.* Wald's political coalitions forged with mayors, congressmen, and the president of the United States set her apart from other nurses. Dickstein (1940) considered Wald one of "America's urban pioneer[s]" and reflected on the many influential guests who had met with Wald at Henry Street. The list of dignitaries included names like the prime minister of England, J. Ramsay MacDonald, New York Governor Alfred E. Smith, and President Theodore Roosevelt. It also included many neighbors in the Lower East Side. All who came to Henry Street were influenced by Wald's commitment to public health.

Birth Control

At different points during the twentieth century, professional organizations and individuals engaged in political activism that attempted to address social ills. During the same period that organized nursing sought social change, the struggle for birth control was lead by Margaret Sanger, a nurse and noted political activist in the twentieth-century birth control movement.

Sanger, like Lillian Wald and Lavinia Dock, understood the importance of political activism for effecting social change. However, unlike Wald and Dock, who sought organized nursing to gain strength, Sanger formed coalitions with other women's groups, labor organizers, and philosophers of the period. Sanger's political strength emanated from her outrage over society's control of women's reproductive process and her belief in reproductive autonomy. This one political issue led Sanger to argue for legalizing family planning and making it accessible and acceptable in the United States.

A brief history of Sanger shows that she worked as a visiting nurse in the Lower East Side in New York City at the beginning of the twentieth century. In 1912, Sanger had an experience that dramatically influenced her work in the area of birth control. A patient, Sadie Sachs, developed septicemia after one abortion and turned to Sanger for help. Unable to assist her in preventing another unwanted pregnancy, Sanger stood by while Sachs died after a second abortion (Bullough, 1988a).

Sanger and her supporters believed that women needed the right to choose whether or not to have children regardless of church or state (Cott, 1987). Sanger hoped to engage the public in a dialog about this issue by starting a newspaper, *Woman Rebel*. Sanger opposed the constraints surrounding birth control for women of all economic backgrounds and sought to provide information on and access to birth control. Feminists who supported Sanger believed that birth control was needed to address the sexual oppression of women. According to historian Ellen Chesler (1992), Sanger viewed contraception as a "tool of liberation" (p. 15).

Sanger politically challenged America's restrictive laws about birth control and personally experienced the untoward effect. For example, in 1912 Sanger wrote an article about

syphilis for the socialist weekly *The Call*. The United States Post Office declared that issue unmailable because of the nature of the material, invoking the Comstock Act of 1873, which deliberately prohibited the distribution of information about contraception and abortion (Reed, 1980). Sanger's crusade to disseminate contraception began in 1914, when Sanger traveled to Europe to seek out safe contraception measures. After returning to the United States, she claimed that women could separate procreation from the sexual act and published her ideas in *Woman Rebel*. Again the Comstock Act thwarted Sanger's efforts. Because of her writings, Sanger was indicted and fled the country in October of 1914. When she returned in 1915, after the death of her daughter, public sympathy led the government to drop the charges against her.

In 1916, Sanger, along with her sister, Ethel Byrne, opened the first birth control clinic in the Brownsville section of Brooklyn, New York. These two women provided mothers in Brooklyn with advice about birth control until the police closed its doors. Sanger again faced arrest, prosecution, and imprisonment. Sanger challenged the legal restriction to distribute information about contraception. Her strong belief and determination led to changes in interpretation of the law and eventually to the founding of the organization known today as Planned Parenthood.

Integration in the Military

The collective action of the NACGN around the issue of racial discrimination toward black nurses in the military during World War II serves as another example of political activism in nursing. The military finally accepted black nurses after a great political campaign waged by the NACGN. Mabel Staupers (1961), executive secretary of the NACGN between 1934 and 1946, wrote of the struggle that black nurses faced in the battle to serve in the U.S. armed forces:

> What frustrations they encountered, solely because of the color of their skin! In World War I, they were not accepted in the Army Nurse

Corps until after the armistice was signed. During World War II, with persistence and cooperation of many white and Negro Americans, they did get into the Army Nurse Corps in 1941; however, they were assigned to segregated units. This was the Army's pattern for the assignment of all Negro Americans. When they finally were accepted in the Navy Nurse Corps in March, 1945, they served, like all other American nurses, without segregation. [p. 97]

Staupers, considered one of the instrumental people involved in the integration of black nurses into the military, did so by preparing the NACGN to engage in the political effort needed to effect change (Hine, 1993). Staupers not only mobilized the NACGN but also sought the "allegiance of sympathetic white nurses within the profession" (Hine, 1989, p. 170). The NACGN used letter-writing campaigns, alliances with the other professional nursing organizations, membership in the newly established National Nursing Council for War Service, meetings with politically significant people, and collective action to forever change the course of events.

In 1945 Franklin Delano Roosevelt proposed a draft of nurses to meet the increasing shortage of professionals. The idea that some nurses would be drafted while other qualified nurses were turned away because of race further fueled the NACGN's campaign to integrate the military. On several occasions, Staupers (1961) met with important political people such as Eleanor Roosevelt and members of various war committees. On one such occasion, Staupers met with the House Military Affairs Committee and presented statistics that supported the argument that segregation and discrimination "had prevented the full utilization of Negro nurses in the military services" (Staupers, 1961, p. 119). In her presentation to the committee, Staupers noted that the 330 Negro nurses accepted into the Army Nurse Corps "represented even less than one-tenth the proportion of Negro soldiers in the Army" (p. 120). The Army Nurse Corps accepted black nurses by using a quota system and denied them equal opportunity once in the service.

Black nurses experienced discrimination in their assignments and in their living conditions in various sections of the country. Black nurses were assigned to care for black soldiers or to prisoners-of-war camps. The Navy Nurse Corps, on the other hand, had refused altogether to admit any black nurse into service.

Yet a shortage of nurses existed, and the NACGN lobbied hard to let the legislature know how discrimination and segregation hurt the war effort. Representative Adam Clayton Powell, of New York City, spoke out against this discriminatory practice and is quoted by Staupers (1961):

> It is further unbelievable that these leaders have become so blindly and unreasonably un-American that they have forced our wounded men to face the tragedy of death rather than allow trained nurses to aid them because these nurses' skins happen to be of a different color. [p. 120]

The NACGN continued to give testimony refuting the idea that there was a representative number of black nurses for the number of black soldiers. Staupers (1961) noted that if the number of Negro nurses accepted into the Army and Navy were of equal proportion to the number of white nurses, then the number of Negro nurses would be 1,520. She testified against the argument that black nurses were less qualified to serve because of an inferior educational background. Staupers argued that all nurses sat for the same state board examinations. Moreover, the written documentation by Pearl McIver, senior nursing officer of the U.S. Public Health Service, reported that no difference in standards existed between the nurse-training schools for Negro nurses and those for white nurses.

Success came in 1945. By the end of World War II, the Army Nurse Corps had admitted approximately 500 black nurses and the Navy Nurse Corps had admitted four. Although the struggle was long and arduous, the NACGN left an important legacy of integration and political activism.

ALLIANCE WITH THE WOMEN'S MOVEMENT, 1960–1990

The women's movement in the second half of the twentieth century raised the level of the American consciousness. Women actively addressed the prejudice they experienced in all avenues of life. Feminism called for activism on the part of women to redress the ills in society and claim an equal place. With time, nurses recognized their need to actively campaign, persuade, and lobby for better working conditions, higher education, and greater access to health care for the public. Nursing's alliance with the women's movement has evolved and gained momentum during the past 30 years. The result has been the inclusion of the feminist perspective in nursing education and practice (Heinrich & Witt, 1993).

In the 1960s the latest women's movement spread throughout the United States. Interest in the rights of women continued, but in the latter half of the century women had the vote. This second wave of activists could conceivably harness the vote and gain equal status for women in the law, at work, and in the home. Although nursing in the latter half of the century remains essentially a profession dominated by women and shares a similar heritage of sexism and oppression, it has taken time to develop an acceptance of the ideas of the feminism espoused in this movement. In the early 1960s, nursing's presence in the women's movement was "obscure" or "notably absent" (Chinn & Wheeler, 1985, p. 74). Political activism frequently associated with feminist groups was not reported to have carried over into nursing. Allen (1985) described an "uneasy" relationship between nursing and feminism. Nursing did not want to be associated with the militant activities of the "bra burning" feminists, and likewise the feminists did not want to have anything to do with the nurses entrenched in one of the traditionally female professions (Allen, 1985; Lewenson, 1996).

By the 1970s some nursing leaders had enumerated the value of developing ties with the women's movement. Wilma Scott Heide (1973),

a nurse and leader in the feminist movement who served as president of the National Organization for Women (NOW) between 1970 and 1974, called for nurses to embrace the ideas of the feminist movement. Heide (1973) believed that nurses and women shared the similar dilemma of being characterized as caring, nurturing, compassionate, tender, submissive, passive, subjective, and emotional. Whereas some of the traits enhanced the professional role, others served to suppress proactive, empowering behaviors. Heide believed that nursing needed to join with the feminist movement in addressing the inequalities that women faced in society.

Another nurse and feminist, JoAnn Ashley (1976), explained that nurses needed to become advocates for consumer health but could not do so as pacifists. Instead, they had to find ways through which to challenge effectively an essentially male-dominated group.

> Professional nursing must begin exerting open and public leadership in meeting consumer health needs. Dominant influences in health care will not yield to the private and quiet pleas of pacifying women: powerful, male-dominated groups, economically motivated, will not be reasonable with their interests and status threatened. Nurses must change their own attitudes toward themselves and their role. [p. 133]

In the 1980s nursing became a metaphor for the "struggle of women for equality" (Diers, 1984, p. 23). Personal and professional empowerment served as essential qualities for gaining political power. Public policy will not change without advocates who can successfully use persuasive, political strategies. Feminism provides nurses with "a world view that values women and that confronts systematic injustices based on gender" (Chinn & Wheeler, 1985). Nursing's acceptance of this definition of feminism has assisted nursing's struggle for equality and can be traced to the early 1970s with the ANA's support of the Equal Rights Amendment; the formation of a group called Nurses–NOW; and the establishment of the Nurses Coalition for

Action in Politics, nursing's first political action committee.

Changes in women's roles mirror society's perceptions of nursing roles. As women in the second half of the twentieth century challenged their inequality and sought political power, nurses did so as well. However, the political savvy of early pioneer leaders was lost to later generations of nurses, and the political tools are gone as well. Too often nurses are not included at the policy table, not involved in policymaking, or just not seen at all (Gordon, 1997a, 1997b). Talbott and Vance (1981) wrote how they had to employ political strategies just to be placed on the agenda of a women's conference on leadership. The nursism that exists within the broader society and at times within the women's movement has lessened, but nursing needs to be vigilant.

CLOSING

Nursing's legacy of political activism altered the course of events for the profession and for health care in this country. Forgetting this legacy has been detrimental to the profession because it denies the opportunity to learn from nursing's visionaries and leaders. Leaders like Nightingale, Dock, Wald, Sanger, and Staupers used strategies like persuasion, the cultivation of political friendships, letter writing campaigns, defiance of the law, and harnessing the collective voice of nurses. In their quest to improve the standards and quality of health care in this country, nurses have had to participate in the political arena. Nurses must remember their past, learn from it, and use it to its best advantage. History lessons from the professional organizations and individuals responsible for political action can provide a road map for political action today. Uncovering the past will begin to address the adverse affect of nursism and will provide important lessons for the future. These lessons are essential for the health of the profession as well as for the health and welfare of the community.

REFERENCES

Allen, M. (1985). Women, nursing and feminism: An interview with Alice J. Baumgart, RN, PhD. *The Canadian Nurse, 81*(1), 20–22.

Andrist, L. (1988). A feminist framework for graduate education in women's health. *Journal of Nursing Education, 27*(2), 66–70.

Armeny, S. (1983). Organized nurses, women philanthropists, and the intellectual bases for cooperation among women, 1898-1920. In E. Condliffe Lagemann (Ed.), *Nursing history: New perspectives, new possibilities*. New York: Teachers College Press.

Ashley, J. (1975). Nurses in American history: Nursing and early feminism. *American Journal of Nursing, 75*(9), 1465–1467.

Ashley, J. (1976). *Hospitals, paternalism and the role of the nurse*. New York: Teachers College Press.

Backer, B. (1993). Lillian Wald: Connecting caring with actions. *Nursing and Health Care, 14*(3), 122–129.

Belenky, M., Clinchy, B., Goldberger, N., & Tarule, J. (1986). *Women's ways of knowing*. New York: Basic Books.

Birnbach, N. (1985). Vignette: Political activism and the registration movement. In D. Mason & S. W. Talbott (Eds.), *Political action handbook for nurses: Changing the workplace, government, organizations, and community*. Menlo Park, CA: Addison-Wesley.

Boykin, A. (Ed.). (1995). *Power, politics, and public policy: A matter of caring*. New York: National League for Nursing Press.

Brieger, G. H. (1985). Sanitary reform in New York City: Stephen Smith and the passage of the Metropolitan Health Bill. In J. W. Leavitt & R. Numbers (Eds.), *Sickness and health in America: Readings in the history of medicine and public health* (2nd ed., rev.). Madison: University of Wisconsin Press.

Bullough, V. (1988a). Margaret Sanger. In V. Bullough, O. Maranjian Church, & A. Stern (Eds.), *American nursing: A biographical dictionary* (pp. 279–283). New York: Garland.

Bullough, V. (1988b). Emma Goldman. In V. Bullough, O. Maranjian Church, & A. Stern (Eds.), *American nursing: A biographical dictionary* (pp. 141–143). New York: Garland.

Burgess, M. A. (1928). *Nurses, patients, and pocketbooks*. New York: Committee on the Grading of Nursing Schools.

Carnegie, E. (1991). The path we tread: Blacks in nursing, 1854–1990. New York: NLN Press.

Chesler, E. (1992). *Woman of valor: Margaret Sanger and the birth control movement in America.* New York: Simon & Schuster.

Chinn, P. (1985). Historical roots: Female nurses and political action. *Journal of the New York Nurses Association, 16*(2), 29–37.

Chinn, P. (1995). *Peace and power: Building communities for the future* (4th ed.). New York: NLN Press.

Chinn, P. L., & Wheeler, C. E. (1985). Feminism and nursing: Can nursing afford to remain aloof from the women's movement? *Nursing Outlook, 33*(2), 74–76.

Choon, G. L., & Skevington, S. M. (1984). How do women and men in nursing perceive each other? In S. M. Skevington (Ed.), *Understanding nurses* (pp. 101–111). New York: Wiley & Sons.

Christy, T. (1984). Equal rights for women: Voice from the past (pp. 63–67). In *Pages from nursing history: A collection of original articles from the pages of Nursing Outlook. The American Journal of Nursing and Nursing Research.* New York: American Journal of Nursing.

Cohen, S. S., Mason, J. M., Kovner, C., Leavitt, J. K., Pulcini, J., & Sochalski, J. (1996). Stages of nursing's political development: Where we've been and where we ought to go. *Nursing Outlook, 44*(6), 259–266.

Cott, N. (1977). The bonds of womanhood: "Woman's sphere" in New England, 1780–1930. New Haven, CT: Yale University Press.

Cott, N. F. (1987). *The grounding of modern feminism.* New Haven, CT: Yale University Press.

Daniels, L. (1987). *American women in the 20th century: The festival of life.* San Diego: Harcourt Brace Jovanovich.

Darche, L. (1894, June). Employments for women. No. 2: Trained nursing. *The Delineator: A Journal of Fashion, Culture, and Fine Arts. 82,* 667–668.

Deans, A. (1910). Proceedings of the Thirteenth Annual Convention of the Nurses' Associated Alumnae [report of the Interstate Secretary]. *American Journal of Nursing, 10*(11), 861.

Dickstein, S. (1940). Lillian D. Wald, America's urban pioneer. *Congressional Record: Proceedings and debates of 76th Congress, third session.*

Diers, D. (1984). To profess—to be a professional. *The Journal of the New York State Nurses Association, 15*(4), 23.

Dock, L. (1897). *First and second annual conventions of the American Society of Superintendents of Training Schools for Nurses,* Harrisburg, PA. [Also found in Birnbach, N, & Lewenson, S. (1991). *First words: Selected addresses from the National League for Nurses 1894–1933.* New York: National League for Nurses, and in Reverby, S. (1985). *Annual conventions 1893–1899: The American Society of Superintendents of Training Schools for Nurses.* New York: Garland.]

Dock, L. (1907). Some urgent social claims. *The American Journal of Nursing, 7*(10), 895–901.

Dock, L. (1908). The suffrage question. *The American Journal of Nursing, 8*(11), 925–927.

Dock, L., & Stewart, I. (1931). *A short history of nursing* (3rd ed., rev.). New York: G. P. Putnam's Sons.

Editorial comment. (1908). Progress and reaction. *American Journal of Nursing, 8*(5), 334–335.

Fitzpatrick, L. (1975). *The National Organization for Public Health Nursing, 1912–1952: Development of a practice field.* New York: NLN Press.

Florence Nightingale's letter of advice to Bellevue. (1911). *American Journal of Nursing, 11*(5), 361–364.

Gardner, M. S. (1933). *Public health nursing* (2nd ed., rev.). New York: Macmillan.

Gordon, K. M., Myers, A. J., & Kelley, F. (1906). Equal suffrage movement [Letters to the editor]. *American Journal of Nursing, 7*(1), 47–48.

Gordon, S. (1997a, February). What nurses stand for. *Atlantic Monthly,* pp. 80–88.

Gordon, S. (1997b). *Life support: Three nurses on the front lines.* Boston: Little, Brown.

Gray, M. (1979). *Margaret Sanger: A biography of the champion of birth control.* New York: Richard Marek Publishers.

Heide, W. S. (1973). Nursing and women's liberation a parallel. *American Journal of Nursing, 73*(5), 824–827.

Heide, W. S. (1985). *Feminism for the health of it.* Buffalo, NY: Margaretdaughters.

Heinrich, K., & Witt, B. (1993). The passionate connection: Feminism invigorates the teaching of nursing. *Nursing Outlook, 41*(3), 117–124.

Hine, D. C. (1989). *Black women in white: Racial conflict and cooperation in the nursing profession. 1890–1950.* Bloomington: Indiana University Press.

Hine, D. C. (1990). The Ethel Johns Report: Black women in the nursing profession, 1925; From hospital to college: Black nurse leaders and the rise of collegiate nursing schools. In C. C. Hine (Ed.), *Black women in United States history* (Vol. 2). *Black women in American history: The twentieth century.* Brooklyn, NY: Carlson.

Hine, D. C. (1993). Staupers, Mabel Keaton (1890–1989). In D. C. Hine (Ed.), *Black women in America: An historical encyclopedia* (Vol. II, pp. 1106–1108).

Johns, E.. (1925). *A study of the present status of the Negro woman in nursing.* New York: Rockefeller Archive Center. [1.1, Series 200, Box 122, Folder 1507, pp. 1–43, Exhibits A-P, Appendixes I and II.]

Kalish, P., & Kalish B. (1986). *The advance of American nursing* (2nd ed.). Boston: Little, Brown.

Katz, E. (1990). Sanger, Margaret Louise (Higgins) (1879–1966). In A. Zophy & F. M. Kavenik (Eds.), *Handbook of American women's history.* New York: Garland.

Lerner, G. (1977). *The female experience: An American documentary.* Indianapolis: Bobbs-Merrill.

Letter to Col. J. H. Lefroy. In M. Vicinus & B. Nergaard (Eds.). (1989). *Ever yours, Florence Nightingale: Selected letters.* London: Virago Press.

Letter from Lucy Hale Topley to the NACGN Tenth Annual Meeting, held on August 21, 1917. Unpublished proceedings, NACGN Records, Schomburg, Box 1, Vol. 2, p. 2.

Lewenson, S. (1994). "Of logical necessity—they hang together": Nursing and the woman's movement, 1901–1912. *Nursing History Review, 2,* 99–117.

Lewenson, S. B. (1996). *Taking charge: Nursing, suffrage & feminism in America, 1873–1920.* New York: NLN Press.

McBride, A. B. (1976). A married feminist. *American Journal of Nursing, 76*(5), 754–757.

Muff, J. (1982). *Socialization, sexism, and stereotyping: Women's issues in nursing.* St. Louis: Mosby.

Munhall, P. L. (Ed). (1994). *In women's experiences.* New York: National League for Nursing.

National Association of Colored Graduate Nurses. Minutes of the Eleventh Annual Meeting, August 20 and 21, 1918. Unpublished proceedings, Association Records, Schomburg, Box 1, Vol. 2.

Palmer, S. (1897). *First and second annual conventions of the American Society of Superintendents of Training Schools for Nurses,* Harrisburg, PA. [Also found in Birnbach, N., & Lewenson, S. (1991). *First words: Selected addresses from the National League for Nurses 1894–1933.* New York: National League for Nurses, and in Reverby, S. (1985). *Annual conventions 1893–1899: The American Society of Superintendents of Training Schools for Nurses.* New York: Garland.

Palmer, S. (1908). [Editorial policy explained]. *American Journal of Nursing, 9*(1), 49–50.

Palmer, S. (1909). State societies: Their organization and place in nursing education. *American Journal of Nursing, 9*(12), 956–957.

Reed, J. (1980). Sanger, Margaret. In B. Sicherman & C. Hurd Green (Eds.), *Notable American women: The modern period* (pp. 623–627). Cambridge, MA: The Belknap Press of Harvard University Press.

Reverby, S. (1987). *Ordered to care: The dilemma of American nursing, 1850–1945.* Cambridge: Cambridge University Press.

Riley, G. (1986). *Inventing the American woman: A perspective on women's history, 1607–1877,* (Vol. 1). Arlington Heights, IL: Harlan Davidson.

Robb, I. H. (1900). Original communications [Address of the president]. *American Journal of Nursing, 1*(2).

Roberts, M. (1954). *American nursing: History and interpretation.* New York: Macmillan.

Rogge, M. M. (1987). Nursing and politics: A forgotten legacy. *Nursing Research, 36*(1), 26–30.

Rosenberg C. E., & Smith-Rosenberg, C. (1985). Pietism and the origins of the American public health movement: A note on John H. Griscom and Robert M. Hartley. In J. W. Leavitt & R. Numbers (Eds), *Sickness and health in America: Readings in the history of medicine and public health* (2nd ed., rev.). Madison: University of Wisconsin Press.

Rothman, S. (1978). *A woman's proper place: A history of changing ideals and practices, 1870s to the present.* New York: Basic Books.

Siegel, B. (1983). *Lillian Wald of Henry Street.* New York: Macmillan.

Snively, M. A. (1897). A uniform curriculum for training schools. *First and second annual conventions of the American Society of Superintendents of Training Schools for Nurses,* Harrisburg, PA. [Also found in Birnbach, N., & Lewenson, S. (1991). *First words: Selected addresses from the National League for Nurses 1894–1933.* New York: National League for Nurses, and in Reverby, S. (1985). *Annual conventions 1893–1899 The American Society of Superintendents of Training Schools for Nurses.* New York: Garland.]

Starr, D. (1974). "Poor baby: The nurse and feminism," *The Canadian Nurse 70*(3), 20–23.

Staupers, M. (1937, November). The Negro nurse in America. *Opportunity: Journal of Negro Life, 15,* 339–341. [Also reprinted in Hine, D. C. (1985). Black women in the nursing profession: A documentary history. New York: Garland.]

Staupers, M. K. (1961). No time for prejudice: A story of the integration of Negroes in nursing in the United States. New York: Macmillan.

Talbott, S. W., & Vance, C. (1981). Involving nursing in a feminist group—NOW. *Nursing Outlook, 29*(10), 592–595.

Thoms, A. (1929). *Pathfinders: A history of progress of the colored graduate nurses.* New York: Kay Printing House.

Vance, C., Talbott, S. W., McBride, A., & Mason, D. J. (1985). Coming of age: The women's movement and nursing. In D. Mason & S. Talbott (Eds.), *Political action handbook for nurses.* Menlo Park, CA: Addison-Wesley.

Vicinus, M., & Nergaard, B. (Eds.). (1989). *Ever yours, Florence Nightingale: Selected letters.* London: Virago Press.

Wald, L. (1915). *The house on Henry Street.* New York: Henry Holt.

Wheeler, C. (1985). The *American Journal of Nursing* and the socialization of a profession. *Advances in Nursing Science, 7*(2), 20–34.

Zophy, A. M. H. (1978). *For the improvement of my sex: Sarah Josepha Hale's editorship of "Godey's Lady's Book." 1837–1877.* Unpublished doctoral dissertation, University of Ohio. Ann Arbor, MI: University Microfilms International [order No. 7819687].

Chapter 4

ORGANIZATION AND DELIVERY OF HEALTH CARE IN THE UNITED STATES:
The Health Care System That Isn't

JANET HEINRICH

CORE VALUES

As a nation, we embrace our diversity and pluralistic approaches to problem solving. We have a historic distrust of "big government" and centralized control, part of our Jeffersonian inheritance, and at the same time we demand government regulations that will level the playing field because we value fairness and equal access to opportunity. We continue to pride ourselves on being fiercely independent, and yet we also expect that neighbors and communities will help each other out in times of need. These basic values have been at the heart of the health care delivery system in the United States since the mid-1800s. In spite of the ever-present danger of death from smallpox, malaria, and other infectious diseases, people still resisted the implementation of basic state government–initiated public health laws incorporating new science and technology into the control of these deadly epidemics (Shattuck, 1850).

HISTORICAL DEVELOPMENT

Social insurance and national systems of compulsory sickness insurance became the norm in Europe, starting with Germany in 1883 (Starr, 1982). In the United States, government was highly decentralized, leaving any actions related to health to private and voluntary action at the state and local levels. There were trade unions, cooperatives, and social reformers who argued for sickness funds, but there was very little political support for any form of national insurance through the 1920s in the United States.

In 1921, Congress passed the Shepherd-Towner Act, which provided matching funds to the states for prenatal and child health centers. This legislation was aggressively supported by Lillian Wald, the founder of the Henry Street Settlement and public health nursing in the United States. These centers, staffed mainly by public health nurses, sought to reduce rates of maternal and infant mortality by teaching women how to care for themselves and their families. By following the rules of basic hygiene, the program resulted in the prevention of many common diseases. This highly successful program was discontinued in 1927 at the urging of the American Medical Association (AMA), whose members considered it to result in excessive federal interference in local health concerns (Starr, 1982).

There was growing concern, however, about the costs and distribution of medical care. Moore, the staff director of the Committee on the Costs of Medical Care (CCMC), described medical services as maldistributed and badly organized, with no coordination beyond the walls of any particular hospital and clinic (Starr, 1982). The final report of the committee endorsed group practice and group payment for medical care but opposed compulsory health insurance.

Instead, voluntary plans were the preferred next step. In spite of the efforts of the CCMC to include leaders from the AMA in the study and development of recommendations, the report was denounced as "socialized medicine" by the AMA and failed in its efforts to achieve consensus even on the recommendation of voluntary health insurance.

Reformers made several more attempts at articulating the health care needs of the American people throughout the Roosevelt "new deal" period, but most of the recommendations were for subsidies to the states to expand public health and maternal and child health services, expansion of hospital facilities, and increased aid for medical care for special populations. Public opinion polls during this time reflected public support for government funds to help pay for needed medical care, but not if this would mean higher Social Security taxes to pay for health insurance (Starr, 1982). A clear public mandate for public national health insurance did not exist. A bill introduced in 1943 by Senator Wagner, Senator Murry, and Representative Dingell created a comprehensive and universal national health insurance system but met with strong opposition from the AMA. Even when President Truman made national health insurance a campaign issue and won the election, his proposal succumbed to charges of socialism from the AMA. The first recommendation of his plan, the Hospital Survey and Construction Act (the Hill-Burton Act), did pass with support from the AMA and the growing hospital industry.

With the federal government pouring money into construction, the development of powerful new antibiotics and other wonder drugs, and the rise of private hospital insurance, hospitals evolved into meccas of biomedical science. Medical specialization increased dramatically with new scientific breakthroughs after World War II, but this also resulted in the fragmentation of medical practice and the segmentation of the patient into specific diseases or body parts. The policy options recommended at the time were for more and better-trained general practi-

tioners; training in "comprehensive care" (e.g., promotion of health, prevention of disease, diagnosis, treatment, and rehabilitation); and group practices with multiple specialists working together. A small and controversial subgroup advocated group practices linked with prepayment of fees or health insurance (Somers & Somers, 1962).

The progressive groups that had once supported a national health insurance system were completely splintered by the 1950s. The middle class could buy private insurance, labor unions used collective bargaining to gain health insurance benefits for workers, and American veterans had their own system of hospitals and clinics. Instead of a universal system, American society provided insurance for the wealthy, the well organized, and those with political influence. The poor were left out. Many cities and counties tried to provide for indigent care with the building or expansion of public hospitals and clinics, the origins of our current and crumbling "safety net."

The 1965 twin Great Society insurance programs, Medicare and Medicaid, gave hospitals and physicians new streams of income for treating elderly, poor, and disabled persons and created new subsidies for academic medical centers. These programs were not the comprehensive coverage of services at reasonable costs or the more efficient use of scarce resources through a rational organization of services that many advocates worked for. But they are public programs, in the case of Medicare, linked with private insurance carriers, to provide payment for acute medical care services to people 65 years of age and older. Medicare, an insurance program that covers acute episodes of illness, is run by the federal government and is supported primarily with tax dollars. Medicaid, with matching state and federal funds, was established to provide health care services for poor persons as defined by the individual states. The state Medicaid programs have contributed to the many long-term care services needed by elderly families, as well as to the essential health care services for mothers and children.

THE TIGHTENING VISE OF THE MEDICAL-INDUSTRIAL COMPLEX

The 1970s and 1980s were decades of continued but unsuccessful efforts to curtail the growth in dollars spent on health care. There were efforts to limit increases in the number of beds and in the use of new technologies in communities through comprehensive health planning. National legislation made it possible for states to establish health planning agencies that had the authority to control the expansion of health care facilities and the building of new ones. Efforts were made to coordinate facilities and health care programs in a geographic area for specific conditions such as heart disease and cancer through regional health planning. In spite of these efforts, hospitals continued to expand, so that by 1995 there were an estimated 5,194 institutions in the United States (American Hospital Association, 1996). These varied by size, by type (generalized or specialized), and by ownership (public, private, not-for-profit voluntary, or for-profit investor owned). Teaching hospitals, associated with universities and medical schools, nursing schools, and other training programs were expanding their capacity as well, providing an environment for education and research. The teaching institutions received increased payments for services from Medicare and Medicaid because of the teaching responsibilities and provision of services to indigent populations. They developed into high-tech tertiary centers, treating patients with the most complex conditions as they developed and tested new procedures, technologies, and treatments. The research institutions were closely linked with pharmaceutical companies and the manufacturing of drugs and devices. The medical-industrial complex arrived, with the focus on new biomedical breakthroughs to prolong life at any cost.

Recently there has been a frenzy of activity in the hospital industry as organizations position themselves to respond to an increasingly competitive market. New acquisitions, hospital mergers, and conversions from not-for-profit, religion-sponsored organizations to for-profit conglomerates are common across the United States (Claxton, Feder, Shactman, & Altman, 1997). Hospitals changed from individually managed and controlled hospitals into systems of jointly managed organizations. This "horizontal" integration was expected to bring about efficiencies and cost reductions. There was also a surge of "vertical" integration, whereby hospital systems bought outpatient clinics, nursing homes, and home care agencies in an effort to better coordinate and manage services across the spectrum of care. Many hospital administrators also bought into the concepts of "reengineering," or restructuring, as a way of improving productivity and decreasing costs. Common strategies include the use of new treatment technologies, the use of new information systems and computerized patient records, reductions in staff and substitution of less highly trained staff for more highly trained staff, the development of "subacute" beds that are not as costly to staff and the closure of acute care bed units, and a decrease in length of hospital stays with early discharge of patients to the home (Steinwachs, 1992).

With health care spending at about 13.7% of the gross domestic product in 1994, health care costs were growing at a rate seen as unsustainable and unacceptable to many employers, who were paying the largest share of health insurance premiums for employees. The cost of health care was also unacceptable to the American public, who still paid a significant percentage of health care costs in "out of pocket" expenditures. In spite of efforts to manage hospital costs differently, the overall health spending in the United States has continued to grow unabated (Reinhardt, 1996a). We have not found an acceptable way to limit patient access to services, to control physician recommendations for new treatments and the use of new technologies, or to generate new sources of revenue (taxes)!

GROWTH IN NURSING HOMES

During the 1960s, there was rapid growth in the number and size of nursing home facilities to care for people 65 years of age and older as well. Nursing homes were essentially unregulated in most states and were governed almost entirely by market forces. This rapid growth and inadequate regulation resulted in substandard care for the most vulnerable older population (Institute of Medicine, 1986). The concern for quality of care in nursing homes continues to this day and is a volatile issue for health care providers and policymakers at all levels of government (Institute of Medicine, 1997; Wunderlich, Sloan, & Davis, 1996).

More than half of nursing home revenues come from state and federal funds, making states and the federal government accountable for the care provided. In efforts to control their budgets, states began to develop mechanisms to control the number of nursing home beds and to develop alternative community-based services for people who require long-term care. A number of regulations were undertaken by states to improve the quality of care that focused on staffing mix, characteristics of the physical facility, and the level of needs and characteristics of residents (patients). At the same time, there were strong efforts in Congress to totally deregulate the nursing home industry. As a result of national legislation passed in 1987, nursing homes are now required to make individual resident assessments and develop care plans that maximize health and functional status. There is strong evidence, however, that these laws are not enough without adequate nursing staff to provide the necessary services (Wunderlich et al., 1996). For the first time in several decades, there has been a 13% decrease in the number of nursing homes in the United States and only a slight increase (4%) in the number of nursing home residents (U.S. Department of Health and Human Services, 1997). This change is attributed to the fact that more people receive needed long-term care in their homes.

GROWTH OF HOME CARE SERVICES

Home care services were first organized under visiting nursing services as philanthropy in many communities. During the 1950s and 1960s the home care programs were often coordinated with general public health nursing services, with the emphasis on generalized services to families. Categorical public health funding changed this broad community approach, as did increased payment for medically focused home care services under Medicare (Gebbie, 1995). With increased financial pressure to shorten the number of days that patients stay in the hospital, there has been new focus on a variety of "high tech" health care services provided in the home.

Home care services are one of the fastest growing components of the health care industry, with many types of for-profit and not-for-profit organizations providing services. The voluntary, not-for-profit visiting nurse service organizations have not grown over the past several decades; hospital-based programs and for-profit proprietary agencies account for the exponential growth. There are an estimated 14,000 to 16,000 home care providers nationally, with fewer than half meeting requirements for Medicare participation. Some provide only skilled nursing services, whereas others provide only social or homemaker services. State requirements for licensure of home care providers vary tremendously. Agencies may be certified by national organizations, but the decentralized nature of monitoring for quality of services delivered in people's homes is of mounting concern. With growing charges of fraud and abuse, many consumer groups are seeking increased regulation at the state level to ensure patient safety. Questions about quality and cost-effectiveness also make home care a target for budget cuts, even though home care may be preferred by patients and families.

THE SHRINKING "SAFETY NET"

Beginning in the 1970s, many communities experimented with neighborhood health centers in efforts to provide comprehensive community health services that were closely linked to the needs of the community. These centers expanded into medically underserved communities, such as isolated rural areas and economically depressed inner-city communities, reaching out to provide access to services for more than eight million medically underserved people (National Association of Community Health Centers, 1995). There are nearly 600 community and migrant health centers providing comprehensive, case-managed primary and preventive care in the United States. There are approximately 2,500 federally designated rural health clinics, with the majority of funding coming from Medicare and Medicaid. With few physicians available to provide needed services, these centers are often staffed with nurse practitioners and physician assistants. Although seen as successful in providing for the care of indigent populations, ongoing federal support for such programs is questioned.

Other freestanding clinics have developed to serve specific needs, such as community mental health centers, drug and alcohol treatment centers, family planning clinics, abortion clinics, clinics for treatment of acquired immunodeficiency syndrome, and free clinics to serve homeless populations. The number of freestanding clinics is not known. They may be staffed with lay people, volunteers, and paid physicians and nurses and may be funded by private donations, foundation support, or local, state, or federal government. They may charge patients on a sliding fee schedule based on the individual's ability to pay.

These clinics, along with services provided by about 1,400 public hospitals financed by local governments, are part of the "safety net" of services available to individuals without some form of medical insurance. In 1994, about 40 million people less than 65 years of age did not have health insurance. An additional 33.4 million people were enrolled in Medicaid, although this number is expected to decrease as states tighten eligibility rules. Some four million illegal entrants to the United States are also uninsured (Robert Wood Johnson Foundation, 1994). Although the population of uninsured is continuing to grow, resources at the local level to provide these "safety net" services are not. Public hospitals continue to close, and local

charities have not been able to keep up with the demand for services.

PUBLIC HEALTH SERVICES: SEAMLESS OR SEPARATE?

Many of the major improvements in the health of our communities can be attributed to the success of public health measures and our public health infrastructure. Every state and territory and many counties and cities have a public health department. Each state and local government is different, and the health departments operate under unique public health laws and regulations. They may be organized as freestanding entities or combined with environmental, mental health, or social service agencies. The diversity of combinations of agencies and legal mandates reflects the fact that the majority of their support is from local tax dollars, with limited support from other sources. Many suggest that the systems in place to guarantee the health of the public are in "disarray" (Institute of Medicine, 1988). Federal, state, and local public health agencies have traditionally been responsible for the control of epidemics, ensuring safe food and water and providing personal and preventive health services to vulnerable and indigent populations, such as mothers and children.

How services and programs are organized at the local level often depends on outside funding sources. As a means of survival, public health agencies became dependent on Medicaid, fees for service for personal care services, and funding for tuberculosis, family planning, and crippled children's programs. These categorical funds paid for public health clinics and are a part of the "safety net" services available for the medically indigent. Funds for personal services, however, do not provide support for community assessment or assurance activities, critical core elements in ensuring the public's health (Conley, 1995). Many organizations are now advocating a return to the basic public health core functions of assessment, policy development, and assurance, as articulated by the Institute of Medicine (1988) study *The Future of Public Health,* and are focusing on the essential public health services. However, many state and local agencies lack the necessary funding to provide these essential services at a time when managed care organizations are competing with them for the personal care service dollars.

Many state and local health departments are developing strategies to collaborate with managed care organizations so that health promotion and disease prevention services, such as prenatal programs for high-risk women, immunization programs, and tuberculosis and other infection control programs, are well coordinated in a community. For example, managed care organizations can provide care to patients with tuberculosis and supervise their medications, but the local health department remains responsible for overseeing contact tracing to find other people in the community with the disease. Everyone in the community will benefit when the focus is not only on the health of individuals and families but also on the health of the total community. The roles and responsibilities of state and local health departments are still evolving to hold managed care organizations and other types of organizations linked with insurance products accountable for clinical outcomes and the health status of the populations served (Lipson, 1997).

EVOLUTION OF MANAGED CARE

The vast majority of insured Americans today are in one of a growing variety of managed care arrangements. Managed care arrangements entail some connection between financing and delivery of care, usually with cost management as a prime goal. They range from tightly controlled staff-model health maintenance organizations (HMOs) to preferred provider organizations (PPOs) and point-of-service contracts (choice of providers not affiliated with an HMO), to managed indemnity plans and other hybrids that incorporate some aspects of traditional managed care, such as utilization review.

Although staff models of managed care organizations were developed in the early 1930s, the AMA fought the idea of physicians' becoming employees of corporations, as opposed to independent providers reimbursed on a fee-for-service basis for more than half a century (Starr, 1982). There was federal government encouragement of the managed care concept and physician group practice arrangements in the 1960s and again in the 1990s as a way to control spiraling health care costs.

In the early 1990s, there were about 40 million Americans enrolled in health maintenance organizations and 50 million enrolled in more loosely organized preferred provider organizations. By 1995, the number of enrollees in HMOs jumped to 60 million, and individuals covered by PPOs nearly doubled, to 91 million (American Association of Health Plans, 1996). Many states are moving individuals covered by Medicaid to some type of managed care plan. Enrollment of Medicaid beneficiaries grew from an estimated 10% in 1991 to nearly 40% in 1996, according to one estimate (Physician Payment Review Commission, 1997). The Health Care Financing Administration is expected to encourage expansion of the enrollment of Medicare beneficiaries in managed care organizations as well.

Managed care organizations use a variety of methods to control utilization and costs. These include utilization of their market power to negotiate discounts from physicians, hospitals, and other provider groups. They may provide financial incentives to "gatekeepers," usually primary care physicians, to reduce the utilization of hospitals, specialists, and laboratory tests. Another popular method of controlling costs is for HMOs to give a provider group a fixed payment per patient, or capitated rate, that is independent of utilization of services. They may also seek out the most efficient providers, based on data collected on previous medical claims histories or provider profiles (American Academy of Nursing, 1993). Although managed care eliminates perverse incentives to inappropriate overutilization, it also contains incentives to control costs and potentially undertreat patients who need care. Critiques of managed care organizations have been concerned about the denial of services to individuals and families as a way of rationing services (Eddy, 1997). Individuals with special health care needs, such as severe mental illness or chronic conditions such as cystic fibrosis, complain that they do not have access to necessary specialists or special technologies. However, there are also incentives to provide cost-effective programs to keep individuals, families, and communities healthy. There is growing interest in self-care and in teaching families about what they can do to enhance their own personal health outcomes. Methods of systematically monitoring and evaluating the quality of care provided by managed care organizations are developing, and there is keen interest at the state and federal levels in the concerns voiced by patients and health care providers alike. In 1996 a special Presidential Advisory Commission of Consumer Protection and Quality in the Health Care Industry was named to address concerns over quality of care.

READY OR NOT . . .

In 1990 a public opinion poll found that close to 60% of Americans believed that fundamental changes in the health care system were needed, and 29% thought that a complete rebuilding of the system was needed (Blendon, Brodie, & Benson, 1995). It is no wonder that then-presidential candidate Bill Clinton made health care reform one of his top issues during his first term in office. His comprehensive health care reform proposals, however, fared no better than Truman's almost a half century before. "Americans are dissatisfied with the cost of their health care, but happy with the access and with the quality of the care they receive" (Blendon et al., 1995).

The health care reform plan that was presented to the 103rd Congress and to the public in 1994 was based on concepts of managed care and managed competition. The plan tried to enfranchise the uninsured and to control health care costs but did not deal directly with the fundamental problems of how care is delivered

in the United States. The proposal was complex and difficult for consumers to understand, including mandated employer insurance coverage, "global" budgets, and health insurance purchasing cooperatives. Opponents sabotaged the plan by labeling it more "big government" and regulation of health care, which would limit the individual's choice of providers. There was continued concern over costs, quality, and access to health care insurance.

Our insurance system has evolved on the basis of private health insurance coverage linked to an individual's job, with job loss meaning loss of insurance and access to usual health care services. Individuals older than 65 years are covered by Medicare, and individuals and families who meet varying state definitions of poverty are covered by Medicaid. Each insurance plan has different services that are paid for and require different levels of copayments. Insurance fees or premiums are also based on the health status of the individual, as opposed to charging everyone the same rate (community rating). Recent federal legislation (Health Insurance Portability and Accountability Act of 1996) has improved access to health insurance for employed people and prohibits exclusion from insurance coverage when an individual has an existing illness. A new revenue stream was identified by Congress in 1997 to provide states options for covering children above the poverty line. But there have been no efforts to address the increasing number of adults in the United States who are uninsured, lacking access to ongoing health care services from the private sector insurance market (Hacker & Skocpol, 1997). Nor have we answered the concern for constraining costs. While spending growth for physicians' services has slowed, other health care sectors such as inpatient hospital services, outpatient services, and home care are projected to grow unabated (Physician Payment Review Commission, 1997). Policies that restrain prices, volume, or access to new technologies and new drugs are not in place. Ginzberg (1997) argues that, in the future, managed care companies will have a marginal effect on future cost trends.

Health care reform legislation did not pass Congress, but the rapid increase in managed care organizations across the United States and the mergers and consolidations of hospitals and other health care institutions have changed delivery systems dramatically. The shift of ownership from traditional not-for-profit institutions to national and international corporate conglomerates answering to stockholders and capital markets is challenging our basic beliefs and values that health care is a basic human right, not a commodity.

The terms *change* and *chaos* are used interchangeably to describe the current state of the U.S. health care system. No one seems to have a clear vision of how health care services will be organized and delivered in the future. Insurers are becoming health plans and providers; providers are becoming insurers; pharmaceutical companies and suppliers are becoming disease state managers; hospitals are now seen as cost centers and are either closing beds or going out of business; and health care education and delivery are moving to the Internet, where consumers find their own information on how best to manage their health problems.

Some people predict a three-tiered system for the future U.S. health care delivery system based on the individual and family's ability to pay for insurance, with rationing at the lower two tiers (Reinhardt, 1996b). Capitated managed care is advocated by corporate leaders as a less costly method of providing health insurance coverage to workers and by politicians for Medicare and Medicaid populations. Managed care is a strategy for rationing care for the population in the middle tier. Rationing in the bottom tier will be through public expenditures for public hospitals and clinics, currently in disarray. Well-to-do Americans in the top tier will continue to have open-ended access to health care services and providers of their choice.

Shortell and Hull (1996) predict that the current state of chaos will evolve into new organized delivery systems. These will have varying forms of ownership and diverse alliances among hospitals, physicians, and insurers that will be designed to capture market share and to provide cost-effective care to a defined population. Key factors for developing these integrated systems include the following:

- Organization culture
- Information systems
- Internal incentives
- Total quality management
- Physician leadership
- The growth of group practices

Characteristics of organized delivery systems include the following:

- A continuum of care, including primary care and short- and long-term care
- Assumption of financial risk
- Clinical and financial outcome data
- Horizontal and vertical integration of services
- Integration of physician services
- Clinical integration of an array of clinical services in a local market

It has been suggested that these integrated systems could develop structures of political accountability in their communities, developing new governance structures that encourage true coordination and tough allocation decisions at the local level (Emanuel & Emanuel, 1997).

Some advocates suggest an incremental approach to reforming the health care system. They support modest insurance reforms, targeting specific populations, such as children, or adding inclusion of specific services, such as breast cancer screening (Hacker & Skocpol, 1997). Others are hopeful that the current chaos will continue to evolve into a single-payer system with significant government regulation to ensure a level playing field for all Americans. Advocates for this approach do not view markets as working well in the provision of health care services. Health care is viewed as a right that should be provided along the lines of a public service. Advocates point to models in other developed countries, such as Canada and the United Kingdom, and to what is considered "the international standard" for health care systems:

- Universal coverage of the population
- Comprehensiveness of principal benefits

- Contributions based on income, rather than individual insurance purchases
- Cost control through administrative mechanisms, including binding fee schedules, global budgets, and limitations on system capacity (Evans, 1997)

What is clear is that economic incentives and concerns will continue to drive future changes, and that business and corporate America will have more of a say in what the future health care delivery system will be in the near term. Perhaps the next wave of change will be influenced even more by informed consumers, who will exert their power over corporate and government payers, insurers and health care providers, and politicians. If this is to occur, the basic information about health plans and coverage, patient satisfaction ratings, access, cost, and quality need to be conveyed to consumers (Isaacs, 1996). We will need to develop better strategies for promoting public accountability and informed purchasing by the American public.

The U.S. health care system is a patchwork of diverse systems that several experts predict will continue to be in crisis. Many see the conflicts inherent in the trends toward declining private insurance and reduced capacity to provide uncompensated care as becoming explosive (Smith, 1997). This nonsystem has not solved the problems of access, cost, and quality. In fact, the problems of access to health care services have been exacerbated according to surveys of families who report worsening access to care, especially if they are low-income families (Lesser & Cunningham, 1997). Costs are continuing to escalate in spite of efforts to use market forces to provide controls through competition. Managed care companies, which once were holding down premiums on insurance policies, are now raising their rates. Many providers and consumers are voicing fears of decreasing safety and quality as we try to decrease costs and capacity in health care.

The existing system is still oriented toward acute care and episodes of illness rather than toward promoting health and comprehensive care. What we have learned is that it is difficult to control costs piecemeal and just as difficult to expand access using an incremental approach. Partial remedies just don't work and often have negative side effects. We have yet to mobilize our political system around a solution that will ensure a rational health care system for all of us.

REFERENCES

American Academy of Nursing. (1993). *Managed care and national health care reform: Nurses can make it work.* Washington, DC: Author.

American Association of Health Plans (AAHP). (1996). *HMO and PPO trends report.* Washington, DC: Author.

American Hospital Association. (1996). *Hospital statistics, 1996–1997 edition.* Chicago: Author.

Blendon, R. J., Brodie, M., & Benson, J. (1995). What happened to Americans' support for the Clinton health plan? *Health Affairs, Summer,* 8.

Cain, H. P. (1997). Privatizing Medicare: A battle of values. *Health Affairs, 16*(2), 185.

Claxton, G., Feder, J., Shactman, D., & Altman, S. (1997). Public policy issues in nonprofit conversions: An overview. *Health Affairs, 16*(2), 13.

Congress of the United States—Office of Technology Assessment. (1993). *An inconsistent picture: A compilation of analyses of economic impacts of competing approaches to health care reform by experts and stakeholders.* Washington, DC. U.S. Government Printing Office.

Conley, E. (1995). Public health nursing within core public health functions: "Back to the future." *Journal of Public Health Management and Practice, 1*(3), 1.

Eddy, D. M. (1997). Balancing cost and quality in fee-for-service versus managed care. *Health Affairs, 16*(3), 169.

Emanuel, E. J., & Emanuel, L. L. (1997). Preserving community in health care. *Journal of Health Politics, Policy and Law, 22*(1), 179.

Evans R. G. (1997). Going for the gold: The redistributive agenda behind market-based health care reform. *Journal of Health Politics, Policy and Law, 22*(2), 433.

Gebbie, K. M. (1995). Follow the money: Funding streams and public health nursing. *Journal of Public Health Management and Practice, 1*(3), 23.

Ginzberg, E. (1997). Managed care and the competitive market in health care: What they can and cannot do. *Journal of the American Medical Association, 277*(22), 1813.

Hacker, J. S., & Skocpol, T. (1997). The new politics of U.S. health policy. *Journal of Health Politics, Policy and Law, 22*(2), 333.

Institute of Medicine. (1986). *Improving the quality of care in nursing homes.* Washington, DC: National Academy Press.

Institute of Medicine. (1988). *The future of public health.* Washington, DC: National Academy Press.

Institute of Medicine, (1997). *Improving quality in long term care.* Washington, DC: National Academy Press.

Isaacs, S. L. (1996). Consumers' information needs: Results of a national survey. *Health Affairs, 15*(4), 33.

Lesser, C., & Cunningham, P. (1997). *Access to care: Is it improving or declining?* Washington, DC: Center for Studying Health System Change.

Lipson, D. J. (1997). Medicaid, managed care, and community providers: New partnerships. *Health Affairs, 16*(4), 91.

Mendelson, D. N., & Salinsky, E. M. (1997). Health information systems and the role of state government. *Health Affairs, 16*(3), 118–119.

National Association of Community Health Centers. (1995). *America's health centers: Value in health.* Washington, DC: Author.

Physician Payment Review Commission. (1997). *PPRC Annual Report to Congress.* Washington, D.C.: U.S. Government Printing Office.

Reinhardt, U. E. (1996a). Spending more through "cost control": Our obsessive quest to gut the hospital. *Health Affairs, 15*, 156.

Reinhardt, U. E. (1996b). Rationing health care: What it is, what it is not, and why we cannot afford it. In S. Altman & U. Reinhardt (Eds.), *Strategic choices for a changing health care system* (pp. 87–91). Chicago: Health Administration Press.

Robert Wood Johnson Foundation. (1994). *Cost containment.* Princeton: Author.

Shattuck, L. (1850). *Report of the Sanitary Commission of Massachusetts, 1850.* Cambridge, MA: Harvard University Press. [Reprinted 1948.]

Shortell, S. M., Gillies, R. R., & Anderson, D. A. (1994). The new world of managed care: Creating organized delivery systems. *Health Affairs, Winter,* 46–64.

Shortell, S. M., & Hull, K. E. (1996). The new organization of the health care delivery system. In S. Altman & U. Reinhardt (Eds.), *Strategic choices for a changing health care system* (pp. 102–105). Chicago: Health Administration Press.

Smith, B. M. (1997). Trends in health care coverage and financing and their implications for policy. *New England Journal of Medicine, 337*(14), 1000–1003.

Somers, H. M., & Somers, A. R. (1962). *Doctors, patients, and health insurance.* Garden City, NY: Doubleday Anchor Book.

Starr, P. (1982). *The social transformation of American medicine.* New York: Basic Books.

Steinwachs, D. M. (1992). Redesign of delivery systems to enhance productivity. In S. Shortell & U. Reinhardt (Eds.), *Improving health policy and management* (pp. 275–285). Chicago: Health Administration Press.

Thorpe, K. E. (1992). Health care cost containment: Results and lessons from the past 20 years. In S. Shortell & U. Reinhardt (Eds.), *Improving health policy and management* (pp. 233–243). Chicago: Health Administration Press.

U.S. Department of Health and Human Services. (1997, January 23). Americans less likely to use nursing home care today. *HHS News.* [Available on line: www:/CDC.gov/NCHS.www/releases/97news/nursehome.hTM.]

Wunderlich, G. S., Sloan, F. A., & Davis, C. K. (1996). *Nursing staff in hospitals and nursing homes: Is it adequate?* Washington, DC: National Academy Press.

Affordable Long-term Care: Nursing Models of Care Delivery

Virginia Burggraf

The gauge on Richard Starr's blood-pressure cuff quit and his self-care monitoring ended as he took two buses to a hospital to have his BP checked. He had been able to monitor his blood pressure with a BP cuff won at a health fair. His self-monitoring ended when he saw an ad for a nursing service called "The Healthy Seniors Project." This project is a partnership with the federally funded nonprofit Living at Home/Block Nurse Program, begun in 1989 (Jamieson, 1989). This program proved ideal for Richard, who lived only one block from the office, and his designated nurse, Mary Kay Stillson, RN, MPH. This 80-year-old man is now a patient in a program based on the belief that the time is right for the community to address health care, cut Medicare costs, and improve the health of its senior neighbors. Richard Starr is typical of the older person in need of health care and living in the community; the only difference between him and the typical older person is that his community is receptive to his health care needs and is able to sustain him in his own environment.

What Is Long-Term Care?

Long-term care refers to a wide range of supportive services and assistance provided to persons who, as a result of chronic illness, frailty, or disability, are unable to function independently on a daily basis (National Academy on Aging, 1997). Whereas slightly more than half of long-term care beneficiaries are aged 65 years or older, recent data suggest that long-term care needs have increased considerably among the nonelderly. The projected reason is that, although survival rates for individuals with traumatic injuries or severe illnesses have increased, survivors are often left with permanent disabilities that necessitate long-term assistance.

Older Persons Needing Long-Term Care

By the year 2000, it is projected that 13% of the total population will be more than 65 years of age, with a life expectancy of 81 years for women and 74.1 years for men (Older Women's League, 1989). In the years 2010 to 2030, many of the baby boomers will reach 65, with an expectation in 2030 that there will be 70 million older adults—more than twice that of 1990. Approximately 3.6 million with be in need of nursing home beds. These increases are due to the improvements in health care, particularly at the beginning of life. The fastest-growing segment of the population is composed of those older than 80 years, with a preponderance of older women. At age 65 and older, there are 1,000 women to every 674 men. Above age 75, the proportion increases to 1,000 women to 548 men (U.S. Department of Commerce, 1992).

Minority populations are projected to represent 25% of elderly persons in 2030, up from 13% in 1990. Between 1990 and 2030, the white non-Hispanic population 65 years of age and older is projected to increase 93% compared with 328% for minorities, including Hispanics (555%) and non-Hispanic black persons (160%); American Indians, Eskimos, and Aleuts (231%); and Asians and Pacific Islanders (693%) (American Association of Retired Persons, 1994).

Chronic Illness

Chronic illness constitutes our nation's "number one malady" (Lubkin, 1995). Chronic illnesses can take on many forms, beginning as a sudden occurrence or being insidious in origin;

they can be disposed to episodic flare-ups or exacerbations or remain in remission. Chronic conditions with the highest prevalence for persons aged 45 to 75 years and older are arthritis and hypertension. Hearing impairments and heart conditions follow in prevalence for ages 65 and older (U.S. Department of Commerce, 1992). Complicating these illnesses is the fact that they will affect more older women. An older woman who is alone must meet the normal challenges of financing and running a household with possibly few resources. Her support system may be limited and may rely mostly on children and friends for assistance (Lubkin, 1995). Minority women may also face additional challenges and need to be studied in the context of the sociocultural impact of chronic illness.

Generally, society's views regarding both aged and chronically ill persons are negative. There is a tendency to look at age and disability in terms of their effect on the national pocketbook (Lubkin, 1995). In 1991, persons aged 65 and older accounted for one third of 1988 health care costs (Binstock & Post, 1991). Projections into the future imply a growth in the amount and percentage of health care dollars for older persons. Unlike investing in children's health, investment in older people brings limited promise of return.

Need for Community Access to Health Care

In 1983 a prospective payment system featuring diagnosis-related groups was introduced to curb the high costs of inpatient care. Its impact on health care provisions for older Americans revealed a "care gap" of crisis proportions in the community-based long-term care system, especially regarding access to nonmedical services (Estes et al., 1993).

At the urging of a number of nursing and health care groups, including the American Nurses Association (ANA) and the People to People Health Foundation (Project Hope), Congress included in the Omnibus Reconciliation Act of 1987 (Section 4079) the Community Nursing Organization (CNO), a 3-year demonstration administered by the Health Care Financing Administration (May, Schraeder, & Britt, 1996). It was in this environment that Richard Starr was able to receive care.

The CNO provides an environment for investigating a health care delivery system based on registered nurses' management of specific health care services for Medicare beneficiaries. Testing prepaid, capitated funding for community nursing and ambulatory care services for these beneficiaries, the project began enrolling members early in 1993. Participating national sites include the following:

- Carle Clinic Association, Urbana, Illinois
- Carondelet Health Services, Tucson, Arizona
- Visiting Nurse Service of New York City
- Living at Home/Block Nurse Program, St. Paul, Minnesota

The CNO demonstration is studying the effectiveness of nurse-managed care in improving access, continuity, and quality of health care for Medicare beneficiaries. The goals include the following:

- Prevention of unnecessary institutionalization through preventive support and health promotion.
- Support and coordination of care.
- Effective use of prospective payment methods.
- Adherence to capitated payment methods.

In 1996 and 1997, these demonstration Medicare programs were approved for funding until December 1999. They may shape the future of Medicare and, consequently, care and wellness for all seniors. The programs test cost capitation (the allocation of a fixed dollar amount to care for a patient/client) and up-front personal nursing care and prevention to keep seniors healthy (Lamb, 1995).

Living at Home/Block Nurse Program

Partnerships with the client and the community are essential to the effectiveness of the Living at Home/Block Nurse Program (LAH/BNP). Neighbors helping neighbors is a basic tenet of the program. This particular program had its beginning with a coffee held in 1981 by one nurse, Marjorie Jamieson. In time a St. Paul (Minnesota) neighborhood community was mobilized to care about its older citizens (Health Link, 1996). The program was initiated and developed by community residents and started with one or two people who took a leadership role to begin a project through volunteer activities that demonstrate concern and caring for elderly neighbors. These volunteer activities take on a multiplicity of tasks, from lawn mowing to providing rides to grocery stores and doctor appointments. Once the volunteer effort is firmly based in the community, a steering committee or board is formed to oversee all the volunteer activities. These simple measures of support eventually lead to the provision of nursing care services and linkages with home care agencies, with in-kind contributions from churches and various local groups. These agency linkages provide for access to private insurance and public entitlement programs and are Medicare reimbursed. A nurse is selected by a community, with the home health agency serving as the vehicle for personnel management, quality assurance, professional liability, and billing. Since the community group undertakes a large portion of the administrative work, it contracts for nursing care at discounted rates.

Services are tailored to the individual. Primary nurses coordinate health care as well as community services and empower seniors to take more responsibility for their care. It is estimated that a primary nurse has a caseload of about 175 persons. Members receiving routine Medicare coverage are assessed every 6 months. The assessment measures members' health and quality of life, as well as level of happiness, isolation or socialization, and activity. Members can volunteer or receive services of volunteers, in addition to, like Mr. Starr, visiting the "Nurse Is In Clinic" with questions about medications, diet, exercise, and other health issues of concern. The average age of the members is 76 years, with more than 70% generally healthy and 30% with well-managed chronic illnesses.

It is estimated that only about 10% of this group needs home care services at a given time. Case management, home care, rehabilitation, social work evaluations, respite care for caregivers, health counseling, and other services that bolster members' health, with no copayments, are some of the services provided to seniors.

The Cost Advantage

A 1994–1995 analysis of LAH/BNP services and cost data in 13 Minnesota communities revealed that 246 elderly residents would otherwise have been admitted to nursing homes; the resulting cost savings was $3.2 million. Data from nine programs in Minnesota providing nursing services describe a typical client as an 82-year-old woman living alone (70%) on less than $650 monthly income, and dependent for daily living activities (50%) because of functional deficits requiring nursing observation (32%) and assistance with personal care (35%). This clearly indicates the effectiveness of a nurse-managed Medicare program (Health Link, 1996). By combining the financing and delivery of health care services to those 65 and older in one package, the CNOs provide mechanisms for addressing patients' needs in an environment of shrinking resources. The capitated model of nurse-managed health care provides community-based health services to the elderly at a predictable and controlled rate by using registered nurses as health educators and care coordinators. Some of the benefits demonstrated by the CNOs include high enrollee satisfaction at lower costs than initially projected, decreased traditional Medicare home care costs, and use of less expensive equipment.

The LAH/BNP uses geriatric nurse case managers who closely scrutinize utilization and cost while acting as advocates who are well versed in health issues. That is an important piece: giving nurses the responsibility for making the assessment and matching the care in the most cost-effective manner. Nurses get to know their clients, and clients know that they can depend on their primary nurse. This trust has developed into an empowerment model for self-care. This program is one that can be replicated in other parts of the country.

Early in the project, LAH/BNP teamed with HealthSpan, which agreed to provide care for 5% less than Medicare costs. At this time the project has provided care for even less than the budget and has demonstrated that it can lower the costs of senior wellness and health care programs.

The concepts of health promotion and disease prevention are not new. Thirty years ago the U.S. Department of Health and Human Services developed health objectives for the decade that were population based. In 1990, Healthy People 2000 Objectives included the older adult (U.S. Department of Health and Human Services, 1990). The CNO demonstration projects can ensure that these objectives are met as we prepare for a larger segment of elderly persons—the baby boomers—in our society.

As we prepare for this "senior surge" (the baby boomers who will need health care as they turn 65 years of age in the next century), a discussion of elder home care coverage under Medicare is appropriate. Long-term care, although reformed from its past identity, was ensured and protected by the passage of the Balanced Budget Act of 1997. A big win accrued in provisions for home care, in the elimination of copayments on home care visits, in the shift of home health–related provisions from Part A to Part B, and in the redefinition of normative and homebound standards. Many more complexities of this act are detailed in the National Association of Home Care's report (722a) of August 1, 1997. There is a defined need to maintain persons in the community in which they live while providing services that are cost-effective and realistic, such as transportation, meals, and medical equipment; home care; and provision for resources that promote self-care.

References

American Association of Retired Persons. (1994). *A profile of older Americans.* Washington, DC: Author.

Binstock, R., & Post, S. (Eds.). (1991). *Too old for health care: Controversies in medicine, law, economics and ethics.* Baltimore: Johns Hopkins University Press.

Congressional Budget Office. (1992). *Projection of national health expenditures.* Washington, DC.: U.S. Government Printing Office.

Estes, C., Swan, J., and Associates. (1993). *The long-term care crisis: Elders trapped in the no-care zone.* Newbury Park, CA: Sage.

Health Link. (1996). Making a difference. *Health Link, 1*(3), 1, 4.

Jamieson, M., Campbell, J., & Clarke, S. (1989). The Block Nurse Program. *Gerontologist, 29*(1), 124–127.

Lamb, G. S. (1995). Early lessons from a capitated community-based nursing model. *Nursing Administration Quarterly, 19*(3), 18–26.

Letsch, S. (1993). National health care spending in 1991. *Health Affairs, 12*(1) 94–100.

May, C. A., Schraeder, C., & Britt, T. (1996). *Managed care and case management: Roles for professional nursing.* Washington, DC: American Nurses Publishing.

National Academy on Aging. (1997). *Facts on long-term care.* Washington, DC: Author.

Older Women's League. (1989). *Failing America's caregivers: A status report on women who care.* Washington, DC: Author.

U.S. Department of Commerce. (1992). *Statistical abstract of the United States.* Washington, DC: U.S. Government Printing Office.

U.S. Department of Health and Human Services. (1990). *Healthy people 2000: National health promotion and disease prevention objectives.* Washington, DC: U.S. Government Printing Office.

Developing and Implementing a Health Promotion Initiative
Hurdis M. Griffith

Put Prevention Into Practice (PPIP) is a disease prevention and health promotion initiative developed by the U.S. Public Health Service to assist primary care providers to improve their delivery of clinical preventive services (screening tests, immunizations, and counseling). Primary care providers were defined to include pediatricians, internists, obstetricians/gynecologists, nurse practitioners (NPs), and family physicians. With a background as an NP and experience in health policy at state and national levels, I served as senior policy adviser in the Office of Disease Prevention and Health Promotion (ODPHP) for 4 years and collaborated with primary health care providers in the development, implementation, and evaluation of PPIP.

Basis and Need for PPIP

PPIP evolved from evidence-based prevention guidelines developed by the U.S. Preventive Services Task Force (USPSTF). Increasingly, evidence-based methods, rather than expert opinion, have been used to develop clinical preventive services (CPS) guidelines (Woolf, 1992). The leader in this trend was the Canadian Task Force on the Periodic Health Examination in the late 1970s (Canadian Task Force, 1979). The next landmark was in 1984, when the U.S. Public Health Service established the USPSTF to develop guidelines for CPS (Lawrence & Mickalide, 1987). The project concluded in 1989 with the release of its first report, *Guide to Clinical Preventive Services* (U.S. Preventive Services Task Force, 1989), which evaluated the clinical effectiveness of 169 CPS and provided age-, sex-, and risk factor–specific recommendations on services that should be considered for inclusion in the periodic health examination. In 1994 the second edition of the *Guide to Clinical Preventive Services* was published (U.S. Preventive Services Task Force, 1996). These scientific guidelines, although controversial, are credible, widely accepted by health care providers, and the driving force in reimbursement for CPS in managed care organizations and among other payers.

Abundant research documents that many deaths among Americans are preventable through CPS that can be delivered by NPs and other primary care providers (McGinnis & Foege, 1993). Delivery of CPS can be improved by the use of evidence-based guidelines, which provide recommendations on who should receive the services and periodicity of performance. Guidelines are a mechanism to improve quality of care as well as reduce costs (Leavenworth, 1994). Yet studies indicate that the majority of primary care providers, including NPs, often do not provide CPS as recommended by major authorities and guidelines. The following are examples of data on delivery rates (routinely delivered to more than 80% of patients who need the service):

1. The *Pneumococcus* vaccination rate for adults aged 65 years and older ranges from 5% to 40%, with the rate for NPs at 33%.
2. Inquiry about tobacco use ranges from 33% to 75%, with the rate for NPs at 51%.
3. Inquiry about sexual practices and sexually transmitted diseases ranges from 13% to 52%, with the rate for NPs at 52%.
4. Cholesterol level screening ranges from 36% to 80%, with the rate for NPs at 45%.
5. Inquiry about alcohol consumption and other drug use ranged from 23% to 63%, with rates for NPs at 45% for alcohol consumption and 43% for other drug use.
6. Inquiry about diet and nutrition and formula-

tion of a plan ranged from 15% to 53%, with rates for NPs at 46% for diet/nutrition and 31% for formulation of a plan.

7. Mammography screening ranged from 53% to 85%, with the rate for NPs at 63% (Griffith, 1993, 1994; USDHHS, 1992).

It was disconcerting that NPs, along with other primary care providers, are not demonstrating a higher rate of delivery of CPS according to scientific guidelines. However, from a policy perspective, it was also troubling to me that the nursing profession did not have official, published recommendations for the delivery of CPS similar to those of the other professional groups represented at the prevention policy table. Guidelines or published recommendations relating to CPS are issued regularly by government health agencies (1988 Joint National Committee, 1988; National Cholesterol Education Program, 1993; National Coalition for Adult Immunizations, 1992; National Vaccine Advisory Committee, 1993), by medical specialty organizations (American Academy of Family Physicians, 1993; American Academy of Pediatrics, 1991; American College of Obstetricians and Gynecologists, 1993; American College of Physicians, 1991; American Society of Colon and Rectal Surgeons, 1992), by professional and scientific organizations (American Medical Association, 1983; American Dental Association, 1982; National Academy of Sciences, Institute of Medicine, 1979), and by voluntary associations (American Cancer Society, 1992; American Diabetes Association, 1993; American Heart Association, 1987). Notably missing from this list are published guidelines for CPS issued by nursing organizations. This lack of an official professional position on the delivery of CPS diminishes the "voice of nursing" (Griffith, 1993, 1994).

After realizing the degree to which this deficiency was adversely affecting the nursing profession, and to address the issue, I met with the American Nurses Association (ANA) Congress on Nursing Practice in 1993. The group unanimously agreed to recommend to the ANA that a panel should be established to develop official, published nursing positions/recommendations on the delivery of CPS, using the scientific evidence of the USPSTF as the basis. The nursing perspective for each of the preventive services would be a unique contribution in the prevention policy arena. To my knowledge, this recommendation has never been acted on.

This issue surfaced again when we were writing chapters for the *Clinician's Handbook*, the manual for providers that is a component of the PPIP kit. In each CPS-specific chapter there is a section presenting the "Recommendation of Major Authorities." The official, published recommendations of professional associations and other organizations are listed, in addition to the guidelines published by the USPSTF. Most professional associations for primary care providers are represented in nearly every chapter. Among 60 chapters, in only three was it possible to add the official, published nursing position, because for the remainder no position had been developed, adopted, or published. This does not accurately represent nursing's contribution to prevention in the practice arena. Yet, until nurses have official, published CPS guidelines to bring to the policy table, they will be the invisible workers in the area of prevention.

The barriers to consistent use of guidelines in the delivery of CPS are multifaceted and include lack of reimbursement, lack of knowledge or uncertainty about the guidelines, lack of time, and poor attitude about the importance of prevention. Another major barrier is the difficulty of converting from an illness-oriented system to a system in which prevention is an integral part of every patient encounter. The need for a systematic approach to the delivery of CPS and for tools to facilitate the development of a good prevention system were recognized by the founders of PPIP. Therefore PPIP was developed to facilitate a systematic approach to the consistent implementation of evidence-based guidelines.

Development of PPIP

PPIP is a kit of tools to achieve a systematic approach to the delivery of CPS whereby prevention becomes an integral part of every health care encounter, rather than an add-on that is often neglected (Griffith, Dickey, & Kamerow, 1995). PPIP was developed as an office- or clinic-based system but can be modified for other settings. PPIP tools are research or guidelines based and are targeted at patients, providers, and the system. Included are pocket-sized patient booklets (*Personal Health Guides* for adults and a *Child Health Guide*), a user-friendly guide for providers (*Clinician's Handbook of Clinical Preventive Services*), and tools to change the office/clinic system (posters for the waiting and examination rooms, flowcharts, temporary and permanent alert stickers for medical records, prescription pads, and reminder postcards).

Initially the adult patient booklet (*Personal Health Guide*) was physician oriented. When representatives of nursing organizations and I objected to the use of the term *your doctor* throughout the booklet, an introductory statement was inserted: "Please note: The word 'doctor' is used in this *Health Guide* to refer to health care providers of all types, including nurses, nurse practitioners, and physician assistants." This was still deemed unacceptable, and we again suggested that the term *your health care provider*, rather than *your doctor*, be used. Physicians involved in the development of PPIP responded that doctors would not use the materials if the term *doctor* was not used. Finally, negotiations resulted in the decision to develop two adult versions of the *Personal Health Guide*—one with a white cover using the term *your doctor* throughout and the other with a green cover using the term *your health provider* throughout. For the development of remaining PPIP materials, the term *health care provider* was used and the issue never surfaced again.

Even with the resolution of the use of the term denoting health care providers, other discipline-related issues surfaced in the development of the materials. One pertained to limiting the inclusion of services to those recommended by the USPSTF in the guidelines. Professional associations with published recommendations, often primarily based on expert opinion rather than scientific evidence, indicated their difficulty in supporting or using PPIP materials unless their specific recommendations were included. This created a dilemma in that those involved in the development of the program were committed to including only services with scientific evidence of effectiveness. At the same time, if the PPIP materials were unacceptable to large groups of primary care providers, such as pediatricians, use would be greatly diminished. Finally, after extensive negotiations, a somewhat more liberal approach was taken and wording developed that allowed for more extensive inclusion of some services without jeopardizing the original intent. Moreover, on the examination room posters, darker colored bars were used to denote recommendations of the USPSTF and lighter bars provided the recommendations of other major experts. As previously mentioned, in each chapter of the *Clinician's Handbook* the published recommendations of all major experts, not only those based on research evidence, were listed. Although this approach addressed the objections of some of the professions, it was not enough to satisfy everyone, including some in nursing who objected to the PPIP program because it is "not sufficiently community-oriented" and "too medical-model." These objections persisted even after it was explained that PPIP was developed as an office- or clinic-focused program, is certainly within the scope of the practice of NPs, and is clearly applicable and adaptable to the practice of nurses in most settings.

Years later, after leaving my position in ODPHP and becoming involved in a conference sponsored by the National Academies of Practice (NAP) and the Agency for Health Care Policy and Research, the issue related to inclusion of more services with a more frequent or liberal time line surfaced again. Ten disciplines comprising the NAP (dentistry, medicine, nursing, optometry, psychology, social work, osteopathy, podiatry, pharmacy, and veterinary medicine) discussed PPIP materials in a 1-day symposium. Much concern was expressed by disciplines such as psychology, social work, dentistry, and optometry about the limited inclusion of psychosocial services and restricted time lines for dental and optometric services. There is no doubt that when inclusion of services is limited to those with scientific evidence of effectiveness, professionals who believe that expert opinion is sufficient will be dissatisfied. Furthermore, professions with a weaker scientific basis for their practice will be at a disadvantage. Disciplines vary in their scientific basis, and this often impedes communication and coordination among them. Clearly, more research is needed to demonstrate effectiveness of many prevention services, but until we have the evidence, the services should not be included. To include services primarily based on expert opinion would jeopardize the credibility of the program with insurers, managed care organizations, and government agencies.

Only after grappling with these issues both in my position with ODPHP and in my involvement with NAP did I fully appreciate some of the underlying reasons for the lack of understanding between disciplines and the importance of a strong scientific basis for practice. The need for nursing to continue to pursue research-based practice also became clearer. Clearly the medical profession has the strongest scientific evidence for its practice, and this is directly related to the distribution of research monies. Nursing needs to continue to fight for more research resources and to ensure the growth of the National Institute of Nursing Research. In like manner, other disciplines, such as psychology, need to continue to pursue support for their research endeavors.

There is a dearth of scientific evidence to demonstrate the effectiveness of counseling to change lifestyle behaviors, prevent disease, and promote health. There is evidence that healthier lifestyle behaviors reduce rates of morbidity and premature death, but there are very few scientifically strong studies demonstrating health care providers' effectiveness in changing personal behaviors to improve health status. Although the USPSTF was relatively liberal in recommending counseling as an intervention for behavioral and lifestyle change, the scientific evidence to substantiate those recommendations was weaker than for other prevention activities. Nursing research and interdisciplinary research is desperately needed in this area.

Dissemination and Implementation of PPIP

PPIP was developed and implemented in phases. First, the passport-sized adult patient care booklet, initially titled *Prevention Passport,* was developed. It was then discovered that the name had to be changed because someone had already patented that title. It was renamed *Personal Health Guide.* As organizations became aware of its availability, it was tempting to view this useful, inexpensive booklet as a "quick fix" to advance prevention among employees. For example, SmithKline-Beecham printed 150,000 copies and distributed them to employees in Christmas letters. The Maryland State Personnel System placed them in more than 100,000 employee mailboxes.

Although these patients booklets have inherent usefulness to promote prevention and increase patient education, their effectiveness when used alone in these ways is much less than when they are part of a program designed to change the office/clinic delivery system. Most patients benefit from reinforcement by health care providers in promoting positive behaviors. For example, if patients are asked to bring in their *Personal Health Guide* each time they come for a clinic or office appointment, and if someone in the office assists them in updating it during the visit, they will value the booklet more than if it is presented once and never referred to again.

Health education materials, including those focused on prevention, are readily available. PPIP patient booklets, standing alone without being part of a system-changing program to ensure that prevention is consistently addressed, would add minimal value beyond the myriad of other patient education brochures and booklets available from federal and private sources. Therefore we attempted to convince those interested in PPIP materials to implement the full range of PPIP materials, rather than printing only adult and child patient booklets. However, "selling" this concept was often difficult because distributing patient booklets was much easier than changing a delivery system.

While completing the development of the numerous components of PPIP, we began marketing them, that is, increasing knowledge and desire to become involved with the program. This involved extensive networking with professional associations, managed care organizations, industries, insurers, researchers, and individual practitioners. We made presentations at major professional meetings and were encouraged by the positive response and enthusiasm for PPIP. Telephone calls into ODPHP inquiring about the program proliferated. We were able to garnish federal resources to develop professional association partners who committed to promoting PPIP among their memberships, printing and marketing the materials, and conducting evaluations of the effectiveness of the program. Professional partners included the American Academy of Family Physicians, American College of Physicians, American Academy of Nurse Practitioners, American Nurses Association, and National Association of Pediatric Nurse Associates and Practitioners. Later, the American Academy of Pediatrics and the American Cancer Association also printed and disseminated the materials. Camera-ready film and printing materials were provided as an incentive to these associations at no cost. We also encouraged these associations, as well as hospitals and other health care organizations, to put the name of their organization and their logo on the cover of the materials. The only restriction was that they could not change the content or remove the official government seal from the back cover. Even

those simple restrictions became problematic at times because some professional groups wanted to change the recommendations in the booklets to reflect their own guidelines. We spent a considerable amount of time negotiating and creating a "win-win" situation by convincing them to support evidence-based recommendations but also allowing some of their language.

One of the most exciting PPIP outreach efforts was the convening of medical directors of the 20 largest managed care organizations at a meeting held in Washington, D.C., and chaired by the assistant secretary of health. It was unusual for representatives of these competing organizations to sit at the same table to problem solve an issue—specifically how to coordinate efforts to change systems of health care delivery to ensure more consistent delivery of evidence-based CPS. Because a certain percentage of enrollees/members in managed care organizations periodically move from one organization to another, and because the "profits," or outcomes, from preventing disease are long term, the incentives to deliver prevention activities is diminished. However, if all managed care organizations implemented a PPIP type of prevention program, it could be seen as a worthwhile investment. Although some patients in whom they invest move to another organization, they gain others who already have received recommended screening tests, immunizations, counseling on lifestyle behavior change, and a copy of the *Personal Health Guide*. Representatives of the managed care organizations at the meeting generally agreed that cooperating in the implementation of a common prevention program could benefit all participants. In addition, many agreed that a system to integrate prevention into everyday practice was probably better than the traditional method of conducting campaigns to increase rates of prevention services, such as campaigns to provide mammograms, "pap" smears, immunizations, and cholesterol screening. These campaigns are often undertaken by public relations departments of managed care organizations rather than by medical or other health care services.

In addition to meeting with representatives of managed care organizations, I made initial attempts to work with the National Committee of Quality Assurance (NCQA), the organization that accredits managed care organizations and develops "report cards" evaluating their services. Working with the NCQA to include PPIP in its accreditation criteria or on its report cards would be another, and probably more efficient, approach to addressing these issues.

Evaluation of PPIP

Five study instruments for measuring effectiveness of PPIP materials were developed by ODPHP staff and external research consultants. The instruments included a provider questionnaire, patient interview schedules, an office manager–office staff questionnaire, a medical record review, and a billing record review. Assuming each group will customize for their setting, we hoped that using these core questionnaires would produce findings that could be compared among the various types of organizations implementing PPIP. The instruments were made available on the PPIP home page.

An evaluation of implementation of PPIP has been carried out in four family practice residency programs and three community health centers funded by the Texas Department of Health. Interviews conducted with staff during the first 18 months showed implementation to be most successful in sites with the following:

1. A high degree of readiness.
2. The presence of a strong program champion with authority to effect implementation.
3. Teamwork among providers and staff.
4. An environment conducive to patient flow that offers opportunity for multiple teaching moments.
5. Technical assistance for dealing with barriers.
6. Open communication among all actors.
7. Appropriate tracking and monitoring systems (Goodson, Gottieb, & Radcliffe).

Research is also being conducted on the implementation of PPIP materials by primary care physicians participating in Keystone Health Plan East, a health maintenance organization in southeastern Pennsylvania modeled as an independent practice association. Preliminary conclusions indicate that on-site office training using PPIP materials provided by plan coordinators or American Cancer Society volunteers is effective in promoting the use of prevention materials (Eisenberg et al., 1997).

Summary

The interdisciplinary implications of PPIP and the involvement of nursing groups are important to the development of the program. Prevention is an excellent area for nurses wishing to increase their interdisciplinary focus and contributions to improve health care.

References

American Academy of Family Physicians, Commission on Public Health and Scientific Affairs. (1993). *Age charts for periodic health examination.* Kansas City, MO: Author.

American Academy of Pediatrics, Committee on Practice and Ambulatory Care. (1991). Recommendations for preventive pediatric health care. *American Academy of Pediatric News* 7:19.

American Cancer Society. (1992). *Summary of American Cancer Society recommendations for the early detection of cancer in asymptomatic people.* Atlanta: Author.

American College of Obstetricians and Gynecologists. (1993). *The obstetrician-gynecologist and primary-preventive health care.* Washington, DC: Author.

American College of Physicians. (1991). Guidelines. In Eddy, D. M. (Ed.), *Common screening tests* (pp. 411–416). Philadelphia: Author.

American Dental Association. (1982). *Accepted dental therapeutics* (39th ed.). Chicago: Author.

American Diabetes Association. (1993). Position statement: Screening for diabetes. *Diabetes Care, 16,* 7–9.

American Heart Association. (1987). Cardiovascular and risk factor evaluation of healthy American adults: A statement for physicians by an ad hoc committee appointed by the steering committee. *Circulation, 75,* 1340A–1362A.

American Medical Association, Council of Scientific Affairs. (1983). Medical evaluations of healthy persons. *Journal of the American Medical Association, 249,* 1626–1633.

American Society of Colon and Rectal Surgeons. (1992).

Practice parameters for the detection of colorectal neoplasms. Palatine, IL: Author.

Canadian Task Force on the Periodic Health Examination. (1979). The periodic health examination. *Canadian Medical Association Journal, 121,* 1193–1254.

Eisenberg, F. P., Lyons, D. C., Ford, S., Rothnev-Koziek, L., Stone, K., & Wender, R. (1997, April). Evaluation of "Put Prevention Into Practice" in an individual practice association health maintenance organization. Atlanta: American College of Preventative Medicine.

Goodson, P., Gottlieb, N. H., & Radcliffe, M. M. Put prevention into practice: Evaluation of program initiation in nine Texas clinical sites. Unpublished manuscript, University of Texas at Austin.

Griffith, H. M. (1993). Needed: A strong nursing position on preventive services. *Image Journal of Nursing Scholarship, 24,* 272.

Griffith, H. M. (1994). Public policy: Nursing's role in the delivery of clinical preventive services. *Journal of Professional Nursing, 10,* 69.

Griffith, H. M., Dickey, L., & Kamerow, D. B. (1995). Put prevention into practice: A systematic approach. *Journal of Health Management Practice, 1*(3), 9–15.

1988 Joint National Committee. (1988). The 1988 report of the Joint National Committee on Detection Evaluation, and Treatment of High Blood Pressure. *Archives of Internal Medicine, 148,* 1–23.

Lawrence, R. S., & Mickalide, A. D. (1987). Preventive services in clinical practice: Designing the periodic health examination. *Journal of the American Medical Association, 257,* 2205–2207.

Leavenworth, G. (1994). Quality costs less. *Business & Health: Special Report on Guidelines 1994, 12*(Suppl. B), 6–11.

McGinnis, J. M., & Foege, W. H. (1993). Actual causes of death in the United States. *Journal of the American Medical Association, 270,* 2207–2212.

National Academy of Sciences, Institute of Medicine, Ad Hoc Advisory Group on Preventive Sciences. (1979). *Preventive services for the well population.* Washington, DC: Author.

National Cholesterol Education Program. (1993). *Second report of the National Cholesterol Education Program Expert Panel on Detection, Evaluation, and Treatment of High Blood Cholesterol in Adults (Adult Treatment Panel III).* Bethesda, MD: National Heart, Lung, and Blood Institute.

National Coalition for Adult Immunizations. (1992). *Standards for adult immunization practices.* Bethesda, MD: Author.

National Vaccine Advisory Committee. (1993). *Standards for pediatric immunization practices.* Atlanta: Centers for Disease Control and Prevention.

U.S. Department of Health and Human Services, Public Health Service, Office of Disease Prevention and Health Promotion. (1992). Study of the delivery of clinical preventive services by primary care providers. Unpublished.

U.S. Preventive Services Task Force. (1989). *Guide to clinical preventive services: An assessment of the effectiveness of 169 interventions.* Baltimore: Williams & Wilkins.

U.S. Preventive Services Task Force. (1996). *Guide to clinical preventive services* (2nd ed.). Baltimore: Williams & Wilkins.

Woolf, S. H. (1992). Practice guidelines: A new reality in medicine. II. Methods of developing guidelines. *Archives of Internal Medicine, 152,* 946–952.

Chapter 5

HEALTH CARE FINANCING

Joyce Pulcini and Diane Mahoney

A patient with newly diagnosed acquired immunodeficiency syndrome (AIDS) enters a major metropolitan hospital for the first time since his diagnosis. He has been working part time as a clerk in a department store and part time as a self-employed musician and is uninsured. He has a small amount of money in the bank and owns a cooperative apartment with a friend. He is not close with his family, beyond his aging mother and a sister who lives 1000 miles away. What are the prospects that this patient will have adequate care throughout the course of his illness, including the most effective medications, long-term care, and home care that will be needed at an unknown later time? Will the available health care resources adequately meet this person's needs now and throughout his illness?

This chapter will describe and analyze the features of the health care financing system in the United States. It will first present a historical perspective to provide a basis for understanding the current system. The chapter will then explore the financial and economic forces that drive the health care system and describe measures to contain costs. The health care financing system will be described, including the public and private sectors. A major focus will be on financing long-term care as well as acute and primary care. Finally, implications for nursing will be discussed.

HISTORICAL PERSPECTIVES

History reveals some dominant values underpinning the U.S. political and economic systems. From its origins, the United States has had a long history of individualism, emphasis on freedom to choose among alternative options, and an aversion as a nation to large-scale government intervention into the private realm. Social programs have been the exception rather than the rule and have arisen primarily during times of great need, such as in the 1930s and 1960s. Health care has its origins in the private sector, and strong resistance has been raised to government intervention in health care, particularly by physician and hospital groups.

During the Great Depression of the 1930s, first, Blue Cross, an insurance plan to cover hospital care, and then Blue Shield to cover physician care were created. Starr (1982) describes the initial reluctance of the American Hospital Association and of the American Medical Association to adopt any form of prepaid hospital or medical expenses. But hospitals in 1933 and physicians in 1938 were hit hard enough by bad debt to endorse plans that laid the foundation for what is now Blue Cross and Blue Shield. The rationale behind instituting such private insurance plans was that persons should pay for their medical care before they actually got sick, thus ensuring some security for both providers and consumers of medical services in time of need. Starr (1982) points out that the development of these plans effectively diffused what had been, at that time, a strong political move to legislate a compulsory health insurance plan. The Social Security Act of 1935 is striking as a comprehensive piece of social legislation in its failure to include health care. This issue never again came up with any real political strength until the 1960s.

Blue Cross and Blue Shield continued to dominate the health insurance industry until the 1950s, when commercial insurance companies entered the market. These insurance companies had been discouraged from entry partially because of discounted room rates negotiated with hospitals by Blue Cross. Moreover, state regulations required Blue Cross/Blue Shield to use "community rating," or rates based on the total utilization of health care services across a whole population or community. One way that commercial insurance companies were able to compete with Blue Cross and Blue Shield in the health care market was to utilize experience rating, which is based on the recruitment of a select and usually low-risk population or community. Experience rating decreases the price of health insurance because high-risk individuals can be excluded from the plan. This distinction between Blue Cross/Blue Shield and commercial insurance companies exists today in some states, but Blue Cross/Blue Shield is increasingly transforming itself to compete directly with managed care plans by diversifying its product.

The United States in the 1960s enjoyed relative prosperity along with a burgeoning social conscience that led to a heightened concern for poor and elderly populations in this country. Another issue at this time was the failure of health insurance to protect persons who had catastrophic illness. The catalyst for a governmental solution to the lack of health care for these populations was the framing of these issues as a series of "crises" that garnered public support and created an atmosphere for change (Alford, 1975). As a result of these forces, Medicaid and Medicare, two separate but related programs, were passed in 1965 as amendments to the Social Security Act. Medicare, or Title XVIII, is a federal program for the aged and disabled, and Medicaid, or Title XIX, is a jointly funded program of both federal and state governments, with eligibility determined by income and resources.

Within years of the passage of Medicare and Medicaid, it became clear that these programs were contributing greatly to escalating costs of health care. The government's and society's inability to react to the escalation of health care costs is one of the root causes of our current fiscal crisis in health care. In fact, it was within a decade after the passage of Medicare and Medicaid that cost began increasingly to dominate all policy decisions in health care.

The health care field has evolved from a rather small and unorganized private enterprise to a large, multifaceted business affected by interrelated forces. The role of third-party payers in the financing of the health care industry has grown tremendously in the past 40 to 50 years. Historically, the majority of payments for health services came from first- or second-party payers or from the patients or their families, respectively. In 1940, 81.3% of health care was paid for by the individual or his family and 18.7% was financed by third-party, or intermediary, payers. Of this last figure, only 2.6% was financed by private insurance companies and 16.1% by public funding (state, federal, local). By 1980, these figures had reversed themselves, with 32.9% of costs borne by the patient or his family and 67.1% of these costs by third-party or public payers. Of this last figure, private insurance companies had financed 27.4% of these costs and public funding, 39.7% (Gibson & Waldo, 1982).

Currently the majority of people are covered by employer-based health insurance. Increasingly, however, full-time jobs with benefits are being replaced with part-time positions without benefit of health insurance. This is occurring particularly in lower-paid positions in the service sectors of the economy. Others who do not have health insurance available through the workplace opt for coverage by purchasing individual insurance or receive government health insurance such as Medicare or Medicaid. Most employers now require some portion of the monthly premiums to be paid by the individual. Generally, about 80% is paid by the employer and 20% by the individual. Two decades ago, most employers offered 100% payment as a fringe benefit; however, with the sharp escalation in costs of health insurance has come a

Table 5-1 National Health Expenditures Aggregate and Per Capita Amounts and Percent Distribution, by Source of Funds: Selected Years 1960–1995

Item	1960	1970	1980	1985	1990	1995
			Number in Millions			
U.S. population	190.1	214.8	235.1	247.1	260.0	273.0
			Amount in Billions			
Gross domestic product	$527	$1,036	$2,784	$4,181	$5,744	$7,254
			Percent of Gross Domestic Product			
National health expenditures	5.1	7.1	8.9	10.2	12.1	13.6
			Amount in Billions			
National health expenditures	$26.9	$73.2	$247.2	$428.2	$697.5	$988.5
Private	20.2	45.5	142.5	253.9	413.1	532.1
Public	6.6	27.7	104.8	174.3	284.3	456.4
Federal	2.9	17.8	72.0	123.3	195.8	328.4
State and local	3.7	9.9	32.8	51.0	88.5	128.0
			Per Capita Amount			
National health expenditures	$141	$341	$1,052	$1,733	$2,683	$3,621
Private	106	212	606	1,027	1,589	1,949
Public	35	129	446	705	1,094	1,672
Federal	15	83	306	499	753	1,203
State and local	20	46	140	206	341	469
			Percent Distribution			
National health expenditures						
Private	75.2	62.2	57.6	59.3	59.2	53.8
Public	24.8	37.8	42.4	40.7	40.8	46.2
Federal	10.9	24.3	29.1	28.8	28.1	33.2
State and local	13.9	13.5	13.3	11.9	12.7	12.9

NOTE: Numbers and percents may not add to totals because of rounding.
From Health Care Financing Administration, Office of the Actuary: Data from the Office of National Health Statistics, 1996. (HCFA, 1997 www.hcfa.gov/stats/Table 1.TXT)

concomitant drive to share these costs with employees.

Cost escalation in health care has created a powerful incentive to alter the system. Table 5-1 provides a graphic picture of the costs of health care from 1960 to the present. As costs rose in the 1970s and 1980s, the balance of power changed in the health care field. More and more groups outside the health field became involved in attempts to contain costs. Leaders from business, large corporations, and labor offered solutions to the problems because they were purchasing or negotiating for health care benefits. Patients also became disillusioned, initially with the quality of health care that they were receiving and later with the high cost of this care. Physicians who had traditionally managed hospitals and health care facilities were increasingly replaced with business executives who focus on cost-containment efforts. By the 1990s the health care arena had undergone radical changes that ultimately revolutionized the financing and delivery of health care.

COST CONTAINMENT IN HEALTH CARE

Efforts toward cost containment have taken on many faces as providers, insurers, employers, unions, and individuals have become alarmed about the current and long-term economic consequences of the escalating costs of health care. A range of strategies have been used to curb these costs.

Regulation Versus Competition

In the 1970s, the preferred solution to the escalating cost of health care was government regulation. Regulation took the form of health planning at all levels of government and included certificate-of-need programs, which were administered by health systems agencies (HSAs) at the federal, state, and local levels. These programs were intended to avoid duplication of new technologies and certain health care services, limit capital expansion, and ultimately cut unnecessary costs. Professional groups, such as physicians, responded to cost containment through self-regulation mechanisms such as professional standards review organizations (PSROs). PSROs were created by the 1972 Medicare amendments to monitor the quality of federally funded care and to ensure its delivery in the most efficient and economical manner (Davis, Anderson, Rowland, & Steinberg, 1990). In 1983, peer review organizations were created and placed under contract to the Health Care Financing Administration for utilization review and quality-of-care assessments of hospitals, health maintenance organizations (HMOs), and some office practices.

Many of the regulatory efforts of the 1970s and 1980s went by the wayside because they did not significantly reduce costs. Although regulation did involve consumers and community agencies in the process of thinking about cost containment, the solution to the problem was beyond its grasp. Local health planning agencies were often controlled by provider groups or consumers with vested interests who were unwilling or unable to curb what was an expanding problem. Professional groups, while giving lip service to decreasing costs, continued to respond to the overwhelming economic incentives inherent in the health care system, and as a result HSAs disappeared or lost much of their influence during the 1980s.

The 1980s brought an emphasis on competition as a mechanism to cut costs. Competition is based on the premise that the health care system has enough similarities to the free market that cost would be controlled by the entry of a large number of competing elements. The problem is that, at least at the level of the patient, the health care system does not act like a free market system and indeed has few similarities to a fully competitive market in economic terms (Pulcini, 1984). Chapter 12, which focuses on economics, more fully describes the mechanisms underlying the market system.

Although not a perfect solution, competition is based on the economic assumption of scarcity—that is, health care is not an unlimited resource, so choices must be made as to how it will be distributed. Competition has allowed us to experience in the health care market the effect of economic incentives on cost control. The 1980s brought attempts to change the existing incentives in health care so that providers and patients could begin to understand the financial effects of high-cost care. Competition has been used effectively at the health plan level, especially with the entry of many new managed care organizations that do compete vigorously with each other. In this realm the purchasers of health insurance tend to be large corporations, businesses, or unions that buy health benefits for their employees or members. The major impetus for cost containment in the 1980s came from these groups, which are indeed the ultimate buyers of health insurance. The problems, of late, are that health care reform efforts based solely on decreasing costs can lead to care that is compromised at the individual patient level. With maturity of the managed care marketplace, one would hope that this competition will be based on quality and access as well as cost.

Other examples of cost-containment mechanisms are copayments, deductibles, and coinsurance, which have the expressed goal of informing consumers of the cost of health care and discouraging unnecessary use. Some argue that although these efforts have had some effect, they have tended to discourage early identification of health problems. One can question whether these efforts have, in effect, decreased access to primary prevention and increased the overall cost of care initiated at later stages in an illness episode. By the end of the 1980s, there was a realization that neither pure competition nor regulation would be effective as a solution but that some combination would be needed. Managed competition, as put forth by President Clinton's Health Security Act, was an example of this concept. At the level of the individual patient, the care that is received is dependent to a great extent on what will be reimbursed by insurance companies and managed care plans. States and even the federal government have begun to pass regulatory legislation in the form of health plan accountability laws to further regulate managed care plans (Kongstvedt, 1996). These laws encompass a variety of areas such as grievance procedures, confidentiality of health information, requirements that patients are fully informed of the benefits they will receive under a managed care plan, antidiscrimination clauses, and assurances that various quality assurance mechanisms are in place so that patient satisfaction is measured and efforts to control costs do not curtail needed care.

Prospective Versus Fee-for-Service Financing

The 1980s brought pressure on the government from corporations and business groups to change financing from fee-for-service, or retrospective, reimbursement to prospective modalities. Because the federal government has direct control only of its own programs, it targeted Medicare Part A by developing in 1983 a prospective payment system (PPS) for hospital care, commonly known as diagnosis-related groups (DRGs). DRGs set a payment level for each of 467 diagnostic categories typically used in inpatient care. The goal was to place a cap on escalating hospital costs. Prospective payment measures have helped to slow the rate of growth of hospital expenditures and have had a major impact on length of stay (Fuchs, 1988). Initially, DRG rates were allowed to increase each year, and payment rates were also adjusted for geographic differences in wage levels. Certain services (such as outpatient and long-term care services) and hospitals (such as children's hospitals, psychiatric facilities, and rehabilitation hospitals) were excluded from the PPS. Capital and training expenses were reimbursed at cost. Since its initial passage, PPS has undergone some changes, but currently, the payment received per hospital discharge is based on what is called the DRG relative weight and a national average cost per discharge (Davis, Anderson, Rowland, & Steinberg, 1990).

The PPS contributed to significantly increased patient acuity in inpatient settings, and resulting gaps and problems still exist. Decreased length of hospital stay caused a ripple effect in the home care industry, which has had to care for more acutely ill persons in the home. Between 1975 and 1996 the number of inpatient hospital beds decreased by 45%. The number of skilled nursing facilities increased rapidly, as did the number of home health agencies (Health Care Financing Administration [HCFA], 1996). As a result of these changes, the health care industry has become reimbursement driven and more focused on individual versus family-centered care in order to control costs (Phillips, Cloonan, Irvine, & Fisher, 1990).

With the enormous federal budget deficit, there has been increased pressure to decrease outlays by cost-saving measures aimed at Medicare Part B. In March 1992, physician payment reform was initiated by means of the Resource-based Relative Value Scale (RBRVS). Its goal was not only cost savings but also a redistribution of physician services to increase primary care services and decrease the use of highly specialized physician care. The RBRVS was developed by William Hsiao and his colleagues (1988) to establish comparable fees for medical services based on time and intensity of effort, with consideration of typical overhead and malpractice costs. Other Medicare Part B cost-saving measures are limitation of home health care services and institution of fixed payments for outpatient care. Other programs such as Medicaid and more recently Medicare are increasingly using managed care arrangements to contain costs. These will be discussed further in the upcoming sections on Medicare and Medicaid.

Although health care expenditures as a percentage of the gross domestic product have been increasing steadily since the passage of Medicare and Medicaid in 1965, this figure stabilized at between 13.5% and 13.6% from 1993 to 1995. This represents the slowest growth rate in health care spending in more than three decades (HCFA, 1996). This growth stabilization is due in part to some of the just described cost-containment measures.

Managed Care

Managed care is rapidly becoming the dominant health care financing and delivery system in the United States. As of 1994, 51.1 million persons were enrolled in an HMO, and this represents a 23% increase from 1992 and a 300% increase from 1988 (Bodenheimer, 1996; Kongstvedt, 1996). As of June 1996, 40.1% of the total Medicaid population, or 13.3 million persons, were enrolled in managed care plans. They represent 35% of all beneficiaries and a 170% increase since 1993. As of January 1997, 4.9 million Medicare beneficiaries, or 13% of the total, were enrolled in managed care plans (HCFA, 1997a). Managed care has its origins in the early prepaid health plans that have been in existence in the United States from at least the 1920s. A managed care system shifts the emphasis of the provision of health care away from the fee-for-service mode toward a system in which the provider is a "gatekeeper" or "manager" of the client's health care. In a managed care system the provider or insurance company assumes some degree of financial responsibility for the care that is given. According to Curtiss (1989), managed care implies not only that spending will be controlled but also that other aspects of care will be controlled and managed, such as price, quality, and accessibility.

In managed care systems, the primary care provider has traditionally been the "gatekeeper" deciding what specialty services are appropriate and where these services can be obtained at the lowest cost. More recently, though, insurance companies themselves are becoming involved in patient care decisions in their attempts to authorize payment for less expensive procedures. Many providers are questioning this type of intervention in direct patient care and are even starting their own plans that leave more of the decisions to the providers themselves.

Many types of managed health care plans exist. They range from models that have increased control, accountability, and operating complexity to plans that incorporate some aspects of managed care but not all. Kongstvedt (1996) places these on a continuum from closed-panel HMOs to managed indemnity plans (Fig. 5-1). HMOs assume responsibility for organizing and providing comprehensive health care services for members in return for a monthly set payment. HMOs incorporate four key concepts:

1. An enrolled population
2. A prepayment of premiums

Figure 5–1   Continuum of managed care. (Reprinted with permission from Kongstvedt, P. [1996]. *The managed care handbook* [3rd ed.]. Gaithersburg, MD: Aspen Publications, p. 35. © 1996 Aspen Publishers, Inc.)

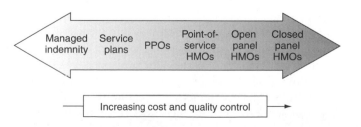

3. Coverage of comprehensive medical services
4. Centralization of medical and hospital services.

Closed-panel HMOs include staff model HMOs, in which physicians/providers are salaried employees, and group model HMOs, which contract with multispecialty physician group practices to provide all physician services to its members. Open-panel HMOs include network HMOs, which contract with more than one group practice, and the individual practice association (IPA) type of HMOs, which contract with an association of physicians to provide services to members. In point-of-service (POS) plans and in preferred provider organizations (PPOs) the patient is allowed to self-refer to a specialist but must pay higher premiums if they do so. The POS plan is distinguished from the PPO in that the enrollee belongs to an HMO and must have a designated primary care provider, or gatekeeper, but can opt to see a provider outside of the HMO at a greater cost to the enrollee. PPOs are entities through which employer health plans and insurers contract to purchase health care services for covered beneficiaries from a selected group of participating providers. In PPOs the insurance company generally accepts the capitation risk rather than the PPO itself, whereas in POS HMOs the provider accepts the risk. The managed indemnity plan is the most traditional model and uses only some managed care mechanisms, such as precertification of elective admissions and case management of catastrophic cases. The service plan may, in addition, have minimal contractual relationships with providers regarding allowable fees (Kongstvedt, 1996).

Provider groups or managed care plans also can incorporate elements of managed care through quality control, utilization review, or bundling of services into units for the purpose of establishing prospective prices (Curtiss, 1989). Many plans attempt to manage quality by providing incentives to increase behaviors that promote a healthy lifestyle such as smoking cessation or exercise programs. Yet capitation seems to be a key element in containing cost. While capitated HMOs have clearly cut the

number of hospital admissions and reduced lengths of stay, other forms of managed care have not yet been proved to have a major cost-cutting effect. One reason may be that fee-for-service systems have taught our consumers to shop around for medical care, and the consumer movement has increased the power of the recipients of health care. Managed care systems are clearly moving in the direction of cost containment but sometimes conflict with the freedom of choice to which consumers have become so accustomed. The issue of quality will be the next competitive battlefield for managed care organizations, particularly if consumers begin to shop around for higher-quality care.

THE HEALTH CARE FINANCING SYSTEM IN THE PUBLIC REALM: FEDERAL LEVEL

The health care financing system is composed of many interrelated parts at the federal, state, and local levels. Both government and private sectors play a role at each level. No one entity oversees or controls the entire system. At the federal level the Medicare and Medicaid programs are administered through the Health Care Financing Administration (HCFA), an agency of the U.S. Department of Health and Human Services. Expenditures from these two programs totaled $317 billion in 1995 and financed 36.1% of all personal health care expenditures in that year. Medicare outlays were $184 billion in 1995, and 37.5 million aged and disabled persons were served. Medicaid outlays in 1995 were $133 billion, with 36.3 million people receiving care through this program (HCFA, 1996). Enrollment projections for 1996 were 38.1 million persons for Medicare, which represents a 95% increase since 1967, and 37.5 million persons for Medicaid, which represents a 275% increase since 1967 (HCFA, 1996).

Smaller federal health care programs also exist to provide services for specific segments of the population. Eligible veterans are covered through the Veterans Administration. Dependent families of servicemen are covered through the Civilian Health and Medical Program of the Uniformed Services (CHAMPUS), a program within the Defense Department. Expenditures for this program are part of the defense budget. The CHAMPUS program is notable because it was one of the first federal programs to reimburse nurses for their services. The Federal Employees Health Benefits Plan is another federally administered plan that has required direct payment to nurse practitioners and physician assistants authorized to practice in their respective states. It is important to remember that just because care is reimbursed through federal policy, it doesn't mean that nurses, as providers of that care, can be covered if state laws interfere. An example would be in states with nurse practice acts that limit nurses' scope of practice.

Medicaid

Medicaid is a jointly funded program of both federal and state governments, and until 1997, eligibility was determined by income and resources. Those eligible included persons receiving Aid to Families with Dependent Children (AFDC), people older than 65 years of age, blind and totally disabled persons who received cash assistance under the Supplemental Security Income (SSI) program, pregnant women, and children born after September 1983 in families with incomes at or below the poverty line. A minimum set of benefits are provided by each state to qualify for Medicaid matching grants, including hospitalization, physician care, laboratory services, x-ray studies, prenatal care, and preventive services; nursing home and home health care; and medically necessary transportation. Medicaid programs are also required to pay the Medicare premiums, deductibles, and copayments for certain low income persons (Bodenheimer & Grumbach, 1995).

ELIGIBILITY AND POPULATION COVERED

In 1997 major changes began to occur in Medicaid, particularly in eligibility requirements. P.L. 104-193, the Personal Responsibility and Work Opportunities Act of 1996, eliminated the AFDC cash assistance program and replaced it with a block grant program called Temporary Assistance to Needy Families (TANF). Under the new welfare law, Medicaid has been disassociated from AFDC and SSI so that automatic coverage is not guaranteed. However, families who met the AFDC eligibility criteria before welfare reform were at least initially still eligible for Medicaid. By September 1997, states were required to redetermine the Medicaid eligibility of many individuals, including children currently eligible for SSI, many noncitizens, and individuals who had been receiving disability cash assistance (SSI) based on alcoholism and drug addiction. Under P.L. 104-193, states are permitted to deny Medicaid benefits to adults and heads of household who lose TANF benefits because of refusal to work. However, this law exempts poverty-related pregnant women and children from this provision and mandates their continued Medicaid eligibility (HCFA, 1997b).

As an optional service, states may continue to cover the "medically needy." These individuals are often poor or have spent down to poverty level after a catastrophic illness but earn too much money to qualify for TANF, AFDC, or SSI and would be eligible for one of these programs by virtue of being in a family with dependent children, more than 65 years of age, blind, or totally and permanently disabled. It is under this medically needy category that many elderly or persons with life-threatening chronic illnesses such as AIDS may qualify for Medicaid (Bodenheimer & Grumbach, 1995). Medicaid is increasingly becoming a long-term care program of last resort for elderly persons in nursing homes. Many of them had to "spend down" their lifesavings to become eligible for Medicaid. In 1995, 68% of those receiving Medicaid were in poor families, but they accounted for 26% of Medicaid's total expenditures, whereas 27% of those receiving Medicaid were elderly or disabled persons living in nursing homes or long-term care facilities and accounted for 72% of Medicaid's expenditures (HCFA, 1997c).

Family nurse practitioners, pediatric nurse practitioners, geriatric nurse practitioners, and certified nurse midwives must also be reimbursed under Medicaid if in accordance with state regulations they are legally authorized to provide Medicaid-covered services.

CURRENT FINANCING

Medicaid is funded partially by a General Fund allocation of the federal budget but is a matching government program with state revenue budget allocations. It was originally intended as a dollar-for-dollar match between state and federal governments on a 50% basis. However, the federal matching formula is calculated on a per capita income base, so many of the poorer states actually pay less than the fifty-fifty match. In 1995, Medicaid served the needs of 24.1 million of the nation's poor, or roughly 75% of those living in poverty (HCFA, 1997b).

As stated earlier, Medicaid programs in the states are increasingly using managed care organizations to provide care for recipients. In many states, waivers afford the state flexibility to (1) develop and implement creative alternatives to placing Medicaid-eligible individuals in medical facilities such as nursing- or community-based facilities (Home and Community Based Waivers), or (2) waive the requirement that beneficiaries may select their own Medicaid providers (Freedom of Choice Waivers). States may also apply for research and demonstration waivers that test new policy ideas related to Medicaid. This will be discussed in greater depth in the State Level section, below. Because of the waivers and the TANF block granting process, many are concerned that state Medicaid programs will be so diverse that we will, in essence, have 50 different Medicaid programs nationwide.

CHILD HEALTH PROVISION OF 1997 BUDGET RECONCILIATION ACT

Another important development in the balanced budget bill was the inclusion of $24 billion in child health block grants over 5 years for the Child Health Insurance Program. Nearly $4 billion of this money will be spent on increased Medicaid spending for several groups of children. States will choose to participate in this grant program and may use the money to either expand Medicaid or create a new state program for children's health insurance, or both. Up to 10% of a state's allocation can be spent on a combination of administrative costs, outreach, direct health services for children, and other health initiatives. Depending on the state, children with family incomes at or below 200% of the federal poverty level may be covered. A state running a child health insurance program must provide, at a minimum, the benefits covered by certain specified, commercial health insurance plans. To receive federal funds, a state must pay matching amounts. The state's matching percentage is 70% of its matching rate under Medicaid (Children's Defense Fund, 1997).

Medicare

Medicare legislation was passed in 1965 as an amendment to the Social Security Act to help older people pay for their health care in retirement. For most retirees, the premium cost of adequate health insurance exceeded their retirement income budgets, and affordable private insurance was available only through group coverage, which excluded retirees (National Commission on Social Security, 1981). Sixty years ago, before Medicare, half of older Americans had no health insurance; today 90% of senior citizens have health care coverage through Medicare. As evidence of Medicare's beneficial economic effect, the poverty rate for older people decreased from 27.9% to 12.9% during the period of 1967 to 1992, whereas the nonelderly poverty rate rose from 11.8% to 14.7% during the same period (Radner, 1995).

ELIGIBILITY AND POPULATION COVERED

Individuals are eligible for Medicare hospital insurance (Part A) at age 65 years on the basis of their own or their spouse's eligibility for Social Security. A person can be eligible for Medicare at less than age 65 if she or he has been a Social Security Disability beneficiary for 24 months or more. A person with permanent kidney failure can be eligible at any age if she or he receives ongoing dialysis or has had a kidney transplant and qualifies for other benefits through Social

Security. A person can apply for Medicare 3 months before the sixty-fifth birthday, even if retirement is not planned at that time. Medicare Part B is optional and, if not elected during initial enrollment, cannot be obtained until the next annual open enrollment period, which runs from January 1 to March 31 each year (Social Security Administration, 1996a).

Medicare Part A helps to pay for 60 days of inpatient care in a hospital or 100 days in a skilled nursing facility after a 3-day hospital stay. There is an annual Medicare deductible, and after 60 days a daily coinsurance is charged for all covered services. To be eligible for Medicare hospice coverage, one must have a terminal diagnosis and a prognosis of less than 6 months to live. Once a person is eligible for hospice care, the traditional Medicare benefits are broadened to include coverage for pain relief and other support services for terminally ill people. Medicare does not pay for custodial care or nonskilled home health care to help with dressing, walking, or eating, nor does it cover routine checkups, dental care, foot care, or visual or hearing examinations (Social Security Administration, 1996a). The following preventive services were included for coverage starting in 1998: mammography screening, pap smears, prostate screening, colorectal screening, bone density measurement, and diabetes training and self-management; the trial coverage of influenza and pneumococcal vaccinations was extended through 2002.

As of January 1, 1998, Medicare will reimburse for services provided by nurse practitioners (NPs) and clinical nurse specialists (CNSs), regardless of their geographic location or practice setting. Under this legislation, the Primary Care Health Practitioner Incentive Act of 1997, which was passed in August of 1997, all NPs and CNSs will be able to bill for direct Medicare reimbursement at 85% of the physician fee schedule for services that they are legally authorized to perform under state law, regardless of whether or not they are under the supervision of, or associated with, a physician (see Chapter 16).

THE TRADITIONAL FEE-FOR-SERVICE PLAN

The traditional fee-for-service plan offers the beneficiary a choice of hospital and provider but requires the payment of an annual deductible, a fee each time a service is used, and the payment of the 20% difference between the Medicare-approved amount for a covered service and the Medicare payment. It requires a well-informed consumer to understand the complex billing practices associated with this plan. A new private fee-for-service plan was created in 1997. Unlike traditional Medicare, this option makes Medicare fixed monthly payments to certain plans from which beneficiaries would purchase private indemnity health insurance policies. The plan, not the provider, would determine the rate of reimbursement, and providers are not allowed to balance-bill Medicare patients more than 15% above the payment level set by the plan.

MEDICARE MANAGED CARE

Prepaid coordinated health plans such as HMOs contract with the Medicare program and generally are one of two types of plans. In risk plans, the beneficiary is required to receive all of their services from within the organization's network of providers. In cost plans, there is no such requirement, and this type of plan may be best for those who travel or live outside a plan service area for part of the year. Most HMOs charge a small copayment each time a service is used, and no additional charges are rendered. Subscribers must be enrolled in Medicare Part B. Benefits vary by HMO, but they usually include preventive care services not covered by traditional Medicare and optional prescription drug coverage for an additional premium (U.S. Department of Health and Human Services, 1996a). The 1998 budget reconciliation bill created a new program called Medicare+Choice. In addition to the HMO option described above, several new managed care options were added. Under Medicare, preferred provider organizations (PPOs) are groups of physicians and hospitals who contract with insurers to serve a group of enrollees on a fee-for-service basis, but the rates charged are lower than those charged to nonenrollees. Provider-sponsored organizations (PSOs) do not contract with insurers but form a network similar to HMOs to enroll and directly treat beneficiaries for a preset fixed amount. All Medicare+Choice managed care plans must institute a quality assurance program that monitors and reports quality indicators and health outcome measures.

CURRENT FINANCING

There are two Medicare trust funds. The federal Hospital Insurance Trust Fund is used to pay for the services covered under the hospital insurance (Part A) of Medicare. This is financed through the payroll tax on current workers that funds Part A. The solvency of this trust fund was of great concern in 1996 because it was projected to run out of funds by 2002. Reform efforts, which will be discussed later, resulted in extending the solvency of this trust fund until 2007.

The Supplementary Medical Insurance Trust Fund finances services covered under the medical insurance (Part B) of Medicare. Social security taxes do not finance this trust fund; rather, revenues come from the General Fund of the Treasury and from enrollee premiums, so it is solvent by definition (Social Security Administration, 1996b).

MEDICARE REFORM

Between 1993 and 1996 the Medicare program took in less money than it paid out in benefits. Serving 38 million older adults and disabled citizens, the program cost $200 billion annually, or 12% of the federal budget. Notably, 5% of the beneficiaries incur 50% of Medicare costs, and 10% incur 70% of the Medicare costs. Persons with end-stage renal disease have the highest costs per person.

Given the political attention that the costs of the Medicare program received in the 1996 elections, the desire for a balanced federal budget, and the need for immediate action to address the Hospital Insurance Trust Fund shortfall, changes to the Medicare budget were certain to occur. On August 5, 1997, President Clinton signed into law the Balanced Budget Act of 1997, the fiscal year 1998 budget reconciliation bill. This act reduces Medicare spending by $115 billion during the period of 1998–2002 and pushes back the trust fund's insolvency date to 2007. The bulk of the budget cuts are targeted to reducing the payment rates to hospitals, doctors, and other Medicare providers. The reform changed the nature of the entitlement process from access to specific benefits regardless of cost to a fixed federal dollar contribution toward the cost of health care (Friedland, 1995).

Provider cuts in payments will disproportionately occur in the fee-for-service sector; thus financial incentives will encourage providers to shift to managed care. Medicare managed care programs have grown only slowly. Approximately 3 million of 38 million Medicare beneficiaries are enrolled in managed Medicare programs. Some researchers have argued that (1) the HMO reimbursement rate, which is based on an adjusted average per capita cost (AAPCC) per enrollee, overcompensates these plans because Medicare's payments do not reflect the better health status of HMO enrollees, and (2) that rates should therefore be lowered by 12% (Riley, Tudor, Chiang, & Ingber, 1996). Since Medicare has increased the number of types of managed care options, one can expect that enrollments, expenditures, and health outcomes from these programs will be closely monitored and AAPCC adjustments made accordingly.

Hospitals on average had a Medicare profit margin of 5% in 1994 and 7.9% in 1995. These figures give an average, and almost one third of hospitals did not make any profit on Medicare reimbursements. Cutbacks aimed at the hospital sector will need to consider the variation in profits and make allowances for facilities serving the underinsured and those with limited access to health care. Home health care is rapidly expanding and costs are escalating, making this an area of concern for Medicare coverage. The FY98 budget bill shifts the coverage for home health visits that do not follow a 3-day hospital stay, and visits beyond 100 a year, from Part A to

Part B of Medicare and institutes a prospective payment system for home health care, skilled nursing care, and outpatient services, to extend the HI Trust Fund solvency.

Medicare beneficiaries will continue to contribute 25% of Part B costs, which will raise their monthly premiums from $45.70 in 1998 to $67 by 2002. (The government has set aside $1.5 billion to help low-income beneficiaries pay their Part B premium.) In addition, the government will increase attempts to reduce provider fraud. The Government Accounting Office estimates that $275 million a day is lost to fraud in the health care system. A centralized Medicare fraud registry was established to encourage beneficiaries to report suspected cases of provider abuse. Harsh penalties are imposed on any health care provider convicted of defrauding Medicare.

Social Security
PRINCIPLES OF SOCIAL SECURITY

Although America has always valued individualism, the Great Depression of the 1930s cruelly taught American workers that they were financially vulnerable because of factors beyond their control. When President Roosevelt signed the Social Security Act in 1935, it provided a base of economic security that allows older Americans to live with dignity and independence. The Act was carefully crafted to distinguish this program from welfare programs and to promote its acceptance as a social insurance by society. Social Security's key principles are as follows:

1. *Individual equity or fairness.* This principle means that the amount a worker pays into the system determines how much he or she will earn in benefits.
2. *Social adequacy.* With this principle, benefits are calculated by means of a weighted formula that ensures a minimum floor of protection for workers with lower average lifetime earnings. Benefits are also adjusted for inflation, which offsets financial erosion with time. The concept of social insurance and protection of individual dignity evolved from this principle. The social insurance

aspect includes three important tenants. First, insurance protection is provided not only to workers but also to their dependents. Second, all eligible workers participate; individuals cannot opt out of the system. (It does not cover about 20% of state and local employees and some federal employees hired before 1984 [National Academy on Aging, 1996].) Third, contributors are protected against destitution by pooling risk of lost income among all contributors.

3. *Efficiency.* This principle dictates that the highest possible benefits be provided to retirees with minimum administrative costs both to the beneficiary and to the nation.
4. *Individual dignity.* A belief in individual dignity dictates that there be no means test for a person to qualify for benefits and that benefits be considered a statutory right.

ELIGIBILITY AND POPULATION COVERED

To be eligible for Social Security, one must earn 40 credits by working and paying taxes into Social Security for approximately 10 years of work. The amount of Social Security benefits received is based on a formula that takes into consideration earnings, wage inflation, and whether the beneficiary is planning to retire early (with reduced benefit starting at age 62) or to wait for full benefits (at age 65 years until 2003). Thereafter the retirement age will gradually increase to age 66 for persons born in 1950 and beyond, up to age 67 for those born in 1960 or later.

Approximately one of every six Americans collect some type of Social Security benefit. The majority (60%) do so because of retirement but others because they are disabled, a dependent of someone who receives Social Security, or a spouse or child of a Social Security beneficiary who has died (Social Security Administration, 1996c).

CURRENT FINANCING

Social Security is financed through the Federal Insurance Contributions Act (FICA), which authorized payroll deductions for Social Security. In 1996, the Social Security part of the tax was 7.65% of gross wages, up to $62,700. Employers match the workers' tax payment. Self-employed people pay taxes equal to the combined employee-employer tax, but half of it is deductible as a business expense. There are four Social Security trust funds: (1) Old-Age and Survivors Insurance (OASI), (2) Disability Insurance (DI), (3) Hospital Insurance Trust Fund (or Medicare Part A), and (4) Supplementary Medical Insurance (or Medicare Part B). The 7.65% Social Security tax deduction is allocated as follows: 5.26% to the OASI Trust Fund, 0.94% to the DI, and 1.45% to the HI. For people who make more than the $62,700 ceiling, they and their employers would continue to pay the Medicare portion of the tax (1.45% each) on all earnings. The Social Security trust funds take in about $5 billion more per month than they pay out. The surplus dollars are invested in U.S. Treasury bonds, the safest but also one of the lowest-paying financial investments. In the year 2000, total tax contributions to OASI is projected to be $397 billion to cover 39 million beneficiaries at an outflow cost of $372 billion. This does not include interest.

For every dollar a worker pays in Social Security and Medicare taxes, 69 cents goes to the trust fund that pays monthly benefits to retirees and their families and to widows, widowers, and the children of workers who have died; 19 cents goes to the Medicare trust fund that covers hospital and health care services for Medicare beneficiaries; and 12 cents goes to the trust fund that covers payments to people with disabilities (Social Security Administration, 1996b). These disability and survivor death benefit payments make Social Security more than a retirement plan and establish a safety net for our individual and societal social security.

Social Security, however, never was designed to be the only source of retirement income in our society. Retirement income is seen as a three-legged stool: one leg comprising Social Security benefits, the second pension income, and the third personal savings and investments. Social Security is seen as replacing about 30% to 40% of a worker's salary; thus it does provide

a safety net—but not a comfortable one for enjoying retirement. For example, the average 1996 monthly Social Security benefit for a retired worker was $720; for a retired couple it was $1215, for a widow(er) $680, and for a disabled worker $682. The critical question to be asked is, If this were your only income, would you be able to maintain your present standard of living? If not, a personal savings plan for retirement is a critical component of future financial security. Most retirement counselors recommend aiming for 70% to 80% replacement of a person's preretirement earnings in order to live comfortably.

SOLVENCY: SOCIAL INSECURITY

The fervor of reform has spread to the third rail of politics—Social Security. Called the third rail because it was thought to be untouchable for political survival, it is now being portrayed by its critics as "social insecurity." The rhetoric of baby boomers' bankrupting Social Security trust funds infiltrates the popular press (Church & Lacayo, 1995; Peterson, 1996). Economic analysts and policy researchers, however, challenge the charges of social insecurity and contend that our society has the ability to make modest changes that will ensure future solvency (Cohen & Beedno, 1994; Kingston & Shultz, 1996; National Committee to Preserve Social Security and Medicare, 1996; Quadagno, 1996). The interdependency of financing Medicare through Social Security trust funds makes it imperative to follow and understand the implications of reform proposals. In the current debate over the solvency of future Social Security trust funds, one hears the following key arguments and counter arguments:

ARGUMENT: Retirement of the baby boomers from 2010 to 2030 will be supported by a relatively smaller work force than in prior generations. We will have a large dependent aged population that will overwhelm the payroll contributions from a smaller work force.

COUNTER ARGUMENT: Starting in 1983, Social Security shifted from a "pay as you go" system to a partially prefunded one; thus the baby boomers contributed to a prefunded surplus that now reduces the burden from future workers to the boomers themselves. Although the baby boomers will receive a lower rate of return than previous retirees, it will be positive. In addition, the dependency ratio will not radically increase because it is based on both child and adult nonworking Americans. Therefore, although the number of adults retiring will increase because of the number of baby boomers, at the same time the percentage of dependent children will shrink.

ARGUMENT: Suggestions have been made that Social Security won't be there when the baby boomers retire, and that it would be better for all citizens to invest their Social Security contributions on their own for a higher rate of return.

COUNTER ARGUMENT: The question of whether workers receive their money's worth from Social Security requires an analysis of four measures: the payback period, the benefit/tax ratio, the lifetime transfer, and the internal rate of return. Interested readers are referred to Leimer (1995) for a detailed explanation of these measures. Typically, most critiques of Social Security focus on only one measure and ignore the individual variations to the "money's worth" question when all the measures are taken into consideration.

ARGUMENT: The most pessimistic projections indicate that the OASI trust fund will be depleted by 2020, and only an optimistic formula suggests solvency beyond the next 75 years.

COUNTER ARGUMENT: Contingency options are available to offset even the most pessimistic calculations. The following are the most discussed options:

1. Include previously exempted workers such as new state employees in Social Security. Along with the new federal employees who recently joined, this would add between 3 and 7 million contributors who won't be collecting payments for a long period.

2. Change the contribution period from 35 years to 38 years or raise the contribution rate 0.15%, or $15 per $10,000 earnings per year.

3. Raise the payroll tax by 2.19 percentage points, to 14.59%. This change alone would ensure solvency for the next 75 years.

4. Tax the amount of Social Security benefits that exceeds one's individual contributions.

5. Invest more aggressively in the stock market. In 1995 the trust funds earned $35 billion in interest, representing an annual interest rate of 7.8%. Shift a small portion of the surplus funds into nontreasury funds with higher interest potentials.

6. The Consumer Price Index is used to calculate the amount of yearly Social Security cost-of-living adjustments and deductions. Reducing this index by 0.5% would save $125 billion over 6 years.

SHOULD SOCIAL SECURITY BE PRIVATIZED?

Job loss in the 1990s occurred for the first time amid a growing economy. Confidence in the concept of lifetime employment and job security was eroded. For the first time when there was no recession, American workers saw their jobs lost because of downsizing, often without regard for seniority. Many workers used their individual retirement accounts to cover financial crises such as mortgage payments and college tuition. If Social Security is privatized, and accessible, policy analysts worry that people may rely on and deplete their contributions and be left without any source of retirement support (Quadagno, 1996).

The mutual fund/broker lobby has a major vested interest in seeing Social Security funds released to the private citizen for investment purposes. They will strongly lobby for this option. Reliance on the markets, however, creates economic insecurity associated with market fluctuations and substitutes individual risk for social security. If privatization were to occur, these key costs would need to be considered: major administrative costs to establish a major new program; massive public education to promote its utilization; massive enticements by the stock promoters would incur new costs that ultimately would be passed onto the consumer in higher broker fees; and loss of the national safety net, which means that unsophisticated and unlucky investors would be on their own. Most important, loss of the following unique and important features of Social Security would occur: cost of living adjustment; portability of earning credits and payments; survivor death and disability benefits paid to each spouse and child; and lower taxation rates than other pension benefits and notably low administrative costs.

We can expect the momentum of reforming the financing of health care to continue into the future. Consequently, it is important for nurses to understand the forces that influence reform proposals so that they will have informed opinions about policy choices. Various proposals will be submitted, each offering different features from the prior proposal. In general, the reader must weigh the suggestions for change against the strengths and uniqueness of the present Social Security system and judge whether or not the benefits of change outweigh the costs of the contingencies discussed. Because there is increasing bipartisan agreement over the need to slow Medicare's growth and incur savings for Social Security, changes will occur. How modest or how radical these changes are will depend on the politics of persuasion. Typically, legislation develops incrementally and does not radically depart from prior legislation. For a more detailed review of the 1997 reform proposals, the reader is referred to Stern's (1997) discussion; for current Social Security information visit the Social Security Administration's web site (Social Security, 1996d).

STATE LEVEL

Some federal health programs, such as Medicaid, are administered at the state level. Another example of state administration of a federal program is the Title V Maternal-Child Block Grant Program, which has as its objective the improvement of maternal, infant, and adolescent health and the development of service systems for children at risk of chronic and disabling conditions.

States also have an important role in setting health policy through health planning efforts and in regulating health care costs and insurance carriers through rate-setting efforts. States take on responsibility for ensuring quality health services through oversight of health care providers and facilities. Local government health services are also authorized at the state level.

In addition, the state insurance regulation agency has a major role in regulating insurance companies through the insurance laws. It is in this capacity that states are increasingly becoming involved in regulating the quality of care provided in health insurance plans or managed care programs.

Individual state decisions around financing for Medicaid are being driven by the overwhelming demands on health care budgets and by the continued pressure on states to decrease taxes. States are often using managed care plans to provide services for Medicaid recipients and are seeking cost-effective solutions to what has continued to be a crisis in health care at the state level as state legislators become more cost conscious. Currently 48 states offer some form of managed care (HCFA, 1997a). A major issue for states is that the Medicaid program has specific requirements for uniformity across the state program and a freedom-of-choice clause, which mandates that to receive matching Medicaid grants, states may not restrict the choice of providers for Medicaid enrollees. States have been required to apply for waivers from the restriction of choice or uniformity requirements that exist in federal Medicaid regulations so that a mandatory managed care initiative can be instituted for their Medicaid programs. Thus many states have applied for waivers so that they can alter their Medicaid programs and cut costs. The federal government grants two kinds of Medicaid managed care waivers. Section 1915(b) waivers, or freedom-of-choice waivers, permit states to waive beneficiaries' rights to select their own Medicaid providers and require beneficiaries to enroll, for example, in managed care plans. Under this waiver program, states may also apply to waive the requirement that services must be comparable statewide in order to adjust the program to needs in different parts of states. Section 1915(c) waivers, or home and community-based waivers, afford states the flexibility to develop and implement creative alternatives to placing Medicaid-eligible individuals in medical facilities such as nursing homes and allow alternatives in home-based or community-based programs. Under this kind of waiver, services may allow the person to stay at home and avoid institutionalization. States may also target these waiver programs to individuals with a specific illness or condition such as persons with AIDS, physical and developmental disability, mental illness, or mental retardation. Section 1115 research and demonstration waivers allow states to test new approaches to benefits, services, eligibility, program payments, and service delivery. States applying for these waivers must demonstrate that the new approaches are budget neutral and do not add costs to the Medicaid program. By January 1997, 96 Section 1915(b) waivers, more than 200 Section 1915(c), and 15 Section 1115 waivers had been approved (HCFA, 1997a, 1997b). As of January 1998, states are no longer required to apply for waivers to mandate managed care for individuals who are Medicaid recipients.

LOCAL LEVEL

Local governments, along with state government, have the ultimate responsibility for protecting the public health. Local governments also may decide to fulfill a responsibility for indigent care by funding public hospitals and clinics. New York City's Health and Hospitals Corporation and Chicago's Cook County Hospital are good examples of this type of control. Even these hospitals, while receiving a subsidy from their local government, tend to get large amounts of operating money from Medicaid and Medicare, so public hospital care is indeed dependent on the decisions made within these two programs. In many areas of the country, public hospitals are in danger of being sold or privatized or are otherwise in jeopardy because of mergers or acquisitions by larger hospitals or networks. As the costs of care have increased and more care has been performed in the home and in the community, competition between hospitals has intensified. Another problem is the increased supply of medical specialists and a decreased supply of primary care providers. The 1997 balanced budget legislation included a nationwide expansion of a program that began in New York City and that offers financial incentives to hospitals that train fewer doctors, especially in the medical specialties (1000 Hospitals . . . , 1997). Ultimately, HCFA believes that savings will occur as a result of reduction of the physician supply. This type of disincentive for residency-training programs may have a major effect on the supply of nurse practitioners and other nonphysician primary care providers.

With the cost constraint strategies of the 1980s and the misconception that infectious diseases were no longer a major threat, population-based health services such as those originating from state and local health departments received proportionately less and less funding (Institute of Medicine, 1988). Traditional public health nursing functions to provide surveillance in this important area were minimized or eliminated in this period because they were viewed as having a lower priority than individual health (morbidity) services, which were also being cut back. The crises in the control of infectious diseases such as measles and tuberculosis have taught us important lessons on the need for strong local public health agencies (Brudney & Dobkin, 1991). The onset of AIDS has greatly escalated the problem and has reinforced the need for primary prevention and basic public health strategies. When public health strategies are superseded by an emphasis on the individual, major health problems can "fall through the cracks" of the system, and the whole of society will suffer.

THE PRIVATE HEALTH CARE FINANCING SYSTEM

The private component of the health care system consists of all nongovernmental sources and, in fact, is the largest component because most health care facilities in this country are run by private for-profit or not-for-profit corporations. The entire health insurance industry is also within the private system. Included as part of what has been called the "medical-industrial complex" are the pharmaceutical companies, suppliers of health care technology, and the various service industries that support the health care system (Meyers, 1970; Relman, 1980). Because so much of the industry is controlled by private sources, it is difficult for cost controls to reach all segments of the health care industry equally. The for-profit health care system is growing in this country, as well as internationally, as public sector health care costs rise and more of the responsibility to deliver health care is relegated to private organizations (Smith & Lipsky, 1992; Young, 1990). The greatest growth in this country has been in the for-profit sector with the sale and consolidation of private not-for-profit hospitals to for-profit firms (Lutz & Gee, 1995). In 1997, Columbia/HCA Health Care was the nation's largest for-profit hospital system, owning 350 hospitals in 38 states while maintaining a 20% gross profit target (Herman, 1997). The health care industry has been transformed in the past 10 years by a business mentality that has and will continue to have far-reaching effects on the overall health care system. Although this chapter has largely described the public sector in health care, one must also recognize the large role the private sector plays in today's health care system.

FINANCING CHRONIC CARE

Unfortunately, much of the public believes that Medicare covers chronic care needs, and many are surprised to discover that only limited benefits are provided for skilled services, with no coverage for chronic care maintenance services. Although Medicare was intended to be a comprehensive program, over the years, as a result of rising health care expenditures, an ever-widening gap between the costs of care that are covered and those that are not covered has become evident. Out-of-pocket expenditures for Medicare beneficiaries have grown to an average of 21% of all home health care charges and 37% of all nursing home costs (U.S. Department of Health and Human Services, 1996a).

"Medigap" insurance, offered by private insurers, developed in response to the widening gaps in uncovered Medicare services. Medigap plans vary in amount, type of coverage, and range of covered services. Some add little if any additional coverage to traditional Medicare coverage, whereas others cover the annual deductibles and copayments and reimburse the difference when Medicare covers only 80% of the approved charge.

Because Medicare does not cover most long-term care costs, private insurers have entered this market. Long-term care insurance generally includes some combination of home care benefits and nursing home care. Growth in the long-term care insurance market has been hindered by low enrollment because of the very high premiums and the lack of public awareness about the need for this type of insurance. Beginning in 1997, people with long-term care policies will not count as taxable income the first $68,875 in benefits received annually. It is hoped that this allowance will increase the incentive to purchase long-term care policies. If more people purchase these products, the premiums will be lowered, making this a more affordable option. Another factor hindering this area is the fact that Medicaid will cover long-term care for those who pass the means test for this program. This creates a major financial incentive for a beneficiary to "spend down" his assets to qualify for Medicaid nursing home coverage. The Health Insurance Portability and Accountability Act of 1996 included a provision that makes it a federal crime to purposefully transfer assets within 3 years of applying for Medicaid. The budget bill of 1997 clarified this provision to include estate planners and lawyers who knowingly assist consumers to transfer or hide assets in order to qualify for Medicaid.

INNOVATIVE FINANCING AND IMPLICATIONS FOR NURSING

Nursing has a major role in creating cost-effective but viable options for patients who are in need, particularly the chronically ill and elderly who need care as well as cure. Consider the community nursing organizations that care for patients with human immunodeficiency virus infection and chronic illness at home. Nursing organizations such as visiting nurse services are providing innovative solutions for patients who need care across a full continuum of services but with a reconsideration of patient needs and costs of care. Technology itself has been harnessed with the use of computers and telehealth to reach patients at home without an actual home visit each time the patient needs a contact. Computerization supplements nursing care in a way that can actually increase the number of contacts that can be made with patients, thus increasing the chances that they will remain stable at home (Mahoney & Tarlow, 1998).

CONCLUSION

During the past 30 years, the health care system in the United States has grown to almost unmanageable proportions and complexity. The "medical-industrial complex" pervades all sectors of our economic system and employs a vast number of citizens. It consumes more than 13% of our gross national product and only recently has begun to level off in any significant way. Health care costs cannot continue to escalate without jeopardizing our total economy. As Friedland (1995) has stated: "Growth in health care expenditures of 9 percent or more per year are not sustainable without reordering federal budget priorities or raising taxes. The question for all of us is: What do we want as a society for our parents and our children?

If unmet needs are not financed collectively, then they must be financed individually, or not provided at all" (p. 16).

Perhaps nursing will find the creative solution of integrating the uncoordinated long-term care and acute care services, creating a continuum of services that everyone is eligible for regardless of setting. Providers need the ability to follow a patient and to integrate their services across hospital, adult day care, home care, and institutional care settings. The present system is a myriad of roadblocks to this integrated care approach. Nurses as providers must decide what the ultimate health product should be and give that message to policymakers. Nurses need not be passive participants in the policy debate about the reshaping of health care and its financing. Rather, they can shape health care policy and the resulting decisions that are made.

REFERENCES

Alford, R. (1975). *Health care politics: Ideological and interest group barriers to reform.* Chicago: University of Chicago Press, 1975.

Bodenheimer, T. (1996). The HMO backlash: Righteous or reactionary? *New England Journal of Medicine, 335,* 1601–1604.

Bodenheimer, T., & Grumbach, K. (1995). *Understanding health policy.* Stamford, CT: Appleton & Lange.

Brudney, K., & Dobkin, J. (1991). Resurgent tuberculosis in N.Y.C.: Human immunodeficiency virus, homelessness and the decline of tuberculosis control programs. *American Review of Respiratory Disease, 144*(4), 745–749.

Children's Defense Fund. (1997). *Summary of the child health provisions in the 1997 Budget Reconciliation Act. August 8, 1997.* [On-line: http://www.childrensdefense.org]

Church, G., & Lacayo, R. (1995, March 20). Social insecurity. *Time, 145*(11), 24–32.

Cohen, L., & Beedon, L. (1994). Options for balancing the OASDI trust funds for the long term. *Journal of Aging and Social Policy, 6*(1–2), 77–93.

Curtiss, F. R. (1989). Managed health care. *American Journal of Hospital Pharmacy, 46,* 742–763.

Davis, K., Anderson, G., Rowland, D., & Steinberg, E. (1990). *Health care cost containment.* Baltimore: Johns Hopkins University Press.

Friedland, R. B. (1995). Medicare, Medicaid, and the budget. *The Public Policy and Aging Report, 7*(1), 1, 2, 14–16.

Fuchs, V. (1988). The "competition revolution" in health care. *Health Affairs, 7*(3), 5–24.

Gibson, R. M., & Waldo, D. R. (1982). National health expenditures, 1981. *Health Care Financing Review, 4*(1), 1–35.

Health Care Financing Administration, Bureau of Data Management. (1996). *1996 HCFA statistics.* Washington, DC: Author.

Health Care Financing Administration. (1997a). *National summary of Medicaid managed care: Programs and enrollment, June 30, 1996.* Washington, DC: Author. [On-line: http://www.hcfa.gov.]

Health Care Financing Administration. (1997b). *Medicaid: Professional/technical information.* Washington, DC: Author. [On-line: http://www.hcfa.gov.]

Health Care Financing Administration. (1997c). *1996 HCFA statistics.* Washington, DC: Author. [On-line: http://www.hcfa.gov.]

Herman, E. (1997). Downsizing government for principle and profit. *Dollars and Sense, 210,* 10–13.

1000 Hospitals will be paid to reduce supply of doctors. (1997, August 25). *New York Times,* p. A16.

Hsaio, W., Braun P., Dunn, D., & Becker, E. (1988). Results and policy implications of the Resource-based Relative Value Scale. *New England Journal of Medicine, 319,* 881–888.

Institute of Medicine. (1988). *The future of public health.* Washington, DC: National Academy Press.

Kingston, E., & Schultz, J. (1996). *Social Security in the twenty-first century.* Cary, NC: Oxford University Press.

Kongstvedt, P. (1996). *The managed health care handbook* (3rd ed.). Gaithersburg, MD: Aspen.

Leimer, D. (1995, Summer). A guide to Social Security money's worth issues. *Social Security Bulletin, 58*(2). Washington, DC: Social Security Administration Office of Research and Statistics.

Lutz, S., & Gee, P. (1995). *The for-profit health care revolution: The growth of investor-owned health systems in America.* Chicago: Irwin Professional.

Mahoney, D., & Tarlow B. (1998, July/August). A computer-mediated intervention for Alzheimer's caregivers. *Computers in Nursing.*

Meyers, H. (1970, January). The medical-industrial complex. *Fortune,* 90–91, 126.

National Academy on Aging. (1996). *Social Security: The Old Age and Survivors Trust Fund, 1996.* Washington, DC: Author.

National Commission on Social Security. (1981). *Social Security in America's future.* Report of the Commission to the President. Washington, DC: Author.

National Committee to Preserve Social Security and Medicare. (1996, May). *Social Security Privatization.* Washington, DC: Author.

Peterson, P. (1996). *Will America grow up before it grows old? How the coming Social Security crisis threatens you, your family and your country.* New York: Random House.

Phillips, E. K., Cloonan, P., Irvine A., & Fisher, M. E. (1990). Non-reimbursed home health care: Beyond the bills. *Public Health Nursing, 7*(2), 60–64.

Pulcini, J. (1984). Perspectives on level of reimbursement for nursing services. *Nursing Economics, 2,* 118–123.

Quadagno, J. (1996). Social Security and the myth of the entitlement "crisis." *Gerontologist, 36*(3), 391–399.

Radner, D. (1995, Winter). Incomes of the elderly and nonelderly, 1967–92. *Social Security Bulletin, 58*(2).

Relman, A. (1980). The new medical-industrial complex. *New England Journal of Medicine, 303,* 963–970.

Riley, G., Tudor, C., Chiang, Y., & Ingber, M. (1996, Summer). Health status of Medicare enrollees in HMOs and fee-for-service in 1994. *Health Care Financing Review, 17*(4).

Smith, S. R., & Lipsky, M. (1992). Privatization in health and human services: A critique. *Journal of Health Politics, Policy and Law, 17*(2), 233–253.

Social Security Administration. (1996a, June). *Medicare.* [SSA Publication No. 05-10043.] Washington, DC: Author.

Social Security Administration. (1996b, July). *Financing Social Security.* [SSA Publication No. 05-10094.] Washington, DC: Author.

Social Security Administration. (1996c, May). *Social Security: Understanding the benefits.* [Publication No. 05-10024.] Washington, DC: Author.

Social Security Administration. (1996d). *Social Security Online.* [http://www.ssa.gov.] Washington, DC: Author.

Starr, P. (1982). *The social transformation of American medicine.* New York: Basic Books.

Stern, L. (1997). Can we save Social Security? Quick fix or radical reform—guide to the upcoming debate. *Modern Maturity, 1*,28–36.

U.S. Department of Health and Human Services. (1996a, April). *Medicare managed care.* Washington, DC: Author. [Health Financing Administration No. 02195.]

U.S. Department of Health and Human Services. (1996b). *Health United States 1995.* Washington, DC: Centers for Disease Control and Prevention National Center for Health Statistics.

Young, D. (1990). Privatizing health care: Caveat emptor. *International Journal of Health Planning and Management, 5*, 237–270.

VIGNETTE

One Nurse's Perspective on Managed Care

Margaret A. Leonard

The whole approach to health care in the United States is evolving, and Medicaid managed care is part of that evolution. Nurses need to be part of this process, advocating for patients' rights and working to ensure nursing's place in this new arena. This vignette explains how one nurse's involvement in her professional nursing organization and her experiences on both the provider and the payer sides of Medicaid managed care afforded her the opportunities to bring about change in organizational and public policy. It is hoped that the examples related here will demonstrate how nurses can bring about positive changes for patients and nursing, illustrate the benefits of professional and political involvement, explain how nurses can prepare themselves for the opportunities that are unfolding in the Medicaid managed care arena, and encourage nurses to become more involved.

New York State Medicaid Managed Care Bill

Decades after its inception, "managed care" still conjures up negative images for many. It was no surprise that when the government proposed implementing managed care for Medicaid recipients (a population considered vulnerable by many), there was a negative outcry from Medicaid recipients, their families and caregivers, and consumer advocacy groups. But why? We all agreed that health care costs in the United States were "out of control," escalating to more than 13% of our Gross Domestic Product, and that we as individual taxpayers or as a nation could no longer afford this unprecedented skyrocketing of costs. Commercial insurers on the West Coast had been successfully containing costs through managed care for several years. Therefore, why shouldn't the government, the largest reimburser of health care expenses, turn to managed care if it could contain costs?

In New York in June 1991, the Statewide Managed Care Act (Chapter 165, Laws of 1991) was passed by the legislature and signed by Governor Mario Cuomo. One of the state's most significant health care initiatives of the past decade, the Act was created to reduce costs while improving the delivery of services to Medicaid recipients. Additionally, it was designed to significantly increase the state's commitment to expanding managed care as a viable alternative for Medicaid recipients.

The purpose of the state's initiative to enroll Medicaid recipients in managed care programs was to improve access, continuity, and management of care to the more than 1.7 million recipients in a fee-for-service system. In July 1997 *The New York Times* reported that more than 3 million Medicaid recipients nationally accessed health care through the traditional fee-for-service model at a cost of $24 billion a year.

The Statewide Managed Care Act included the following policy objectives:

- Enhance access to mainstream medical care and services for Medicaid recipients.
- Ensure that managed care programs offer Medicaid recipients as wide a choice of primary care and other medical service providers as possible.
- Promote more rational patterns of medical and health service utilization by Medicaid recipients.
- Ensure quality of care.
- Establish cost-effective programs.

The concepts of Medicaid managed care were in line with nursing's health care agenda by providing for accessible, quality health care for all Medicaid recipients and shifting the emphasis to primary care. However, nurses were concerned about how Medicaid managed care would be implemented and how it would be regulated. They were also concerned about how these recipients would be ensured quality care. After all, the idea of Medicaid managed care, from the outset, was plagued by negative publicity and consumer skepticism. Sometimes skepticism can be healthy, and in this case it promoted consumer and provider involvement in the managed care process and inquiry into what safeguards would be provided to program participants.

Political Journeys

In my role as patient service manager in the managed care unit of the Visiting Nurse Service of New York (VNS), I heard first hand about the problems that nurses and consumers were experiencing with new managed care operations and procedures. Many of these problems were caused by the inappropriate use of agents and processes employed by some of the managed care organizations (MCOs). Managed care was affecting how my agency would be reimbursed for services rendered by nurses. Care that nurses deemed necessary was seen by the MCOs' utilization review agents (URAs) as unnecessary or unreimbursable. Even more frustrating, these URAs were denying service because they weren't notified within 48 hours of the start of care, even if that care was delivered over a weekend and the insurance company was closed. Often these URAs were clerical staff who made care decisions from a printed list of criteria, without professional knowledge. In addition, the MCOs were setting the rules but were not letting VNS know what the rules were. What types of care would they reimburse us for? How much service would they approve? Could we appeal the denials we were receiving? It is very difficult to play the game when you don't know the rules. I saw all of this as appalling. When the New York State Nurses Association (NYSNA) asked if my name could be submitted to Senator Michael Tully's office for consideration as an appointee to the newly forming New York State Senate Committee Task Force on Quality Care, I jumped at the chance. (Senator Tully at the time was the chair of one of the most powerful committees, the Health Care Committee.)

I was also asked by NYSNA to present testimony for the regulation of utilization review practices in MCOs before the chairs of the New York State Assembly and Senate health committees and insurance committees. NYSNA selected me for both assignments because of my volunteer work as chair of the Director Care Practitioners Functional Unit and as a leadership fellow with the organization. Fortunately for me, the Senate committee was looking for someone with managed care provider experience, and I was already involved! I attribute my appointment to three factors: (1) I was employed by the largest freestanding not-for-profit home care agency in the United States, (2) I was recommended by the state's professional nursing organization, and, last but not least, (3) I was a member of the political party in control of the legislature.

Much to my delight, I was appointed. The task force was charged with examining "managed care," its effectiveness, and opportunities for improvement. Some of the areas that were addressed were utilization review, notification timeframes, and the denial/appeals process. Although my female voice was often not heard above the "old boy" voices of the task force members, it could not be ignored because it was the voice of the 35,000 nurses who were members of NYSNA. The results were extremely positive. The Senate bill that was drafted as a result of the task force's recommendations addressed several issues, including qualifications of URAs, expansion of the time frame for notification by providers to insurers for services rendered, and development of an appeals process. This bill called for URAs to be licensed professionals with expertise, specifically in the areas in which they deny and authorize service.

Organized nursing was supportive of this bill and was anxious to see a companion bill introduced into the Assembly. Assemblyman Richard Gottfried, the chair of the Assembly Health Committee, introduced a bill that addressed these same issues. Neither one of these bills passed during the session, but they did lay the foundation for what would evolve into a more comprehensive "managed care bill" that NYSNA lobbied for and would become law in 1997.

This experience heightened my interest in politics and public policy, so I submitted my name for nomination to the NYSNA Legislative Council and was appointed. I was appointed because I was actively involved in my district nurses association (NYSNA) as chair of the public policy committee; I was successful in my local grassroots organizing efforts; I was from the second largest district in the state; I had gained some experience in the workings of state politics; I knew some of the key players (e.g., Senator Tully); and I was a hard worker.

During this time, other problems were arising for nurses and nursing in my area. Medicaid managed care was causing hospitals to rethink how they were doing business. As a result of mergers and acquisitions that engulfed the health care industry, there were massive layoffs of nurses caused by "reengineering," "downsizing," "rightsizing," and the use of unlicensed assistive personnel. As president of the Nurses Association of the Counties of Long Island, District 14 of NYSNA, I was hearing that Medicaid managed care was presenting other issues as well for the nurses in New York State.

Again, my involvement with NYSNA afforded me the opportunity to be part of the evolutionary process by presenting testimony before the chairs of the New York State Assembly committees on education, labor, and social services. In this testimony, I emphasized the need to have educational funds available for nurses to retrain them for the positions they were being "reengineered" or "downsized" into.

Meanwhile, back on the job, my frustrations continued to grow as it became more evident that the managed care organizations were "calling the shots." I decided that I wanted to be on the side that was "calling the shots." I wanted to be on the payer's side of the fence. I accepted a position with a newly formed Medicaid managed care company as director of quality assurance and improvement. I hoped that there would be opportunities for me to influence policy—and there were. Collaboratively with the medical director, I designed and oversaw the implementation of all the utilization management policies, the appeals and denials policies, and the credentialing policies. Registered nurses staffed our utilization review phones, and disputed authorizations were referred to me or to the medical director for resolution. All of our policy and procedure manuals were written using the word *provider,* not *physician.* I was making a difference. I was making the changes for patients that I had been advocating for, and I was doing my part to ensure nursing's place in the Medicaid managed care world.

American Nurses Association Task Force

My new position made me a prime candidate for yet another task force, the American Nurses Association (ANA) Task Force on Regulations and Standards for Managed Care. Here I examined managed care from a regulatory and standards perspective. The task force committee met for the first time in Washington, D.C., in

April 1995 and consisted of five members, all nurses from across the United States.

The task force was charged with the following:

- Reviewing the standards and regulations of 12 public and private regulatory/accrediting bodies for managed care
- Identifying nursing's recommendations for the essential elements of managed care regulation
- Preparing a policy briefing paper that identifies areas not addressed in current regulations
- Preparing a report to the ANA Congress on Nursing Practice

The task force identified elements that it deemed essential to a managed care system, such as an adequate, accessible provider network; quality assurance programs; provider credentialing criteria; fiscal soundness; ability to track, trend, and report data; enrollee participation through board-of-director membership, enrollee input, or both; utilization policy and procedures; and an appeal and denial policy. We then categorized these elements into three areas: structure, process, and outcomes (patient, provider, and system) and analyzed the 12 regulatory and accrediting bodies to see which ones addressed these elements of a managed care system.

The task force found the following:

- There were numerous overlapping regulatory bodies, creating a situation of "too much" regulation or "too many" regulatory requirements.
- With one exception, all essential elements are fully covered by one or more regulatory or accrediting bodies.
- The health care industry is still in transition from a fee-for-service/indemnity insurance payment mechanism to a capitated/prepaid managed care system, and the regulatory/accreditation process will continue to mature.
- Health maintenance organizations (HMOs) are heavily regulated through state licensure and federal legislation.

- Preferred provider organizations (PPOs) and other discounted fee-for-service entities are largely unregulated, or where regulations exist, they are less stringent in areas of fiscal solvency and quality accountability than are the regulations applied to HMOs.
- Several good options exist for voluntary accreditation of managed care organizations or their contracted providers through private accrediting bodies, such as the National Committee for Quality Assurance.

The report also identified the demand for outcome studies, accountability for cost and quality, and fiscal responsibility.

The task force offered the following suggestions for ANA participation in policymaking:

- Advocate for continued funding of existing federal and state managed care regulatory bodies during the transition to mature managed care systems in all markets.
- Promote regulation of all provider/insurer organizations in the areas of consumer protection, quality accountability, and fiscal solvency.
- Work to develop partnerships with consumers to ensure access to comparative health outcome data.
- Promote outcome-based research about the effectiveness of preventive and health maintenance services.
- Use the list of essential elements outlined in this report to evaluate managed care organizations, benefit packages, or regulatory or accrediting schemes.
- Support and expand programs that encourage state nurses associations and other groups to assist registered nurses in making the transition into the managed care environment (ANA, 1995).

The task force also recommended that the ANA actively seek to ensure that nurses receive support to make necessary transitions in our changing health care system by directing its resources to helping nurses prepare for the emerging roles in managed care systems. These recommendations have been used to develop platforms for legislative and educational programs for nurses and nursing.

Conclusion

Medicaid managed care is an evolving program, and nurses are in a position to take an active role in its evolution. To be effective, we must understand the issues, processes, and politics surrounding it. We must become politically involved at some level where we work and where we live. There are many levels of involvement, ranging from telephoning your legislator to express your views on a particular issue, to running for an elected office. Your level of involvement is up to you!

Nurses must realize that Medicaid managed care will be presenting them with many employment opportunities as direct care providers, utilization review agents, case managers, benefits analysts, regulators, and government liaisons. Through education, advanced training, and a varied skill base, nurses must be prepared to assume these positions. Additionally, it is the responsibility of nurses to continue to be patient advocates to ensure that the policy objectives outlined in Medicaid managed care legislation are realized, so that our patients have access to and receive quality care.

UNIT I CASE STUDY

Moving a Vision: The Vietnam Women's Memorial

Diane Carlson Evans

BACKGROUND

The Vietnam Women's Memorial was dedicated on the National Mall just yards from the Vietnam Veterans Memorial, *The Wall,* on November 11, 1993, in Washington, D.C. One may think that the approval, placement, and financing of a statue for such a just cause would be a relatively simple process—after all, this was the first memorial on the Mall of our nation's capital to honor the military service of women. To the contrary, the process was long and arduous and included two separate pieces of Congressional legislation and approval of three federal commissions. The dedication of the Vietnam Women's Memorial (VWM) represented the culmination of a 10-year struggle by thousands of volunteers who overcame controversy, rejection, and challenge by those who thought that a women's memorial was not needed. This case study is about the passion, the process, and the politics of turning a vision into reality and how one former army nurse made a profound difference in women's history (Vietnam Women's Memorial Project, 1993).

MOVING A VISION

When this monument is finished, it will be for all time a testament to a group of American women who made an extraordinary sacrifice at an extraordinary time in our nation's history: the women who went to war in

I am grateful for the unstinting help from so many who gave their time, expertise, and talents to make the Vietnam Women's Memorial a reality. Special thanks to Colonel A. Jane Carson, USA, Ret. (Army Nurse Corps), and Diana Hellinger, whose wisdom, inspiration, and encouragement helped make this case study possible.

Vietnam. . . . You went. You served. You suffered. . . . And yet your service and your sacrifice have been mostly invisible for all these intervening years. When you finished what you had to do, you came quietly home. You stepped back into the background from which you had modestly come. You melted away into a society which, for too long now, has ignored the vital and endless work that falls to women and is not appreciated as it should be. [Powell, 1993]

General Colin Powell's words rang with passion and purpose on the day of groundbreaking for the Vietnam Women's Memorial, July 29, 1993. In listening to his every word on that historic day, one couldn't help but drift and digress to many years before. Thousands of women left the comforts of America to find themselves in the midst of guerilla warfare. Having volunteered, they served in helmets and flak jackets, spending long hours easing the pain and suffering of wounded soldiers.

On July 1, 1980, President Jimmy Carter signed legislation granting the Vietnam Veterans Memorial Fund (VVMF) authorization to construct a memorial on a site of two acres in Constitution Gardens near the Lincoln Memorial in Washington, D.C. The legislation read that the memorial would honor men and women of the armed forces of the United States who served in Vietnam. Two years after authorization was received, the design and plans were approved and construction was under way. The Vietnam Veterans Memorial, designed by Maya Lin and commonly referred to as "the Wall," was formally dedicated on November 13, 1982.

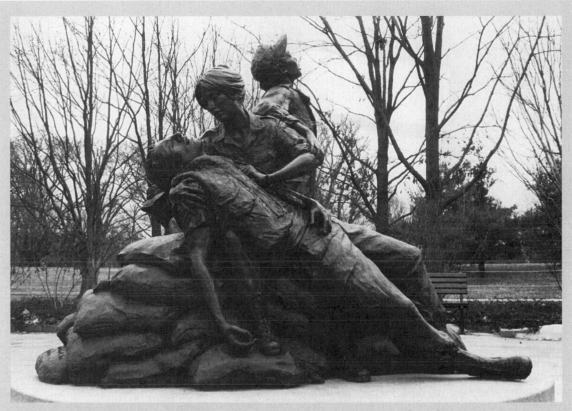

Vietnam Women's Memorial. Glenna Goodacre, sculptor. Gregory Staley, photographer. (© 1993 Vietnam Women's Memorial Project, Inc.)

Just as the Vietnam war had divided our nation, the veterans themselves were divided on the design of their memorial. Some argued that the V-shaped wall was inadequate and demanded something more heroic. Some called it a big black scar, a black gash of shame, a hole in the ground. A compromise was struck to settle the dispute. Former Secretary of the Interior James Watt had refused to authorize construction of the Wall unless a statue of an American soldier was added to it. The directors of the VVMF agreed to commission the highest-ranking sculptor in the design competition, Frederick Hart, of Washington, D.C. He would design a bronze sculpture of three infantrymen to accommodate concern that the Wall lacked specific symbols of the veterans and their patriotism. Mr. Hart described his design as follows:

> The portrayal of the figures is consistent with history. They wear the uniform and carry the equipment of war; they are young. The contrast between the innocence of their youth and weapons of war underscores the poignancy of their sacrifice. There is about them the physical contact and sense of unit that bespeaks the bonds of love and sacrifice that is the nature of men at war. And yet they are each alone. Their strength and their vulnerability are both evident. Their true heroism lies in these bonds of loyalty in the face of their aloneness and their vulnerability. [Vietnam Veterans Memorial Fund, 1982]

In 1983 a photograph of a bronze statue portraying three military men appeared in

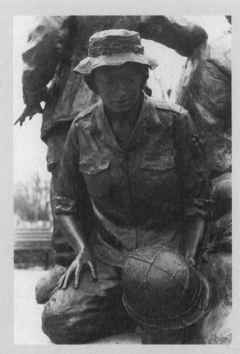

Vietnam Women's Memorial. Glenna Goodacre, sculptor. Gregory Staley, photographer. (© 1993 Vietnam Women's Memorial Project, Inc.)

national newspapers, raising painful personal awareness that our country did not and might not ever know the women who served alongside those depicted.

"Consistent with history." These words crystallized for me the need to change that consistency, that image. In 1983 when I saw the design commissioned by Mr. Hart, I was moved by what I did not see. His account that the "portrayal of figures was consistent with history" reflected the belief that only men serve and therefore are portrayed. The names of eight women nurses who died in Vietnam are etched on the granite wall. The Wall, in its minimalistic concept and simplicity, was complete—as Maya Lin had described it. The names of men and women who died in Vietnam were etched together in granite for eternity. With the dedication, Americans began to learn about the lives

and losses of the male and female soldiers. They were able to begin their healing journey. I was struck by a personal belief that the addition of the Hart statue honoring the living implored another point of view, and another healing element. Although people would see men in bronze, a whole and true portrait of the women who served during the Vietnam War, depicting their professionalism, dedication, service, and sacrifice, had yet to be seen—their stories yet to be heard. Women, too, needed a healing place and a healing process. Historically, women who have served humanity during America's struggles and wars are not included in the artistic portrayals. They slip into history unrecognized and forgotten, compounding the myth that either they did not serve or their service was not noteworthy. They, too, had disappeared off the landscape of the Vietnam era.

Although many thought that the addition of the statue portraying three servicemen completed the Vietnam Veterans Memorial, it is paradoxical that it rendered an incompleteness. A piece of history remained missing. By all public accounts, the profound legacy of women's service in Vietnam was sealed, closed from view, and dispensable. The time had come. The norm of leaving women out of the historical account of war had to change.

Believing that people would support a memorial honoring women if given the information and the opportunity, I gave my first speech in 1983 at a Lions Club. My anxiety grew as I looked out on the room and thought about the public, which had once been hostile and unappreciative. Reexperiencing my feelings when I stepped off the plane in the United States on my return from Vietnam and was greeted by angry war protesters, my knees went limp and I started to shake. I was reluctant to speak experientially, to open myself up to strangers. I talked about the other women and said that more often than not it was an American nurse who a soldier looked to during the last moments of his life. I talked about the Vietnam Veterans Memorial—how beautiful and fitting it is, but that women needed to be honored and remembered as well. There were many questions about my own service. The speech ended with a standing ovation. I was stunned and realized I would have to overcome fear and personal anxieties and share some of my own stories. I remembered what Eleanor Roosevelt said: "You gain strength, courage, and confidence by every experience in which you really stop to look fear in the face. . . . You must do the thing you think you cannot do."

Perhaps it was fate that year when I attended my first veterans reunion in my home state of Minnesota. It included an exhibition of war art by veterans. No images of women were depicted. There I saw a work of sculptor Rodger Brodin entitled *The Squad*, a realistic depiction in bronze of 13 "grunts" on patrol. I was instantly taken back to Vietnam. I felt compelled to call and ask Rodger whether he had ever thought of sculpting a woman soldier. We met, and over the course of 5 months Rodger listened to my stories of the women who had served and those of the war: the deaths, weariness, frustration, and seeing young American men and Vietnamese mutilated. Using a 21-year-old model, he created a 33-inch bronze composite of a military nurse. She was to become the galvanizing force and symbol affectionately named "the Lady" by former GIs. To Rodger she was *The Nurse*.

Having never been involved in political action, raised funds, or spoken to the media or the public, and with a suspicious view of government and the press because of my personal experience in the Vietnam War, I now had to find the courage to work toward justice. Hard work did not frighten me. Failure to achieve rightful honor for women did. I had an unsettling feeling of powerlessness reminiscent of wading into uncharted territory—not unlike stepping off a helicopter in Vietnam, entering a field hospital, and asking, "Where do I start?"

Anxiety was justified. Little did I know that realizing this vision would require a full-time, 10-year campaign convincing government agencies, Congress, journalists, and the public. Some engaged in vilifying our service and undermined our intent to honor women. Little did they know who they were up against. It took time for them to understand us—a core of nurses, veterans, and others who had profound stories to share and a firm belief in a common cause. We would be misjudged and our motives challenged, questioned, and discounted. It would be our role to teach, move the mission forward, and create a national consensus while overcoming ignorance and denial. We would not be rebuked, censured, or deterred. Thomas Jefferson said, "When things get so far wrong, we can always rely on the people, when well informed, to set things right."

DEVELOPING THE STRATEGY

Our first core meeting was held in February 1984 with sculptor Rodger Brodin and four people, all veterans. Soon thereafter I made telephone calls, wrote letters, and extended invitations to other veterans, lawyers, and a representative from the Minnesota Nurses Association. Nine people attended the second meeting. In the words of Margaret Mead, "Never doubt that a small group of thoughtful, committed citizens can change the world; indeed, it's the only thing that ever has." Together we decided to organize a national nonprofit organization for the purpose of fund raising and moving the vision forward. Officers and a board of directors were elected, and the organization was named the Vietnam Nurses Memorial Project. Later we changed the name to the Vietnam Women's Memorial Project (VWMP) to embrace all the military and civilian women who had served during the Vietnam era in our education and recognition efforts. We laid the groundwork, developed a mission statement that included objectives, wrote bylaws, filed articles of corporation, applied for an Internal Revenue Service nonprofit tax status, and wrote a policy and procedures manual filled with guidelines for meeting our objectives.

We began building the team and the coalitions that could help meet our three objectives: (1) to identify the women who served during the Vietnam era and facilitate research, (2) to educate the public about the contributions of these women, and (3) to erect a monument on the grounds of the Vietnam Veterans Memorial in Washington, D.C., ensuring a place in recorded history for women Vietnam veterans. On identifying advisory members, we recruited them to serve on the corporate advisory board, the education council, and the monument council. We looked for individuals who would lend their name and those who could do the work. We were all volunteers.

Three months after our first meeting, we organized a special event to unveil Rodger Brodin's statue, *The Nurse.* We invited the press and made our first official public announcement that we wanted to place this statue honoring women veterans at the Vietnam Veterans Memorial in Washington, D.C. We were an intrepid group! We had yet to feel the heat of the backlash or experience the entanglements inevitable in government bureaucracy. And, unknown to us, a new law was in the making—the Commemorative Works Act, enacted in 1986—after the Project's signed agreement with Rodger Brodin making it necessary for the VWMP to meet the requirements of federal regulatory review and approval.

A Minneapolis corporation donated a small office space used by the core group of volunteers and later by staff. We created management and organizational systems for daily operations, including mail and phone logs, form letters for "thank yous," general information responses, an annual budget, and financial accountability systems. We set up a regional infrastructure of volunteer coordinators who would assist in publicizing the mission of the VWMP, solicit funds, amass additional volunteers, and seek endorsements from politicians and organizations. The American Nurses Association donated a small space in its Washington, D.C., office for the use of our national volunteer coordinator.

Still with some stage fright, I found on the speakers' circuit that I was influencing people simply by sharing the stories of women's service and placing the tangible symbol, *The Nurse,* in front of them. Many were moved and wanted more information. They wanted to know names of books on the subject, to procure a bibliography. They wanted to know whether women had been affected by Agent Orange, and whether they suffered from posttraumatic stress disorder, as did their male counterparts. I began to learn the enormous scope and responsibility of our undertaking. And I realized how much I needed to learn so that I could adequately answer questions and better represent the service of women. I became acutely aware of the nonnurse veterans, such as physical therapists, dieticians, administrators, air traffic controllers, Red Cross workers, USAID workers, and others who asked to be equally honored and remembered.

I was not ignorant, however, of burgeoning foes. At times I was described as a radical feminist—one who so described me said I was using the Vietnam dead to further my cause. With increased public awareness of the vision, there were those who insisted on changing it—or in opposing it altogether. It triggered hate mail, threats, and angry phone calls. Some said women had not been in combat, did not suffer, and were too few in number to be honored. Many people were comfortable with the popular stereotype of the all-male American military. For adversaries we were providing a new emblematic definition of women they were eager to impugn.

In February 1985 a meeting was held in the Old Executive Office Building of the White House. We met with the associate director of the Office of Public Liaison to discuss the subject of recognizing the contributions of women in service to our country. Here we met women from the Pentagon and the Veterans Administration, representatives of military service and other overseas service by civilians (Red Cross), and the woman who served as campaign director for the building of the Vietnam Veterans Memorial and as an independent fund-raising consultant. People brought their divergent views of how to go about recognizing women. Some left with an interest in a presidential proclamation honoring all women veterans and others with an interest in building a memorial to all women who served throughout America's history, in war and peace. It was an important meeting. For us it led to funding connections, volunteers, and visibility. For others, it led to an all-encompassing memorial to military women. Subsequently, in March 1985, legislation was authorized to build a memorial to all women who had served since the time of the American Revolution. It would be called the Women in Military Service for America (WIMSA) Memorial and would be built at the entrance to Arlington Cemetery. We sent testimony from VWMP to Congress, supporting the legislative effort. Later a federal commission would use the WIMSA Memorial as an argument against the efforts of the VWMP. We continued on in our mission to complete the Vietnam Veterans Memorial with the addition of a sculpture portraying women.

By the fall of 1985 we had four 33-inch bronze replica statues of *The Nurse* traveling across the country and exhibited in California, Connecticut, Delaware, the District of Columbia, Florida, Illinois, Indiana, Iowa, Kentucky, Louisiana, Maryland, Minnesota, Missouri, New York, Oregon, Texas, Washington, and Wisconsin. Accompanying the statue were VWMP press releases with photographs of *The Nurse*, brochures, and information packets with requests for donations. The statue became

the primary focus and vehicle through which women veterans came out of hiding. At war's end, many had gone their separate ways, getting on with their lives and careers. Unknown within their communities and even among each other, they joined with their sister veterans—many for the first time—and with their male counterparts. A decade after the war's end, the cathartic process of healing began. The outpouring of interest and the offers to volunteer were phenomenal. Our office was flooded with letters of inquiry and letters from veterans and families expressing appreciation. And there were those who doubted that the effort was worth fighting. One letter from a former military nurse asked, "Do you think anyone will give a damn?"

At the Project's small Minneapolis headquarters, we developed short- and long-range plans of action for grassroots and national support, fund raising, education, and public relation activities. We wrote fact sheets, position papers, media advisories, and press releases and designed brochures. Our plan included action steps: a checklist; time lines; and who would do what, when, and where. At the outset, garnering national support seemed like an overwhelming and formidable task. We broke it down into manageable lists. We targeted the audiences we wanted and developed the message in keeping with our mission that would motivate them to respond. For example, we designed a flyer with the slogan "A Small Donation Makes a Monumental Difference" and sent copies to volunteers to distribute at civic organizations. We began with small action steps focused on veterans and nurses.

For the short-range plan, I determined to start at the grassroots level and visit the local posts of veterans service organizations: Veterans of Foreign Wars, the American Legion, Disabled American Veterans, Paralyzed Veterans of America, and the Vietnam Veterans of America. I was also "testing the water." There were a lot of unknowns regarding interest or potential support within this community, but, if moved, they could take ownership and meet the many challenges ahead with us. Galvanizing them now would ignite their energy and unleash the collective strength needed for a nationwide campaign.

On successfully gaining local support and with a formal resolution in hand, I went up the ladder to the district and state conventions. The language of the resolutions was fine tuned in committees, voted on, and forwarded to national offices. As hoped, veterans and their auxiliary members were excited and proud to be a part of the process. They lobbied long and hard within their groups to defend what they had supported. After researching each of their unique procedures and parliamentary rules, I requested time to speak from the floor of their national conventions in 1985. Individuals behind the "con" microphones lined up much longer than those behind the "pro." Comments were heated and some questions laced with barbed cynicism. Miraculously, having engaged strong and powerful support early on, the pros won. By the end of that year, we had the support of the five major veterans' organizations, with their 6 million members behind us.

I became active in those veterans' organizations and remained highly visible during the 10-year effort. It was important for the VWMP to establish a reputation of trust and credibility. Using the strategy model of the veterans' organizations, we asked nurses who were politically active in their nurses' and other organizations to represent the Project and employ their influence. More than 100 did so with pride and enormous success.

In the long-range plan, we targeted a variety of civic and humanitarian groups with a clear intent to co-opt both genders and the age groups before and after the Vietnam era. We worked toward that end because numbers would count. The grassroots appeal gained national momentum.

Our first highly visible major fundraiser was held in September 1986 in Washington, D.C., near the Lincoln Memorial. It was cosponsored by Senator Edward Kennedy and the William Joiner Center of the University of Massachusetts. About 300 people gathered in a tent. Senator Kennedy took the podium, commending those "gallant and courageous women who served our country in Vietnam" and stressing the need to "recognize those women who served under the colors of our flag and who lost their lives." Senator John Kerry followed, saying, "Any of the names on the Wall could be any of us that are here. Our mission is to remember, and no one can remember in the way we ought to remember until there's a statue that reflects the service of women in Vietnam." A year later we would need the help of these senators in Congress to ask their fellow members to put these words into action.

We were on our way. Our media plan went into action, heightening awareness across America. Volunteers received official status to represent the VWMP and spoke at local and national association conferences, conventions, and civic organizations. Radio, television, and newspapers called asking for interviews. After a while, I found that the most predictable statement was, "I didn't know there were women who served in Vietnam." The most predictable question was, "Were you ever rocketed or attacked?" We would negate the myth and defy the stereotype on both counts. Yes, women were there, and, yes, they were wounded and killed. After what seemed a long media blackout, the journalists were finally interested in the real-life stories of women veterans.

Simultaneously, we appealed for contributions of goods or services from businesses and organizations. Two major corporations printed thousands of brochures for the Project pro bono, and another prepared a short documentary for fund-raising purposes. We asked supporters to help us identify and approach corporate sponsors and private foundations.

Northwest Airlines agreed to provide air cargo free of charge for the 150-pound *Nurse* as it made stops around the United States. We sought professional counsel from an advertising agency. The slogan "A Small Donation Makes a Monumental Difference" made a poignant appeal in fund-raising materials and advertisements. By July 1987, $250,000 had already been raised from corporate gifts, individual donations, appeals at veterans' meetings and conventions, and special fundraisers. More than $100,000 worth of in-kind services (management consultant services, legal fees, rent) had been received. A pharmaceutical company approached us for a market tie with a surgical scrub used by medical personnel that subsequently netted the Project a half-million dollars.

Armed with a clear vision, a tangible symbol, public support, and preliminary funding and grounded with a legitimate nonprofit corporation, we were ready to ask for the endorsement of the Vietnam Veterans Memorial Fund, the organization that built the Wall and placed the bronze statue of three servicemen. VVMF founders Jack Wheeler (chairman) and Jan Scruggs (president) offered an official endorsement, as required by the Memorandum of Conveyance, in the spring of 1986.

The ensuing months were filled with fund raising, education, public relations, sister search activities, and plotting the strategies for seeking formal approval from federal agencies. However, in 1986, in view of the rapidly diminishing outdoor sites in the nation's capital that are suitable for the erection of commemorative works, Congress enacted the Commemorative Works Act (CWA). We read it with trepidation. The regulations were new—and very complicated. We saw loopholes—language that was left up to the interpretation of the reader. We believed that our proposal was simply an addition to an existing memorial and therefore not subject to the CWA, which did not speak to additions but to new memorials intended as a commemoration of an individual, group, or event and which can be authorized only by an Act of Congress. We sought legal counsel and asked a lot of questions. Unanimous formal approval for a commemorative work—including additions to existing memorials—was needed from the Secretary of the Interior, the Commission of Fine Arts, the National Capital Planning Commission, and the National Capital Memorial Commission. Subsequently, we spent inordinate hours researching the role and authority of each. This knowledge alone should have been enough to deter even the most hearty and committed of souls. Indeed, that was the Act's intent—to stop the proliferation of memorials in Washington, D.C.

With the endorsement of the VVMF in hand, we proceeded as planned and took our first major step. In September 1987 the Secretary of the Interior approved our proposal to add a statue representing women at the Vietnam Veterans Memorial. This permission was based on his conclusion that our proposal was an addition to an existing memorial and thus not subject to the CWA. The Secretary forwarded the proposal, bearing the Department of Interior's official approval, to the Commission of Fine Arts. Elated, we requested a hearing with the Commission of Fine Arts. As the "gatekeeper" to memorials in Washington, the Commission's purpose is to supply artistic advice related to the aesthetic appearance of Washington, D.C., and to review the plans for all public buildings, parks, and other architectural elements in the capital (Kohler, 1985). While waiting for the hearing date, we prepared testimony and informed our supporters and the public at large of the upcoming hearing.

On October 22, 1987, we went before the Commission of Fine Arts. We listened to impassioned testimony from the opposition, letters of dissent from members of the public, and discussion and comments from the six presidentially appointed commissioners. We were thunderstruck that some minds and powerful pens in

Washington, D.C., had already been made up before we had an opportunity to testify before the prestigious and powerful Commission. Minutes before we entered the hearing room, someone handed us a copy of the October 22, 1987, *Washington Post* with an article by Benjamin Forgey, "Women and the Wall Memorial Proposal: Honor Without Integrity."

> It has the lofty ring of a just cause, but the proposed Vietnam Women's Memorial, which has been approved by the Secretary of the Interior and which will be considered today by the Commission of Fine Arts, is not a very good idea. To be precise, it's a bad one. This is not to say that the women who served in the U.S. armed forces in Vietnam were not brave, did not perform essential duties, do not deserve our respect. It is simply to point out that if our female veterans deserve more conspicuous honor than they already have received at the Vietnam Veterans Memorial in Constitution Gardens, where the names of the eight female dead are inscribed along with those of their male counterparts, then they should be given such honor elsewhere. To add a statue of a nurse to that extraordinary memorial—the central feature of this misguided proposal—would create a serious symbolic imbalance in one of the nation's preeminent commemorative places.

As I took my seat I thought: *So! Nurses and women aren't good enough for this sacred ground!* I knew we were in trouble before we entered the door, and soon the words out of the commissioners' mouths would echo those of Mr. Forgey. Backroom discussions had unmistakably taken place.

Our testimony included facts on the lack of other memorials to women in our nation's capital. Of the 110 memorials in Washington, D.C., only three were to women, and none of these honored military women. We addressed the history of women's service and issues of compatibility, dignity, need, simplicity, completeness, honor, healing for all veterans to include women, and the merits of a statue. Members of a prestigious Washington, D.C., landscape architectural firm testified in support of our site and design.

Opponents to the concept insisted that an addition would encourage other groups and ethnic minorities to claim statues as well. One antagonist said that the Wall was complete "as is" and that attempts to depict everyone literally can only diffuse its symbolic power and weaken the memorial. Maya Lin, artist of the original design, protested further, concerned about "individual concessions" to special interest groups. "I am as opposed to this new addition as I was to the last," Lin concluded. "I cannot see where it will all end" (Minutes, 1987).

There were derisive and heated remarks by commissioners. Frederick Hart, sculptor of *Three Fighting Men* (who disqualified himself from casting a vote), argued against the addition by insisting that the statue of three men stood for the whole veteran population regardless of gender. He held that his work had created a "fragile balance" with the Wall, a balance likely to be disturbed by the intrusion of added elements. Another commissioner called it an "unneeded clarification." J. Carter Brown, Chairman of the Commission, delivered the coup de grâce. He declared that the three male figures by Hart were already "symbolic of humankind and everyone who served." He asserted that a proliferation of statues would be uncontrollable, saying, "The Park Service has even heard from Scout Dog associations." He referred to the VWMP statue as "an afterthought, sort of a putdown, almost a ghettoization." Mention was made of a statue already dedicated to nurses—the Nurse's Monument, which overlooks the graves from the top of a hill in Arlington National Cemetery. We were urged to believe that this was quite enough for nurses. I knew from my research that this monument had been placed in honor of Army and Navy nurses in 1938. It was rededicated by the chiefs of the Army, Navy, and Air Force in 1971.

The Commission voted 4 to 1 to reject our proposal. Their comments seemed to mirror those in the *Washington Post* column by Benjamin Forgey, who had branded the project a "bad precedent," saying, "*The Nurse* in answer to Hart's statue has no psychological or physical relationship with the memorial as a whole" (Forgey, 1987).

Minutes after the vote, some of us talked to waiting members of the press. When asked about the hearing, I stated matter-of-factly that the Commission ignored the support of thousands of Americans and treated women veterans with arrogance and insensitivity, and I said that we would be back. One journalist asked me what it would take to place a statue of a woman at the Wall. Quite spontaneously, I said, "an act of God and an Act of Congress." Carter Brown also talked to the press: "It could be a work of art done by Michelangelo, which it isn't, and it would still detract from the enormous power of the memorial" (*Washington Times*, 1987).

"What Brown neglects to specify, however, is precisely how much *The Nurse* might dilute the power of the Wall as compared to how much the existing statue on the site—*Three Fighting Men*—already compromises the Wall's inclusive embrace by its omission of women" (Marling & Wetenhall, 1989).

I knew we were in for a long, tough road ahead. We would need legislation in our hands to challenge a hostile Commission of Fine Arts again. Navigating a twisted bureaucratic path would require researching the laws and using them to our advantage, activating an even larger segment of the American people to use their voices and power, cultivating relationships with federal agency and legislative staff, finding more money, compromising, and plotting a good map. Hours after the Commission hearing, we regrouped and started charting the map. We would use our nursing skills to practice patience, diplomacy, and advocacy and would exercise the art of grace. Above all, we would need perseverance and a good sense of humor to keep ourselves balanced amid an endless barrage of irrational opposition. We viewed the roadblocks and setbacks as detours.

Before us loomed the tremendous responsibility to the people of America who shared our fervent hope that a memorial would find its way to its appropriate place of honor. We could not let them down. And, we were soon to learn, they would not let us down. Morley Safer, of the television program *60 Minutes*, learned of the Commission of Fine Arts hearing. Featuring our efforts on one of the programs, Safer interviewed five military nurses who had served during the Vietnam war. He placed their extraordinary and compelling stories of service and our mission to build a memorial in front of several million households for 14 minutes. This was to be a major turning point.

Our first strategy was to win the support of the American people. We built coalitions of varying interests and groups. We had a strong infrastructure of dependable, reliable, and enthusiastic volunteers. We accomplished our long-range goal of achieving the endorsement of 40 national organizations. Because we did not believe that this was a special interest "nurse" or "women's" movement, we appealed to people of all ages, both genders, veterans of all wars, and peacetime soldiers—in other words, to all citizens of America. Through efforts such as the *60 Minutes* program and numerous interviews with the electronic and newsprint media, we built a large audience of American citizens who became a strong and effective constituency of loyal supporters. We had evidence of this support. A clipping service we used sent us copies of hundreds of heart-rending, supportive letters to the editor, editorials, opinion pieces, and stories from newspapers around the country. Many of them were in response to negative pieces written about the Project's efforts. More evidence arrived in the form of donations: thousands of dollars in small amounts poured in, many with a note attached saying that the giver wished it could be more.

These constituencies were integral in the success of **our second strategy—lobbying Congress.**

- In November 1987, just 1 month after the rejection by the Commission of Fine Arts, Senator Dave Durenberger introduced SJ 215 in the Senate.
- Congressman Sam Gejdenson introduced companion bill HR 3628 in the House, authorizing the building of a Vietnam Women's Memorial at the Vietnam Veterans Memorial.
- Consultation with a Washington, D.C., insider and former lobbyist helped to familiarize us with the political process and prepare us for future hearings.
- The VWMP office was moved from Minnesota to Washington, D.C., facilitating our national and legislative efforts.
- In February 1988, we testified at hearings on the bill (changed to SJ 2042) before the Senate Subcommittee on Public Lands, National Parks and Forests.
- The bill was received favorably and marked up to the full committee.
- In June 1988 the Senate passed SJ 2042 by a vote of 96 to 1.
- In June 1988, we testified at a hearing held before the House Subcommittee on Libraries and Memorials. Management and financial questions were posed. Preparation equals performance, and we were prepared. Questions were answered honestly, clarifying and identifying the actions taken that met the committee's concerns. However, having our day in court brought out a myriad of contentious old conflicts, including a woman's place, tensions left over from the Vietnam war, and flare-ups of the original controversy regarding the design of the Vietnam Veterans Memorial. We were dealing with more than just a memorial proposal. We were confronted with political and sociological undercurrents.
- After extensive debate between the House and the Senate over the language of SJ 2042, the House rejected Senate language and on September 23, 1988, passed another version of the bill.
- On October 12 the Senate passed an amended version of SJ 2042 as passed by the House.
- A week later the House rejected the Senate's amendment. The Senate then receded to the House position.

We unhappily settled for a watered-down version of the original specific language regarding site and design. At the eleventh hour, as Congress adjourned on November 14, 1988, Public Law 100-660 authorized "the Vietnam Women's Memorial Project to establish a memorial on federal land in the District of Columbia or its environs to honor women of the Armed Forces of the United States who served in the Republic of Vietnam during the Vietnam era." **It was important for what it did not say.** It was not specific enough regarding placement of the memorial on the Mall. Although the sense of Congress stipulated with respect to location that it would be most fitting and appropriate to place the memorial within the 2.2 acre site of the Vietnam Veterans Memorial in the District of Columbia, it was *our* sense that, being subject to the standards of the CWA, the three federal governing agencies would yet have the last say—the leverage to place our memorial anywhere in the *environs* to the exclusion of the Vietnam Veterans Memorial. We had yet to face the hostile Commission of Fine Arts, whose members made it clear that they did not wish to see anything added within the 2.2 acre site of the Vietnam Veterans Memorial. Moreover, although the Senate bill penned the word *statue,* the House of Representatives bill would not. It would not dictate design by specifying "statue" but opted for the more generic term *memorial.* We determined to go back to Congress during the next session and start the legislative process over—and get the bill we needed that would firmly secure the site at the Vietnam Veterans Memorial. However, the word *memorial* would remain.

Within a month of the passage of our first bill, we initiated a second and more powerful legislative campaign to put our strategies again into play. We hired a public relations consultant who helped us generate thousands of stories across America from the women who served, asking them to share in their own words their personal experiences with the public—the veritable substance behind the quest for a Vietnam Women's Memorial. The response was phenomenal.

Over the course of 1989, members of our board and staff met frequently with congressional members and the staff of legislative committees. We adopted a policy always to go in pairs or more, depending on the circumstances. This allowed us to debrief, compare notes about what was said, discuss any conflicting messages, and subsequently write a summary for later reference—our own as well as for the full board of directors. When deemed necessary, we set the record straight by sending a memorandum of understanding to legislative staff. Together we formulated a new slate for the 101st Congress and worked to identify panels of witnesses representing different organizations and interests for the hearings. In addition, I again spoke before committees and testified at four congressional hearings in the House and Senate.

Throughout the duration of the legislative process, we were successfully employing the "Seven Rules for Testifying Before Congress" before Thomas E. Harvey's work of the same name was published in the fall of 1989! We had used common sense, respect, and assorted advice from experienced sages in the veterans' and nurses' organizations and from trusted legislative staffers. And we used a plan. For its good merits, I offer Harvey's pertinent rules:

It is important to remain courteous even under hostile questioning. Think of the hearing as a positive experience, and approach it with a tolerance for the opinions of others.

1. Know why the hearing is being called.
2. Meet with committee members and staff in advance.
3. Prepare and provide your testimony as far in advance as possible.
4. Arrive early.
5. Be brief and to the point.
6. If you don't know, say so.
7. Be courteous, and tell the truth. [Harvey, 1989]

A third strategy was to activate our supporters. Using the volunteer network, we initiated a massive campaign asking supporters to contact congressional members by telephone, mail, or personal visits. As the bills progressed through the political process, these efforts were targeted to specific legislators. One by one, they signed on. We accomplished this strategy by the dissemination of information through the national newsletters of endorsing organizations, through local newsletters whose mailing lists we were fortunate to have obtained, through highly active telephone trees designed by the volunteers, and through appeals to the public through media relations activities. We sent press releases and fielded questions at press conferences.

It was critical for our supporters to know the goal, the progress of lobbying stages with the Congress, and what was expected of them. With updates and the dissemination of information, we kept the vision of the VWMP before them and provided a guiding force. Information is powerful. We found that our weakest links in the networking chain were those who had not been given the information. Not only could they not act, but some lost faith because they felt overlooked or abandoned. At every national convention of the veterans' organizations, I gave briefings and asked specific action steps of the members. VWMP board members and more than 150 official volunteers performed these same duties at nurses' associations, women's organizations, social clubs, patriotic and civic organizations, schools, universities, and other forums. Mobilizing them and hundreds of unofficial volunteers toward action required articulating expectations through consistent distribution of information. Giving them something tangible to work with proved enormously successful.

With the help of an ad agency, we designed a promotional poster for the legislative effort that read, "Not all women wore love beads in the '60s." It depicted a woman soldier's name imprinted on dog tags connected to stainless steel beads. On the reverse side, hundreds of signatures petitioned lawmakers to appeal on behalf of Vietnam's forgotten veterans. Thousands of these petitions and pallets of cardboard tubes were sent to volunteers and supportive coalitions across America. At shopping malls, veterans' clubs, nurses' meetings, and street corners, Americans were asked to sign the petitions and forward them to their senators and representatives. More than 25,000 posters and tubes were sent to the national veterans' conventions alone in one summer. Legislators became so tired of receiving the tubes they said "no more!" They had gotten the message. Later, we learned that many posters never made it to their appropriate designations because the unique design was so well liked they ended up in frames on office walls.

THE BACKLASH

When knowledge of our prolific and unrelenting lobbying efforts reached newspapers and their readership, the backlash was fascinating if not vicious.

> Congress should resist efforts to tinker with one of the most effective and powerful memorials built in this country—the Vietnam Veterans Memorial in Washington's Constitutional Garden. . . . It's hard to vote against the flag or

Army nurses. But, in this instance, congressmen should. The Vietnam Veterans Memorial is as close to perfection as it can be. To add anything to it would only be to detract from the powerful memorial it has become. [*Indianapolis News*, 1988]

We pressed on.

Our legislative strategy won. On November 28, 1989, President George Bush signed legislation authorizing Area 1, the central monumental core of the Capital City, the site for the Vietnam Women's Memorial. The explicit criteria of the CWA had still to be met. We had yet to win the approval of the federal authorizing agencies to place the memorial near the Vietnam Veterans Memorial or prove that the "subject of the memorial is of pre-eminent historical and lasting significance to the Nation" (*National Capital Memorials ETC*).

Before these agencies, I asked:

> Is not the selfless service of 265,000 women, all volunteers, who served during the Vietnam era around the world, 10,000 of them—the majority of whom were nurses—in Vietnam under grave and life-threatening conditions, saving the lives of 350,000 American soldiers, of the greatest historical significance and worthy of this nation's eternal gratitude?

Supported by drawings, sketches, mockups, and reports from engineers, planners, and landscape architects, in a 5-month process of informal and formal hearings, we finally gained the approval of regulatory agencies for our preferred site within Area 1. Site review ensured that the site selected was relevant to the subject and did not interfere or encroach on existing memorials or features. In April 1990 the Commission of Fine Arts voted to accept a recommendation to locate the Vietnam Women's Memorial on the Mall near the Vietnam Veterans Memorial. We held fast to the vision, and our determination was vindicated. We now had a site worthy of the women who had served.

Because our first design, *The Nurse,* had been rejected in 1987, we launched a national open one-stage design competition for the design of the Vietnam Women's Memorial to solicit a new design. A competition would provide us with the opportunity to discover the most creative and appropriate work of art. It was an exciting way for Americans to participate in designing a national memorial that honors forever the heroic spirit of more than 265,000 American women. We had to be confident that a jury of eminent architects, renowned members of the arts community, and highly regarded Vietnam veterans would select a design worthy of the women who served. Ultimately, however, the VWMP board would make the final decision. With the guidance of a professional competition adviser, site feasibility consultants, technical advisers, and legal counsel, we developed the design standards, rules, and procedures to be used by the design competition applicants for the Vietnam Women's Memorial. We put out the call for the memorial design entries and required that they be received between August 1990 and the end of October 1990.

The design phase was arduous and demanding, and required hundreds of hours of time from August 1990 through March 1993 by committed individuals. In the weeks and months that followed the design competition results, we worked with the artists who won first place to develop their designs further. Ultimately the board of directors of the Vietnam Women's Memorial Project decided to move forward with the design offered by Glenna Goodacre, of Santa Fe, New Mexico. She had won an honorable mention in the design competition. We did not schedule meetings with the federal agencies to review her design until we had solicited the opinions of representatives of several of the Project's endorsing organizations: the American Legion, Veterans of Foreign Wars, Vietnam Veterans of America, Paralyzed Veterans of America, and Disabled American Veterans. Again, it was a part of our overall philosophy and strategy to be inclusive and to inform our supporters, seek their valued input, and ask their counsel. In quiet celebration while meeting together in Washington, D.C., they unanimously embraced the design placed before them as fitting, appropriate, and worthy of the women who served. With their positive consensus on the Goodacre design, we were ready for the last phase.

During 1991, we met with the National Capital Memorial Commission, the Commission of Fine Arts, and the National Capital Planning Commission to present and review Ms. Goodacre's bronze model of a multifigure sculpture-in-the-round depicting three Vietnam era women, one of whom is tending to a wounded male soldier. By fall 1991, after many staff meetings, hearings, and unsuccessful bureaucratic attempts to alter the concept, the design was approved by all three commissions. In Santa Fe, Ms. Goodacre proceeded to build the life-size monument in clay for its final review. On March 11, 1993, the clay sculpture-in-the-round was approved by all the regulatory agencies. The monument would now be cast in bronze.

By this time the news media neither helped nor hindered the approval efforts. Opinions continued to be voiced by well-known syndicated columnists and small-town journalists, but there was no turning back. "Monumentitis is making the Mall in Washington a monument to mars and to irritable factions" (Will, 1991). In addition, most of the media were now on the side of building the memorial. They would be the chief catalyst for informing the country, and foreign countries, of the upcoming dedication.

Finally, on November 11, 1993, women veterans were thanked by a grateful nation during the dedication ceremony, entitled "A Celebration of Patriotism and Courage." The Vietnam Women's Memorial statue was unveiled on the grounds of the Vietnam Veterans Memorial 300 feet southeast of the statue of three servicemen near the Wall of names. Many tears were shed, and many thoughts and sentiments were shared. Former Chairman of the Joint Chiefs of Staff Admiral William Crowe noted: "This moving monument finally completes the Vietnam circle by honoring the spirit and achievements of the women who participated in that effort. But more important, it will serve as a shining beacon for future generations of American women." A wounded Marine said, "I would not be alive today without the super professional service of the American women the memorial honors" (DB). From a woman who served in Vietnam came the statement: "I'm so grateful for your perseverance, commitment, and passion to make the women's statue become a reality. . . . My heart is still overflowing with feelings from my experiences in D.C. You have given each of us women a priceless gift—the gift of hope and healing. For us to be recognized, honored, appreciated, and united was unbelievable" (Gail Hager). For the VWMP's commemorative book, *A Celebration of Patriotism and Courage,* Charles T. Hagel said: "The dedication of the Vietnam Women's Memorial will complete the long march toward universal recognition of all who served their country in Vietnam. This memorial honors the commitment and inspiration of the American women whose service during this turbulent and difficult time cannot be overstated."

Vision, that picture of desired results, is just that—a vision. Although I provided the vision and leadership, accomplishment was achieved with the help of many who provided the complex combination of necessary abilities. Keeping the vision clearly out in front of the American people, a board and staff committed to written policies and speaking with one voice, and commitment to strategic planning and results—these helped realize the victory. Moving the vision of the Vietnam Women's Memorial Project forward is truly a testament to the will of the people. It took a creative team of

diverse talents and personalities. Many came and went at critical junctures, offering expertise and guidance; all made a difference. It was important to listen. Ultimately, it was collective persistence and determination in using political action that moved a nation. Eleanor Roosevelt said: "It is deeply important that you develop the quality of stamina. Without it, you are beaten. With it, you may wring victory out of countless defeats." Her words rang true more than once.

It is easy to be intimidated by the mysteries of politics, by politicians, and by the political process. Yet this is where action, driven by our personal aspirations, values, and beliefs, can force change—and even alter the way people view the world. The secret to the process isn't all that mysterious after all. Demystifying it is analogous to breaking the intricacies of nature down into understandable parts. "By viewing Nature, Nature's handmaid Art, Makes mighty things from small beginnings grow" (John Dryden, as cited in a reproduction of his work, 1995).

A small group grew to the thousands of veterans, other Americans, and people from around the world who went to Washington, D.C., on Veterans Day 1993 to dedicate the Vietnam Women's Memorial and say "thank you" to women who served our nation. Vice President Al Gore, a Vietnam veteran, praised his sister veterans during the dedication ceremony. He stated, "Let's all resolve that this memorial serve as a vehicle for healing our nation's wounds. Let's never again take so long in honoring a debt" (Gore, 1993).

We wrote the final chapter of the Vietnam Veterans Memorial with a legacy that will long be remembered. It was a matter of honor and, yes, a matter of justice. According to the British thinker Eric Ashby, to effect positive change, it is necessary to go beyond saying that "something must be done" to doing "the hard work of showing just how it can be done" (Annual Report, 1993). As nurses work more closely with bureaucrats in addressing the social, economic, and other myriad problems of the human condition, then let them see our efforts as worthy of recognition in national memorials, works of lasting art, and other forums. This will validate the profound worth of women, the profound worth of their contribution, and the need to learn from them and see them as protagonists, mentors, role models, leaders, and, perhaps, great humanitarians.

LESSONS LEARNED

"Delay is preferable to error," wrote Thomas Jefferson in a letter to George Washington on May 16, 1772. The original target date for dedication of the Vietnam Women's Memorial was 1988—four years after the founding of the organization. Ultimate success would require 5 more years. During wakeful nights and stress-filled days, it was difficult not to become discouraged and wonder whether the struggle was worth it. There was a path of less resistance. Would settling for something else be another and perhaps even better choice? We had faced delays. We had received many offers of pared-down memorial concepts and different sites. We could have accepted them and gone on with our lives. The aim of the opposition is to win by demoralizing you and diminishing your work—to wear you down so you will quit. Admittedly it was frustrating, even painful, when others asked why the effort was taking so long. We lost volunteers, we lost some support, and some of us lost friends. There were gains and losses. The personal price and the price to the organization had to be weighed. Our particular crusade required waiting; working harder, longer; and taking new risks. Externalizing the destructive criticism and skepticism, which became part of the norm, was critical to maintaining harmony amid the balancing act of family and Project responsibilities. The Project's inner circle gradually came to view delays as an inevitable part of the process. They were preferable to taking

less than our mission called for. The error would have been choosing the easier path of acquiescence. The delays, in fact, were to our advantage.

It became crystal clear that to succeed the achievement of the vision before us would require some compromise, but giving up was not an option. We would find a new design but would not concede on the choice of site. I often had to remind myself of my own words before the national veterans service organizations in 1988 when requesting their legislative support:

> We wish to stand near the Wall of names of those we cared for in death and the bronze statue portraying the men we helped come home. We were with them in the war and we want to be with them now. I want the women who served to know that they are not forgotten, that there is a special place for them, too, on honored ground.

The legislative and approval effort, although daunting, moved forward efficiently and successfully largely because of the extraordinary role played by a strong executive director hired by our board of directors during the introduction of the legislation in the fall of 1989. Her remarkable ability to juggle many responsibilities at once and interface effectively with key legislative and agency staff, her keen and perceptive sense of timing, and her being at all times the eyes and ears for the board of directors were essential if not critical. Staff and volunteer efforts were augmented by the active involvement and expertise contributed by the Project's board of directors. Because members of the board lived in different states, time and money were saved by holding teleconference board meetings as needed. We combined board meetings in Washington, D.C., with hearing dates. The Project became a strong organization, driven by an effective goal-oriented board whose policies were implemented by an able and conscientious executive director. It was important to have the Project well established in the nation's capital during this critical phase.

PROFILE OF THOSE WHO SERVED

The major source for the following information is the tables from the *National Vietnam Veterans Readjustment Study* (Department of Veterans Affairs, 1988).

1. Population
   a. More than 265,000 women served in the military during the Vietnam War. Although an accurate number of the women who were actually stationed or performed military duty in Vietnam is not available, it is estimated that 10,000 to 11,000 served "in country."
   b. Within the total population of military women, 85% were enlisted. However, 90% of the women stationed in Vietnam and the adjacent waters were officers. The majority (87%) were military nurses.
2. Service Specialties
   a. In addition to nurses, women served in a variety of military positions, including intelligence, public affairs, supply, air traffic control, special services, administration, finance, occupational therapy, physical therapy, and dietetics.
   b. Although it is difficult to determine the exact number of civilian women who served in Vietnam, their contributions are no less important. These women served as news correspondents and workers for the Red Cross, the USO, the American Friends Service Committee, Catholic Relief Services, USAID, and other humanitarian organizations.
3. Casualties
   a. Eight military women (seven army nurses and one air force nurse) lost their lives in Vietnam. Their names are engraved on the Vietnam Veterans Memorial, the Wall, along with 58,209 other military personnel who made the ultimate sacrifice for their country. More than 50 civilian women died in Vietnam.
   b. Fewer then 2% of the casualties treated in Vietnam died. However, more than 350,000 casualties were treated and 75,000 were permanently disabled.
   c. Other facts about the women who served in Vietnam:
      (1) 5.8% were wounded in Vietnam.
      (2) 1.3% were wounded in combat situations.
      (3) 1.2% received the Purple Heart.
      (4) More than 20% have service-connected disabilities.

POSTSCRIPT

Many women veterans who volunteered to go to Vietnam to help save lives and who experienced the carnage of war on a daily basis came home to the same hostile treatment as did the returning combat soldiers. They suffered posttraumatic stress disorder with all the accompanying problems, pancreatic and uterine cancer, and other diseases related to combat, and yet only recently have major studies been initiated and medical support provided. More than a decade of research and numerous publications looked at the psychobiological consequences of combat on male theater veterans, but no biological trials with women Vietnam veterans in the theater of operations have been published. Research has provided some basic information, but much more is needed to understand the complex issues surrounding combat theater assignment of female military personnel (Department of Veterans Affairs, 1996). In 1996 the first major female veterans study with a national outreach was commissioned by the Department of Defense and the Veterans Affairs Department.

References

Annual Report of the Commonwealth Fund. (1993). Innovators: The president's essay. New York: Margaret E. Mahoney.

Bartlett's familiar quotations (14th ed.). (1968). Boston: Little, Brown.

Commemorative Works Act. Public Law 99-652-H.R. 4378 40 U.S.C. 1001.

Department of Veterans Affairs. (1988). *National Vietnam Veterans Readjustment Study.* Washington, DC.

Department of Veterans Affairs. (1996). *Vietnam Nurse Veterans Psychophysiology Study Information Sheet.* Washington, DC.

Dryden, J. (1995). *Songs of the earth.* Philadelphia: Running Press.

Flikke, J. O. (1996). In P.M. Donohue (Ed.), *Nursing, the finest art* (2nd ed.). Nurses in action, wars of the twentieth century. St. Louis: Mosby–Year Book.

Forgey, B. (1987, October 22). Women and the wall

memorial proposal: Honor without integrity. *Washington Post,* E1, E11.

Gore, A. (1993). Dedication speech, Vietnam Women's Memorial, Washington, DC.

Harvey, T. (1989, September). Bearing witness: A practical guide to testifying on Capitol Hill. *Government Executive, 29.*

Indianapolis News. (1988, February 19). Additions that detract (editorial).

Kohler, S. (1985). *The Commission of Fine Arts: A brief history, 1910–1984.* Washington, DC: U.S. Government Printing Office.

Marling, K. A., & Wetenhall, J. (1989). The sexual politics of memory: The Vietnam Women's Memorial Project and "The Wall." *Prospects: An annual of American cultural studies.* New York: Cambridge University Press.

Minutes of the Commission of Fine Arts. (1987, October 22). Washington, DC.

National Capital Memorials, ETC., 40 USCS. National capital memorials and commemorative works (Chap. 21). Washington, DC: U.S. Government Printing Office.

Naythons, M. (1993). *The face of mercy: A photographic history of medicine at war.* (Prologue by William Styron.) New York: Random House.

Powell, General C. (1993, July 29). Groundbreaking ceremony remarks. Washington, DC.

Ratzloff, T. (1993). Return from the front. *Minnesota Nurse, 1*(14), 6.

Roosevelt, Eleanor. Quote on bookmark. Reel Images, Inc., No. 7113.

Scruggs, J. C. (1985). *To heal a nation: The Vietnam veterans memorial.* New York: Harper and Row.

Senate Joint Resolution 2042, 100th Congress, November 15, 1988.

Senate Joint Resolution 207, 101st Congress, November 28, 1989.

Vietnam Veterans Memorial Fund (1982). *National salute to veterans.* Program souvenir of events of November 10–14, 1982. Washington, DC.

Vietnam Women's Memorial Project (1990). *Vietnam Women's Memorial National One-Stage Open Design Competition Program, Design Standards, Rules and Procedures.* Washington, DC.

Vietnam Women's Memorial Project, Inc. (1993). *Celebration of patriotism and courage.* Washington, D.C.

Washington Times (1987, November 11). Vietnam women veterans' statue now going the legislative route. (Quote by J. Carter Brown.)

Will, G. F. (1991). Monumentitis is making the mall in Washington a monument to Mars and irritable factions. *Newsweek,* August 26.

Women in Military Service for America Memorial Foundation, Inc. Washington, D.C.

Unit *II*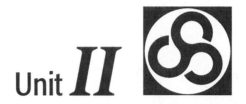

POLICY AND POLITICS: Knowing the Process, Using the Power

Unit II

analyzes the key concepts of policy, politics, power, and conflict, as well as related strategies and issues. Chapter 6 describes the policy process and policy analysis, whereas Chapter 7 discusses how to conduct a political analysis and the strategies that are available to nurses who want to influence policymaking in any sphere. The vignette that follows this chapter examines networking as an essential skill for the politically astute nurse. Chapter 8 brings these concepts alive, describing the political dynamics of the policy process through two case scenarios illustrating the strategies that nurses used to effectively move policy and practice issues.

Conflict is an inherent part of policy development and political action. Chapter 9 explores different kinds of conflict and presents strategies for managing it.

One of the premises of this book is that collective action is often more effective, innovative, and stimulating than individual action. Chapter 10 outlines strategies for organizing and mobilizing nurses and others for collective action. The vignette that follows describes a group of nurses and physicians that has formed to respond to a health care system that they view as more concerned with profits than with patients.

Several other strategies for influencing policy are explored in this chapter. The role and nuances of research as a political and policy tool are examined in Chapter 11. During a cost-conscious time in health care, nurses' understanding of the economics of health care is paramount. Models for analyzing the economics of policy decisions are discussed in Chapter 12. Chapter 13 examines the role of the media in influencing policies. Two vignettes augment this chapter. The first discusses the use of letters to the editor and call-ins to talk shows as ways to get free media coverage. The second vignette describes the New York State Nurses Association's highly effective media campaign around the theme of "Every Patient Deserves an RN."

The ethical dimensions of policy, politics, and power are complex and often difficult. These issues are explored in Chapter 14. This theme is carried through as it applies to public policy and rationing in the Unit II Case Study. This end piece describes nurses' participation in the development of one of the most controversial state health policies in recent years–the Oregon Basic Health Care Act. This health policy embodies the ethical dilemmas confronting society as it makes tough decisions about how to allocate scarce resources.

Chapter 6

POLICY DEVELOPMENT AND ANALYSIS

Barbara E. Hanley

The restructuring of the health care industry into managed care models has increased the need for integration of policymaking knowledge and skills into nursing roles. Understanding the concepts, approaches, and strategies in policymaking and having basic skills in policy analysis are essential. The purpose of this chapter is to provide a theoretical and rational approach to the study of policy development, a process that may frequently appear chaotic.

Policy encompasses the authoritative guidelines that direct human behavior toward specific goals, in either the private or the public sector. It includes the broad range of activities through which authority figures make decisions directed toward a goal and levy sanctions that affect the conduct of affairs. *Private policy* is made by health care agencies or institutions; it includes directives governing conditions of employment and guidelines for service provision. *Public policy* refers to local, state, and federal legislation, regulation, and court rulings that affect individual and institutional behaviors under the respective government's jurisdiction, such as state licensure for professional practice and federal Medicare legislation. However, there is a close link between the two as institutional policy frequently reflects the means to implement or comply with public policy. *Health policy* refers most often to public policies directly related to health care service delivery and reimbursement, although it may include policies in the private sector as well. *Policy analysis* is the systematic study of the content and anticipated or actual effects of standing or proposed policies. The

process through which policies are analyzed is therefore applicable to any setting.

PUBLIC POLICYMAKING

J. E. Anderson (1990) describes public policy as a purposive course of governmental action to deal with an issue of public concern. A policy may therefore refer to a specific governmental decision or a course of action—or inaction—to deal with the issue (Helco, 1972). The decision of an authoritative body *not* to take action is as important as a decision *for* action. To exemplify, Congress' failure to enact some form of the Clinton Health Security Act in 1994 left a policy vacuum rapidly filled by the for-profit restructuring of the health care system into managed care models.

Policy formulation occurs in a number of ways: the enactment of legislation and its accompanying rules and regulations, which have the weight of law; administrative decisions in interagency and intraagency activities, including interpretative guidelines for rules and regulations; and judicial decisions that interpret the law. In short, public policy encompasses anything a government chooses to do or not to do (Dye, 1987).

Public policy is characterized by its application to all members of the society and involves prescribed sanctions for failure to comply. Rather than being limited to a specific law, regulation, legislative proposal, or organizational decision, policy is a dynamic phenomenon; its analysis serves as a means to stop the action, a snapshot. What is visible to the observer at any point is therefore a stage or phase in an ongoing sequence of events in formal policy development or in governmental action and inaction (Dye, 1987; Jones, 1978). It is important, therefore, to clarify the context in which the term *policy* is used and the meaning intended.

An additional definition is that of *policy stakeholders,* which includes those elected or appointed officials, interest group representatives, and individuals who are directly involved in shaping a particular policy and may be directly affected in some way by its outcome. Stakeholders are also relevant in private sector policymaking, although they may not be as highly visible.

Public policymaking begins with "We the people . . . ," who, through the Constitution, give the authority for decision making to the three branches of government—the executive, the legislature, and the judiciary, which serve as a system of checks and balances. The judicial process is costly and reserved for resolution of dispute, so in practice the basic policy loop includes the "Iron Triangle" of the executive, the legislature, and interest groups. Policymaking thus has many points of access through which legislators, agency officials, constituents and interest groups, and media representatives may exert influence at local, state, and federal levels. The input of substantive experts on behalf of these players is also increasing. Interest group activity is diversifying to include data gathering, mass marketing, and wholesale lobbying (Petracca, 1992). Finally, there is increasing interaction between the public and private health policymaking sectors because of the corporate takeover of health care. State legislatures and Congress are attempting to regulate the practices of managed care organizations (MCOs) for the purpose of protecting the rights of MCO enrollees through enactment of legislation such as for a mandated minimum length of stay for deliveries and breast cancer surgery (Hellinger, 1996).

An area of particular and growing importance is intergovernmental relations that focus on the interrelationship between federal, state, and local governments (Sabatier, 1991). All three levels function interdependently in resolving complex policy issues such as dealing with underinsured and uninsured persons and medically indigent persons. Federalism refers to the shared power between federal and state governments based on the Constitution: all powers not specifically granted to the federal government reside with the state. The federal role in health and social policy was greatly enhanced during the Great Depression, when states were unable to provide for the basic needs of citizens. The next spurt occurred in the 1960s with President Lyndon Johnson's "Great Society," including the enactment of Medicare and Medicaid to ensure health care for elderly and poor persons. As health care costs have consumed an increasingly greater proportion of the gross domestic product, Republican proposals to reform Medicaid have focused on block grants, thereby limiting federal financial responsibility and shifting the struggle among interest groups for increasingly scarce dollars back to the state and local governments.

A policy trend illustrating the interrelationship of federal and state policymaking with major implications for nursing is the movement of the Medicaid population into managed care. Medicaid is a federal program administered by the state with joint federal-state funding. State Medicaid costs exploded in 1991, fueled by an increase in federally mandated benefits under the program and by the loss of private health insurance as people lost jobs during the recession. Since 1994, encouraged by President Clinton, states have increasingly applied for Section 1115 waivers from Title XIX of the Social Security Act. These Medicaid waivers allow states to develop demonstration projects, primarily to move their Medicaid populations into managed care, thereby saving money—and in some cases expanding the number of people they can cover.

Approaches to Public Policymaking

Political scientists have established a number of conceptual models that provide varying perspectives on public policymaking (Dye, 1987).

They enable one to organize one's thinking in relation to the policy process as applied to a particular case, and they offer explanations for its dynamics. Adherents to each model may therefore identify different variables or view the same variables differently in conceptualizing the way in which specific policy decisions are made.

The *rational* approach to policy decisions reflects an ideal world. Here policymakers define the problem; identify and rank social values in policy goals; examine each policy alternative for positive and negative consequences, costs, and benefits; compare and contrast these factors among all options; and select the policy that most closely achieves the policy goals (Anderson, 1990; Dye, 1987). However, because the rational model holds the possibility of sweeping policy change, it is an unrealistic, if not impossible, approach to policymaking. Its importance lies in its striving for the ideal solutions in the face of political pressures. Again the failed Clinton Health Security Act in 1994 provides a clear example. The Clinton plan proposed a total revision of the health care industry through a blend of market competition and regulation. However, the magnitude of the proposed change enabled those with a vested interest in the status quo to target numerous pieces, mobilize public fear, and ultimately defeat the proposal. Health care reform was relegated to the state level, where small changes have been made primarily in insurance law to increase citizens' access to private insurance. Policy changes in the United States are most often made *incrementally*, with small changes at the margins as opposed to sweeping restructuring of ineffective or dysfunctional systems. Proposals begin with the status quo and reflect the turf, goals, and politics of policy stakeholders, such as elected officials, interest groups, and bureaucratic administrators. The political dynamics among these actors are so important that policy options developed without addressing them would have little or no chance for success. Lindblom (1996) terms this approach as "the science of muddling through." Consider the success of the Kassebaum-Kennedy Health Insurance Portability and Accountability

Act (HIPAA) of 1996, in contrast to the Clinton plan. As an incremental step in increasing access to health insurance, HIPAA directly addresses the problem of job lock when one has a preexisting health problem.

To address specific policy decisions over time, analysts must also consider the substantive input from researchers, specialist reporters, professional associations, and institutional policy specialists (Sabatier, 1991). The growing role of these policy subsystems underscores the importance of nursing research; nurse legislative and political action at local, state, and national levels; and the presence of nurse policymakers and analysts. Coalitions of nursing groups such as the Tri-Council for Nursing (American Nurses Association, National League for Nursing, American Association of Colleges of Nursing, and Association of Nurse Executives) ensure a unified nursing approach in key policy debates.

Failure of the Clinton Health Security Act has shifted reform to the state level, where both private and public health care financing systems are being overhauled. Battles regarding nursing roles as primary care providers and network panel members, as well as prescriptive authority, will be fought in 52 venues. Development of Health Care Financing Administration (HCFA) Section 1115 waivers to move state Medicaid populations into managed care provided nurses a vital avenue to serve as patient advocates and to ensure key roles in primary care and health care management. Nursing's Agenda for Health Care Reform, established during the Clinton initiative, provides criteria for nurses to evaluate health care reform legislation.

The Policy Process

The *policy process* refers specifically to the steps through which a policy moves from problem to working program. Here we look at two models of how this has been conceptualized. The first, *Kingdon's "Policy Streams" Model*, is briefly described because of its dynamism. Next, more attention is given to the Stage-Sequential Model, a chronological nuts-

and-bolts approach, as described by Ripley (1996) and Anderson (1990), that may be more helpful to neophytes.

KINGDON'S POLICY STREAMS MODEL

Kingdon's model is based on Cohen, March, and Olsen's (1972) "garbage can" model, which describes the process as a series of options floating around seeking a problem. It contains three streams of activities:

1. *Problem stream,* dealing with the complexities in getting policymakers to focus on one problem out of many facing the constituency, such as the lack of access to health care faced by uninsured persons.
2. *Policy stream,* addressing policy goals and ideas of those in policy subsystems, such as researchers, congressional staff, agency officials, and interests groups. These ideas float around policy circles in search of problems, as in the garbage can model.
3. *Political stream,* including factors in the political environment that influence the policy agenda, such as an economic recession, special interest media campaigns, or a pivotal election such as the 1991 Thornburg-Wofford special U.S. Senate race in Pennsylvania. Interpreted as a rejection of Bush Administration policies when former U.S. Attorney General Dick Thornburg was soundly defeated, Harris Wofford's espousal of health care reform had a pivotal effect on focusing the Bush Administration and later the first Clinton Administration on the need to address the problem.

Kingdon sees these streams as floating around and waiting for a "window of opportunity" to open through a change in the political stream. "Couplings" of the policy and problem streams lead to new opportunities for policy change. An application of this approach can be seen in the evolution of the community nursing organization (CNO) model. CNOs provide capitated care to ambulatory elders to facilitate independent living, promote maximal wellness despite age-related health problems and chronic illness, and

prevent or delay institutionalization. This practice model had long been advocated by nursing, but lack of reimbursement structures precluded their development. The political debate over reducing prohibitive Medicare cost inflation opened a window of opportunity for nurses to offer a cost-saving alternative for community care of elders. Legislation to authorize CNO demonstration projects was enacted in the Omnibus Budget Reconciliation Act of 1987; however, the HCFA did not issue its Request for Proposals for CNO demonstrations until 1991. The delay was due to administrative opposition to implementation related to fear of additive costs. Four demonstration projects were developed and operational by 1994—seven years from legislation to a working program.

THE STAGE-SEQUENTIAL MODEL

Many political scientists have described a systems-based model that views the policy process as sequential or as a series of stages in which a number of functional activities occur (Anderson, 1990; Anderson, Brady, & Bullock, 1984; Ripley, 1985, 1996). In this model a group's policy problem is identified and placed on the policy agenda, and then a policy is developed, adopted, implemented, and evaluated. The process is dynamic and cyclical, with policy evaluation and oversight to identify either a well-functioning program or new problems, thereby restarting the cycle. Once established, programs are rarely terminated. Figure 6–1 provides Ripley's (1996) model, which includes stages, activities, and products.

Stage 1: Policy Agenda Setting. The first step in setting a policy agenda is identification of a *policy problem,* a "situation which produces needs or dissatisfaction . . . for which relief is sought" (Anderson, 1990, p. 79). There are many public problems, but only those that are brought to policymakers' attention for action by a spokesperson qualify as policy problems. Jones (1977) terms this the "Problem to Government" phase, or "getting the government to consider action on the problem" (Anderson et

Stages (Functional Activities)

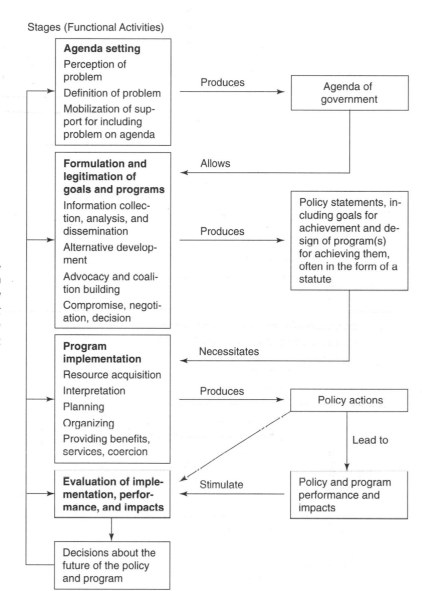

Figure 6–1 The flow of policy **stages,** functional activities, and products. (From Ripley, R. B. [1996]. Stages of the policy process. In D. D. McCool [Ed.], *Public policy theories, models and concepts: An anthology* [p. 158]. Englewood Cliffs, NJ: Prentice-Hall.)

al., 1984). Ripley (1985) cautions that there may be competition here among groups trying to attract governmental attention to their problems and competition over the definition of specific problems.

Next, the problem is refined to a *policy issue,* a problem with societal ramifications of concern to a number of people on which there are conflicting opinions for resolution. Values of the involved stakeholders play a large role here and

determine the amount of political interest the issue will generate, the identification of policy options, and the analysis that should follow. Operationally, it is useful to frame the issue as a question: What could/should be done about this problem?

In practice, Wildavsky (1979) cautions, it is only through analysis that the true underlying issue is identified. For example, at the institutional level, hospitals have been developing policies for how unlicensed assistive personnel (UAPs) should be utilized. Comprehensive analysis of the problem reveals that the underlying issue is whether or not technical nursing functions should be delegated. A critical component is identification of the short- and long-term implications of delegation to a new group of technical providers for both patient care and professional practice, as well as the fiscal impact on the institution. Once the discussion is limited to how UAPs will be utilized, the importance of the underlying issue, and alternative strategies for its resolution that could be more beneficial in the long run, may be overlooked.

Problem and issue definition and mobilization of support produce a governmental policy agenda that includes those issues being addressed by public policymakers. It is vital to identify the appropriate policymaking body with jurisdiction over the matter, as well as individuals and groups who might be interested in working toward a positive resolution. Agendas convey the notion of issue prioritization by policymakers, particularly in the first two stages. The *discussion agenda* includes issues that merit the attention of policymakers on the basis of the input from involved interest groups, consumers, or policy elites in stage one. The *action agenda* designates which issues receive active attention. Media coverage plays a major role in broadening public interest, enlisting group support, and alerting policymakers to the issue. Finally, the *decision agenda* reflects policy issues in the last stages of legitimation by policymakers.

The issue of MCOs' overt rationing of care through setting truncated length-of-stay parameters for maternity and postmastectomy cases has been sensationalized in the media. Evidence of these problems produced a target for consumer backlash against perceived MCO threats to quality care. It galvanized both the public and policymakers in seeking legislative redress in response to growing frustration with perceived interference with patient-provider decisions. As a result, the issue moved to action and decision agendas nationwide at both state and federal levels, despite lack of concrete evidence that harm has been done (Friedman, 1997).

Stage 2: Policy Formulation. Here policymakers determine the type of policy options to be developed, responding to questions such as, "What could or should be done to deal with 'X'?" This is a technical phase in which legislative or regulatory language is drafted. Information on the issue is collected, analyzed, and disseminated. Various interest groups and policymakers may develop alternative proposals, each of which must be evaluated in terms of its costs and benefits to the target group and the "spill over" effects on those external to it—the externalities (Gwartney & Stroup, 1987). Anderson (1990) cautions that care should be exercised in addressing concerns raised by interest groups and those to be regulated because they frequently seek loopholes when implementation begins.

Policy proposals now move through the appropriate legislative or regulatory process, and the policy decision is made. A critical component here is the development of a program budget and the funding appropriation process. This phase is characterized by input from all those holding a stake in the issue: interest groups, policymakers, and target groups; however, the final decision will be made by the legitimate authority. Public pressure must be continued or increased to advance the issue's priority rating until resolution is achieved in the form of a policy document such as a statute or regulation. Ripley (1985) stresses the importance of compromise and negotiation to reach a decision. As a result, policy and program design may be vague and sketchy; details will be defined in the less contentious regulatory process. Jones (1987) describes this as the "action in government" stage.

Stage 3: Program Implementation. In this stage the government's policy is aligned with the problem (Anderson et al., 1984; Jones, 1977). The executive or regulatory body charged with implementing the program develops the guidelines and regulations necessary for a functioning program. In effect, the implementing body translates the authorizing policy into a workable program. Although less contentious than the legislative process, implementation activities of legislative interpretation, planning, and organizing are still very political (Ripley, 1985). In this phase, criteria must be identified for use in evaluation to determine whether a program has met policy goals and objectives.

Interested nursing groups must monitor the *Federal Register* and corresponding state publications for notices of proposed rule making and publication of rules, regulations, standards, and guidelines to ensure that these reflect the original intent of the legitimating body, and to assess their impact on health care delivery and professional practice. Administrative agencies and interest groups frequently use the regulatory process to include program elements they were unable to put into legislation, thereby undermining legislative intent.

Stage 4: Policy Evaluation. This "program to government" phase addresses the question, "Did the policy work?" (Anderson et al., 1984; Jones 1977). The program's implementation, performance, and impact are evaluated to determine how well the program has met its goals and objectives. Evaluation should identify whether a program has satisfactorily met the original concerns and should be continued, or whether segments of the original policy goals remain unmet or new issues have surfaced, thereby restarting the cycle. A program that has met its objectives or is superseded by a newer policy and is no longer necessary may be terminated. An example is the policy of deinstitutionalization of mentally ill persons and the subsequent closure of state mental institutions.

Dye (1987) argues that although the "stages" model offers a rational and systematic schema for policymaking, it fails to explicate "who gets what and why" in policy decisions. Nevertheless, its usefulness lies in simplifying the "how" of a frequently confusing process.

POLICY AND ISSUE ANALYSIS

Policy analysis is the systematic "description and explanation of the causes and consequences of government action" and inaction, not just its goal-oriented activity (Dye, 1987). Historically, a wide range of social science disciplines and professions have focused their research activities on governmental policies as system outputs. More recently the study of policy science theory and methodology has become an interdisciplinary subspecialty, with programs in most major universities. Formally, policy analysis is conducted in universities and policy research firms, which utilize principles and analytic tools from economics, probability theory, and statistics, as well as in legislatures, governmental agencies, or organizations. On the basis of the institution's function, the analyst roles vary from the academically oriented "objective technician," to the more politically oriented "issue advocate," who promotes societal welfare, to the "client advocate," whose role is to develop the best case for the employer (Jenkins-Smith, 1982). Nurses tend to function as issue advocates.

Nurses have a unique perspective for policy decision making because of their clinical knowledge and advocate orientation. They are increasingly visible as stakeholders in health policy debates through policy positions in both legislative and executive branches of government, and as a special interest group. The role of the nurse policy analyst has been identified as a distinct advanced-practice role because it includes components of research, leadership, and change agency (Stimpson & Hanley, 1991). Nurses now receive formal policy preparation in master's and doctoral programs; however, nurses in clinical practice roles also participate in the policy debate and need a format to analyze policy decision making in either the clinical or governmental setting.

Analyst Values and Inherent Bias

Any issue or policy analysis holds the inherent bias of the originating group based on their values, frame of reference, and ideology. Although the analyst strives for objectivity, the truth will be filtered through the stakeholder's values, ideology, perspective, and goals (Dunn, 1981). As a result, the same data may be used to support opposing points of view; only the

Table 6–1 Issue Analysis for Decision Making

CONTEXT (DEFINITION)	POLICY OPTIONS	EVALUATION OF OPTIONS	RECOMMENDED SOLUTION

Policy problem
Background
  Social
  Economic
  Ethical
  Political/legal
Stakeholders
Issue
	Identify policy goals/
	  objectives
	Specify policy options
	  (include "do nothing")
		Set criteria to meet objectives
		Evaluate each option on
		  basis of criteria
		Compare options (use
		  scorecard)	

perspective in viewing the data changes. Nevertheless, analysts within the legislature and administrative agencies sometimes develop proposals not supported by data. Throgmorton (1991, p. 174) addresses the persuasive quality inherent in all policy analyses and suggests that "analysis should stimulate and maintain a conversation among scientist, politicians and lay advocates" to mediate rather than polarize their communication and perspectives.

Approaches to Analysis

Policy analysis comprises a structured approach to problem solving and decision making that is useful in any setting. Stokey and Zeckhauser (1978) offer a useful five-point framework:

1. Establish the context, including definition of the problem and specific objectives.
2. Identify alternatives for resolving the issue.
3. Project consequences for the identified options.
4. Specify criteria for evaluating options' ability to meet objectives.
5. Recommend the optimal solution.

The policy-issue-paper format, the first step in the policy analysis process, serves as a valuable tool in these situations. Table 6–1 outlines a model of the issue analysis process.

SAMPLE ISSUE PAPER

Policy issue papers provide a mechanism to structure the problem at hand and identify the underlying issue. This step is essential to identification of stakeholders and specification of alternatives with both positive and negative consequences. It identifies the variables to be included in full analysis models such as cost-effectiveness or cost-benefit analyses (Hatry, Blair, Fisk, & Kimmel, 1976). Issue papers help to specify arguments to support one's cause, recognize those of opposing stakeholders, and develop strategies to advance the issue through the policy cycle.

This section provides an abbreviated outline of a policy issue paper. It addresses the problem of MCOs' policies determining length of hospital stay because of its implications for both the public and private sectors and its effect on nursing roles.[1]

Problem Identification

Problem identification clarifies the underlying problem. It includes facets such as the causes of the problem, the current and future effects of the

---

[1]The purpose of this example is to illustrate the process of analyzing policy options. It is noted that the Newborns and Mothers Health Protection Act reflects the input of the mother in the length of stay (LOS) decision.

problem on the community, those who raised the issue and those now interested in it, and how the problem moved to the public agenda (Hatry et al., 1976).

The U.S. health care system is dominated by MCOs. As the fee-for-service model declines, managed care models such as health maintenance organizations (HMOs), preferred provider organizations (PPOs), and provider-sponsored organizations (PSOs) increase. By definition, MCOs integrate both finance and delivery of health care services. Because of this link, escalating hospital costs are a major focus of MCO cost containment. Length of stay (LOS) is a specific target, as evidenced in the widely publicized cases of the discharge of mothers and newborn infants in less than 24 hours after birth and of women who have undergone mastectomy on an outpatient basis. Broad media publicity of this change in care standard, based on the publication of a guideline developed by Milliman and Robertson, a Seattle actuarial firm ("More HMOs order . . . ," 1996), has led to the introduction of federal and widespread state legislation: in 1996, more than 1000 bills were introduced (Hellinger, 1996). Although this guideline was intended for routine, uncomplicated cases, such decreased LOS is rapidly becoming the norm, with the potential for inadequate care for some individuals. However, many patients may do well if given adequate support services.

Background

Exploration of the background of the problem provides the context of the issue and should include social, economic, ethical, and political factors.

Social Factors. Many institutions provide supportive care programs such as home visits the next day and 24-hour call lines to reach a registered nurse. However, these programs are not yet the norm. There is potential for people lacking family and environmental support structures to be negatively affected. Blanket early discharge policies do not reflect individual differences in physical condition, circumstances, education, knowledge, and ability to obtain needed care or to identify emerging problems.

Economic Factors. Hospital costs provide strong economic incentives for third-party payers to require discharge of clients as soon as possible. MCOs' failure to use birthing centers for low-risk deliveries, which would lower costs, raises the questions of role perception and control. Physicians are still perceived as the primary providers; advanced practice nurses must market their services to MCOs on the basis of quality of care, cost savings, and client satisfaction.

Ethical Factors. The key principles in conflict here are justice as fairness (each receiving care according to need) versus autonomy (payers' right to determine the amount of care for which they will pay). The drive to reduce costs has the potential effect of denying access to needed care. Additional ethical concerns are infringement on provider autonomy in using professional judgment to determine care that is needed by clients, and clients' autonomy in determining their needs.

Political and Legal Factors. Public pressure on state legislators has led to the introduction and enactment of numerous legislative proposals addressing "drive through" births and mastectomies. At the federal level, President Clinton signed an amendment to P.L. 104-91, the Kassebaum-Kennedy "Health Insurance Portability and Accountability Act" (HIPAA), which ensures new mothers the *option* of 48 hours in the hospital after normal delivery and 96 hours after cesarean delivery ("President signs bill . . . ," 1996).[2] This law amends the Public Health Service Act and, importantly, the Employment Retirement Income Security Act (ERISA).

---

[2]This law is part of the Veterans Administration–Housing and Urban Development appropriation bill (H. R. 3666).

Enactment of such a law at the federal level is technically critical because ERISA exempts self-insured companies, which employ over half of insured individuals, from regulation under state insurance law. State insurance mandates therefore do not apply to over half of the insured population. Further, 52 different laws would create implementation nightmares.

The HIPAA amendment also addresses the need for oversight of implementation. It mandates the U.S. Department of Health and Human Services (DHHS) to initiate an advisory committee to guide the conduct of a DHHS study of issues related to maternity and postmaternity care. The DHHS must report its findings back to Congress in two interim reports and a final report to be made in 2001.

Several state legislatures have also introduced and enacted legislation mandating specified lengths of time for hospitalization after breast cancer surgery. The move toward outpatient mastectomies and lumpectomies is based on Milliman and Robertson's development of an MCO guideline that modified radical mastectomies should be classified as an ambulatory procedure ("Managed care and breast cancer . . . ," 1997).[3] Federally, DHHS Secretary Donna Shalala has issued a policy letter banning managed care mandatory outpatient surgery and limits on hospital stay for breast cancer surgery ("Managed care plans . . . ," 1997). Although there is a growing body of research demonstrating that quality of care and patient satisfaction can be maintained on an outpatient or up-to-23-hour-discharge basis (Burke, Zabka, McCarver, & Singletary, 1997; Gazmararian et al., 1997), such outcomes require comprehensive preoperative teaching and a network for follow-up care.

Issue Statement

The issue statement, usually a question, should be phrased in a way that recognizes the underlying problem and conflicting values and

seeks to identify options. The use of questions, such as "How could/should 'X' be addressed?" removes the focus from a specific policy proposal and allows for objective analysis of the issue. To maintain focus, the analyst must keep the issue statement in mind through each stage of the analysis.

In our example, the issue statement would be: *Who should determine hospital length of stay?*

Stakeholders

Stakeholders are the parties who have a stake in the outcome of the policy debate, such as policymakers with specific proposals to deal with the issue, those who would be potentially affected by the policy, special interest groups (who may or may not be included with the previous group), and those with a position on the issue.

In the LOS case, the key stakeholders are the MCOs. Although they have a distinct economic incentive to reduce stays, they also need to maintain a positive public image so that they can be competitive and attract customers. Physicians have a stake both in preserving their clinical autonomy and in "first do[ing] no harm" to their patients. As the primary hospital care providers, nurses' stake is in protection of patients as well as in protection of their jobs. The public has a stake here because limited LOS policies have the potential for negatively affecting them. Finally, legislators, as representatives of constituents, have a need to demonstrate concern for voters, who put and keep them in office. Further, there is a backlash against MCOs as working and middle-class voters increasingly find their health care options narrowed. Widespread anecdotal reports have persuaded legislators that "something needs to be done." Taking a stand on protection of women, mothers, and babies gives them something positive to tell constituents.

Policy Objectives

The overall objective of the policy should be stated succinctly. It is useful to keep policy objectives foremost when developing policy

---

[3]Milliman and Robertson is a Seattle actuarial firm that sets standards of care for many managed care organizations.

options, to ensure that alternatives could potentially meet the objective and resolve the underlying issue.

In our example, the goal of an LOS decision is to provide consumers with cost-effective care based on their individual need. Objectives toward this end could include the following:

1. To ensure cost-effective care in the most appropriate setting
2. To protect the provider-client relationship in care decision making
3. To protect the rights of both health care workers and clients

Policy Alternatives

Wildavsky (1979) defines policy alternatives as hypotheses: if x is done, then y will be the result. Resources necessary for programs are included, along with program objectives and criteria. In identifying policy alternatives, one may consider any number of proposals under current consideration, including an alternative that the analyst may wish to put forth. It is frequently useful to consider and analyze the "do nothing" option, because there is frequently pressure to preserve the status quo.

Policy alternatives for LOS decisions include the following:

1. Legislative mandate for MCOs to allow providers discretion in determining length of hospital stay
2. Legislative mandate for MCOs to allow providers, in consultation with clients, to determine length of hospital stay
3. Allow MCOs to determine length of hospital stay ("do nothing")

Evaluation of Options

Next, criteria must be identified by which policy options may be evaluated to ensure achievement of the policy goals and objectives. General criteria for evaluation of health policy options include areas such as quality, access, fairness, cost, and administrative and political feasibility. Analysts may identify other criteria

that may be of particular relevance for the policy or the group sponsoring the analysis (e.g., inclusion of reimbursement for nonphysician providers when analyzing proposals for health care and health insurance reform).

Criteria identified for the LOS example include the following:

1. Cost containment
2. Quality
3. Protection of patient rights
4. Protection of provider's professional autonomy
5. Political feasibility

Following is an example of an analysis of Option 1 for illustrative purposes.

OPTION 1: LEGISLATIVE MANDATE FOR PROVIDER DISCRETION IN DETERMINING LENGTH OF HOSPITAL STAY

Cost Containment. The double-digit inflation level of medical costs began a decline in 1991 that brought it just below the consumer price index in 1996. The initial cost savings of managed care, which shadowed prices in the fee-for-service market, although MCOs had enrolled a generally well population (Light, 1997), are thought to have bottomed out. Analysts believe that medical costs will again begin to rise, placing new stress on profit margins for insurers and providers ("Employers should expect . . . ," 1997). These industry pressures increase the need for cost containment wherever possible.

PRO: In general, mandated provider discretion in determining length of hospital stay would increase costs. However, in cases where complications could be prevented, there may be some cost savings.

CON: A legislative mandate for provider discretion in determining LOS could limit the autonomy of MCOs in controlling care delivery and reduce their ability to contain costs.

Quality of Care. There is a growing body of research since the mid-1980s on the outcomes of shortened maternity and breast cancer LOS. Findings reveal that, in general, patients do well as long as they have comprehensive prehospitalization education and posthospitalization services such as 24-hour access to professional consultation and home visits as needed (Burke et al., 1997; Gazmararian et al., 1997).

PRO: A legislative mandate may offer increased quality of care, particularly for patients who have complex problems or who may be at risk of complications.

CON: Many institutions have developed comprehensive programs for maternity and breast cancer surgery patients and caregivers, including preoperative teaching and posthospitalization follow-up services, and have demonstrated high patient satisfaction and quality outcomes. A legislative mandate may impede development of such programs.

Protection of Patient Autonomy. Autonomy is a basic principle of medical ethics. It addresses the patient's right to make choices in health care (Bodenheimer & Grumbach, 1995). Although there was a strong emphasis on patients' rights during the decade of the 1980s, the current emphasis is increasingly on patient responsibility (Mason, McEachen, & Kovner, 1993). Restriction of consumer freedom of choice is essentially a defining characteristic of managed care.

PRO: Patients' rights to perceived needed care would be protected, as long as those who want early discharge can have it. Such legislative mandates can be viewed as consumer protection initiatives to counter profit-driven insurer policies.

CON: None.

Protection of Provider Professional Autonomy. The link of primary care providers with MCOs leads to infringement on the providers' ability to make medical decisions, which may increase costs. MCO-dictated LOS is an example.

To counteract the public backlash against MCOs, the American Association of Health Plans (AAHP) developed a series of principles to "reaffirm the central role of physicians in directing medical decision-making" ("AAHP sets 'physician-central' policies," 1997). Member MCO plans are required to include physicians in programs such as quality assessment and improvement and utilization management.

PRO: A legislative mandate specifying an option for an increased LOS would increase provider autonomy.

CON: A mandate specifying LOS would interfere with provider autonomy.

Political Feasibility

The criterion of political feasibility refers to the likelihood of political support for enactment of the policy. Maternity and mastectomy LOS may be viewed as "motherhood and apple pie" issues strongly endorsed by voters. Even conservative legislators may therefore be wary of voting against them, especially if facing reelection in the near future.

PRO: In general, more liberal legislators tend to support regulation of health care delivery. Further, anecdotal reports of care limitations by MCOs publicized by the media have fed a public backlash against restrictive MCO policies, leading to development of such legislation.

CON: As more economically conservative, probusiness legislators have been elected in recent years, enactment of additional insurance mandates may not be politically feasible.

Comparison of Alternatives

After analysis of all the identified policy options, the findings are evaluated and summarized. The analyst may then make a recommendation for the best policy to deal with the issue. The *scorecard* format is a useful way to summa-

Table 6–2 Policy Alternatives Scorecard

CRITERIA	MAND PRO	MAND PRO/PT	SELF-REG
Cost containment	–/+	–/+	++
Quality of care	+	++	–/+
Patient autonomy	–/+	++	–
Provider autonomy	++	++	–
Political feasibility	+	+	–/+

MAND PRO = Mandatory provider determination of LOS; MAND PRO/PT = Mandatory provider/patient determination of LOS; SELF-REG = Allowing MCO industry to self-regulate ("do nothing"); ++ = Strongly positive; + = Positive; – = Negative.

rize analysis findings. This includes a two-dimensional grid, with the evaluation criteria on the left column and the alternative policies on the horizontal. A summarizing notation on each criterion is made for each alternative. The policymaker is then able to compare the strengths and weaknesses of each alternative side by side. A scoring system is established, such as the plus-minus system used here, designation of "high, medium, and low," or brief verbal descriptions. In the model scorecard shown in Table 6–2, hypothetical "scores" are included for the other alternatives for illustrative purposes.

Results of Analysis

The results of the analysis depicted in Table 6–2 indicate that Option 2 (Mandatory MCO Provider/Patient Determination of LOS) scores highest, with Option 1 (Mandatory MCO Provider Determination of LOS) a close second when compared across criteria. MCO self-regulation scores strongly positive only in cost containment. It scores –/+ on quality because it may stimulate development of care models that enhance quality of care; however, the implementation of a shortened LOS policy before safeguards, such as comprehensive preoperative teaching and home follow-up networks, are in place could be potentially harmful. Patient autonomy is directly addressed only in Option 2. As patients take increased responsibility for their

care, it is fitting that they have input into LOS decision making. Provider autonomy is directly addressed in Options 1 and 2; Option 3 receives a partial positive score because of the industry (AAHP) initiative to reaffirm the centrality of physician decision making. Finally, political feasibility is comparable for Options 1 and 2 because of the current backlash against MCOs.

CONCLUSION

Nurses' participation in the policy process through their primary roles as analysts or their secondary roles as clinical/professional advocates through their institutions or organizations will ensure the inclusion of their unique perspective in private sector and governmental policy decisions. The definitions, sequential model of the policy cycle, and outline of a policy issue paper as described herein offer tools to facilitate nurses' participation. Issues such as LOS decision making directly impact nursing practice and demonstrate the need for nurses' input into the policymaking process. Decision making in any professional situation requires clear, systematic thinking; the analytical approach described here is directly applicable.

REFERENCES

AAHP sets "physician-central" policies, latest initiative in patient campaign. (1997, May 19). *BNA Health Care Policy Report, 5*(20), 800.

Advisory panel on maternity stays still pending Shalala appointments. (1997, January 6). *BNA Health Care Policy Report, 5*(1), 5.

Anderson, J. E. (1990). *Public policymaking.* Boston: Houghton-Mifflin.

Anderson, J. E., Brady, D. W., Bullock III, C. S., & Stewart, Jr., J. (1984). *Public policy and politics in America.* Monterey, CA: Brooks/Cole.

Bodenheimer, T. S., & Grumbach, K. (1995). *Understanding health policy: A clinical approach.* Norwalk, CT: Appleton & Lange.

Burke, C. C., Zabka, C. L., McCarver, K. J., & Singletary, E. (1997). Patient satisfaction with 23-hour "short stay" observation following breast cancer surgery. *Oncology Nursing Forum, 24*(4), 645–651.

Cohen, M. D., March, J. G., & Olsen, J. P. (1972, March). A garbage can model of organizational choice. *Administrative Science Quarterly, 17,* 1–25.

Dunn, W. N. (1981). *Public policy analysis.* Englewood Cliffs, NJ: Prentice-Hall.

Dye, T. R. (1987). *Understanding public policy.* Englewood Cliffs, NJ: Prentice-Hall.

Employers should expect gradual climb in medical costs over next few years. (1997, May 19). *BNA Health Care Policy Report, 5*(20), 801–803.

Friedman, E. (1997). Managed care, rationing and quality: A tangled relationship. *Health Affairs, 16*(3), 174–182.

Gazmararian, J. A., Koplan, J. P., Cogswell, M. E., Bailey, C. M., Davis, N. A., & Cutler, C. M. (1997). Maternity experiences in a managed care organization. *Health Affairs, 16*(3), 198–208.

Gwartney, J. D., & Stroup, R. L. (1987). *Microeconomics: Private and public choice.* Orlando, FL: Harcourt Brace Jovanovich.

Hatry, H., Blair, L., Fisk, D., & Kimmel, W. (1976). *Program analysis for state and local governments.* Washington, DC: The Urban Institute.

Hayes, M. T. (1992). *Incrementalism and public policy.* NY: Logman.

Helco, H. H. (1972, January). Review article: Policy analysis. *British Journal of Political Science, 2,* 83–108.

Hellinger, F. J. (1996). The expanding scope of state legislation. *Journal of the American Medical Association, 276*(13), 1065–1070.

Jenkins-Smith, S. (1982). Professional roles for policy analysts: A critical assessment. *Journal of Policy Analysis and Management, 2,* 88–93.

Jones, C. O. (1977). *An introduction to the study of public policy.* North Scituate, MA: Duxbury Press.

Kingdon, J. W. (1995). *Agendas, alternatives, and public policies.* Boston: Little, Brown.

Light, D. W. (1997). The restructuring of the American health care system. In T. J. Litman & L. S. Robins (Eds.), *Health politics and policy* (3rd ed.). Albany, NY: Delmar.

Lindblom, C. E. (1996). The science of "muddling through." In D. C. McCool (Ed.), *Public policy theories, models and concepts: An anthology* (pp. 142–157). Englewood Cliffs, NJ: Prentice-Hall.

Lindblom, C. E. (1987). Still muddling, not yet through. In D. L. Yarwood (Ed.), *Public administration politics and the people* (pp. 222–233). New York: Longman.

Managed care and breast cancer: Questions and strategies. (1997, January). *NABCO News.* National Alliance of Breast Cancer Organizations.

Managed care plans may not mandate certain breast cancer treatment limits. (1997, February 17). *BNA's Health Care Policy Report, 5*(7), 271.

Mason, D. J., McEachen, I., & Kovner, C. T. (1993). Contemporary issues in the workplace. In D. J. Mason, S. W. Talbott, & J. K. Leavitt (Eds.), *Policy and politics for nurses* (pp. 223–240). Philadelphia: W. B. Saunders.

More HMOs order outpatient mastectomies. (1996, November 16). *Wall Street Journal,* B1, 8.

Nelson, B. J. (1978). Setting the policy agenda. In J. May & A. Wildavsky (Eds.), *The policy cycle* (pp. 17–42). Beverly Hills, CA: Sage.

Petracca, M. P. (1992). The rediscovery of interest group politics. In M. P. Petracca (Ed.), *The politics of interests* (pp. 3–31). Boulder, CO: Westview Press.

President signs bill to expand maternity, mental health coverage. (1996, September 30). *BNA Health Care Policy Report, (4)*36, 1531–1532.

Ripley, R. B. (1985). *Policy analysis in political science.* Chicago: Nelson-Hall.

Ripley, R. B. (1996). Stages of the policy process. In D. C. McCool (Ed.), *Public policy theories, models and concepts: An anthology* (pp. 157–162). Englewood Cliffs, NJ: Prentice-Hall.

Sabatier, P. A. (1991). Toward better theories of the policy process. *PS: Political Science and Politics, 24*(2), 147–156.

Simon, H. A. (1955). A behavioral model of rational choice. *Quarterly Journal of Economics, 69,* February. (As cited in Lindblom, 1968, *The policymaking process.* Englewood Cliffs, NJ: Prentice-Hall.)

Stimpson, M., & Hanley, B. (1991). Nurse policy analyst: Advanced practice role. *Nursing and Health Care, 12*(1), 10–15.

Stokey, E., & Zeckhauser, R. (1978). *A primer for policy analysis.* New York: W. W. Norton.

Stone, D. (1992). *The policy paradox: The art of political decision making.* New York: W. W. Norton.

Throgmorton, J. A. (1991). The rhetoric of policy analysis. *Policy Sciences, 24*(2), 153–179.

Wildavsky, A. (1979). *Speaking truth to power.* Boston: Little, Brown.

Williams, C. H. (1991). Doing critical thinking together: Applications to government, politics and public policy. *PS: Political Science & Politics, 24*(3), 510–516.

Chapter 7

POLITICAL ANALYSIS AND STRATEGY

SALLY S. COHEN, JUDITH K. LEAVITT, MARY ALICE LEONHARDT,
AND DIANA J. MASON

If policies are the outcomes or choices that public or private entities make to achieve certain goals, then politics is the means to those ends, or the interactions among players that result in certain outcomes. Harold Laswell's classic definition of politics as "who gets what, when, and how" (Laswell, 1958) still holds true today. Analyzing the politics of an issue can enhance an understanding of the stakes, players, and strategies needed to achieve certain desired outcomes. Unraveling the politics also sheds light on the substance of the debates and critical bargaining points. All these are important for nurses and others who are looking to influence policy, especially the course of policy deliberations.

Political scientists have developed numerous models for analyzing the politics of policy formation and implementation. These models may help nurses interpret political events surrounding issues such as funding for nursing education and research, achieving Medicaid reform, obtaining direct Medicare reimbursement, family planning, and providing community-based care for elderly and disabled persons.

This chapter presents a framework for political analysis. It covers key political concepts, including power and conflict, and offers ways to analyze political situations. It concludes with strategies for enhancing ways in which nurses can be effective as political players.

POLICY ARENAS AND THE POLITICS OF POLICYMAKING

Theodore Lowi (1964) developed what has become a somewhat classic scheme of policy arenas. He claimed that the pluralist model (based on groups as the major unit of analysis) failed to acknowledge that most players interacted primarily with people on their own side, not with all groups involved with a particular issue. Furthermore, there was little evidence that legislators were swayed by interest groups, one way or the other. Lowi also claimed that C. Wright Mills' elitist model (based on the notion that a handful of business, political, and military interests dominate political and social structures) failed because only a small number of business groups were ever aligned with one side; military groups were hardly ever involved; and power in Congress was too fragmented to depend on a small group of people to make important national decisions.

Lowi based his work on the notion that "the types of relationships to be found among people are determined by their expectations—by what they hope to achieve or get from relating to others" (Lowi, 1964, p. 688). Politically, people's expectations are based on governmental outputs or policies. "Therefore, a political relationship is determined by the type of policy at stake, so that

This chapter draws on two excellent chapters in the second edition of this book: Vernice Ferguson's chapter "Perspectives on Power" and Susan Talbott's "Political Analysis: Structure and Process." We are grateful for their vision, insight, and analysis in this work.

for every type of policy, there is likely to be a distinctive type of political relationship" (p. 688). In short, the type of policy determines the *politics.*

On the basis of these ideas, Lowi identified three major policy arenas: *distributive, regulatory,* and *redistributive.* These categories provide a context for understanding the current political issues. According to Lowi, each arena "tends to develop its own characteristic political structure, political process, elites and group relations" (Lowi, 1964, pp. 689–690). It is useful to review their meanings because they provide a way of understanding politics and analyzing political situations.

In the distributive arena, decisions are made almost as if there were unlimited resources. They are often referred to as "pork barrel programs" that tend to "produce only winners, not losers, and involve a high degree of cooperation and mutually rewarding logrolling" (Newman, 1995, p. 145). Distributive policies are characterized by patronage and tend to maintain the status quo. In a sense, distributive policies "keep larger social questions from becoming issues of public policy" (Lowi & Ginsberg, cited in Newman, 1995, p. 148). Although there may be many groups involved, there is little need for coalitions because all the individuals or groups manage to succeed with their political aims. An example of a distributive program is federal scholarships for nurse practitioners who agree to practice in underserved areas. Few would oppose such an initiative (Weissert, 1996).

The regulatory arena is one that most resembles the pluralist model. Many groups, often organized or forming coalitions around certain issues, are typically involved. However, the coalitions are often short lived because of the changing dynamics and interests of the groups. Unlike distributive policies, regulatory policies "involve a direct choice as to who will be indulged and who deprived" (Lowi, 1964, pp. 690–691). Regulatory policies typically involve "formulating or implementing rules imposing obligations on individuals and punishment for nonconformance." Regulatory agencies tend to be small but to have significant influence in their "particular sector of regulation" (Newman, 1995, p. 145). Examples of regulatory policies include insurance and regulation of health professions.

Redistributive policies entail the reallocation of resources or rights among groups or social classes. Policies regarding health, welfare, labor, and many education programs are considered redistributive. They tend to affect society on a "larger scale" than the other arenas, and they often generate conflicts between the rich and poor, old and young, or employed and unemployed, or among racial and ethnic groups, as with affirmative action policies. The policymaking process is characterized by high levels of visibility and conflict and often upsets the status quo (Newman, 1995, p. 146). Many of the social and health policy issues on federal and state agendas today are redistributive in nature.

What can we learn from these arenas of policy? First, they provide a framework for understanding different types of policy discussions. Recognizing, for example, that a policy is redistributive enables one to expect a certain intensity of interactions and political conflicts. Second, identification of the type of arena can enhance one's ability to develop political strategies. For example, when engaged in regulatory deliberations, one would tend to form coalitions, recognizing that they are short term in nature, and to forge ahead with strategies that focus on administrative agencies involved with specific policies. This contrasts to the more expansive policies of the redistributive arena regarding issues such as health care or welfare reform, which entail significant vying among groups and the use of language that focuses on winners and losers.

One political scientist recently studied how Lowi's typology of federal policies applies to the work environment of state agencies and to female involvement in those policy arenas. For example, policies, such as health and welfare, that typically interest and involve women tend to be redistributive and characterized by a high degree of conflict (Newman, 1995, p. 161). Because nurses who are active in policy typically focus on health and welfare issues, they can expect that much of the political work they engage in will be characterized by power and conflict struggles.

THE CONCEPT OF POWER IN POLITICAL ANALYSIS

Power is one of the most complex political and sociological concepts to define and measure. It is also a term that politicians and policy analysts use freely, without necessarily giving thought to what it means. One of the most widely used definitions of power is Max Weber's:

> Power . . . is the probability that one actor within a social relationship will be in a position to carry out his own will despite resistance, regardless of the basis on which this probability rests. [quoted in Duke, 1976, p. 40]

Power can be a means to an end, or an end in itself. Power also can be actual or potential. The latter implies power as undeveloped but a "force to be reckoned with" (Kelly & Joel, 1995, p. 367). Many in political circles depict the nursing profession as a potential political force given the millions of nurses in this country and the power we could wield if most participated in politics and policy formation.

There are no absolute or definitive models of power, and at times, aspects of power can seem contradictory. That is, power may be considered a prerequisite for social or political action, or it may be an indicator of behavior or a result of a certain action. Sometimes power is asymmetrical, as when one person or group has more control than another. In other circumstances, power is more symmetrical, involving reciprocal influences between two parties, such as between leaders and followers (Duke, 1976). Finally, power can be considered a zero-sum entity in which one person or group's possession of power precludes possession by another. In other cases, power is a less restricted and more "sharable commodity," with its benefits being

distributed among many parties (Duke, 1976, p. 42). All these perspectives illustrate the dynamic nature of power and ways in which nurses can analyze and use power to their advantage.

French and Raven (1959) developed a frequently cited typology of sources of power, which Hersey, Blanchard, and Natemeyer (1979) subsequently expanded to seven power bases:

1. *Coercive power,* rooted in real or perceived fear of one person by another
2. *Reward power,* based on the perception of the potential for rewards or favors by honoring the wishes of a powerful person
3. *Legitimate (or positional) power,* derived from an organizational position rather than personal qualities
4. *Expert power,* based on knowledge, special talents, or skills, in contrast to positional power
5. *Referent power,* emanating from admiration, charisma, or belief and some type of mutual identification between people with similar backgrounds
6. *Information power,* resulting when one individual has (or is perceived to have) special information that another individual desires
7. *Connection power,* granted to those perceived to have privileged connections with individuals or organizations (Ferguson, 1993; Kelly & Joel, 1995).

These bases of power provide a framework for understanding the dynamics of power in political situations, whether in work, community, organizational, or government settings.

Some feminist scholars claim that these bases of power assume "masculine norms as the standard of behavior" and fail to account for the complexity of the "gender power and leadership nexus" (Kelly & Duerst-Lahti, 1995, p. 46). The term *gender power* focuses on the sources of power available to women, based on structural, individual, organizational, interpersonal, and symbolic factors. In the contexts of politics and government, "the gender power balance has been in men's favor" (Kelly & Duerst-Lahti,

1995, p. 47), although there is evidence that this is slowly changing. Understanding the ways in which power affects women politically is important for nursing.

Politically, there is ample evidence that nurses have succeeded in flexing their political muscles and have demonstrated the power behind their political effectiveness. Examples include direct Medicare reimbursement for advanced practice nurses as part of the 1997 budget bill; legislation creating the National Institute of Nursing Research in the early 1990s; breakthrough enactment of legislation establishing the National Center for Nursing Research in 1985; and numerous collaborative efforts with other groups in areas such as advancing women's health and protecting patients' rights under managed care at state levels of government.

Nurses can also benefit from looking at the headway made by women politicians. These trend setters demonstrate the value of working with other women to enact certain health and social welfare policies. For example, in early 1997, the nine women senators formed a bipartisan coalition advocating legislation regarding mammograms. They pushed their bill through the Senate by a vote of 98 to 0 and identified other issues important to women, such as educating homemakers on establishing their own individual retirement accounts ("Gender power," 1997).

Women and nurses have a lot of potential power to execute in increasing the number of elected and appointed positions they hold. The "avenues to influence legislation have been opening for women lawmakers" and their supporters, but recent studies show that "it is not enough to be elected" if women want to exert influence in political decision making (Norton, 1995, p. 117). The way to broaden one's power base is to achieve power through many methods, including obtaining legitimate stature as elected officials, aligning oneself with candidates who hold positions on issues similar to one's own, and joining coalitions with other groups. These and other strategies are discussed in more detail at the end of the chapter.

CONFLICT IN POLITICAL ANALYSIS

Conflict is an inherent part of the political process, especially as people vie for power. Conflict occurs whenever an individual's or group's "action is oriented intentionally to carrying out the actor's own will against the resistance of the other party or parties" (Max Weber, cited in Duke, 1976, p. 43). Another way of looking at conflict is to understand that it arises when there are limited resources or rewards such that one individual or party gains at the expense of the other (Duke, 1976, p. 43). Thus, in many ways, conflict is inevitable because in every society there is always a scarcity of some type of good or service (Duke, 1976). The ubiquitous nature of conflict should help nurses realize that, like power, conflict is unavoidable and something to be addressed rather than avoided.

A renowned political scientist, E. E. Schattschneider (1960), developed a useful framework for understanding the role of conflict in political situations. He described how expanding the scope of a conflict, or what he called the "contagiousness of conflict," could affect the outcome of political deliberations. As he explained, "competitiveness is the mechanism for the expansion of the scope of conflict" (Schattschneider, 1960, pp. 17–18). The loser may call in outside groups to shift the balance of power. New scope and balance can make possible many things and can also make many things impossible.

According to Schattschneider, every conflict has two parts: the individuals engaged and the audience attracted to the conflict. The audience is never neutral. Once people become involved, they take a side and influence the outcome. Therefore the "most important strategy of politics is concerned with the scope of the conflict" (Schattschneider, 1960, p. 3).

Schattschneider also pointed out the importance of visibility. One can't expand scope without making issues visible to one's constituency and outside audiences. As he explained, "a democratic government lives by publicity" (p. 16). According to Schattschneider, "politics is the socialization of conflict." Moreover, as long as the conflict remains private, the political process is limited, if initiated at all. "Conflicts become political only when an attempt is made to involve the wider public" (Schattschneider, 1960, p. 39).

The significance of these words to nurses looking to exert political influence is that, first, expanding the scope of conflict can be a strategy for achieving political change, used by one's friends and foes alike. Second, when the scope of conflict is expanded, it is important to engage the media and other avenues of publicity. Of course, this doesn't ensure that the outcome will be as one hopes. The outcome is dependent on many other factors, including "which of a multitude of possible conflicts gains the dominant position" (Schattschneider, 1960, p. 62).

Thus, power and conflict can be seen as critical features of the political process. With a sound understanding of the political environment, nurses are well equipped to engage in political work involving any aspect of government, organizations, the workplace, or community.

POLITICAL ANALYSIS OF SITUATIONS

The best approach to accomplish change must include a thoughtful analysis of the politics of the problem and proposed solutions (Gerston, 1997). Although this chapter explores the *political* analysis of a problem and proposed solutions, the reader is referred to Chapter 6 for an in-depth discussion of *policy* analysis. These two analytic processes should actually be done simultaneously. In fact, the impact of not doing so was exemplified in the demise of President Clinton's Health Security Act. Much attention and praise was given to the policy process of developing the president's plan for health care reform. Many small groups met to analyze the various dimensions of the problems in health care and possible solutions; however, a comparable process was not used for the political analysis of how to move the issue until the opposition had been mobilized.

A *political* analysis should include the following steps: (1) identifying and analyzing the problem and proposed solutions; (2) taking into account the various environments where the issues matter; (3) identifying the arenas where nursing's political clout can be best utilized to accomplish change; (4) evaluating the stake holders; and (5) recognizing the resources available, both financial and human, to win nursing's issues. Once this type of political assessment has been performed in relation to the problem, strategies for moving proposed solutions can be designed and successfully implemented. The section that follows uses advanced practice nursing issues to highlight the process of political analysis and strategy development (see examples below).

Problem and Solution Identification

The first step in conducting a political analysis is to identify the problem clearly (Backer, 1991). What is its scope, duration, history, and whom does it affect? What data are available to describe the issue and its ramifications? Is the stated problem the true issue? Is this a public issue (i.e., one for government to address), is it a workplace issue, or can it be a workplace issue that has relevance to government officials, such as health and safety precautions related to the transmission of human immunodeficiency virus?

Sometimes what appears to be the problem is not. For example, proposed mandatory continuing education for nurses is not a problem; rather, it is a possible solution to the issue of ensuring the competency of nurses. After an analysis of the issue of provider competence, one might review the policy options and establish a goal that includes legislating mandatory continuing education. The danger of framing solutions as problems is that it can close off creative thinking about the underlying issues, and the best solution may remain uncovered.

Both the problem and the proposed solutions need to be clearly and concisely defined; however, such clarity requires immersion in the details and nuances of the issue. Preliminary analyses may suggest that more research is needed.

There are many problems confronting advanced practice nurses (APNs):

The expanding roles of nurses, particularly of APNs, have developed through a patchwork of legislation, regulations, judicial interpretations, agency rulings, advisory opinions, and practice standards. Because the definition of nursing practice for all levels varies from state to state, what constitutes nursing practice at each level of licensure in various practice settings is inconsistently determined and often inappropriately restricted. The most common issues confronting nurses today include educational preparation; prescriptive authority; ability to practice without physician supervision; reimbursement; and the acquisition of credentials and privileges in the context of managed care organizations, provider-sponsored networks, and integrated service networks.

Clearly, there are many issues or problems that one could focus on just in relation to advanced practice nursing. In-depth information on various problems, their ramifications, and their context will facilitate establishing priorities, designing creative solutions, and developing an effective plan for action.

Environmental Context

Understanding the environmental context in which the problem and its proposed solutions occur is the next critical component of a political analysis. It enables those attempting to move an issue along to become aware of the forces that will support or obstruct them. In addition, an assessment of the environment provides an understanding of the values that may need to be addressed through the solutions or political strategy. Points of analysis might include the following:

• What are the current *values, priorities, and concerns* in the environment? What are the issues and concerns related to ethnicity and class? Is this a community that embraces for-profit, venture businesses? If so, a proposal to ban for-profit hospital takeovers is likely doomed to failure. If cost concerns are a priority, one will need to frame the arguments accordingly. Sometimes it may be a stretch to do so, but even a token gesture to acknowledge the importance of this value may assuage those who are concerned about financial constraints. For example, any change that is being proposed within an organization undergoing downsizing must address either the revenues that will be enhanced by the project or the cost savings that will be generated. (For a discussion of how to conduct a cost analysis, see Chapter 12.)

• What *history* might be playing out in the current environment? For example, in the United States, one would not be successful in moving social welfare legislation that was associated with high taxes because of our culture of individualism, which is less dominant in countries with a socialist philosophy, such as the Scandinavian countries.

• What is the current *sociopolitical* context operative in the environment? What are the dominant groups in the community? What is the dominant political party? Is this a community or group that needs to be organized, or is it one that is actively engaged around issues? What are the "hot" issues of concern? What is not of concern or is missing from the community's or organization's agenda? For example, approaching the head of the hospital to support a publicly sensitive venture is inappropriate when the institution has just made the front page of the local newspaper for questionable financial practices.

• What are the *trends* in the community? Answering this question requires knowing the demographic characteristics of the community or organization, as well as anticipated national and global trends that may play out at the local level in the near future. For instance, is long-term care an unmet need that you can respond to in a community faced with an increasingly older population with inadequate support services? Or is your issue something that can be part of the overall plan for "empowerment zones" (communities targeted by the federal government for financial and business development)?

An example of how the sociopolitical climate must always be ripe for any effort to change nursing practice and reimbursement was demonstrated by Koch, Pazaki, and Campbell (1992) when they performed an exhaustive study of nursing practice in the mid 1980s. They documented how history, psychology, sociology, politics, and economics have helped to crystallize and perpetuate physician dominance over nursing practice. They concluded that the social, political, and economic position of nurses, particularly of nurse practitioners, was cemented by the interrelated factors of labor market competition and professionalism. Several factors have contributed to an expansion of nurses' roles in health care delivery toward more autonomous practice and their growing conflicts with the traditionally male-dominated medical profession. These factors include (1) the success of the women's and civil rights movements; (2) focus on access to care as a political concern; and (3) the perceived shortage of primary care physicians (Phillips, 1985; Safriet, 1992; Stolberg, 1997). Nevertheless, nurses' efforts to pierce through the numerous barriers to autonomy and sovereignty (Heffernan, 1995; Inglis & Kjervik, 1993; Pearson, 1998) continue to be met with fierce resistance by physicians against what they perceive as intrusions on their turf. When nurses try to eliminate these barriers, they can expect hostility and often retaliatory conduct from physicians and others within their own workplaces and from medical societies. On the other hand, environments such as community-based clinics or physician practices may welcome linkages with nurse practitioners and can serve as favorable demonstration sites. The current societal focus on reducing costs and emphasizing prevention has created a supportive context for policymakers to be open to innovative delivery systems that can demonstrate these goals, including cost-effectiveness. According to one study (Bissinger, Allred, Arford, & Bellig, 1997), if APNs were used to their full potential, an estimated $6.4 to $8.75 billion would be saved on an annual basis. Other studies show cost savings to using APNs, too (Nichols, 1992). The inescapable reality in the 1990s is that the current health care economics and consumer demand for quality care are fostering a more nurse-friendly environment in all health settings.

The political forces at play in any environment will provide a good gauge for determining whether any effort to effect change will succeed. They also point to the sources of power and conflict.

Political Arenas

Once the problems and solutions have been clearly identified and described, the appropriate *political* arenas for influencing the issues need to be analyzed. Most often, this begins by identifying the entities that have jurisdiction and responsibility for the problem and proposed solutions. For instance, is this a public issue, a private issue, or one that involves both sectors? A common mistake that nurses sometimes make is to approach a state legislator with a federal issue over which he or she has no jurisdiction. Some nurses look to public officials to "fix" a workplace issue that would seldom, if ever, receive governmental attention. On the other hand, issues that appear to be the jurisdiction of only the private sector can become public issues. For example, many maternity nurses and pediatricians became concerned about premature discharges of postpartum women and newborn infants. Although they fought this issue in the workplace, media attention on distressed new mothers led to its becoming an issue of concern to the public. States, and eventually the Congress, took up the issue. Legislation (public sector) was passed that required insurance and managed care organizations (private sector) to cover 48-hour minimum maternity stays if the mother and her provider deemed it necessary.

Another example of identifying the appropriate arenas for moving an issue is "entry into practice." Although there have been legislative and regulatory decisions that define APNs' licensure requirements and scope of practice, the profession has not been able to move legislation (except in North Dakota) that defines educational requirements for entry into professional nursing practice. One "entry into practice" option would require a minimum of a baccalaureate degree for licensure as a registered nurse. State legislators see this as a professional issue, rather than an issue to be dealt with in the public arena. They claim that until there is consensus from within the nursing community, they are hesitant to become involved. With few exceptions, nursing has been reluctant to push this issue because it has been so divisive in the past. As a result, the entry-into-practice bills have never been adopted by most states.

At an institutional level, once the relevant political arenas are identified, the formal and informal structures and functioning of that arena need to be analyzed. The formal dimensions of the entity can often be assessed through documents related to the organization's mission, goals, objectives, table of organization, constitution and bylaws, annual report (including financial statement), long-range plans, governing body, committees, departments, and individuals with jurisdiction. In the government arena, one needs to know the legislative and regulatory processes as described in Chapters 22, 24, 25, and 26. In addition, many states and local governments have publications describing their organizational structure and processes.

Questions that should be included in any analysis of the political arenas include the following:

- What is the organizational structure? Is it a public or private entity? Is it a for-profit or a not-for-profit entity? Is it a state or local government? Is it the legislative, executive, or judicial branch that has primary jurisdiction over the issue at this point? Which legislative chamber has primary jurisdiction (e.g., some political appointments are approved by only one chamber of the legislature)? What are the stated mission, goals, and objectives of the entity? For example, a nurse working in women's health in a Catholic hospital should not expect to get support for a new abortion service.

- What subgroups or committees have jurisdiction over the issue? Committees can be important places in which to influence an issue. Nurses should seek committee appointments in

> **TIPS ON COMMITTEE INVOLVEMENT**
>
> - The person who chairs a committee and sets the meeting agenda has a major influence on the direction of the committee's work.
> - The person who takes minutes influences the manner in which the committee activities are recorded.
> - The committee secretary can keep the participants focused on the agenda by alerting the chair when the group's attention strays. She might also offer to summarize the discussion to help the committee determine a plan of action.
> - A committee member can influence action on an item of concern by lobbying other members before the meeting.
> - Sometimes a member's initial efforts to influence action fail, but will be successful the second time.
> - A member who wants to work on a particular committee should seek out the chair to find out details of the committee's work and then ask to be appointed.

their workplaces and elsewhere. See the box above for tips on committee involvement.

- What are the formal methods of communication? What is the table of organization and the chain of command?

- What are the informal processes and methods of communication? A well-known example of the power of informal processes and communication is the case of the business lunch or the golf game, which in the past may have excluded women. It is just as likely that informal communication occurs at cocktail parties, dinners, or other social situations in which personal connections are important.

- What financial and human resources are available?

- What is the budget process? How much money is allocated to a particular cost center or budget line? Who decides how the funds will be used? How is the use of funds evaluated?

How might an individual or group influence the budget process?

• Does the entity use parliamentary procedure? Parliamentary procedure provides a democratic process that carefully balances the rights of individuals, subgroups within an organization, and the membership of an assembly. The basic rules are outlined in *Robert's Rules of Order Newly Revised* (Robert, 1990) (see also Nichols, 1985, pp. 149–150).

The following APN example demonstrates the importance of first identifying the appropriate political arena(s) for moving an issue:

EXAMPLE

APNs have focused on the legislative arena for moving their issues and concerns. This focus was warranted because nurse practice acts in most states actually provided legal barriers to APN practice; however, regulatory reform may be a more expeditious route to remove some barriers to practice. For example, changes in health, insurance, social service, or other state departmental regulations can address issues such as naming APNs as providers in regulations that previously specified "physicians." Several years of effort by nurses in Connecticut directed at expanding Medicaid reimbursement for APN service culminated in the issuance of revised regulations by the Connecticut Department of Social Services, allowing for all types of APNs in any geographic setting to be reimbursed at 90% of the physician-based payment level for services provided to Medicaid beneficiaries. These efforts required a working knowledge of the executive branch of state government. Most other states have approved similar regulations after enactment of federal legislation in the late 1980s requiring states to pay for services of certain APNs (Hoffman, 1994).

Stakeholders

Once the issue and political arenas have been analyzed, the overt and potential "stakeholders" must be identified. The stakeholders are those parties who have influence over the issue or who could be mobilized to care about the issue. In some cases, stakeholders are self-evident. For example, nurse practitioners are stakeholders in issues concerning reimbursement of primary care providers under Medicare. In other situations, stakeholders can be created by helping them to see the connections between the issue and their interests.

Careful consideration should be given to the following questions:

• Who are the overt stakeholders in this issue?

• Who could be turned into stakeholders by virtue of their interests and values? Nursing has increasingly realized the potential of consumer power in moving nursing and health care issues. For example, nurses have worked with the American Association of Retired Persons on long-term care, with the Children's Defense Fund in advocating for child health, and with the American Cancer Society on tobacco issues.

• Who has power in relation to the issue and other stakeholders? Who brings a powerful voice or presence to the issue? For example, before running for office, Congresswoman Carolyn McCarthy became a respected and powerful spokesperson around gun control because of the media coverage of the fatal shooting of her husband (see Chapter 30). Certainly, she was able to mobilize other victims of gun violence (stakeholders) during her campaigns for gun control and for Congress.

• What kind of relationships do you or others have with key stakeholders? For example, who is playing golf with the chair of the insurance committee in the legislature that has jurisdiction over bills related to reimbursement of nurses? Or whose children are in the same class as the chair's?

• Which of these stakeholders are potential supporters or opponents? Can any of the opponents be converted to supporters?

• What are the values, priorities, and concerns of the stakeholders? How can these be tapped in planning political strategy?

- Are the supportive stakeholders of the issue reflective of the constituency who will be affected by the issue? For example, one of the failures of entry into practice legislation was its lack of support by ethnic minority nurses who were concerned that financial and other barriers would prevent their attainment of a baccalaureate degree.

A variety of potential stakeholders must be taken into consideration when one is developing a strategy for advanced practice nursing issues:

EXAMPLE

The cascade of recent national and state-level managed care reform legislation, passed largely in response to the **consumer** outcry against health care policies that put profits before patient needs and safety, demonstrates the tremendous political clout of consumer groups. Because consumers are generally strong advocates of nurses, they are among the most powerful allies that nurses can rely on to accomplish nursing's agenda. Building relationships with individual consumers, as well as consumer groups, who will speak in support of legislative and regulatory initiatives benefiting nurses will significantly enhance the likelihood of successful outcomes. Legislative efforts proposed by nurses will "catch fire" when nurses make consumers and their advocates their teammates.

The American Medical Association, state medical societies, most **physicians,** and other physician-based professional organizations, reeling from the harsh reality that managed care is driving down reimbursement levels and struggling to maintain their traditionally large piece of the pie, will continue to wage fierce battles against nurses' autonomy. Though their objections are usually based on quality and safety concerns, many studies have repeatedly documented the quality and value of nursing services, particularly those of APNs (Brown & Grimes, 1995; U.S. Congress, Office of Technology Assessment, 1986). More disconcerting is that many legislators are often reluctant to alienate physicians and their professional organizations, even though they recognize the substantive merit attendant to the advancement of the nursing profession. Nurses can, however, diminish the impact of the opposition from the physician community. It is well known among the nursing profession that many physician specialty groups are supportive of nurses and the autonomous roles they seek. As nurses divide physician groups and create conflict between the medical specialties, some of whom readily support collaborative working relationships with nurses, the medical profession's opposition will be conquered.

Payers (e.g., insurance companies) are still clinging to the misperception that empowerment of APNs and continued utilization of nurses instead of unlicensed assistive personnel in health care settings will cost them more money. Many managed care organizations have come to believe in nursing's crusade to broaden practice opportunities, and they support the notion that nurses can be utilized in a broader fashion to accomplish the goals of health care reform. However, they have not yet fully committed to actively supporting the advancement of nurses. This "holding back" posture acts as an impediment to nursing's legislative efforts. Legislators often use the lack of enthusiastic support and active participation of these players in nursing reform efforts as an excuse to withhold their support and affirmative vote.

Although these payer sources and their representatives, whose lobbying power rivals that of the American Medical Association and other medical organizations, have buttressed the opposition to full utilization of nurses across health care settings, they may soon become supporters of nurses with focused encouragement and lobbying efforts (Mason, Cohen, O'Donnell, Baxter, & Chase, 1997). These alliances can and will be built as more patient care is delivered under the "managed care" model.

Health policy analysts are opposed to expanding the fee-for-service system to other provider groups besides the medical profession because they believe it will lead to greater escalation in the cost of health care (Enthoven & Kronick, 1991). A detailed business plan with demonstrated cost cutting that emphasizes the long-term savings accomplished by nurses will eventually win over these skeptics.

Many **employers** lack an understanding of the savings that can be obtained through greater and more efficient utilization of nurses, and so they are also resistant to joining nursing efforts. Hospitals and other health care institutions, represented by their politically influential national and state organizations, often oppose nurses' initial efforts to secure direct reimbursement. This is partly because physicians dominate these administrative structures and because the institutions are reluctant to lose the revenue that would go directly to nurses who contract for their services. Employers in nontraditional settings may already be supporters, having abandoned many of the stereotypical misperceptions against nursing's broad professional capabilities. They can be extremely effective in supporting nurses' efforts to change policies, laws, and regulations when they vocalize their recognition of nurses' value to the delivery of health care.

Other professions competing with nurses for a larger piece of the health care pie may also assist the medical profession's battle to thwart nursing's professional advancement efforts. For example, as psychologists aggressively pursue prescriptive authority, legislators may be less willing to promote autonomy for APNs, believing that their vote to eliminate barriers to independent APN practice will inappropriately cast the die for other professions. To the extent that nursing can neutralize these groups when an issue important to nursing is in debate, the likelihood of a successful outcome will be greater. Moreover, these groups may even be allies for nurses when an issue addresses common concerns. For example, national and state legislative efforts to achieve "parity" for mental health conditions were lobbied for by professional groups from many different health care specialties.

Resources

An effective political strategy must take into account the resources that will be needed to move an issue successfully. Resources include time, money, people, positional connections, and intangibles such as creative ideas.

Analyzing the resources thus requires both a long-term and a short-term view.

- What resources (financial and other) are needed to build nursing's political power over the long run versus what resources are needed to influence an immediate issue?
- What are the human resources available? Are there sufficient numbers of people who will work on the issue? Can a diversified coalition be formed to support the issue?
- What will be the costs of accessing the media or other publicity efforts, copying, telephone use, and other office supports? Can an organization donate these resources?

- How much creativity is evident among the stake holders? How can creativity be stimulated and channeled?

EXAMPLE

Financial resources will continue to play an important role as nurses advance their issues. Legislators and local politicians often look for financial support from nurses as individual constituents as well as from their formal nursing organizations. Implicit in these expectations is, for the most part, a view that lawmakers and nurses, working toward the common good, require financial support to accomplish the more specific goals. Therefore, although nurses should always keep consumers as the top priority, they need to keep in mind the significance of lending some level of financial support to those lawmakers whom they expect to spearhead efforts on their issues, such as reimbursement. In addition, it is often wise for nursing groups to employ the services of one or more lobbyists to advance their issues. Funding of lobbyist support can require a substantial commitment. Money may also be needed to conduct research—for example, to conduct studies that demonstrate the positive outcomes of APN practice. Funds for political strategies, such as a media campaign to publicize APNs as providers of choice for primary care, may be essential to gaining public acceptance.

STRATEGIES

Strategy is the identification of specific objectives and the formulation of a plan to achieve the established goals. Political strategies are integrated throughout this book. This section will highlight generic strategies that should be considered when one is devising any plan for developing a policy or moving an issue. They are framed as political principles or axioms (Talbott, 1993).

Look at the Big Picture. The prior section on political analysis provides the basis for nurses to understand the context in which an issue occurs. It is human nature to view the world from a personal standpoint, focusing on the people and events that influence one's daily life. Political strategy requires that one step back and take stock of the larger environment. It can provide a more objective perspective and increase nurses' credibility as broad-minded visionaries, looking beyond personal needs. Staff nurses who are trying to implement a wellness program will be more likely to succeed if they can address the need for their organization to decrease its expenditures for employee health care and then expand their proposal to cover all employees.

Do Your Homework. As discussed above, make sure the issue is well defined.

- Clarify your position on the problem and possible solutions.
- Gather data and search the literature.
- Prepare documents to describe and support the issue.
- Assess the power dynamics of the players and context.
- Assess your own power base and ability to maneuver in the political arenas.
- Plan a strategy and assess its strengths and weaknesses.
- Prepare for the conflict. Where is it anticipated and how will you respond?
- Line up support. Are your supporters ready to act?

It's Not What You Say, It's How You Say It. Contrary to what this axiom suggests, the content of an issue *is* important, but it may be secondary to how the message is framed and conveyed to stake holders. Learn to use strong affirmative language to describe nursing practice. In addition, adopt lawmakers' and managers' lingo and the "buzz words" of key political and administrative proponents. Appealing to a variety of stake holders often requires developing rhetoric or a message to frame your issue that is succinct and appealing to the values and concerns of those you want to mobilize or defeat. For example, "Cut Medicare" was an ineffective political message that the Republicans used to try to gain public support for decreasing spending on Medicare. When the

message was changed to "Preserve and Protect Medicare," the public was more supportive, even though the policy goals were the same. How you convey your message involves developing rhetoric or catchy phrases that the media might pick up and perpetuate (see Chapters 8 and 13). Nurses need to develop their effectiveness in accessing and using the media, an essential component of getting the issue on the public's agenda.

It's Not What You Know, It's Who You Know. The power that results from personal connections is often the most important strategy in moving a critical issue. Sometimes it comes down to one important personal connection. For example, a nursing reimbursement bill in a Southern state was passed because the director of the state nurses association was best friends with the chair of the committee responsible for moving the legislation to the full voting body. Or consider the nurse who is the neighbor and friend of the secretary to the chief executive officer (CEO) in the medical center. This nurse is more likely to gain access to the CEO than will someone who is unknown to either the secretary or the CEO. Networking is an important long-term strategy for building influence; however, it can be a deliberate short-term strategy, as well (see the vignette on networking following this chapter).

United We Stand, Divided We Fall. Collective action is almost always more effective than individual action. Besides having one's own group organized and ready to be mobilized, what other networks do you have or can you develop? Can coalitions be formed around the issue (see Chapter 10)? Sometimes, diverse groups can work together on an issue of mutual support, even though they are opponents on other issues. Public and private interest groups that identify with nursing's issues can be invaluable resources for nurses. They often have influential supporters devoted to advancing any cause they commit to, or they may have research and other information that can help nurses to move an issue along on the substantive arguments alone. Rallies, letter-writing campaigns, activism, and grassroots efforts by these groups can turn up the volume on nursing's issues and create the necessary groundswell of support to overcome what is often fierce opposition to nursing's agenda.

Nothing Ventured, Nothing Gained. Nurses have always been risk takers. Margaret Sanger fled to England after she was sentenced to jail for providing women with information about birth control (Chesler, 1992). Clara Maas lost her life while participating in research on malaria. More recently, Helen Miramontes, of California, volunteered to be among the first healthy subjects for a study of the first vaccination against the human immunodeficiency virus. Such thoughtful risk takers weigh the costs and benefits of their actions. They consider possible outcomes in relation to the expenditure of available resources. For example, a nurse may decide to run for Congress, knowing that she has little chance of winning. She risks losing, but running will give her the opportunity to bring important health issues to the public's attention and will gain name recognition for her next race.

Get a Toe in the Door, or Half a Loaf Is Better Than None. Incremental changes or actions may have a better chance of success than a project of major proportions. Resistance to change can often be overcome if a pilot or demonstration project is created to test an idea on a small scale. For example, when nurses wanted to get government support for nurse-managed centers, they proposed that Congress support four community nursing organizations (CNOs) to provide care to older adults under capitated arrangements with Medicare. The CNOs have received ongoing Congressional support for evaluating their outcomes. With these data, it is expected that support for expanding CNOs will be forthcoming.

Many times we are confronted with situations in which we may not get all we want. It pays to figure out acceptable solutions or alternatives. Identification of alternatives represents a good way to test one's convictions and to consider what the long- and short-term goals are. The failure of Clinton's health care reform legislation, which would have overhauled health care in the United States, was partly attributed to the fact that policymaking in this country is usually incremental rather than revolutionary. Some state nurses associations have opposed legislation that would provide third-party reimbursement for one group of nurses (such as nurse midwives) rather than for all nurses. In most cases the associations have been unsuccessful in securing passage of the broader bills.

Quid Pro Quo. "Something for something." "You scratch my back, I'll scratch yours." Some say these phrases represent a cynical view of human or organizational relationships, whereas others acknowledge that they represent a realistic approach to life. Because nurses interface with the public all the time, they are in excellent positions to assist, facilitate, or otherwise do favors for people. Too often, nurses forget to ask for help from those whom they have helped and who would be more than willing to return a favor. In Washington, D.C., getting and returning favors is socially accepted and expected behavior. Consider the visiting nurse who is asked by the director of purchasing for the home care agency to look in on her aging mother, who has seemed depressed recently. The nurse works a visit into her day's schedule, evaluates the mother, and recommends a referral to a community support group for widows and widowers. The director of purchasing later reports to the nurse that her mother loves the group and is doing so much better. As the director leaves, she says, "If there are any supplies or equipment that you ever need, just give me a call and I'll fix you up." Interchanges like this occur every day and create the basis for "quid pro quo."

Walk a Mile in Another's Moccasins. A successful political strategy is one that tries to accommodate the concerns of the opposition, insofar as morally feasible. It requires disassociating the emotional context of working with opponents—the first step in principled negotiating (see Chapter 9). The person who is skillful at managing conflict will be successful in politics. The saying that "politics makes strange bedfellows" arose out of the recognition that long-standing opponents can sometimes come together around issues of mutual concern, but it often requires creative thinking and a commitment to fairness to develop an acceptable approach to resolving an issue.

The other dimension of this axiom is creating opportunities for your opposition and power holders to gain firsthand experience with your issue. The many "Walk a Mile With a Nurse" campaigns have provided hospital executives and public officials with the opportunity to understand the complexities of a nurse's daily work, the barriers he or she confronts, and possible solutions (McEachen, Mason, & Jabara, 1992). Media coverage of your issue can also help to accomplish this end, particularly when personal stories are used to illustrate the conflicts or concerns raised by an issue.

Strike While the Iron Is Hot. A well-thought-out plan may fail because the timing is off. Judging the right time to act is not always easy. For example, a nurse on the board of directors of a nursing association plans to resubmit a proposal for a media campaign about the value of nurses that was first proposed several years ago but rejected because it would be expensive and would stretch the resources of the organization. The growing concern among nurses about their job security in a managed care environment has led the board to believe that it must respond proactively to the members' concerns. The proposal is resubmitted and supported unanimously because the timing is right.

This political axiom suggests that solutions that did not work at one time should be kept at hand for future opportunities. Bills can be introduced to the legislature without movement for years until the right conditions are created for passage. One can deliberately strategize to "turn up the heat" on an issue. The media are often used to get an issue on the agendas of the public

and policymakers (see vignette on "Whistle Blowing," Chapter 19).

Read Between the Lines. Communication theory notes that the overt message is not always the real message (Gerston, 1997). Some people say a lot by what they choose not to disclose. When legislators say they think your issue is important, it does not necessarily mean that they will vote to support it. The real question should be, "Will you vote in support of our bill?" What are the hidden agendas of the stake holders concerned with the issue? What is not being said?

The Best Defense Is a Good Offense. When the opposition is gaining momentum and support, it can be helpful to develop a strategy that can distract attention from the opposition's issue or that can delay action. For example, one nurses association continually battled the state medical society's efforts to amend the nurse practice act in ways that would restrict nurses' practice and provide for physician supervision. Nurses became particularly concerned about the possibility of passage during a year when the medical society's influence with the legislature was high. Working with other professions' organizations engaged in similar battles, the nurses proposed a bill that would go after the physicians' practice act by removing all oversight authority from it. The physicians knew that a large coalition backing this bill would divert their energies from focusing on the nurse practice act to fighting the coalition's proposal.

Do to Others As You Would Have Them Do to You. Although successful political operatives may resort to Machiavellian strategies to win their issue, increased public scrutiny of politics is limiting this type of behavior. This is where politics gets its negative connotation. On the other hand, effective politicos can often be found among those individuals who have impeccable reputations for honesty, fair play, and commitment. Certainly, nurses have a trustworthy reputation in the public's eye and are seen as credible stake holders. This is where the ethics of politics becomes most critical. Will nurses be successful if they take the high road in politics? Some feminists believe that there are other, more positive frameworks for resolving conflicts around issues, such as consensus building and principled negotiating. At the very least, those in power need to know that you are honest and committed to resolving conflicts fairly. For example, one of the principles of lobbying legislators is to be honest if one does not know the answer to a question. Following up with accurate information will further your reputation with them. It is even more effective to convey the position of the opposition and then to dispute it with logical arguments.

Rome Was Not Built in a Day. Change can take a long time. The effectiveness of any effort can be reinforced if nurses build on their successes and learn from their failures. For example, efforts to change workplace policies may take an extended period, requiring many committee meetings and approvals. Each discussion of the issue offers insight on how to pursue the issue successfully at the next presentation. Similarly, legislative or regulatory initiatives often take years of sustained effort.

Political work requires patience, perseverance, and an exquisite sense of timing. Failure to recognize these requirements can result in nurses' getting discouraged and feeling inadequate as political operatives. The following are helpful ways to minimize the frustrations that can accompany political work:

- Have a well-defined political plan with both long-term and short-term objectives.
- Evaluate one's progress and modify the plan as needed.
- Identify how to turn seeming defeats into victories.
- Celebrate the small gains.
- Acknowledge, thank, keep informed, and otherwise actively support collaborating stakeholders.

A House Divided Is a House Defeated. Achievement of nursing's agenda can be accom-

plished only through activism by a united front. It is in nursing's best political interest to end the seemingly endemic divisiveness among nurses and professional nursing organizations, and to foster ways for nurses to become flexible and politically responsive. On the other hand, nurses are so diverse that perhaps we should no longer expect to agree on everything. Instead, we should look for opportunities to reach consensus or remain silent in the public arena on an issue that is not of paramount concern.

Ignorance Is NOT Bliss—It's Stupid! It is critical that nurses stay abreast of the issues affecting their professional practice and the societal context in which they occur. A number of sources are available to stay informed on issues, including briefing materials from national and state organizations and political information from the Democratic, Republican, and other political organizations. Read a reputable national and local newspaper or news magazine that analyzes emerging policy issues, political discussions, economics, and other relevant developments. Letters to the editor can provide an analysis of public opinion, support, or opposition. Organizational newsletters, position statements, and advisories can also be helpful.

EXAMPLE

Managed care legislative initiatives throughout the country presented excellent opportunities for nurses to insert themselves in a more significant fashion into the health care debate. Public hearings on the array of issues incorporated in sweeping managed care reform bills gave many nurses an opportunity to speak up in favor of measures that would protect patients' safety, enhance access to care, and ensure proper reimbursement for services. For example, in 1997 in Connecticut alone, there were almost a dozen bills introduced at the commencement of the legislative session that were aimed at ensuring appropriate lengths of stay and treatment for breast cancer patients. These bills eventually culminated in a comprehensive anti-drive-through mastectomy law similar to those passed in other states. Nurses also spoke up in favor of measures requiring "parity" in coverage for mental health and addictive disorders. Support of managed care legislation that mandates proper patient appeal mechanisms from coverage and treatment decisions by payers also gave nurses an opportunity to insist on legislation that would facilitate access and reimbursement for their services.

Active participation in this fashion enabled nurses to build relationships with legislators and other provider groups, gain respect as a profession among lawmakers, and recognition as an important resource to be consulted as legislation is developed and acted on. At the same time, the focus on managed care legislation also offered nurses an opportunity to advance their issues through specific legislative initiatives. In Connecticut a coalition of nursing groups initiated legislation to eliminate mandatory physician direction over APN prescriptive practice. Consideration of the proposed bill was timed in relation to the heating up of the debate between physicians and insurers concerning sweeping managed care reform legislation that legislative leadership was determined to pass. Physicians, with a lot at stake in the managed care bill, were focused on that legislation, and their ability fully to engage in an effort to oppose the APN legislation was limited. As a result, the APN effort advanced at a much faster pace than was anticipated by nursing's opponents. Though the bill did not pass on the first round, it gained considerable momentum and support while the physicians were busy on other fronts. This is a superb example of nurses' taking advantage of a favorable political and business climate to advance an important issue and timing the initiation of the effort to the disadvantage of their opponents.

CONCLUSION

The future of nursing and health care may well depend on nurses' skills in moving a vision. Without a vision, politics becomes an end in itself—a game that is often corrupt and empty. Political analysis and strategizing become means to an end, if nurses master relevant knowledge and apply it to their political situations.

REFERENCES

Backer, B. A. (1991). You can get there from here: Guide to problem definition in policy development. *Journal of Psychosocial Nursing, 29*(10), 24–28.

Bissinger, R. L., Allred, C. A., Arford, P. H., & Bellig, L. L. (1997). A cost-effectiveness analysis of neonatal nurse practitioners. *Nursing Economics, 15*(2), 92–99.

Brown, S. A., & Grimes, D. E. (1995). Meta-analysis of nurse practitioners and nurse-midwives in primary care. *Nursing Research, 44*(6), 332–339.

Chesler, E. (1992). *Woman of valor: Margaret Sanger and the birth control movement in America.* New York: Anchor Books.

Connecticut Public Act 97–99.

Duke, J. T. (1976). *Conflict and power in social life.* Provo, UT: Brigham Young University Press.

Enthoven, A. C., & Kronick, R. (1991). Universal health insurance through incentives reform. *JAMA, 265*(25), 32–36.

Ferguson, V. D. (1993). Perspectives on power. In D. J. Mason, S. W. Talbott, & J. K. Leavitt (Eds.), *Policy and politics for nurses: Action and change in the workplace, government, organizations, and community* (2nd ed.) (pp. 118–128). Philadelphia: W. B. Saunders.

French, J. R. P., & Raven, B. (1959). The basis of social power. In D. Cartwright (Ed.), *Studies in social power.* Ann Arbor: University of Michigan.

Gender power. (1997, February 17). *U.S. News and World Report,* 25–26.

Gerston, L. N. (1997). *Public policy making: Process and principles.* Armonk, NY: M. E. Sharper.

Heffernan, L. F. (1995). Regulation of advanced practice nursing in health care reform. *Journal of Health and Hospital Law, 28,* 2, 73.

Hersey, P., Blanchard, K., & Natemeyer, W. (1976). Situational leadership: Perception and impact of power. *Group Organizational Studies, 4,* 418–428.

Hoffman, C. (1994). Medicaid payment for nonphysician providers: An access issue. *Health Affairs, 13*(4), 140–152.

Inglis, A. D., & Kjervik, D. K. (1993). Empowerment of advanced practice nurses: Regulation reform needed to increase access to care. *The Journal of Law, Medicine & Ethics, 21*(2), 193–205.

Kelly, L. Y., & Joel, L. (1995). *Dimensions of professional nursing* (7th ed.). New York: McGraw-Hill.

Kelly, R. M., & Duerst-Lahti, G. (1995). The study of gender power and its link to governance and leadership. In G. Duerst-Lahti & R. M. Kelly (Eds.), *Gender power, leadership, and governance* (pp. 39–64). Ann Arbor: University of Michigan Press.

Knox, R. A. (1996, July 24). State legislatures take on HMOs' managed care policies. *Boston Globe,* p. A12.

Koch, L. W., Pazaki, S. J., & Campbell, J. D. (1992). The first 20 years of nurse practitioners literature: An evolution of joint practice issues. *The Nurse Practitioner: The American Journal of Primary Health Care, 17,* 62–71.

Laswell, H. (1958). *Who gets what, when and how?* (with postscript) (2nd ed.). Cleveland: World Publishing.

Lowi, T. J. (1964). American business, public policy, case studies, and political theory. *World Politics, 16,* 677–715.

Mason, D. J., Cohen, S. S., O'Donnell, J., Baxter, K., & Chase, A. (1997). Managed care organizations' arrangements with nurse practitioners. *Nursing Economics, 15*(6), 306–314.

McEachen, I., Mason, D. J., & Jabara, I. (1992). Walk a mile with a nurse. *Nursing Spectrum, 4*(3), 5.

Newman, M. A. (1995). The gendered nature of Lowi's typology: Or, who would guess you could find gender here? In G. Duerst-Lahti & R. M. Kelly (Eds.), *Gender power, leadership, and governance* (pp. 141–164). Ann Arbor: University of Michigan Press.

Nichols, L. M. (1992). Estimating the cost of underusing advanced practice nurses. *Nursing Economics, 10,* 343–351.

Norton, N. (1995). Women, it's not enough to be elected. In G. Duerst-Lahti & R. M. Kelly (Eds.), *Gender power, leadership, and governance* (pp. 115–140). Ann Arbor: University of Michigan Press.

Pear, R. (1996, September 5). Clinton to name health-care panel, with eye on second term. *New York Times,* p. A20.

Pearson, L. J. (1998). Annual update of how each state stands on legislative issues affecting advanced nursing practice. *The Nurse Practitioner: The American Journal of Primary Health Care, 23*(1), 14–16, 19–20, 25–26, 29–33, 39, 43–46, 49–50, 52–54, 57–58, 61–62, 64–66.

Phillips, R. S. (1985). Nurse practitioners: Their scope of practice and theories of liability. *Journal of Legal Medicine, 6*(3), 391–414.

Robert, H. M. (1990). *Robert's rules of order newly revised.* Reading, MA: Addison-Wesley.

Safriet, B. J. (1992). Health care dollars and regulatory sense: The role of advanced practice nursing. *Yale Journal on Regulation, 9*(2), 417–487.

Schattschneider, E. E. (1960). *The semi-sovereign people.* New York: Holt, Rhinehart & Winston.

Stolberg, S. G. (1997, August 10). Now prescribing just what the patient ordered. *New York Times,* p. 8.

Talbott, S. W. (1993). Political analysis: Structure and process. In D. J. Mason, S. W. Talbott, & J. K. Leavitt (Eds.), *Policy and politics for nurses: Action and change in the workplace, government, organizations, and community* (2nd ed.) (pp. 129–148). Philadelphia: W. B. Saunders.

U.S. Congress, Office of Technology Assessment. (1986). *Nurse practitioners, physician assistants, and certified nurse-midwives: A policy analysis* (HCS 37). Washington, DC: Author.

U.S. Department of Health and Human Services. (1996). *The national occupational research agenda* (publication No. 96-115). Cincinnati, OH: National Institute for Occupational Safety and Health.

Weissert, C. S. (1996). *Governing health: The politics of health policy.* Baltimore: The Johns Hopkins University Press.

VIGNETTE

Networking

Belinda E. Puetz and Linda J. Shinn

Networking is nothing new; it has always existed. Men traditionally establish "old boy" networks in business, a source of information that permits them to move ahead more rapidly.

Women did not begin to network until they started to enter the business world in greater numbers and discovered they were not moving up the corporate ladder as rapidly as their male counterparts. These women soon realized there was no "old girl" network to which they could turn for assistance as they encountered "glass ceilings" in business and industry. Thus they began to establish their own networks. Viewed by many as the "mother" of women's networking, Mary Scott Welch (1980) defined networking as "the process of developing and using your contacts for information, advice, and moral support as you pursue your career" (p. 15).

Advocates of networking enthusiastically describe its benefits. These benefits—information, feedback, referrals, improved self-esteem, and a sense of collegiality with others—are available to nurses as well as to women and men in general who network. Many nurses know about networking but either do not perceive its value to them or, worse yet, disparage the contribution networking can make to professional accomplishment and success.

Benefits of Networking

Information, the major benefit of networking, is necessary at all points in an individual's career path. Information is necessary for those seeking to get ahead in a field of practice as well as for those who wish to remain where they are. Information is useful to learn about job opportunities, changes in the employment setting that will have an impact on a nurse's practice, upcoming professional events, and more.

Nurses in an employment setting who network with others can learn about possible acquisitions and mergers, downsizing and restructuring plans, and other, similar information that allows nurses to be prepared for a possible job change—or loss. For example, a colleague of one of the authors counts a human resources department staffer among those in her network. From that individual, she learned that layoffs at the middle management level were imminent. Thus she has stripped her office of personal belongings and non-hospital-related professional activity files. She has also determined her severance requirements and assessed her financial condition should she be without employment for a time. Most important, she has passed the word among the contacts in her network that she is actively seeking other employment.

Obtaining information about upcoming professional activities can be of invaluable assistance in this time of uncertainty and change in the health care environment. Another colleague of the authors is a nurse who is uncertain about his future in an acute care setting. He has attended a workshop on making a transition to home care to prepare for the eventuality that he may lose his job. A nurse seeking to change from one specialty area of practice to another because of the perception of more security in the latter specialty area may choose to attend the convention of the specialty organization, not only to explore the knowledge and skills needed for the new practice area, but also to begin to establish a network consisting of individuals already in the field and perhaps to learn about potential job opportunities.

Nurses wishing to abandon traditional health care employment settings altogether in favor of becoming entrepreneurs might join a business organization or chamber of commerce in a local area, or may contact a small-business development center associated with a nearby college or university (Puetz & Shinn, 1997). The authors, both entrepreneurs after years of employment in health care institutions and organizations, credit networking for their ability to get started, find clients, market their services, grow their businesses, and attain success.

Networking relies on contacts. Contacts are individuals from whom an individual can obtain advice, information, or business. Individual contacts in both professional and personal networks can help the nurse achieve career goals.

Identifying Networks

It is wise for nurses to include in their networks the following: people who are less experienced, those at the same level (colleagues and peers), and those more experienced than the nurse (Puetz, 1983; Smith, 1993). The first group are those who will learn from the nurse—those the nurse will nurture and mentor. The nurse's colleagues and peers can function as a support group, and the older, wiser individuals are those whom the nurse will seek as mentors.

The initial step in identifying networks is to make lists of individuals who are in the three spheres described above: the vertical, downward network (less experienced individuals); the horizontal network (peers or colleagues); and the vertical, upward network (more experienced persons). The lists should include those individuals with whom the nurse currently is in contact and others such as former employers and co-workers. Many times individual contacts in the latter group have eventually been lost. In this case the nurse must determine whether it is important to try to reestablish contact in the hope of adding these individuals to an existing network.

The list of individuals in a network should include those in nursing, in health care–related

professions, and in other professions as well. It can be advantageous at times to have an attorney or an accountant in one's repertoire of contacts. One of the authors recently had the occasion to refer a colleague to a nurse attorney practicing in another city when the colleague's employment was unfairly terminated and immediate advice was needed from a trusted professional.

Once these contacts have been identified and placed in relation to the three networks described above, the next step is to identify their contribution to the nurse's networking. For example, review of the three networks may reveal that the nurse spends a great deal of time advising, coaching, and otherwise assisting individuals in the vertical, downward network—perhaps even neglecting other, more productive and more profitable activities as a result. In another example the nurse may spend time with colleagues in the horizontal network, engaging in gossip or idle conversation, neither of which will accomplish any business purpose. It is important to strive to balance networking activities among all three networks.

Organizing Networks

Networking efforts must be organized: Not every contact will be helpful. The 80/20 rule applies here: 80% of the results will come from 20% of the contacts. Figuring out exactly how to use contacts most effectively will make the most efficient use of the 20%.

Organizing and keeping track of contacts can be expedited by using a system such as business cards, a Rolodex file, or a computer software program. All these systems are similar; they are a means of tracking names and other important information about contacts.

Information about a potential contact can be organized in a variety of ways to facilitate retrieval of the information. For example, business cards received at an educational event can be filed under the name of the meeting or the individual's name; by topic heading, such as continuing educator, researcher, grant writer; or by area of practice, such as pediatrics, home care, or oncology. In some cases it may be necessary to classify the individual into more than one category: by area of interest and by location of the conference. The type of organizing mechanism used is not as important as the ability to retrieve the information when needed.

Networking Effectively

To network effectively, one must follow the "rules." The nurse should initially identify the specific purpose for networking. The next step is to identify who can help the nurse achieve this purpose and decide how to meet those individuals, if they are not already in the nurse's network. When a nurse decides to seek a promotion, the obvious individuals to meet are those who will be making the decision about who will be promoted. The nurse should make those contacts and also seek to meet individuals who have held the desired position to learn about what characteristics are needed for the position. Then, in conversation with the decision makers, the nurse can display or discuss the needed skills.

Follow-up with contacts is important; it is essential to keep in touch with them. Deep and Sussman (1990) suggested sending personal notes to colleagues who have accomplished something, such as publishing a book, a chapter in a book, or an article, making a presentation, or otherwise achieving something noteworthy. Information about these accomplishments can be found in newsletters of professional and trade associations or learned from contacts in conversations.

Other ways to keep in touch involve sending notices of position changes, mailing postcards from conventions that the contact has previously attended, and sending clips from newspapers or articles on topics of interest to the contact.

Finally, offer help. Is there something the nurse could do in exchange for what the nurse is seeking from the contact? People tend to remember helpful individuals. Perhaps the nurse seeking a promotion can offer to assume one of the tasks associated with that position, thus relieving someone else of the responsibility and, at the same time, proving that the nurse can do the job.

Being Gracious

Leslie Smith (1995) offered advice to individuals who wish to network effectively: never fail to be gracious. Smith suggests that gracious networkers:

- Do not focus exclusively on what they will get from networking but, rather, focus on how they can help the other individual in a reciprocal exchange that meets both individuals' needs.
- Do not focus on their own self-importance but turn the conversation to the other individual.
- Send a note or make a phone call no later than 10 days after meeting a new contact.
- Join professional organizations and get involved with the organization's activities.
- Do not contact someone only when they want something but, rather, stay in touch with contacts on an ongoing basis.
- Give as much as they get through networking.
- Give thanks when they have received some assistance and pass along the assistance they have received.

Being gracious is an integral part of all interpersonal relationships. Nurses who wish to be effective at networking must be able to socialize successfully with a variety of others. Networking involves more than socializing skills, however. An individual who wishes to network effectively must have expertise in a field of practice, both to be credible and to be able to offer that expertise to others.

Organizational Networking

Networking works for organizations as well as for individuals. Organized nursing is replete with instances of the effectiveness of networking. Whether a homogeneous collection of nursing organizations or a heterogeneous web of people with the same interests, nurses have participated in myriad groups to accomplish something that would not be possible alone.

This collective action is networking—which involves information, feedback, reaction, referral, collegiality with others, and connecting for results.

When Networking Does Not Work

Sometimes networking does not appear to work: the nurse does not get what is needed from contacts. An objective view, however, may reveal that the individual is not networking correctly. For example, networking is not one sided—it is a reciprocal arrangement in which individuals "trade" favors. Networking must be perceived as valuable to both parties, not simply a case of "I hear from her only when she wants something."

Even when one is unable to repay another with a favor of the same magnitude, she has the responsibility to pass the favor on and to notify the original party that she has done so.

Nor does networking work if, for example, the nurse uses an elected or appointed position in a professional organization solely as a platform for self-promotion. These behaviors are generally transparent.

Obviously, networking will not work if the nurse becomes a people "user," thinking only of what the contact can supply, rather than what mutual benefits can accrue. Networking will not work, either, if the nurse fails to attend to the social rules such as planning for more formal interactions with older individuals than with younger ones and at all times being gracious.

Conclusion

Networking does work if the nurse practices skills in meeting people and talking with them and if the nurse treats contacts in the same manner as the nurse wishes to be treated. Networking with honesty and integrity, as well as common courtesy, will set the nurse apart from many others and ensure success.

References

Deep, S., & Sussman, L. (1990). *Smart moves.* Reading, MA: Addison-Wesley.

Puetz, B. E. (1983). *Networking for nurses.* Rockville, MD: Aspen.

Puetz, B. E., & Shinn, L. J. (1997). *The nurse consultant's handbook.* New York: Springer.

Smith, L. (1993, January/February). Do the right people know you? *Executive Female,* p. 56.

Smith, L. (1995, September/October). Never fail to be gracious. *Executive Female,* p. 74.

Welch, M. S. (1980). *Networking.* New York: Harcourt Brace Jovanovich.

Chapter 8

DYNAMICS OF PUBLIC POLICY: Community-based Practice Meets Managed Care

JULIE SOCHALSKI, MELINDA JENKINS, AND ROSEMARY L. AUTH

The effects of public policy are easy to find. The pleas from fund-raising drives on public television are the outcome of governmental decisions to reduce their funding levels. The bus fumes that greet pedestrians crossing busy avenues are the result of years, and some may argue the failure, of contentious public transportation and air pollution control policies. The flight attendant's voice reminding everyone that the flight has been designated as nonsmoking is an example of a surgeon general's sweeping public health directive. Each of these policies embodies an iterative, often protracted, and invariably complex process that ended in a series of actions that affect many lives.

History has shown that the values of those who participate in the policymaking process dictate how the public's interest is protected (Kunin, 1987). As health care providers and responsible citizens, nurses have a strong interest in ensuring that health care policies provide for an effective health care delivery system, now and in the future (Butterfield, 1990; Milio, 1989). Involvement in policymaking is the only way to ensure that nurses' views are represented in health policy. Choosing to become involved, and in what way, are important decisions for each nurse. The outcome of these decisions will be reflected in the nation's health policies. If the views of nurses are not reflected in the resulting policy, it is for one of two reasons: either nurses were not involved in the process or, if they were

involved, more influential participants in the process did not share the nurses' views.

In her thorough review of policy analysis in Chapter 6, Hanley dissects public policy, explaining each step in the process of its development. This chapter picks up where Hanley leaves off and moves from the "classroom" to the "laboratory." On first appraisal, this laboratory appears impossibly complex and reserved for experienced policy mavens and the cognoscenti. This appraisal is only partially true. The process is complex but not impossibly so. And though experienced policy mavens have advantages over the uninitiated, with opportunity and experience one can eventually join their ranks. On the basis of the policy frameworks conceptualized by Kingdon (1984) and Anderson (1984, 1990), we depict the policymaking process in three phases: the stimulus or the idea phase, referred to as the policy formulation phase; the response, or legislative enactment, phase; and the dissemination phase. Within each phase a number of activities and intricate dynamics occur that can overwhelm the unprepared individual; the key is in being prepared (Diers, 1985). In this chapter the policymaking process comes to life through two case studies in which community health nurses and nurse practitioners (NPs) decide to enter the fray and build primary care services in their local communities. These experiences are drawn from actual events, but names and places have been fictionalized.

THE STIMULUS: A GOOD IDEA

CASE EXAMPLE   Dolorosa

The idea of a nurse-run primary health care network in Dolorosa to care for mothers and children came from a group of community health nurses and NPs who worked in the area. Dolorosa was a densely populated, crime-ridden, poor, ethnic-minority, inner-city core of a large metropolis. Primary care had not flourished there for a number of reasons, principally the inability to attract providers into this deteriorating community to deliver badly needed services. The services that were available were fragmented, leaving many gaps in even basic care. Local residents traveled a considerable distance to the nearest medical center to use its clinic services for primary and follow-up care. Dolorosa residents did not like to use the medical center, where there were long waits and they were treated impersonally. The nurses proposed the creation of a health network of clinic services using existing community centers such as schools and vacant stores. The nurses would organize a nursing independent practice association (nursing-IPA) to provide these services, with a staff of NPs and primary care physicians, some of whom were in the community and others of whom would have to be recruited

---

The idea of building a community health network in Dolorosa did not originate in lofty discourse in the halls of Congress; it came from nurses who saw a need. Policy has its origin in the ideas of people. The tuna boycott in the United States, which led to federal intervention to safeguard dolphins from being killed by tuna fishermen and contentious trade negotiations (Noah & Davis, 1994), began as a class project in a small school district. Ideas are seeds that can grow into policy when given the right audience—a person or group with the power to turn an idea into public policy.

Ideas often spring from problems, especially crises, and they become the impetus for policy (Paul-Shaheen, 1990). Examples include the calls for mandatory testing of health care providers for infection with human immunodeficiency virus after several patients of one infected dentist in Florida were found to be HIV-positive, and

the development of national centers for diabetes research and training after one influential senator's diabetic niece was unable to get safe and appropriate treatment. Other ideas defy the odds and eventually result in policy. A good example is Ralph Nader's impact on auto safety policy in this country after he took on General Motors with his thorough exposé of the hazards of the Chevrolet Corvair. And some ideas are put in motion to address more narrow concerns, but in practice the impact is felt much more broadly. The changes in physician licensing requirements and the subsequent consolidation of medical schools, aided by the 1910 Flexner Report, were ideas that fundamentally transformed the education of physicians as well as the delivery and financing of health care in this country (Starr, 1982).

In addition to nursing's own wellspring of ideas, the ideas of others provide valuable opportunities for nurses to take action on policy concerns. In the early 1980s in Michigan, the state nurses' association joined a coalition of groups that was working for the reform of Blue Cross and Blue Shield of Michigan, one part of which was the reconstitution of its board. As a result of nursing's efforts, a new position for a registered nurse on the board of directors was statutorily created—the first in the country. This move provided nurses in the state with a significant opportunity to address critical health policy concerns in a new and influential forum.

In Dolorosa the idea—a primary health care network—sprang from a definite need in the community identified by a group of nurses. On the face of it, the idea provided a novel yet reasonable response to a glaring and very difficult problem. Novel ideas don't often receive a fair hearing, though, let alone get enacted. An integral part of developing an idea, therefore, should be to target an influential audience with similar interests and to incorporate its views into the proposal. Many potential policy ideas compete for an audience, and a number of these ideas compete for the same audience. The competition often becomes fierce because the number of people who can effectively advance an idea is limited. Indeed, health policy ideas are most effectively moved by legislators on health committees; if the legislator does not sit on such committees, getting an idea off the ground may be more difficult. Even if he or she is on a relevant committee, each legislator has limited time and energy. Others' requests may be in line first. Fortunately, the terrain in public policy shifts regularly, and new audiences emerge that can influence policy. Different forms of the same idea can be proposed to more than one audience at a time. For example, in one state, reimbursement was sought for all advanced practice nursing groups through the state legislature; at the same time, one large employer was approached regarding the provision of and payment for psychiatric nurse clinical specialist services.

CASE EXAMPLE Dolorosa *(Continued)*

The nurses of Dolorosa identified two things that they would need to carry out their idea: (1) start-up funding and (2) primary care providers who would be willing to come to Dolorosa. Funding was available through the state health department for developing new primary care services in underserved areas. They were confident that if they met with their local legislator, he would be sure to see the merits of the idea and work with them to obtain funding. They paid a visit to Assemblyman Goodman from Dolorosa and his staff in their state office, and much to their delight, the idea of expanding services in the community received very favorable reviews, in principle, from the assemblyman. However, the nurses also learned that the medical center that Dolorosa residents were currently using was developing a proposal to expand primary care services on its campus, and officials from the medical center had already come to seek support from Assemblyman Goodman. It was likely that only one of the proposals would be funded. To support the nurses' idea, the assemblyman and his staff wanted to be sure that key community groups endorsed the project, that it had a reasonable chance of success once it got started, and that the doctors in the community would not oppose it.

The proposal for a primary health care network through a nursing-IPA would be going up against a formidable counter proposal, one that was already fully developed, supported by an influential constituency, and moving ahead for funding. If the nurses were to have any chance for success with their own idea, they would need to move quickly with their response, the development of a proposal backed by the community, the local legislator, and others. The nurses did learn something valuable from their meeting with Assemblyman Goodman: he strongly supported the notion of developing services in the community, in contrast to the "on campus" approach offered by the neighboring medical center. Developing a proposal that emphasized this feature would favorably position nurses to obtain his support.

THE RESPONSE: DEVELOPING POLICY FROM A GOOD IDEA

Shaping the Idea

Shaping an idea into a policy proposal requires assembling a select and committed planning committee. The process of involving others to help shape the idea and build a larger base of support serves several functions. The more an idea is talked about, albeit with a select and undoubtedly sympathetic group, the clearer its strengths and weaknesses become. The goal is to obtain valid criticism that will help in the design of a successful plan. Addressing the potential pitfalls improves the chances that others will support the project. A broader base of support always makes a proposal appear more attractive to policymakers. It also increases the likelihood of creating a "winner," a project with a better-than-average chance of succeeding.

CASE EXAMPLE Dolorosa *(Continued)*

After the meeting with Assemblyman Goodman, the nurses from Dolorosa scheduled an intensive planning session with several other influential and knowledgeable resources: the director of government affairs for the nurses' association, a friend of one of the nurses who was on the local school board and an ardent community activist, and a health policy professor from the neighboring university. During this session, two main policy objectives were identified as critical to the success of the community health network proposal. The first was the authority to exist. Under the public health code for the state, certain entities were recognized as providers that could deliver and receive payment for services. These providers must meet certain minimum requirements for safety and accountability. The nursing-IPA model was a new concept that would need to be recognized under the public health law. Provider status would need to be sought from the state's department of health. The law was worded broadly enough so that a nursing-IPA could reasonably fit within it. However, if a successful challenge were mounted against the nurses, they realized they would need to have an amendment to the law, sponsored, they hoped, by Assemblyman Goodman. The second objective was start-up money to enable the community health network to get off the ground and resources to recruit providers to Dolorosa.

The members of the planning committee selected by the nurses filled several important roles in this stage of the process. The government affairs director brought expertise in the current legislative/regulatory environment and advice on alternative strategies. The school board member had her finger on the pulse of the community and provided critical information on the political dynamics of the community that would need to be navigated. The health policy professor, a long-time advocate of community-based health care, helped the nurses step back and assess the implications of the direction they were pursuing for themselves and the system at large. For example, if the project did get off the ground but failed for reasons out of the nurses' control, what impact would such an experience have on any future initiatives by nurses? The committee also raised a number of technical issues that needed to be considered: the source of start-up money, fee structures, and plans for

recruiting and retaining providers. Addressing these issues raised by the committee made what was once just an idea into a program that was taking shape.

CASE EXAMPLE **Dolorosa** *(Continued)*

The best source for start-up funding was money set aside by the legislature for primary care initiatives, administered by the state health department. Additional resources would be sought for recruiting providers to Dolorosa in the form of housing, travel, and continuing education allowances and coverage of malpractice insurance costs. A 2-year employment commitment would be required in exchange for the resource allowances. It was decided that fees under the Medicaid program would be accepted, despite their historically low levels, and the same fees would be paid to nurses and physicians. Special provisions to cover the costs of serving the uninsured would also be put into place.

Building the Base of Support

The planning committee becomes the foundation on which is built an elaborate network of support. Looking for support is an essential and continuous effort that begins with having a clear idea of the goal and carefully identifying other advocates. Each person contacted has the potential to become both an ally and the source of more allies.

There are as many ways to build support for an idea as there are people who will potentially promote it. Other individuals and groups can become advocates, each for their own reasons. Building advocacy is rooted in translating the idea for others. The successful translation of the issue into the language of a possible constituent is the hallmark of an astute planning group. In one state where nurses were trying to obtain reimbursement for nurse midwifery services, local labor leaders were contacted as a potential source of support. In addition to the usual arguments of high-quality and low-cost services, the issue was framed specifically in the context of free trade: the ability of nurse midwives to practice freely and without restraint. Much to the nurses' surprise, the free trade context brought a negative reaction from the labor leaders. They believed that if they did not support the idea, they would be in the position of supporting "poor labor practices," and this was viewed as threatening. It was clear that they did not want to feel boxed in to supporting the proposal, so the issue was refocused in terms of *choice:* giving union members the right to choose the practitioner they wanted. The support from labor quickly followed.

Support should never be taken for granted. A community health network may sound as though it is something that the local chapter of social workers would unequivocally embrace; yet they may prefer centralizing the services in the medical center because it would allow them easy access to clients. In contrast, the county medical society may welcome an effort that would take the pressure off the medical center emergency departments and outpatient clinics, as long as physicians retain supervising authority. Support must be conscientiously sought, cultivated, cajoled, and continually reinforced. With each step taken to build support, the idea becomes clearer—and perhaps somewhat altered. It can become a struggle to maintain the integrity of an idea while trying to enlist others to take up the fight.

Potential supporters can be identified by asking these questions:

- Who might favor this idea? There are, first, the usual or obvious candidates, but new constituencies may be unearthed by thinking about what they might gain from this initiative. Discussions with potential supporters should be focused from their perspective. Some other reasons for advocating the idea may not be relevant or important to them and should often be left out of the conversation.
- Who might support this method? Certain groups might like the idea but prefer going about it another way. Their approach may be too far from the goal to consider them to be supporters of the idea.

- What is their reason for supporting this? Have they supported nurses or other health care initiatives in the past, or are they sufficiently opposed to competing proposals that they would support this idea by default? Answering these questions helps to gauge how strong their support is and will continue to be.
- What are the consequences of their support? There are some individuals and groups that the idea's supporters would rather not have associated with their initiative, and every attempt should be made to avoid involving them.

In soliciting support, nurses should identify both advocates and opponents, and the reasons for their stances. This information can be used to both strengthen the proposal and sharpen the arguments that may be needed when the opposition goes to work.

CASE EXAMPLE   **Dolorosa** *(Continued)*

Support for the nurses' proposal came from a variety of places. The local merchants were very much interested in having vacant buildings occupied; they believed the clinics would improve the image of the area and, they hoped, business. Local community- and city-wide activists wholeheartedly endorsed efforts that would improve area services and the community as a whole. Rebuilding the community's infrastructure was in line with their objectives for the area. A number of area physicians were also supportive of an initiative that would include them, as well as rid the area of the Medicaid mills. The local school board was enthusiastic about a service that would fill a great void. The area universities favored the clinic initiative, which, in addition to improving the general welfare of the area residents, would provide badly needed clinical placement sites for primary care nursing and medical students.

The Dolorosa proposal was competing for the set-aside funds for primary care initiatives with a number of other proposals, including one from the neighboring medical center that some thought was in a much better position to provide the services. Separately, the nurses solicited and received seed money from a local foundation. This partial funding sent a powerful message to the project reviewers in the department of health that this project was worthwhile.

The provider recruitment plan had its advocates and its skeptics. The advocates came from the providers and community activists who saw no other way to attract providers to the area. The skeptics included those who had endured the broken promises of the National Health Service Corps—a federal program of grants given to students training in medicine in exchange for a service commitment, a number of whom never served—wondering if this approach would turn out any differently. A quick survey of nurses and physicians in the area showed that the proposed prerequisites would be enough to persuade them to join the network and consider a longer commitment.

Barriers to Implementing Ideas

Once an idea has been carefully crafted, tested on a selected group of knowledgeable and influential supporters, refined, and given initial support from a diverse set of groups, it is ready to be launched. As this phase of the process begins, overt and covert forces can derail the best efforts to move an idea forward.

RHETORIC

Rhetoric, the art of persuasive arguments, is a powerful tool used to shape discussion and prevent action. Skillful rhetoric influences opinion by speaking to the core prejudices of an issue and is only loosely, if at all, based in fact. Physicians have long used the rhetoric of "second-class care" when opposing the use of specialty nurses, although definitive data have been produced to rebut these arguments (Eddy & Billings, 1988; Safriet, 1992). Rhetoric establishes the framework for the issue being discussed; it is steeped in history, often anecdotal, and very difficult to overcome. It is also a deliberate tactic to control discussions, which acts as a barrier to change. Because it is not based in fact, rhetoric is difficult to fight with facts. What is really being fought are impressions, long-held beliefs, or persuasions. When in combat with rhetoric, refocusing the argument, unrelentingly, becomes the chief line of defense.

INERTIA

Where rhetoric leaves off in burying policy initiatives, inertia picks up. There are always many more forces that support inaction, or very cautious action, than those which stimulate change. Inertia, like rhetoric, is often deliberate. Slowing the pace of change can create windows of opportunity to derail initiatives or create time to develop a response. One of the parallel paths of activities pursued to obtain third-party reimbursement for nurses in specialty practice in one state was an attorney general's ruling on the legality of denying reimbursement to one class of providers. This opinion took more than 2 years to be written; during that time, multiple requests for data were made, and countless conversations with staff from the attorney general's office transpired. The final ruling, though generally favorable, provided evidence that, during this long process, opposing groups were able to get their wishes reflected in the opinion.

Inertia can also mean that those in a position to make decisions are unsure about the path they want to take and are weighing the familiar, less controversial, and more predictable position against blazing the new, uncharted path. If action on an issue can be stalled, policymakers can take more time to weigh the pros and cons of their position. Inertia may also be a signal that the idea has come up against an impermeable, or nearly impermeable, barrier. The resulting inaction suggests the need to change course somewhat to get over the hurdle. It does not mean abandoning the chosen path altogether, but an adjustment may be needed.

PRECEDENT SETTING

Red flags routinely go up when any plan is viewed as precedent setting. Changes to the old order, especially actions that create a new order, are generally viewed cautiously. In the debate over the creation of the National Institute for Nursing Research at the National Institutes of Health, many legislators were torn between continuing the administration of nursing research monies through the Division of Nursing—where there would be no start-up costs, no disturbance of any of the historical relationships among the other institutes or of their funding, and no setting of a precedent for other groups wanting to establish a new institute—and responding to the requests of nurses across the country for full recognition of their legitimate research activities. If the precedent being set is viewed negatively, which often happens when sensitive power arrangements are disrupted, barriers to the proposal can be erected quickly (Lindblom, 1980). Precedent setting is probably the single largest factor that can alter the shape of any plan, and it dictates a steady refocusing of the debate so that its effects can be overcome. Refocusing includes such arguments as noting the broad base of support enjoyed by the idea and the high likelihood of achieving objectives.

COMPETING FORCES

Success is proportional to how effectively the opposition is neutralized. Competing forces can and do come from almost anywhere, not just from where they are expected. Overcoming the influence of competing forces on the audience and potential supporters can involve a series of battles, the outcome of which rarely depends on one person's efforts alone. Each potential supporter has many other connections, and some of them are the competition. Despite sympathy for the new project, not all potential supporters will be willing or able to promote the plan, at least not publicly. Anticipating the competing forces and the messages they will convey will help in preparing to neutralize the arguments. At some point there may be a showdown, and the people best positioned—with all their forces lined up—will prevail.

TIMING

Timing plays an important role in ensuring success. A good idea can die on the vine if the timing is wrong. Timing does not have to be perfect for an idea to succeed, but those advocating the project often have to work harder, and sometimes get less than they wanted, when timing is not in their favor. Assessment of tempo-

ral events should be a part of developing an idea and shaping the plan of action for its enactment.

The Final Pursuit

The creation of public policy requires endurance, patience, and hard work, in greater amounts than one envisions at the outset. From photocopying to public speaking, many different tasks are a part of such an effort, and consequently many different people and talents are necessary for success. Only a small cadre of people will be in the limelight, leading the effort to advance the objective. Their role is to ensure that the key players follow through on their pledges, to secure backup support when necessary, and to keep the effort moving forward. Countless details need to be attended to during this process, though, and strong commitment from everyone involved is essential to success.

There comes a point when there is no turning back. Yet, while going forward, it is important to look in both directions continually: What has been learned? How might it change the direction being taken? With time, a good sense develops of when to keep going, change direction, or take what has been gained. There are no hard-and-fast rules on how to decide what to do; it is basically a testing-feedback process. A good part of this decision has to do with the energy that can be mustered and the support that is there to keep the fight going. Sometimes just taking a brief pause allows the dust to clear enough to reevaluate progress and strategy. The balance between taking time and moving forward is something, like the entire policymaking process, that is learned (Levin & Ferman, 1985). A critical part of policymaking is to watch for unraveling within the ranks and to send in reinforcements that will ensure that progress will continue.

In preparing to defend an issue, it is wise to hold back a few key arguments that can be used when all else fails. It is tempting to try to level the opposition with everything, in the hope that it will go away. That, unfortunately, never happens. The opposition can be tenacious. As the rhetoric flows, the most persuasive arguments can be restated. Only when nothing else seems to be working should a new argument be introduced. Moreover, the same arguments can be used with new audiences, with the hope that they may also start using them against any opponents. Sometimes an opponent hearing the same argument from a new person will rethink his or her opposition.

Finally, fortitude is critical to pursuing goals. The rewards will be a long way off and sometimes will seem out of proportion to the energy expended. Often when the project succeeds, people come out of nowhere to celebrate and, of course, take part of the credit. It is important to give them the opportunity to celebrate and take part of the credit—and then sign them up for the next adventure.

CASE EXAMPLE **Dolorosa** *(Continued)*

The reticence of the health department in granting provider status to the nursing-IPA, despite the detailed responses and information sent to the authorities to address each concern, began to hinder the progress of the project. Assemblyman Goodman's office was asked to make a strategic telephone call to check on the application's standing in the approval process. It turned out that there were concerns about the scope of reproductive health services that would be offered. Supplemental information was promptly provided, outlining the services and addressing these remaining concerns. This step appeared to clear the way for the application for provider status.

Things were beginning to look promising, and from the nurses' perspective, the timing could not have been better for their proposal. The city had just issued its community mortality report, and Dolorosa headed the list. The health status of its citizens had been deteriorating over the past decade, and the erosion of primary care services had been painfully registered. The medical center proposal had not been viewed as the best solution but until now had been the only solution. The mayor had publicly committed himself to take action in Dolorosa and was looking for a way to ensure adequate primary health care services to silence his critics.

But the battle had not yet been won. As expected, organized medicine opposed the community health network proposal. The area physicians who supported the concept remained silent, though their voices would not have made much difference, given the full effort that organized medicine had launched. The physicians were backed by the medical center that had presented a competing proposal, and the voices of the two groups were loud. The rhetoric of "second-class care" raised its head, and it seemed to resonate with community activists. Physician consultation was suggested as one way to ensure that quality care standards were met, but this would push up the cost of the project, negating one of its strongest advantages. Another key element of the proposal—the ability to recruit and retain providers—was being attacked as naive and unrealistic.

The nurses of Dolorosa feared that all their hard work was evaporating before their eyes. The opposing forces had grown in number and strength, and the nurses found themselves fighting on every front. An emergency caucus of the leadership was held to survey the prospects for success, and it resulted in the following plan. They scaled back the scope of the community health network to a more modest network of satellite clinics affiliated with the local public health agency. The scope of services and nursing's role in managing the IPA would be maintained. However, an advisory committee was created, made up of community members and prominent physicians from the medical center. The committee would not have any voting authority or financial ties to the IPA but would exercise an important advisory and consultation role. With these steps, the nurses secured the support of the community and Assemblyman Goodman, and opposition from the physicians was successfully muted. The nurses breathed a collective sigh of relief and joy—their efforts had paid off.

DISSEMINATION AND REPLICATION

The efforts of the nurses in Dolorosa went beyond that of establishing a network of satellite primary care clinics managed by nurses. They also initiated nursing as a new entrant into the policymaking arena for the configuration of primary health care services, laying the groundwork for future activity in Dolorosa and in other communities. By establishing their right to exist as a service provider, nursing faced down much of the rhetoric and political malaise that had hampered previous efforts, they challenged physician hegemony in health care decision making in communities, and they sought out and worked with an array of policy vehicles to achieve their objectives. These were not small steps, but they were only the beginning. Disseminating and replicating these activities would have to follow if nursing's vision for health care service delivery would be realized. In a rapidly evolving health care delivery system, nursing's role in structuring that system will be directly proportional to nurses' involvement in shaping the policies that govern it. Further, as the players in the policymaking process continue to evolve, nursing's role must also evolve.

One of the principals seated at the policymaking table today (some, arguably, would say at the *head* of the table) is managed care. Throughout the decade of the 1990s, managed care has done more to transform the landscape of health services than almost any other single entity (Ginzberg & Ostrow, 1997). In this nation's unceasing effort to reduce the growth in health care costs, the payers of care have turned to managed care as the mechanism for extracting cost savings while ensuring appropriate care. Managed care has altered the traditional power arrangements in health policy, particularly those of providers such as physicians. This shifting terrain creates both opportunities and new hurdles for nursing in policymaking circles. We describe here how nurses in Hampton Woods seized the opportunity presented them to organize primary care services in this needy community as Medicaid managed care came to town, replicating many of the steps taken by their comrades in Dolorosa.

CASE EXAMPLE   **Hampton Woods**

Hampton Woods was no ordinary public housing community. Situated in the southwest corner of a large city, Hampton Woods was made up of housing units erected directly after World War II for returning servicemen. Its conversion to public housing, along with the decline in the surrounding neighborhood, was accompanied by a gradual deterioration of the grounds and a substantial increase in crime and drug

dealing in the immediate vicinity. Yet, rather than resolutely accommodating their lives to the seemingly endemic problems of their community, the residents of Hampton Woods chose a proactive route. They instituted a tenant management program, hired security to help root out crime, and organized residents to begin a cleanup program for the grounds.

These activities were noticed by Rosemont Human Services (RHS), a nonprofit human service agency that organized, managed, and funded a wide range of human services projects in the larger metropolitan area. When a request for proposals from the federal government for establishing federally qualified health centers in public housing communities arrived at RHS, Hampton Woods was seen as an ideal candidate for lodging such a service. The RHS approached the members of the tenant council at Hampton Woods to assess their interest in submitting a proposal to develop a health center on the grounds, and the reception was positive within the council. Residents of Hampton Woods had been dissatisfied with the services they received at the medical center, the main source of care in the area, and the opportunity to have a convenient alternative was appealing. RHS then contacted a family nurse practitioner (FNP) consultant, with whom it had worked on another project, to see whether she would be interested and willing to set up an NP-managed health center at Hampton Woods. "What progress we have made," mused the FNP as she accompanied representatives from RHS to continue discussions with the tenant council for developing the health center. After years of effort to establish nursing's legitimacy in providing and directing health services, communities were now coming to nurses to address their needs.

The FNP recommended a community partnership primary care model as the structure for the health center, which would link existing community services under the auspices of the new health center to ensure comprehensive, accessible services to residents. Members of the tenant council and representatives of the RHS were taken on a site-visit to another nearby NP-managed clinic serving both private and Medicaid patients that was organized in this fashion. The visit demonstrated the success of such an organizing structure to all in attendance, and proposal development ensued. Several primary care nursing faculty from the local university with expertise in grant writing were called on to help with developing the proposal. The tenant council members, RHS, and the NP consultants met with key members of the administrative and medical staff at the nearby hospital to review the proposal with them and to obtain their agreement to serve as the predominant referral destination for patients requiring specialty or inpatient care. With that agreement in hand, a legal contract was then drawn up between RHS and the tenant council to define the roles and responsibilities of each in the administration and oversight of the NP health center, and the proposal was submitted. Within 3 months the parties learned that the proposal had been favorably reviewed—and the Hampton Woods Health Center got under way, with the FNP as its new director.

Indeed, as noted by the FNP here, nursing had made "progress" toward the goal of decisive involvement in the making of health care policy. In Dolorosa, nurses took their ideas for filling the primary care services gap to the community and worked with their leaders and other key individuals in the process to have their ideas adopted as a part of the solution. In Hampton Woods, nurses were sought out as a part of the solution. This transition for nursing was the result of several factors. First, nurses, by gradually and increasingly inserting themselves into the policymaking establishment, were successful in shaping a more responsive health care delivery system in which they achieved a vibrant role. This role was the outgrowth of assessing the full slate of barriers, identifying the necessary policy "fixes," and diligently pursuing the changes with the help of a growing group of supporters. Second, by taking on such activities, nurses were introduced to a much wider audience than previously—their state representative and his staff, community leaders, and activists, as seen in the Dolorosa scenario—who gained a clear understanding of the common ground between them in their health care policy objectives. This knowledge would serve both nursing and the policymaking community well in future activities. Third, as a by-product of their involvement, the nurses uncovered previously uncharted health policy terrain—other individuals, initiatives, and state agencies influencing primary care service delivery—that presented strategic opportunities for future involvement. Finally, nurses gained a stronger foothold in their communities, directly positioning themselves to be seen as a part of a solution to the communities' health care needs.

The importance of nursing's policy involvement to the "progress" achieved in primary care services delivery cannot be overstated. The success of community health centers in improving the health of the public, and especially that of some of our most vulnerable populations, has been well established (Sardell, 1988; Starfield, 1992). Studies have demonstrated favorable quality care outcomes at these centers compared with the outcomes in private physicians' offices and hospital outpatient departments (Starfield et al., 1994). Nurses have been the fabric of these centers that dot the countryside, bringing care to populations chronically underserved in our health care system (Physician Payment Review Commission, 1994). Yet despite their central role in addressing the health care needs of communities through the successful intervention of health centers, nursing has not been able to assert its role in directing and shaping these endeavors. To move from passive participant to active leader, nurses needed to broaden their role to encompass policymaking activities.

CASE EXAMPLE **Hampton Woods** *(Continued)*

It was not long after the Hampton Woods Health Center opened that the state acted under its federal waiver to move Medicaid patients into managed care plans. Most patients seen at the health center were covered by Medicaid and opted to join one of the HMO offerings. Since the NPs were not listed as primary care providers with the HMO plans, their patients were assigned to one of the listed physician primary care providers, though they continued to seek care from the NPs. With that assignment, though, went the monthly capitation payments, resulting in a rapid drain in revenue away from the Hampton Woods Health Center. Consequently, RHS and the health center director set off to negotiate contracts for the center with the HMO plans covering their patients. The first HMO they approached requested an exclusive contract with the center, which meant that the center would not establish contracts with any other plans, and the HMO offered a premium in exchange. The NPs and RHS believed that their patients would not be well served by limiting the scope of plans with which they would do business; yet they were concerned that if they passed up this opportunity to negotiate a contract, they might have no viable contracts at the end of the process. They ultimately decided against accepting the offer of exclusivity with the first plan and in the end were pleased to have negotiated contracts with all the plans.

Medicaid managed care comprises one of the most intricate sets of policy and regulatory issues that nurses working with underserved populations have faced in some time, and it is further complicated by the introduction of a whole new cast of characters. Generally speaking, the locus of authority for most issues previously resided at the state government—for reimbursement from the Medicaid program and for scope of practice from the state licensing board and practice act. In the new world order, managed care plans have much more to say about both sets of issues, and the messages are not necessarily consistent across plans. The NP center at Hampton Woods was in one of the best positions to respond to the shift to Medicaid managed care, and even that center was nearly caught in an unfortunate tailspin. A clear understanding of the regulations undergirding the operations and financial arrangements of managed care is essential to the viability of nursing centers, together with a careful eye to unfolding policy actions that have affected and will affect future statutes and regulations. Alliances with key interest groups, such as the National Health Law Program on Medicaid managed care issues, can aid nurses in keeping abreast of the issues likely to affect them.

NP centers offer several advantages to managed care plans as they seek to expand their health care markets, and these advantages can serve as bargaining chips in contract negotiations. To begin with, in an increasingly competitive marketplace, NP centers offer plans an opportunity to enroll insured populations at a relatively low cost. Furthermore, the health center at Hampton Woods began receiving quarterly reports on patient costs and utilization from the HMO plans that showed notable cost-per-member savings for the health center compared with the physician practices also having contracts with the same HMO plans. Collecting data for tracking these trends and other measures of quality and patient outcomes provides nurses with another critical tool for policy debates on nursing's role in ensuring high-quality, low-cost care for needy individuals and families.

CASE EXAMPLE **Hampton Woods** *(Continued)*

After some time, the All-Health HMO, which covered most of the NPs' patients, made a decision that uncovered a regulatory issue of utmost importance for NP centers. All-Health had been operating its Medicaid plan under the HMO license of another managed care organization and decided to discontinue this arrangement and seek its own HMO license with the state. The state department of health (DOH), after reviewing its provider panel as part of the license application, informed All-Health that the regulations governing the definition of primary care providers did not allow for the listing of NPs in this capacity. With its HMO license application in jeopardy unless it terminated or radically restructured its relationship with the Hampton Woods Health Center, All-Health immediately contacted the center's director, who conferred with the NPs and contracted with a health lawyer to assist in the review and interpretation of these regulations. A letter was sent to the director of the Bureau of Health Care Financing, who administered the regulations, requesting a meeting to review their interpretation and to seek a ruling on the issue. In response, the bureau's director paid a visit to the health center to review patient charts and determine whether DOH quality-of-care standards were being met. After this visit, a large meeting was held at the DOH offices. It was attended by the NPs from the Hampton Woods Health Center and other NPs from across the state, the center's director and attorney, representatives from a number of the HMOs providing services under managed care contracts, leading members of the physician community, and officials from the DOH and the Bureau of Health Care Financing. The meeting offered a forum for all parties to share their views with government officials. Support for a clear ruling that allowed NPs status as primary care providers was surprisingly strong, with opposition coming only from several of the physicians in attendance.

The DOH promised a quick ruling on the issue; yet shortly after the meeting the director of the bureau vacated the position unexpectedly, and an acting director was put in his place. The hearts of the NPs sank at the news because they had left the meeting feeling optimistic for a quick and favorable ruling. Furthermore, without a quick ruling, the health center was facing a depleted stream of revenue and the possibility of closing. To their surprise, however, after just a few weeks the health center's director was contacted by DOH and was asked to attend a smaller meeting, where the issue could be reviewed once again. The health center's director and its attorney met with the bureau's acting director and counsel to explore the issues to be considered for a potential ruling. During this meeting a provision in the regulations was found that allowed for the granting of "exceptions" that would permit the extension of primary care provider status to NPs. A technical advisory memorandum was developed by DOH as a guideline for HMOs to use in requesting an exception to the regulations. The memorandum noted that establishing NP centers for primary care in underserved areas would constitute a condition under which listing NPs as primary care providers may be approved. This ruling allowed the doors of the Hampton Woods Health Center to remain open for all patients, and subsequently three additional NP centers in neighboring underserved areas were able to establish contracts with HMOs and expand their services.

Despite a wellspring of savvy and considerable attention to detail, the health center at Hampton Woods was nearly derailed once again. Here the regulations governing managed care were dictating the scope of authority of NPs by essentially withholding the designation of "primary care provider." Without this authority, NP centers for the underserved would not survive in their current form—and perhaps not at all. By marshaling resources, policy skills, experience, and supporters, the NPs went on to affix yet another brick in the regulatory foundation on which their practices could safely rest—for now. Vigilance will be required to ensure the integrity

of this foundation. The issue of "participating providers" has become enormously contentious for physicians as well as nurses, as evidenced by the spate of "any willing provider" bills that have been introduced in state legislatures across the country (Bodenheimer, 1996; McCarthy, 1997). These debates pose both opportunities and pitfalls for nurses, and as their experience in policymaking grows, so does nursing's ability to potentiate the opportunities in lieu of the pitfalls.

The Hampton Woods story underscores many of the lessons learned from the Dolorosa effort. For the Hampton Woods Health Center, the timing and circumstances were nearly perfect for setting up the service, and many of the hurdles that blocked previous efforts had been cleared. Yet even after the establishment of a health center that was remarkably successful on both cost and quality grounds, the rhetoric of "second-class care" once again reared its head. Only after a site visit to the health center were officials assured that quality standards were being met. Clearly the state officials were cautious about the precedent they were setting regarding the designation of NPs as primary care providers. The "exception" provided a mechanism through which the regulations could accommodate the reality of practice settings, and each circumstance could be reviewed and individually approved. Without the exceptions clause, though, the ruling by the bureau may have looked decidedly different.

CONCLUSION

Bismark once said, "Politics is the art of the impossible." Indeed, that which seems impossible at the outset can, through the art of the policymaking process, become possible. Through careful planning, tenacious effort, and commitment, success can be achieved. Yet how does one judge success? Each of these two case studies would be judged as having met with success but for somewhat different reasons. The nurses in Dolorosa may not have opened the community health network they had originally set out to open, but they were successful in achieving provider status as a nursing-IPA, which would be key in leveraging future projects. The NPs in Hampton Woods were able to open and maintain a thriving health center that enjoyed strong ties to the community, only to have it nearly snatched from their grasp. In each case the nurses relied on careful assessment of the unfolding events, rallied the necessary resources, never lost sight of the objective, and responded to each challenge with increasing precision and confidence.

These case studies are also emblematic of what is ahead for nurses in effecting public policy in health care. The fundamental organization and financing of health care services is being rapidly transformed, as policymakers increasingly turn to the marketplace for solutions to rising health care costs and inefficiencies in service delivery. These organizational arrangements, and the policies that direct them, are evolving continuously and in many different ways. The resulting labyrinth presents a daunting challenge to nurses and others who seek to implement strategies aimed at configuring a health care system responsive to the needs of consumers, especially the most vulnerable. While the nurses at both Dolorosa and Hampton Woods were finding avenues of success, they were barely keeping up with the ever-growing set of regulations, business arrangements, and public policies that could significantly affect their practices. Nevertheless, the skills and supporters they had gained at each step along the way would help them on their journey.

REFERENCES

Anderson, J. E. (1990). *Public policymaking.* Boston: Houghton Mifflin.

Anderson, J. E., Brady, D. W., Bullock, C. S., III, & Stewart, J., Jr. (1984). *Public policy and politics in America* (2nd ed.). Monterey, CA: Brooks/Cole.

Bodenheimer, T. (1996). The HMO backlash—righteous or reactionary? *New England Journal of Medicine, 335,* 1601–1604.

Butterfield, P. G. (1990). Thinking upstream: Nurturing a conceptual understanding of the societal context of health behavior. *Advances in Nursing Science, 12*(2), 1–8.

Diers, D. (1985). Policy and politics. In D. J. Mason & S. W. Talbott (Eds.), *Political action handbook for nurses* (pp. 53–59). Menlo Park, CA: Addison-Wesley.

Eddy, D. M., & Billings, J. (1988). The quality of medical evidence: Implications for quality of care. *Health Affairs, 7*(1), 19–32.

Ginzberg, E., & Ostrow, M. (1997). Managed care: A look back and a look ahead. *New England Journal of Medicine, 336,* 1018–1020.

Kingdon, J. W. (1984). *Agendas, alternatives, and public policies.* Boston: Little, Brown.

Kunin, M. (1987). Lessons from one woman's career. *Journal of State Government, 60*(5), 209–212.

Levin, M. A., & Ferman, B. (1985). *The political hand.* Elmsford, NY: Pergamon Press.

Lindblom, C. (1980). *The policy making process* (2nd ed.). Englewood Cliffs, NJ: Prentice-Hall.

McCarthy, D. (1997). Narrowing the provider choice: Any willing provider laws after New York Blue Cross v. Travelers. *American Journal of Law & Medicine, 23,* 97–113.

Milio, N. (1989). Developing nursing leadership in health policy. *Journal of Professional Nursing, 5*(6), 315–321.

Noah, T., & Davis, B. (1994, May 23). Tuna boycott is ruled illegal by GATT panel: Blow to U.S. policy to save dolphins may escalate attacks on trade pact. *The Wall Street Journal,* p. A2.

Paul-Shaheen, P. A. (1990). Overlooked connections: Policy development and implementation in state-local relations. *Journal of Health Politics, Policy and Law, 15*(4), 833–856.

Physician Payment Review Commission. (1994). *Annual report to Congress.* Washington, DC: Author.

Sardell, A. (1988). *The U.S. experiment in social medicine: The Community Health Center Program, 1965–1986.* Pittsburgh: University of Pittsburgh Press.

Safriet, B. J. (1992). Health care dollars and regulatory sense: The role of advanced practice nursing. *Yale Journal on Regulation, 19*(2), 417–488.

Starfield, B. (1992). *Primary care: Concept, evaluation, and policy.* Oxford: Oxford University Press.

Starfield, B., Powe, N. R., Weiner, J., Stuart, M., Steinwachs, D., Scholle, S. H., & Gerstenberger, A. (1994). Costs vs. quality in different types of primary care settings. *Journal of the American Medical Association, 272,* 1903–1908.

Starr, P. (1982). *The social transformation of American medicine.* New York: Basic Books.

Chapter *9*

CONFLICT MANAGEMENT

ALMA YEARWOOD DIXON

CASE EXAMPLE   **Organizational Conflict**

She knew it was going to be a difficult meeting. Each year when the schools of nursing and the clinical agencies gathered to allocate sites for students, the tension always existed because of limited placements and the divide between education and practice. This year the meeting was expected to be even more tense because of increased demands on staff time and the unwillingness of staff to take on another role—mentoring students.

She knew that baccalaureate programs would argue for more community sites because they believe that only their students are educated to care for clients, groups, and communities. Because of downsizing in institutional settings and the need to expand to noninstitutional sites, she expected the other nursing programs to disagree.

Historically the hospitals and other clinical agencies always bargained for students to assist with daily care to help with staffing. They exhibited minimal interest in theory and prolonged assessments and planning. She definitely was not looking forward to a meeting of professionals who overtly would try to reach a compromise as long as it did not interfere with their separate agendas. As chairperson for this Education-Practice Clinical Site Committee, she wondered whether there could be a creative way to reach an agreement.

When the meeting began, it was apparent that everyone came prepared with a list of demands. Quickly, positions were stated and lines drawn in the sand. Everyone spoke from a position of authority and knew what was right for the profession and, of course, the client.

Whenever two people interact, the potential for conflict exists because of the unique way that each person perceives the situation, processes information, and forms an opinion. Conflict within the work setting is a natural occurrence as people define and work toward common goals. The need to work for a "common good" facilitates conflict resolution. However, the current environment in health care has resulted in increased discord among staff, who are being engulfed by changes dictated by socioeconomic forces outside the profession. These changes are driving nursing education and practice in profoundly different ways. Consensus building and teamwork are more difficult because the players and the playing field are unfamiliar. Therefore nurses need to acquire new skills in conflict resolution and the art of negotiation.

TYPES OF CONFLICT

Conflict can be defined as the internal discord that occurs as a result of incongruity or incompatibility in ideas, values, or beliefs of two or more people. As opposed to a misunderstanding, conflict is more than a failure in interpretation; it usually represents some combination of a perceived threat to power or social position, scarcity of resources, and differing value systems. Conflict induces incompatible or antagonistic actions between two people or among groups.

Conflict can take many forms and occur in a concentric fashion, beginning with incompatible personal thoughts, values, perceptions, or actions (intrapersonal conflict), and can radiate to differences in relationships between people (interpersonal conflict) or groups of people (intergroup conflict) and in organizational demands, policies, or procedures (organizational conflict).

Intrapersonal Conflict

Intrapersonal conflict occurs within the individual nurse and represents an internal struggle to clarify values, perceptions, or needs. "Intrapersonal conflict exists in the cognitive and affective domains of an individual. There are no overt behavioral changes at this point, and yet the problem may eventually cause physiological or emotional stress. If intrapersonal conflict persists, it will manifest itself in some type of behavior that will precipitate interpersonal conflict" (Booth, 1993, p. 152).

This type of conflict can occur when a nurse is challenged to behave in ways that are not consistent with felt beliefs about professional ethics and practice, although the action may achieve organizational goals. For example, no matter where they practice, nurses are constantly challenged to question what they personally believe about health care and the practice of nursing with questions such as the following:

- Is quality care sacrificed with shortened hospital stays?
- Can you really do more with less?
- If I say no, will I have a job?
- Does a person's right to die influence my practice?
- How can I teach what I don't know?

Intrapersonal conflict can serve as the impetus for personal growth and change. According to Kritek (1994), conflicts are teaching experiences that call forth a commitment to courage, self-honesty, and learning. Recognizing that conflict resolution requires an exploration of alternatives, "one is divested of the illusion of a belief in 'the one right way,' the doors open to a myriad of ways, each with some truth and some distortion" (Kritek, 1994, p. 21).

Interpersonal Conflict

Conflict between people can be manifested by angry, hostile, or passive behaviors. These behaviors may be verbal, nonverbal, or physical. According to Brinkman and Kirschner (1994), interpersonal conflict occurs when the emphasis is placed on differences between people, and as a result, "united we stand, divided we can't stand each other" (p. 38).

Interpersonal conflict can impair working relationships, hinder productivity, and damage morale. Brinkman and Kirschner (1994) suggest strategies of blending and redirecting to resolve conflict in a timely and efficient manner. Blending involves reducing differences by finding common ground and mutual understanding, and redirecting is a process of using the rapport to change the trajectory of the communication toward a positive outcome.

To accomplish these strategies, one must be able to communicate and to listen until the issue is understood. The following steps are suggested:

1. Demonstrate listening and understanding by posture, voice volume, and action.
2. Backtrack or repeat some of the words used.
3. Clarify meaning and intent.
4. Summarize what was heard.
5. Confirm to find out whether understanding was reached.

These steps to careful listening and understanding facilitate conflict resolution by enabling the participants to define the problem clearly and by setting a climate for cooperation.

Intergroup Conflict

Intergroup conflict occurs between two or more groups of people, departments, or organizations. When intergroup conflict occurs, the participants form into cohesive teams that "circle the wagons" against the other teams who are perceived as the enemy with opposing views. Each of the teams tends to recognize only the positives within its membership and only the negatives within the other teams. Behaviors exhibited include "we-they language," gossip and blaming, back stabbing, and sabotage.

The resolution of intergroup conflict involves a process of identifying shared goals, focusing on the benefits of differences and diversity, valuing the input of all team members, and clarifying misperceptions.

Organizational Conflict

Organizational conflict can reflect intrapersonal, interpersonal, and intergroup conflict. According to Marquis and Huston (1994), this form of conflict is perceived as being either vertical or horizontal. Typically, vertical conflict occurs between superiors and their subordinates, or between staff and management. It usually concerns policy, power, and status. In contrast, horizontal conflict involves individuals with similar power and status in the table of organization. It usually occurs over discord related to authority, expertise, or practice issues.

Organizations are large, complex social systems with interacting forces that exert influence on nursing in all practice and education settings. These influences include the constant pressures of shrinking resources and financial constraints, the expanding needs and expectations of clients, the increasing militancy of nurses and students, and the persistent problems of interprofessional competition. These influences add to the prevalence of organizational conflict.

Nurses are required to function with political astuteness and prudent skill in identifying the subtle forces that have an impact on practice. They are required to make a realistic assessment of the circumstances, discern the obvious, and grasp and comprehend the obscure. Effective nurses have an astute grasp of the situation, with a logical shrewdness. However, when faced with conflict, too many nurses resort to a spontaneous emotional response without thinking of circumstances or consequences.

Effective organizations are composed of competent individuals who are able to practice in environments where differences are valued and serve as the impetus for constructive change. Organizational conflict that is not resolved can result in warring factions, reduced productivity, and disruption of teamwork.

CASE EXAMPLE   **Organizational Conflict** *(Continued)*

Within a short time the committee members were unwilling to change positions. The chairperson needed to achieve a resolution to the stalemate. The baccalaureate position involved more clinical time in the community while maintaining the same time in the hospitals. The stand was immutable because, they argued, the demands of the current health care system required more graduates with a bachelor of science in nursing degree, not associate degree nurses and certainly not licensed practical nurses.

The associate degree programs, larger in number of faculty and graduates, intended to win by sheer force of numbers and past practice.

The institutions, feeling harried and overworked, clearly wanted students to augment their staffing. Their pleas were for an "extra pair of hands."

Faced with these conflicting demands, the chairperson wanted to reach a lasting resolution to the conflict without resorting to the win-lose strategies of the past.

CONFLICT RESOLUTION

Conflict resolution involves a process of negotiation toward a mutually acceptable agreement. Methods for resolving conflict may result in win-lose solutions or, ideally, in win-win solutions.

Win-Lose Solutions

According to Roe (1995), win-lose solutions can be categorized in the following manner:

1. Denial, or withdrawal, involves attempts to get rid of the conflict by denying that it exists or by refusing to acknowledge it. If an issue is not important or if it is raised at an inopportune time, denial may be an appropriate strategy. However, if the issue is important, it will not go away and may grow to a point where it becomes unmanageable and builds to a greater complexity.

2. Suppression, or smoothing over, plays down the differences in the conflict, and the focus is placed on areas of agreement rather than on differences. Smoothing over may be appropriate for minor disagreements or to preserve a relationship. It is especially inappropriate when the involved parties are ready and willing to deal with the issue. It is important to note that the source of the conflict rarely goes away and may surface later in a more virulent form.

3. Power or dominance methods to resolve conflict allow authority, position, majority rule, or a vocal minority to settle the conflict. Power strategies result in winners and losers; the losers do not support the final decision in the same way that the winners do. Although this strategy may be appropriate when the group has agreed on this method of resolution, future meetings may be marred by renewal of the struggle.

4. Compromise is considered a mutual win-lose method of conflict resolution that involves each party's giving up something (losing) to gain and meet midway (winning). In our culture, compromise is viewed as a virtue. However, bargaining has serious drawbacks. For example, both sides often assume an inflated position because they are aware that they are going to have to "give a little," and they want to buffer the loss. The compromise solution may be watered down to the point of being ineffective, and there is often little real commitment to the solution. Further, compromise may result in antagonistic cooperation because either or both parties perceive that they have given up more than the other. Despite these drawbacks, compromise can be useful when resources are limited, when both sides have enough leeway to give, and when it is necessary to forestall a total win-lose stance.

CASE EXAMPLE   Organizational Conflict *(Continued)*

It was clear to the chairperson that the associate degree and allied health programs intended to win their bid for clinical sites by power and dominance. In the past, their requests were difficult to deny because of the need to place large numbers of students. As a baccalaureate faculty member, she was also aware that programs like hers had inflated their demands so that they would have a bargaining point to give up.

She also anticipated that the clinical sites would make every effort to compromise and appear neutral in order to maintain their relationships with the educational programs. With the shift in staffing patterns and the uncertain recruitment future, they could not afford to antagonize anyone at the table.

Despite the inherent problems, she was determined to develop a positive climate for conflict management and a resolution of the problems. The acrimonious debate resulted in a meeting that ran overtime. Forced to reschedule another time for the meeting, she was glad for the opportunity to plan another strategy for conflict resolution.

Win-Win Solutions

The goal of win-win solutions is to manage discord so that the conflict is a constructive impetus for growth, innovation, and productivity. Two win-win strategies are collaboration and principled negotiation.

COLLABORATION

The goal of collaboration is for everyone to win—no one has to give up anything. According to Marquis and Hurston (1994): "In collaboration, both parties set aside their original goals and work together to establish a supraordinate goal or common goal. Because both parties have identified the joint goal, each believes they have achieved their goal and an acceptable solution. The focus throughout collaboration remains on problem solving, and not on defeating the other party" (p. 290).

This approach to conflict resolution requires that all parties to the conflict recognize the expertise of the others. Each individual's position is valid, but the group emphasis is on solving the problem rather than on defending a particular position. All involved expect to modify original perceptions as the work of the group unfolds. The belief is that ultimately the best of the group's collective thinking will emerge because the problem is viewed from varied vantage points rather than one limited view.

Collaboration takes time and commitment to the problem-solving process. It requires mutual respect, listening skills, and an environment in which facts, assumptions, and feelings are verbalized and heard.

PRINCIPLED NEGOTIATION

Principled negotiation is a method of conflict resolution that is used as an alternative to positional bargaining. It was developed at the Harvard Negotiation Project and can be summarized in four basic steps, as identified by Fisher, Ury, and Patton (1992):

1. Separate the people from the problem. This step recognizes that all players in the negotiation are human beings with emotions, felt needs, deeply held values, and different backgrounds, experiences, and perceptions. Therefore the world is viewed from a selective vantage point, and perceptions are frequently confused with reality.

Because conflict is a dynamic process that begins on an intrapersonal level and expands to include relationships between people, it is easy to understand that negotiations are often clouded by the problem and the relationships. Therefore conflict resolution that results in a battle over wills and positions fosters identification of the positions with personal egos as those positions are defended against attack and become nonnegotiable. Saving face becomes necessary to reconcile future decisions with past positions. Moreover, arguing over positions endangers ongoing relationships and entangles the relationship with the problem.

In separating the people from the problem, one must pay careful attention to perception, emotion, and communication. Attempts are made to see the situation as the "other" and to have an empathetic understanding of the other point of view. This includes suspending judgment and actively listening. The parties work to avoid blaming each other for the problem or putting the worst interpretation on each action and instead discuss each perception. Emotions are valued and creative ways are sought for their expression.

2. Focus on interests, not on positions. Interests define the problem, and the conflict in positions is usually a conflict between needs, desires, concerns, and fears. Interests are the motivators behind positions, and identifying them allows for alternative positions that satisfy mutual interests. Dirschel (1993) wrote: "Identify the facts and feelings behind each side's desires and concerns. Behind opposing positions often lie shared and compatible interests. If the focus is on positions rather than interests, the parties will have difficulty brainstorming other options, because they will be intent on keeping their bottom-line positions" (p. 164).

3. Invent options for mutual gain. One answer to a dispute is counterproductive and leads to negotiations along a single dimension. Wiser decision making involves a process of selection from a large number of possible solutions. The more options identified, the more chances there are for creative, productive solutions for all parties concerned.

Successful negotiations that result in several options are often impeded by seeking the single answer because it is believed that resolution to discord requires narrowing the gap between positions rather than broadening the options available. Negotiations that are bound by a fixed-pie approach also dictate win-lose battles because there are only a few good options to go around.

The process of brainstorming is one method used to invent options without judging them. Participants in the exercise are encouraged to identify as many ideas as possible without judgment or criticism. Attempts should be made to invent ideas that meet shared interests. These interests need to be explicit and stated as goals.

4. Insist on using objective criteria. To ensure a wise agreement between opposing wills involves negotiation on some basis of objective criteria. These criteria need to be based on a fair standard and, ideally, be prepared in advance of the agreement. Discussion of the criteria, rather than of positions to be gained or lost, allows for deferment to a fair solution instead of bruised egos and hurt relationships.

Fisher et al. (1992) conclude: "In contrast to positional bargaining, the principled negotiation method of focusing on basic interests, mutually satisfying options, and fair standards typically results in a wise agreement. The method permits you to reach a gradual consensus on a joint decision efficiently without all the transactional costs of digging in to positions only to have to dig yourself out of them" (p. 14).

CASE EXAMPLE **Organizational Conflict** *(Continued)*

No one expected the facilitator to have a picnic lunch ready and to move the meeting to a more informal setting. They were especially surprised by the seating arrangement, which placed them side by side in different pairings from their co-workers. The reason, she said, was for them to tackle a common problem together, as a group—not as different agencies. As the facilitator she would guide the discussion. Everyone would be heard without criticism. Everyone knew each other's positions and points of disagreement. Therefore the purpose of the meeting was to elicit interests and to produce as many ideas as possible to address the problem at hand.

In this meeting there would be no good gals or guys in white hats and bad ones in black. The issues were too complicated and deserved more than simple answers. She challenged her colleagues to see the others as a resource rather than as the cause of the problem. The only bottom line to this meeting would be a fair agreement that was advantageous to everyone.

The settings in which nurses practice and teach will continue to require expertise in conflict resolution as the challenges of transforming health care move into the twenty-first century. According to Kritek (1994), negotiating often occurs at an uneven table at which some participants are at a disadvantage that others do not acknowledge. Uneven tables represent situations in which the assurance of justice, equity or fairness is uncertain or unlikely. The nurse is challenged to recognize conflict as an impetus to change that requires personal growth. Choosing a method of conflict resolution will depend on

---

> **STEPS TO CONFLICT RESOLUTION**
>
> 1. Whose conflict is it?
> 2. What is the common denominator?
> 3. Set a climate of trust.
> 4. Separate the people from the problem.
> 5. Stay in the present and the future.
> 6. Stick to the topic at hand.
> 7. Brainstorm options.
> 8. Develop objective criteria for evaluating options.
> 9. Look for consensus.

personal style and the situation. The choice can be facilitated by a few considerations that are outlined in the box above.

According to Rhode (1996), the steps to reaching a positive solution begin with identifying the parties involved in the conflict. It is important to get all parties to list, in writing, their positions (what is wanted) and interests (why it is wanted). This fosters understanding of positions taken because of vested interests and hidden agendas. Shared interests can serve as common denominators in the resolution process. A climate of trust can be established by open communication, with parties using "I" statements as personal ownership of positions and problems. Rules that prohibit zapping, back stabbing, and sarcasm enhance trust. Yelling and aggressive body language violate that trust.

Separating the person from the problem allows for addressing the problem without attacking the person involved. Personal attacks impede communication and conflict resolution. Past injustices and hurt feelings have no place in resolving present conflicts; therefore stay in the present and focus only on the problem at hand. Use the process to identify ways to make sure the problem does not reoccur in the future.

The temptation may be to tackle more than one problem at a time. However, success depends on the ability to stick to the topic at hand and handle only one conflict at a time. Finally, in looking for consensus, it is useful to remember that if 75% of the parties involved agree, and

25% or less dissent but agree to support the solution, a resolution can be reached.

CASE EXAMPLE **Organizational Conflict** *(Continued)*

The meeting began with everyone's stating his or her position and interest, which were then recorded on a flip chart for all to see. That part was easy— everyone wanted more clinical time. The reason that an increase in time was needed was more difficult to ascertain. However, she made sure that everyone's position and interest were listed.

To arrive at a win-win solution, she encouraged the participants to think of possible alternative clinical sites. In effect, the options were being expanded and new resources found. She chose this method because the initial conflict was based on a shortage of resources.

She was also aware that basic conflicts in philosophy about nursing education and practice were still an issue for the participants. Therefore she suggested a future summit meeting on this issue to resolve this conflict. This allowed her to reformulate the problem of the shortage of clinical sites by addressing only the key interests of all parties.

This chapter was not meant to suggest one method of conflict resolution. Instead, varied strategies were presented to assist nurses in coping with intrapersonal, interpersonal, intergroup, and organizational conflict. The nurse will need to be able to reduce disharmony within her internal set of values, needs, and perceptions as they are called into question by an increasingly complex, differentiated system of health care delivery. Competence in managing interpersonal and organizational discord will be essential as work groups become more diverse and the chance for differing viewpoints increases. Nurses can play a pivotal role in facilitating an environment in which conflict is used to enhance the exploration of new approaches and alternatives to problems.

REFERENCES

Booth, R. (1993). Dynamics of conflict and conflict management. In D. J. Mason, S. W. Talbott, & J. K. Leavitt (Eds.), *Policy and politics for nurses* (2nd ed). Philadelphia: W. B. Saunders.

Brinkman, R., & Kirschner, R. (1994). *Dealing with people you can't stand.* New York: McGraw-Hill.

Dirschel, K. (1993). Dynamics of conflict and conflict management. In D. J. Mason, S. W. Talbott, & J. K. Leavitt (Eds.), *Policy and politics for nurses* (2nd ed.). Philadelphia: W. B. Saunders.

Fisher, R., Ury, W, & Patton, B. (1992). *Getting to yes: Negotiating agreement without giving in* (2nd ed.). New York: Penguin Books.

Kritek, P. B. (1994). *Negotiating at an uneven table.* San Francisco: Jossey-Bass.

Marquis, B., & Hurston, C. (1994). *Management decision-making for nurses* (2nd ed). New York: J. B. Lippincott.

Oesterle, M., & O'Callaghan, D. (1996). The changing health care environment. *Perspectives on Community, 17, 78–81.*

Rhode, H. (1996). *Conflict resolution and confrontation skills.* Boulder, CO: CareerTrack.

Roe, S. (1995). Managing your work setting: Positive work relationships, conflict management, and negotiations. In K. W. Vestal (Ed.), *Nursing management: Concepts and issues* (2nd ed.). New York: J. B. Lippincott.

Chapter *10*

COALITIONS FOR ACTION

JUDITH K. LEAVITT AND JANE B. PINSKY

A coalition is one of the most important and effective political strategies for creating concerted action to reach a defined goal. Coalitions arise when a group of people create a situation where it is to everyone's benefit to work together. The results can be far greater than if each individual or group worked alone. A good coalition proves the adage that the whole is greater than the sum of its parts.

This chapter will discuss coalitions as a political strategy to influence public and private policy, to elect candidates, to gain political appointments, to improve the workplace, and to gain visibility and recognition for professional organizations. It will highlight different types of coalitions, how they work, and their strengths and limitations. Examples of short-term coalitions and one lasting many years will be shared. The reader will find guidelines to facilitate participation in and creation of effective collective action.

COALITIONS: AN OVERVIEW

The word *coalition* comes from the Latin word *coalescere,* which means to grow together. Most commonly a coalition is an alliance, a coming together of groups or individuals for a limited period. It can also be a combining— a union—of people, groups, factions, parties, or nations. Coalitions exist because people or organizations share a common concern or goal. For political parties it may be to gain power; for neighborhood associations, it may be to get stop signs; in a professional association, it may be getting an individual elected as president; in a

town it may be to open a community health facility.

There are three reasons to use coalitions as a political strategy. The first is to borrow power (that is, a recognition that an individual or group lacks the power to confront an issue alone). Second, it can be the vehicle to build a base of support. And third, coalitions can prevent another group from challenging a plan. Whatever the reason, it is essential that the goal be clearly defined before groups or individuals are willing to join in collective action. The process of defining the problem may be hard work. Initially a goal may be only vaguely defined by the organizers; however, as groups begin to work together, the goals become clearer and more reflective of the diverse perspectives of members.

A **long-standing, formal coalition** in the United States is the American Federation of Labor–Congress of Industrial Organizations (AFL-CIO). It has changed from a very loose amalgam of labor unions to a highly formalized organization with elected leadership, a large staff in Washington, and chapters in every state. The AFL-CIO has established rules for operating and maintaining a balance of power and momentum. Ongoing coalitions with such stability and breadth of interest are unusual and in the early stages require a huge commitment to a common goal, an unshakable idealism, and an incredibly strong and charismatic leader.

Once a formal coalition is established, changes take place in the kind of leadership and the goals and strategies of the group. One like the AFL-CIO needs an ongoing commitment to common goals, strategies, and tactics. The leader must change from one who is a high-energy, strong-willed person to one who can maintain the organization as it grows. Growth requires the creation of an atmosphere in which groups can compromise and be willing to subjugate individual goals to the overall goal of the coalition. Such a large organization requires considerable resources to meet the diverse needs and maintain the involvement of many constituencies.

A different kind of **long-standing coalition** is the National Federation of Specialty Nursing Organizations (NFSNO). This is a formal coalition of specialty organizations created as a forum to discuss common interests and concerns. They were particularly active and involved during the health care reform debate. The combined strength of more than 70 organizations, along with that of the TriCouncil (American Nurses Association, National League for Nursing, American Organization of Nurse Executives, and American Association of Colleges of Nursing), created an impressive and unified message to President Clinton and the policymakers that the nursing community supported the Health Security Act.

Another example of a **loose coalition of national organizations** was created in the early 1980s by the leaders of major national women's organizations, most of whom are based in Washington, D.C. They met regularly to discuss issues affecting women: key legislative initiatives; policies for which women members of Congress, state governors, and other elected officials needed help in garnering support; women contemplating running for elective office; and political appointments for women. These regular meetings provided a basis for mobilizing around issues like pay equity, women's health, and reproductive issues. It also provided the origin for a more formal coalition, the Women's Federal Appointment Task Force (see Chapter 27: Political Appointments).

The task force was created to find and support qualified women for federal appointments. Starting with the Reagan presidency, the goal of the coalition was to exert collective action by the women's organizations to choose women nominees recommended by the members of the coalition. Originally the list was small and suggestions for appointees were made informally. Then the coalition realized that, to have credibility and be inclusive, it must develop a formalized process for soliciting candidates and collectively recommending women from a selected list of candidates. By the time President Bush was ready to create "short lists" of candidates for appointments, the task force had created extensive background information and support for their suggested candidates. Once the bulk of appointments was completed, the task force became inactive until the next presidential election.

The most common type of coalition is an **ad hoc, issue-oriented coalition.** It forms around a specific issue. When the issue has been resolved, the group disbands. For instance, the National Health Care Campaign was formed in 1993 during the national debate on health care reform. Organizations representing health professionals, consumers, policymakers, and not-for-profit health care institutions wanted to create a strong voice for a system of universal and accessible health care. Once health care reform was no longer on the public agenda, the coalition's goal became unattainable, resources became scarce, and the coalition disbanded.

Coalitions are proliferating as groups recognize the value of working together on specific issues. It is easier, often more expedient, and less expensive to work together through coalitions than to form a new organization. The coalition can be disbanded or realigned as issues are resolved and new ones develop. This approach allows for changes in membership, leadership, and strategies as goals change. As a result, coalitions can be the most effective, economical, and efficient vehicle for achieving collective action.

PRINCIPLES OF ACTING COLLECTIVELY

As different as coalitions may appear, they share some basic principles:

- Coalitions are formed because *the whole is*

greater than the sum of the parts. Strength in numbers and in diversity create a group process that reflects the broadest perspective and creates an outcome that is likely to be more innovative and comprehensive than if individual members acted alone. Coalitions also send a strong message of cohesive support to those who are targeted for influence. Coalitions are proof of the old adage that "though twenty sticks may be broken separately, it is almost impossible to break them as a bundle." The most effective, but often the most challenging, coalitions are those which bring race, gender, ethnicity, regionalism, age, and different values to an issue. Finding common ground can be arduous and is sometimes impossible. Yet in such diversity lies a strength—that so many different voices share a common goal and are intent on reaching it.

- *The process of creating coalitions is largely the same.* It is essential to be attentive to the structure and process of coalitions. To be effective, the coalition must create a structure that encourages and supports involvement in all aspects of decision making. They work well when all members of the coalition believe that they share in the development of goals and strategies.

- *Coalitions work best when the purpose and strategies are clear and simple.* It is always easier to keep a coalition going and minimize the infighting when there is one explicit goal. For example, if a coalition is formed by alumni and community members to keep the nursing program of a local college open, the end point will occur when the board of trustees votes. A clear and simple strategy might be to get alumni and friends to lobby the trustees about the contribution that the program makes to the college. Simple slogans keep people working together and focused. For example, the slogan for a Children's Defense Fund initiative to get the nation to focus on the needs of children was "Stand (up) for Children." The message and the goal for organizing activities were readily understood by participants and the policymakers whom they were trying to influence.

- *All politics is local.* The true strength of coalitions comes from the numbers of people they reach and the level of their active involvement. To be most effective, it must influence and include the people who best know the community and the issues—those who vote, write checks, and are committed to solving problems. "Outside experts" may be used in an advisory capacity but cannot lead the effort and expect to generate strong and sustained dedication.

- *All collective action involves a challenge to the power structure and results in an effort to take or share power.* As with any aspect of changing the balance of power, conflict is inherent in the process. As a result, one can expect resistance and to be perceived as threatening to those in power. It is incumbent on visionary coalitions to be prepared for the conflict by developing strategies that both can be proactive and can refute arguments of the opposition. The ultimate goal of acting collectively is to empower individuals for participation in public and social policy decisions. To do so means that power needs to be shared, mentoring of new and inexperienced members needs to occur, and communication needs to be interactive. In the best of coalitions, participants learn new skills, make new connections, and leave with a willingness to be involved again.

GUIDELINES FOR FORMING AND MAINTAINING COALITIONS

Coalitions need to have a clear vision to generate initial and ongoing support. Most often a few individuals, acting alone or as representatives of a group, will informally come together for the purpose of solving a problem, supporting or defeating a policy, or acting on behalf of or in opposition to a candidate for elected office. Once there is a realization that collective action must be taken to resolve the issue, the formation of a coalition will occur. The following are guidelines to create and maintain coalitions:

1. Identify an issue of concern.

A GUIDE FOR BUILDING COALITIONS

Following is a list of questions that can serve as a guide for forming and maintaining coalitions:

1. What is the goal of this coalition?
   a. Know precisely what you expect to accomplish or what problem needs a solution.
   b. Do you want it to
      (1) Pressure/lobby/persuade elected officials, a board of trustees, a TV network, scholars, educators, researchers, developers?
      (2) Build community awareness or support?
      (3) Raise money to help pay for a solution?
2. What is the expected time frame for the coalition to exist?
   a. When must the issue be resolved?
   b. When must the coalition begin to act?
   c. Must specific tasks be accomplished by certain dates?
   d. What are the repercussions if these benchmarks are not reached?
3. What resources are needed?
   a. What can organizations and individuals bring to the coalition?
   b. What are the priority resources?
   c. How will the coalition function if resources are not available?
4. Who are supporters?
5. Who is the opposition?
6. What groups need to be included? Why?
   a. If two groups don't get along, is the leadership willing to go through the mediation and negotiation needed to keep them in the coalition?
   b. Are there groups who need to be involved solely because they will cause more trouble if they are not included?
   c. What prominent groups or individuals can lend their support and credibility to the coalition?
7. What are the hidden agendas?
8. What are the reasons that each member is willing to join?
9. What is the best structure for the coalition?
10. Who should take leadership roles?
11. What can members take away from their participation?
    a. Specific skills?
    b. A sense of empowerment?
    c. New networks?
12. Is there a logical next step for the coalition? A reason to keep it going? Is there a reason to disband?

---

2. Identify all the groups that share an interest in the issue. Broad thinking is important to be as inclusive and creative as possible. Think of who will be affected by an issue and who can be part of the solution. What are the ties that would bind groups to the issue? For example, a long-term care coalition must include more than those representing the elderly population. It might include groups for disabled persons, for families needing respite, or for staff from public health services, offices for the aging, and social services departments, as well as for groups interested in creating housing for independent living.

3. Define a clear goal. The clearer and simpler the goal, the easier it is to generate support and create strategies for implementation. The greatest "buy in" will occur when members participate in creating the goal.

4. Invite participation through networking with friends, colleagues, and others. To keep a coalition functioning, it is necessary that participants be as committed to the goal as they are to members of the group.

5. Timing is an essential aspect of working in coalitions. It is vital to consider when to recruit participants and when to plan action. Judicious timing enhances the ability of the collective to develop proactive rather than reactive strategies and to create media advocacy to gain public awareness and support.

6. A well-organized, caring, and charismatic leader who can motivate others to be involved is necessary to maintain collective action. Although different people may assume aspects of running the coalition, it takes one leader to unify the group. At different times the leader must act as recruiter, supporter, strategist, agitator, teacher, and spokesperson. Excelling in communication skills and group process is more important than understanding all the nuances of an issue. Skilled leaders know their limitations and recognize when to seek help. The attitude of the leader sets the tone for the members of the collective. Being positive through the process maintains momentum. Being realistic when temporary setbacks occur and seeking input when strategies need revising keep members involved and committed. It is the leader who creates an atmosphere of trust and acceptance of diversity.

7. Establish ground rules that clarify the choices members have in working together. Some members may disagree with one aspect of a planned action but still support the overall goal and long-term strategy. For example, a coalition of nurse practitioners worked collectively for reimbursement. However, there was disagreement about the reimbursement rate; some groups insisted that it be at 97% of a physician's rate, whereas others were willing to accept an 85% rate to achieve the larger goal of direct reimbursement. The disagreement was based on the belief that setting a reimbursement rate lower than that of physicians could jeopardize those nurses employed in group practices whose income would be inadequate to justify their participation. In such a situation, the group wanting "full" reimbursement was willing to lend its name to the coalition's overall goal but chose not to lobby policy makers for the lower rate. The ground rules enabled them to "agree to disagree." They were able to remain involved and could be counted on *not* to oppose the efforts of the full coalition.

COALITIONS IN ACTION

The National Committee on Pay Equity (NCPE) was founded in 1979 by a group made up of representatives of organizations and individuals whose goal was to achieve pay equity for women in the United States. The initial strategy was to publicize the issue and aid in a lawsuit; however, in the 18 years since its founding, it has evolved far from such a simplistic objective. It is now a separate organization with full-time staff and a board of directors—and the goal of equity has not yet been achieved.

Along the way, there were a series of power struggles. Some involved issues of leadership, and others involved issues of responsibility for different tasks. Members struggled with balancing the needs of their individual organizations with the needs of the coalition. Sometimes the decisions were easy, whereas at other times, compromises worthy of Solomon had to be resolved. Occasionally it was worth allowing one member of the coalition to garner publicity or take the lead on a specific strategy, even though such concessions were not always in the best interest of NCPE. In the end, everyone in the coalition managed to make the adjustments necessary to serve both the goal and the organization. Unfortunately, pay equity is still not a reality for most women in the United States.

Coalitions can be short-lived and informal and can form around a "simple" issue. One of the authors was involved early in the 1970s with women in San Francisco who worked in an office building that did not have tampon or sanitary napkin machines in the ladies' rooms. Though the situation was not life threatening, it was annoying and time-consuming to travel down 30, 50, or 60 floors to the drugstore on the ground level. For clerical staff it required getting permission from their supervisors to leave. Several women from one of the offices tried to talk to the building managers, without success. The managers did not want the machines in bathrooms because they marred the design. The next step was to talk to leasing management, who didn't see the issue as important. So the women placed flyers inside the stalls in ladies' rooms to encourage the women to speak to their bosses and persuade them that having the machines in the bathrooms would save time away from work. Eventually, enough tenants pressured the building management that the goal was reached. The power of the women—their numbers and the cost of lost work time—created the pressure needed to reach the goal.

A SUCCESS STORY: THE FAMILY AND MEDICAL LEAVE COALITION

Successful coalitions don't just happen. They require clear goals, careful planning, and careful management. In the early 1980s, children's advocates, sociologists, feminists, employers, and others started talking about ways to reduce stress on families and to help keep workers, especially women, in the work force. One of the greatest stresses they identified was the pull between work and family, particularly when there was an ill family member—a child, spouse, or parent. Another stress occurred when parents needed time at home after the birth or adoption of a child. As the group members looked at the need for "time off from work," they compared the problems that working parents face in the United States with those in other countries. They found that, in other countries, family leave was not only available, it was paid—and the worker was guaranteed the same or a comparable job on return to the work force.

To get family leave of any sort in the United States was a major undertaking. During the Reagan era, "pro family" values favored mothers' staying home to care for children while Dad went to work, something that fewer and fewer families were able to afford. It was also a time of decreasing government involvement in people's lives. Social policy was supported that placed responsibility for solving family issues on the family. Family and medical leave was not supported by many members in Congress nor by the Reagan Administration. As a result, it was clear that garnering support would require a broad-based, diverse movement. In early 1985 the group that evolved became known as the Family and Medical Leave Coalition.

The early organizers put it together thoughtfully and carefully. They analyzed what kind of legislation was needed and whether it should be targeted at the federal or state level. Because most work- and workplace-related legislation (e.g., wage and hour regulations, child labor laws, standards of the Occupational Safety and Health Administration) was under federal jurisdiction, the decision was made to focus efforts on Congress.

The original goal was to propose federal legislation that would accomplish the following:

- Provide family leave to all workplaces with more than 15 employees (the number needed to invoke federal law)
- Cover an employee who worked more than 1000 hours in a year and had been employed for at least a year
- Guarantee paid leave

Although the organizers believed that the goal seemed achievable, it was created to be broad enough to enlist support from a wide assortment of organizations. Many were interested in specific aspects of the issue, rather than the broad goal. For instance, the goal did not originally define a specific time for taking leave. Organizations representing child development experts joined the coalition because they wanted the leave to be for a minimum of 6 months. Other groups were more concerned that the leave be paid, even if it meant that the time would be shorter.

The next task was to develop the membership. In recruiting coalition members, the organizers selected groups whose issues could help refute arguments of the anticipated opposition. They planned their recruiting to bolster the most positive arguments and to counteract the greatest objections. Because of the nature of the issue, there were a number of natural constituencies—women's groups, labor unions, child development experts, pediatricians, and pediatric nurses. There were also a number of groups that did not immediately come to mind but who became key to the success of the legislation: religious groups, like the National Council of Jewish Women and a number of church groups; groups concerned with diseases, like cancer victims and their families; others such as those representing people with chronic diseases; retired, elderly, and older citizens; and educators. Recruiting older Americans brought in the American Association of Retired People, with its financial resources and a constituency that could be activated. Working with child development experts and pediatricians helped attract noted pediatrician and writer Dr. T. Berry Brazelton, who served as a media draw as well as a reliable and credible expert. Whenever groups joined the coalition, it was made clear that the coalition was temporary (it lasted 8 years) and that it had *one* goal—the passage of federal family and medical leave legislation.

The one mistake that the coalition initially made had to do with the involvement of Congressional staff people, especially those who worked for the prime Congressional sponsors. The staff members were integral to the coalition, particularly in developing strategies and priorities; however, their first loyalty was, understandably, to their Member of Congress, not to the coalition. Often the needs and goals of the two were different, and this led to considerable friction. It was not until the staffers were moved from involvement with the overall coalition to focusing on broad legislative strategy that the tension in the coalition diminished. Unfortunately, the conflict consumed precious time, energy, and good will, and recovery took a long time. There were other areas of conflict between the goals and needs of the coalition and the goals and needs of the members, but none was as divisive.

Once the coalition had a critical mass of members, the leadership created a careful structure so that the lines of communication were clear and understood by all members. They also established an explicit decision-making process that was key to the success of the coalition. Numerous coalitions have failed because all the members believed that they each had to know everything. The resulting confusion and paralysis can lead to a lack of success in achieving the desired goal.

A board of directors was formed to serve as a coordinating clearinghouse and central decision-making body. Working groups and task forces were created with clearly defined goals and an understanding of their relationship in the hierarchy of the coalition. Each task force and working group had its own leaders, as well as one or two members who acted as a liaison to the board and to other working groups. Each working group developed its own decision-making process. Generally, it was a combination of consensus and, sometimes, "benign dictatorship."

The legislative task force was the largest and overall the most active, because the goal of the coalition was passage of federal legislation. The needs of this task force drove the rest of the coalition. It was initially where the conflict with Congressional staff was felt, and it remained the group with the most dissension. Several of the members rebelled against the coalition leadership, the task force's leadership, and the Congressional staffers. That meant that some members were sometimes working on their own rather than working in concert.

The strategy and tactics that developed emanated from the political agenda in Congress. As it changed, so, too, did the strategies for garnering support and thwarting the opposition. Members of Congress, who acted as cosponsors of the legislative proposal, helped guide the political strategies. Their insight helped the coalition know which Members needed to be lobbied and where support was forthcoming. The legislative task force of the coalition decided which constituents would lobby, when to use a paid lobbyist, and when to mobilize through phone calls, letters, and postcards.

Because responsibilities were clearly delineated and each group played to its strength, turf battles were infrequent. The working groups met as needed; for the legislative task force, that meant weekly when Congress was in session and once a month when Congress was not. Other working groups met far less often or did so by conference calls. (A mistake coalitions frequently make is to meet too often.) The executive committee tried, not always successfully, to keep all members informed of what each working group was doing and what progress had been achieved.

Eventually the Family and Medical Leave Act passed in Congress three times. Unfortunately, President Bush vetoed it twice; however his veto motivated the coalition to continue a concerted effort until the goal was achieved. Because Congress had twice passed the proposal, the group believed that was positive proof that pressure needed to be continued.

The battle was finally won. Eight years after the coalition started, President Clinton signed the Family and Medical Leave Act on February 5, 1993. The bill was not exactly what the coalition originally envisioned, but it was close enough to provide all the members with a great sense of success. It was a battle whose outcome had been worth the effort.

WHEN COALITIONS DO NOT WORK

Sometimes coalitions are not effective, such as when quick action is needed. Coalitions require consensus and a process for sharing information, which can consume excessive time when a swift response is needed in a rapidly changing situation. For instance, an intergenerational coalition that formed for instituting an after-school program in a senior center disbanded when the center itself was threatened with closure and the coalition's leaders were focused on responding to daily charges of mismanagement. Not only did the leaders of the coalition have to respond quickly to the attacks, but they were forced to become reactive rather than proactive. In such situations, coalitions become an ineffective strategy for reaching a goal.

Second, a coalition may not work well when negotiations must be secret. For instance, during labor disputes, members of a coalition must enable their leaders to negotiate both freely and secretly. If there is a lack of trust in the coalition's representatives, coalition members may withdraw. To prevent such occurrences, coalition negotiators must keep members informed as much as possible.

A third situation when coalitions are not effective occurs when members become polarized over goals, issues, strategies, leadership, or even personalities. Sometimes conflicts can be so divisive and struggles over control of leadership so destructive that the only recourse is to disband the coalition. Two groups with the same goal can have philosophies that are so different that they have great difficulty working together.

Last, coalitions cannot survive if enough resources are unavailable to sustain the needs for meetings, communication, and general operations. Resources may include money but may also include individuals who have the time and commitment to provide in-kind support. Without such resources, a coalition cannot continue.

SUMMARY

This chapter has discussed the use of coalitions as a strategy to mobilize for action. Whether that action is support or opposition for a political candidate, a health policy issue, a workplace policy, or an organizational or community issue, the process is the same. Most nurses have been involved in some type of collective action, often unrelated to a professional issue. However, purposefully creating and leading coalitions become increasingly important as nurses become involved in politics and policy. Nurses have all the skills needed to use coalitions to effect change: leadership, communication, organization, and management. One need only to practice using them by participating in collective action to realize how effective and challenging the use of coalitions can be as a political strategy.

VIGNETTE

The Ad Hoc Committee to Defend Health Care: A Collaborative Nurse-Physician Effort

Betsy Todd

The health care reform efforts of the early 1990s were the first threat in more than 20 years to the people who profit the most from our private insurance–based health care system. When reforms could not be *legislated,* grassroots activists found a new approach to fit a dramatically altered health care climate.

In 1993 the single-payer national health insurance bill proposed by Congressman and physician Jim McDermott (1994, 1995) had more Congressional cosponsors than any other reform bill but was eclipsed in media coverage by President Clinton's more expensive and less comprehensive plan. At the same time, there was renewed interest, albeit limited, in Congressman Ron Dellums' sweeping and progressive proposal for a national health *service.**

Powerful players in the medical-industrial complex took note of all three bills. The surprising Congressional support for Dr. McDermott's bill, in particular, along with its endorsement by a wide range of health and civic groups, suggested that national health insurance was once again a possibility in the United States. On the other hand, President Clinton's weaker but much-ballyhooed reform bill kept private insurance at the center of health care in this country. To many observers, the President's message to the insurance industry was clear: "Your domination of U.S. health care is safe on my watch."

Without the passage of *any* reform legislation, the direction set by the President held sway. During the next 4 years, there was a rapid restructuring of health care services and of the health care workplace as for-profit corporations aggressively bought both insured lives and nonprofit hospitals.

While for-profit health maintenance organizations (HMOs) and other entities cut care to increase profits, nonprofit hospitals and clinics downsized in attempts to contain costs and remain "competitive." However, the real causes of health care inflation—high administrative costs, the inefficiencies of private insurance, and soaring profits—were not addressed, and costs continued to rise.

People's need for care, of course, did not go away; in fact, hospitalized patients were more acutely ill than ever. Short staffing and increasingly limited resources left nurses angry, exhausted, and often stunned by their inability to hold the line for expert and compassionate patient care.

In February 1997 doctors in Boston, outraged at the for-profit takeovers of local nonprofit hospitals, joined together to form the Ad Hoc Committee to Defend Health Care. The committee was chaired by Dr. Bernard Lown, a Nobel Peace Prize recipient for his previous work in organizing physicians against nuclear war. The doctors, convinced that a joint nurse-physician effort was essential to bring about change, then contacted Dorothy McCabe at the Massachusetts Nurses Association (MNA).

MNA nurses had begun a statewide Safe Care Campaign 4 years earlier to address increasingly alarming evidence of unsafe care in the new profit-driven environment. They saw the Ad Hoc Committee effort as another way to bring their concerns to the public. The MNA mobilized nurses around the state.

---

*Mr. Dellums had introduced this bill—written in close collaboration with community activists, progressive clinicians, and "regular" citizens—in every Congressional session for nearly two decades.

Significantly, the Ad Hoc Committee's effort stepped aside from the goal of universal health care to address the immediate crisis brought about by the explosion of for-profit corporations and their dramatic effect on the quality of health care. Many doctors and nurses who were not yet familiar with the remarkable health and economic benefits of universal health care (and therefore not ready to support national health insurance or a national health service) were outspoken critics of the "failed experiment" of profit-driven care. By focusing on what was immediately, desperately wrong without prescribing a long-term solution, the organizers of this effort were able to attract a much larger group of health care professionals to the reform effort.

The Ad Hoc Committee (1997) drew up a *Call to Action*, calling for a dialog between clinicians and the public on the future of health care. Specific goals were to petition local, state, and federal officials for a moratorium on for-profit takeovers of hospitals, insurance plans, HMOs, and other health care institutions, and to initiate an ongoing series of forums, teach-ins, and public meetings to discuss the health care crisis.

Word of the Boston effort quickly spread among reform advocates across the country. Well-known physicians and nurses joined the

---

THE *CALL TO ACTION*

An excerpt from the Ad Hoc Committee's document:
We differ on many aspects of reform, but on the following we find common ground:
- Medicine and nursing should not be diverted from their primary tasks: the relief of suffering, the prevention and treatment of illness, and the promotion of health.
- The pursuit of corporate profit and personal fortune has no place in caregiving.
- Financial incentives that reward the withholding of services should be prohibited. Patient needs, not corporate profit, should determine patient care.
- The right to choose a physician or nurse must not be curtailed. Access to comprehensive, affordable, and quality health care must be the right of all.

---

effort, helping to spark media interest. A lengthy article (Kilborn, 1997) appeared in July 1997—a feat in itself, because the *New York Times* was a strong opponent of health care reform. (Typically, however, the *Times* made no mention of nurses' role in the effort.)

Later that summer, a national conference call for interested doctors and nurses attracted more than 200 professionals in more than 40 states. The multistate conference call was an activist support technique used frequently by Physicians for a National Health Program. For a small fee, the group organizing a call arranges to host it at an appointed time, and conference participants call a designated number at that time. Each person is charged for the call as a regular long distance call (charges appear on her or his bill), with the cost being generally less than $10 for 1 hour. In this way, activists have the opportunity for regular dialog with front-line colleagues in other states, and the costs of the call are shared and therefore not prohibitive for nonprofit groups with small budgets.

As a result of the first conference call, ad hoc committees quickly formed in a dozen states, and new voices calling for health care reform joined activists who had long worked for national health insurance. The effort remained a state-based coalition effort. Though the Boston group played an informal leadership role at times, there was no national organization.

There were many reasons for the strengths of the Ad Hoc Committee's effort. The movement was led by experienced grassroots leaders with good organizational skills. The nurse-physician collaboration struck a chord with many who remembered more collaborative times in the clinical area *and* offered the public the joint leadership of the two professions most associated with health care and caring. The focus on the current crisis brought many more professionals into the reform effort, agreeing to stand together against market-driven care even though many disagreed on long-term solutions. Moreover, the state-based effort, tied together into a coalition without a hierarchical national structure, allowed various regions of the country to focus on their particular problems with for-profit corporations.

The United States is the only industrialized country without a system of national health insurance. As costs continue to climb while fewer and fewer people are able to get the care they need, it is almost certain that Congress will enact some form of national health insurance. To get to this point sooner rather than later (and with important basics intact), activists need to incorporate three strategies:

- **Maintain a clear vision and principles.** Strategies change, but the goal of a just and equitable health care system has to be maintained. Compromise is useful when it enhances progress toward a goal; when *principles* are compromised (which tends to happen when movement leaders get caught up in personal power politics), goals are rarely attained.
- **Seek out opportunities for collaboration.** The power of mega-corporations over the daily lives of individuals has grown at an astonishing rate. Advocates for change will never have the financial resources or access to global communications that are held by the corporate elite. It is only the strength of our numbers that will move any humane agenda forward.
- **Value grassroots action.** A mistake often made by grassroots groups is to compete on "corporate" terms. Many try to raise huge sums of money for media campaigns, for example, despite the fact that the enormous expense merely to enter that arena is pocket change for corporations. We need to hold fast to a strength that corporations will never have: the ability to inspire through person-to-person communication. Door-to-door canvassing, community meetings on the community's terms, tireless educational efforts, and continuous reflection and open debate are key grassroots values. Grassroots action ended slavery, brought women the vote, and attained many basic civil rights. Considering the enormous imbalance of power between industry decision makers and the general public, it is probably the only way to resolve the health care crisis.

References

Ad Hoc Committee to Defend Health Care (1997, December 3). A call to action. *Journal of the American Medical Association, 278*(21), 1733–1738.

Kilborn, P. T. (1997, July 1). Doctors organize to fight corporate intrusion. *The New York Times,* p. A12.

McDermott, J. (1994). Evaluating health system reform: The case for a single-payer approach. *Journal of the American Medical Association, 271*(10), 782–784.

McDermott, J. (1995, January 18). The first step. *Journal of the American Medical Association, 273*(3), 251–253.

Chapter *11*

RESEARCH AS POLICY/POLITICAL TOOL

Donna Diers

Personal Values Get in Way of Bridging Science, Policy

By Abram Katz, Register *Science Editor*

Translating science into effective public policy would be simple if everyone agreed on the best ways to stop AIDS.

But they don't. No amount of science can convince some politicians to support controversial programs; nor will many scientists defer to emotional or moral persuasion.

A federal panel of scientists has concluded that needle exchange programs and safe-sex education are effective in preventing the spread of AIDS. The panel also is critical of policymakers who it says ignore the scientific evidence while people are dying from the disease.

State Sen. Thomas F. Upson said he's not sure why policy-makers should heed scientists.

And he doesn't see the logic in trying to prevent the spread of HIV through needles by giving away needles.

Upson, a Waterbury Republican and deputy minority leader, sponsored bills this year to repeal the state's needle exchange programs.

One bill stalled in the judiciary committee; the other is before the public health committee.

"Taking of drugs is illegal in Connecticut. We're providing something illegal," Upson said. "We don't provide set-ups for alcoholics or masks for bank robbers. It's a slippery slope," he said.

Injection drug users should be offered drug counseling. "If they can afford drugs, they can afford to buy their own needles," he said.

That attitude greatly disturbs public health officials.

"We have really been far too slow in implementing prevention programs," said Dr. Michael H. Merson, chairman of epidemiology and public health at Yale University School of Medicine.

Merson, an internationally known expert on AIDS, was one of 15 scientists who addressed the federal panel in February.

"First and foremost, this is a public health problem. While we must respect each other's morals and culture, we're dealing with a serious public health risk. AIDS is the leading cause of death in people between 25 and 44" Merson said.

"We need to set policy first and foremost on science . . . not just what we think," he said. "We have a Victorian heritage. We stigmatize people with HIV. It's disgusting, it's sexual, it happens in marginalized groups," Merson said.

There's no way Jane Salce, executive director of the Christian Coalition of Connecticut, will be convinced by scientists that needle exchange programs or explicit sex education are the right way to prevent HIV infections.

Salce said teaching the general biology of reproduction is appropriate. Sexual relationships should be discussed at home, she said.

"Now we're getting explicit in school under the guise that teenagers will bumble into sex. Abstinence is the way. We're sending them a mixed message. 'You shouldn't do this, but here's a condom in case you do,'" she said.

"That's like saying, 'We don't do drugs, but here's a clean needle.'"

Salce said no amount of scientific evidence would change her mind. "Some might say I'm living in a fantasy world. If you teach children right from wrong at an early age, we'll see a lot of problems lessened by a major degree."

When science slams into skepticism, where does that leave officials responsible for protecting public health?

"I don't have an answer to that question," said Beth Weinstein, director of AIDS programs in the state Department of Public Health. "It has to do with how we set public policy. I can't begin to figure out what to do," she said.

"We've danced around preventive issues in this country since the beginning," she said.

"In the end there's no substitute for political courage. There's going to be resistance to these programs. We need to educate the public and policy-makers on the facts," Merson said. [From the *New Haven Register*, April 6, 1997]

This story shows the complicated relationship between research and policymaking and how data do not necessarily have the same meaning for different people.

The National Institutes of Health (NIH) Consensus Conference actually held that "needle exchange programs 'should be implemented at once,'" which provoked a moderated response by Donna Shalala, Secretary of Health and Human Services, saying that needle exchange programs "can be an effective component of a comprehensive strategy to prevent HIV [human immunodeficiency virus] and other blood-borne infections" (Editor's note, 1997). The NIH report followed, by 2 years, a well-distributed report by the National Academy of Sciences (Normand, Vlahov, & Moses, 1995), which had found that "well-implemented needle exchange programs can be effective in preventing the spread of HIV and do not increase the use of illegal drugs." But a Congressional ban on funding needle-exchange programs remains in effect.

From the point of view of the quality of the science, the peer review, and the consensus of the scientific community, the policy action to be taken in Connecticut is clear. But the political consensus isn't quite cooked.

"Health services researchers must not imagine that research findings are sufficient to determine the course of health policy," Tanenbaum (1996, p. 517) whinges.[1] She had studied the Canadian and U.S. policy response to studies of medical ineffectiveness and found very different responses based on the *same data*. Therefore, she says, the data must be ambiguous because they do not seem to lead to the same implications for action.

As Tanenbaum recognizes, research all by itself does not make policy. Politics intervene. The research doesn't get to the right people. Policy agendas shift. In Tanenbaum's study an equally viable conclusion is that the U.S. and Canadian medical systems are so different that it is not surprising that different responses follow from the same data. Whether the research is really any good is not the question.

Research may be a tool to help carve policy, in the right hands, carefully sharpened and skillfully applied. But because research design is never perfect, probabilistic reasoning does not satisfy legislators who want a quick and simple "does it work?" answer, and the time may not be ripe, the role of research in policymaking is more complicated than it looks. Even the best designed and conducted research will not move policy if powerful political forces stand in the way.

What makes policy decision making such a fertile field for analysis is that it is so difficult to shape and even more difficult to control.[2] That is exactly what makes it frustrating to action-oriented disciplines such as nursing, and so tiresome to analysts like Tanenbaum, for whom the action that should follow from the data is obvious. The making of *public* policy is even more involved because, by definition, it includes

---

[1]"Whinge" is a peculiarly appropriate verb often used in political commentary in Australia, Canada, and the United Kingdom. It means to whine with a petulant, needy edge, beyond "complain" but short of "snivel." It is not in U.S. dictionaries, more is the pity.

[2]For an example in health care, see Eric Redman's book *The Dance of Legislation* (1973), which is about the creation of the National Health Service Corps. He writes as a medical student and junior staffer at the federal level. He survived with his sense of humor intact.

the acts of government or governmental agencies shaped by the will of the people, whether by formal vote, lobbying, or contributions to political campaigns. Finally, public policymaking, at least in the United States, is *public* to some degree, inviting the participation of all who wish a piece of the action, no matter how ignorant or biased.

To understand research as a policy tool, one must know that timing is everything, as we shall see.

SHAPING AGENDAS

The first step in policymaking is shaping the agenda. As Morone put it,

Interested groups, public officials and the media all maneuver to define the issues we fight over (and those we overlook); the framing of an issue, in turn, shapes potential solutions, allies and enemies, political fights and eventually . . . public policies. [1991, p. 213]

Much of this work occurs behind the scenes, made public strategically by involved parties or accidentally by the media. The work of the American Medical Association (AMA) in shaping the agenda for gun control and tobacco regulation on the basis of research is instructive as examples.

Gun Control as Public Health

The leadership in advocating unrestricted access to purchasing and using guns is the National Rifle Association (NRA). The NRA's agenda combines an interpretation of the Bill of Rights "freedom to bear arms" clause with the interests of people who hunt for sport or food, with an as yet small but highly visible set of militarists, separatists, and paramilitary groups not necessarily united on their own policy agendas.[3]

The federal Centers for Disease Control and Prevention (CDC) has a small unit that tracks statistics on causes of injuries, including product failures, car crashes, and injuries from guns. Their data come from hospital data, in which reasons for hospitalization and emergency treatment from injuries are coded for computer use (E codes in the *International Classification of Diseases* [ICD-9-CM]) and transmitted as reportable to CDC, much as infectious disease is reported. Research, some funded by CDC, began to link the availability of handguns to homicide, suicide, crime, and accident epidemiology (Sloan et al., 1988; Sloan, Rivara, Reay, Ferris, & Kellerman, 1990). The NRA demanded that the researchers be investigated for lapses of scientific integrity (Kellerman, 1993), the most serious allegation possible in academic circles. The complaint was dismissed after internal review at CDC. As more studies were done, with similar findings, the politics escalated and CDC's injury control program was threatened with loss of funds (Kellerman, 1993). The studies were labeled "pseudo-science" in NRA literature ("Medical journals . . . flawed," 1989) and vilified in letters to the editor in several state medical association publications and the *New England Journal of Medicine (NEJM)*. The letters from physicians on both sides of the issue made fascinating reading as research critique mixed with deeply felt political attitudes.

The AMA put a toe in the water when its executive director signaled a gun control position in a letter to Congress (Todd, 1991) on one piece of legislation, the Brady bill, which simply proposed a waiting period for gun purchase. Later the AMA Council on Scientific Affairs (1992) took a formal position on assault weapons as a public health hazard, reflecting, perhaps, then Surgeon General C. Everett Koop's use of the "bully pulpit" of the office and the forum of the *Journal of the American Medical*

---

[3]In spring 1997 the actor Charlton Heston has easily won a seat on the NRA board on a platform the media report as his wish to bring the organization back to center, away from the "right," separatist end of the spectrum.

Association (JAMA) and its editor, George Lundberg (Koop & Lundberg, 1992).[4]

Throwing the clout of organized medicine behind gun control, if only assault weapon control and a waiting period, as a *public health* issue changed the political field (Blendon, Young, & Hemenway, 1996). The public health and health-care perspectives shifted the agenda from NRA's definition of the issue as possession of guns to their use, which is much more subtle and complicated and less easy to regulate. Death and injury from gun use are irrefutable—and impossible to put to a public test through referendum or vote.

Smoking and Policy

The health effects of tobacco smoking have long been debated as a matter of the quality of the research, with the questioning led by the tobacco industry itself but joined by researchers who disputed methods and statistics. The link between smoking and lung cancer in humans was and still is a correlation, not a randomized, controlled clinical trial, which would require prescribing smoking to one group and not to another, followed out 25 years or so. The

tobacco industry took advantage of the methodological problems to hold off health warnings for years.[5]

In July 1995, *JAMA* published an analysis of previously secret tobacco industry documents in which the addictive properties of nicotine and the carcinogenic effects of smoking were revealed to have been known to the industry for 30 years (see Glantz, Fox, & Lightwood [1997] for review). This information has had a major effect on transforming the ways suits against tobacco companies can be litigated and on providing new interest, under state Medicaid programs, in pursuing such suits ("Turning a new leaf," 1997).[6]

The entry of organized medicine has had a chilling effect on acceptance of political contributions from tobacco companies. With the acknowledgement that the effects of smoking were known to industry researchers as a result of their own studies, their credibility has been seriously compromised. The methodological issues are no longer on center stage. The political and economic forces are revealed.

GETTING ON THE AGENDA

Much of the work—and the success—of nursing in policymaking to date has been less in shaping the agendas than in casting nursing issues to match existing policy agendas. Nursing has just begun to participate in setting the agenda for health policy "beyond issues that would be more traditionally defined as relevant to nursing" (Cohen et al., 1996, p. 263).

---

[4]*JAMA* and *NEJM* are remarkably editorially free from their respective sponsoring organizations—AMA and the Massachusetts Medical Society. How free any journal is depends on its relationship with its sponsor and on its editor. Lundberg at *JAMA* and Franz Inglefinger, then Arnold Relman, and then Jerome Kassirir at *NEJM* have all taken positions and used their editorial resources to espouse points of view not necessarily subscribed to by their sponsors. Kassirir (1997) has even said in print, "I believe that the decision of the American Medical Association to back [a bill] was a serious mistake." Because both journals have such huge international circulation, are so important to advertisers, and so significant in fields other than medicine, they have enormous weight in the policy community. In addition, *JAMA* and *NEJM* make available cutting-edge scientific advances to the media before publication, which helps make public perception of the science more accurate and helps make media people happy. Win-win.

[5]Julius Richmond, a child psychiatrist, was the surgeon general who implemented the warnings on cigarette packages. I served on a committee with him, and he would graciously autograph cigarette packages where they said, "The Surgeon General has determined . . ." He always wore a tie with the no-smoking logo.
[6]The tobacco controversy has found another voice in fiction in John Grisham's *The Runaway Jury* (1996), which is an interesting scenario of how to make policy change happen.

Cobb, Ross, and Ross (1976) distinguish among three models for agenda building: the outside initiative model, the mobilization model, and the inside initiative model. In the first, the idea first reaches the public agenda, and only then does it make the formal, or governmental, agenda. This is the "hit 'em on the head to get their attention" model, and it depends on media coverage. Because the public media are more often hooked by anecdote than data, the most effective information for shaping the formal agenda in this model is the sound bite. An example of an issue that fits this model might be the groundswell of public opinion to do something about "drive-through deliveries"—limitations imposed by insurers on postpartum hospitalization ("Deliver," 1995; "Maternity leave," 1996).

If data exist to speak to the policy/political agenda, this is the time to get them in. A sound bite opening has happened. Legislators do not wish to be taken for fools and need to position themselves to respond to something that is engaging the attention of their constituents, as reflected in the newspapers and on television.

Several states have considered and usually passed legislation to curtail drive-through deliveries, and the federal government has also passed legislation. But not on the basis of data. There actually aren't any data on the best postpartum length of hospital stay for the (normal) mother and (normal) baby, which is why insurers got by with the 1-day stay provision to start with. But the accounts of new mothers were so embarrassing to a civilized society, including insurers, that they could not defend the insurance practice.

The use of the research on the public health effects of unregulated guns turned the "outside initiative" model to federal legislation. But the anecdote that started it was the accidental shooting of James Brady, when the shooter was aiming for President Reagan. Sarah Brady and, to the extent he is able to appear publicly, her husband have made gun control a cause, and their credibility is unquestioned.

In the second model, the policymakers have already decided on an agenda and a course of action and now need to sell it. Here, the trick is to figure out what the agenda really is and, if possible, associate nursing's interest to it. Bringing along media attention reinforces nursing's contribution when possible.

The work of nursing in Tennessee to insert nurse practitioners (NPs) into TennCare, the state's managed Medicaid system, is instructive. The governor had already decided on a managed Medicaid plan, but it depended on having an adequate supply of primary care providers. The Tennessee Medical Association (TMA) tried to stonewall. TMA members would not accept Medicaid patients under TennCare. Tennessee NPs seized the opportunity to insert themselves and their own agenda—changing a very restrictive practice act and prescribing language—and appear to be the good guys. They did, and it worked (a much longer story, of course) (Bonneyman, 1996; Gold, 1997; Mirvis, Chang, Hall, Zaar, & Applegate, 1995). The Tennessee nurses received a lot of good publicity for being ahead of nurses in many other states in moving into the managed Medicaid primary care arena. In fact, however, only one small restrictive provision—site-specific prescribing authority—was changed. Still, in the smoke and mirrors of advanced practice, the law and legislation count less than the public perception. In Tennessee, NPs were portrayed as out there where doctors feared to tread.

The inside model proposes that there are some issues that never go "outside" the internal governmental sphere because they are too arcane, controversial, or complex. Many of these issues deal with regulatory change rather than legislation. Here, research and other forms of lobbying information go straight to the legislators and their staffs without playing to the public media.

The creation of the National Center (now Institute) of Nursing Research (NINR) is an example of this model. There was no particular public interest in nursing's having its own place in the federal research funding system. In fact, there was no consensus in nursing that this ought to happen, either ("Commentary," 1984; Dumas & Felton, 1984). A committee of the Institute of Medicine (IOM) had been assigned by Congressional action to study the federal role in nursing education. A draft report midway into the IOM committee's work was circulated by nurse members. An important contribution was Ada Jacox's policy analysis of the composition of the IOM committee and how it was working (it was perceived as being stacked with individuals and interests that might not have understood modern nursing nor nursing research) (Jacox, 1983).[7]

Eventually the IOM committee issued a number of recommendations, among which was one for nursing research to have its own place in the federal funding system (Aiken, 1983; IOM, 1983). An opportunity surfaced with the reauthorization of the NIH funding bill. White and Hamel (1986) describe the work that nursing did to make NINR happen. Public attention outside the internal NIH and nursing communities surfaced in an important article by Barbara Culliton (1983), a science reporter, published in *Science.* She linked nursing's wish to have a place in NIH to the scientists whose fields were important but not "sexy"—rheumatology (arthritis), for example. She essentially argued that nursing's science deserved a place in NIH as much as that of others. Nursing rode in on a Republican administration's wish to attract women voters; the slogan "1 in 44 women voters is a nurse," by the American Nurses Association (ANA), got political attention. Jacox (1985) helped the cause along again with another policy analysis, discussing how nursing might fit within the NIH, which were not welcoming.

The NINR has been remarkably effective in promoting nursing research—so effective that

there are contemporary worries that, in NIH belt tightening, NINR's success in increasing its budget from $16.2 million when it began to $59.5 million in fiscal year 1997 may work against nursing. Some critics believe that the results are inadequate to justify this "special" money.

NURSING ON THE AGENDA

Where nursing has made progress on issues that have to do with our parochial interests such as licensure, scope of practice, third-party reimbursement, and prescriptive authority, the progress has generally been made by sophisticated political minuet rather than data-based argument. On these issues, we have not had sufficient data and still do not. For example, there is very little literature on the effect of granting advanced practice nurses (APNs) prescriptive authority. If nurses can prescribe, do we do it? Do we do it right? How often do we consult a physician, even with full-scope prescribing authority? Yet prescribing authority in one form or another exists in most states (Pearson, 1997) over the opposition of physicians and pharmacists and essentially without data.

An important exception to the lack-of-data rule is in nurse-midwifery, where data collected now for more than 50 years on the safety and effectiveness of nurse-midwifery practice has been used to enact legal authority for practice in all 50 states, Guam, and Puerto Rico (Diers & Burst, 1983; Varney, 1996).

Nurse-midwifery made important progress when it attached its interests in legal authorization to the existing public agenda in implementation of Medicaid. Because much of the research showed the effects of nurse-midwifery in underserved populations, and because the Medicaid program targets women and children, that strategy made sense. It also built on a carefully crafted strategy that began at the federal level when Sen. Daniel Inouye caused legislation to be passed to allow direct payment to nurse-midwives under Medicaid in jurisdictions with legal

---

[7]Lucie Kelly was then editor of *Nursing Outlook,* which was then the official journal of the National League for Nursing. She solicited the commentary on the draft proposal (which argued both sides of the issue) and made the publication of the Dumas/Felton and Jacox proposals timely.

authorization for practice.[8] The literature on effectiveness was used to demonstrate the willingness of nurse-midwives to care for poor women and babies and to counter the allegations of lack of safety made by organized medicine (Diers, 1992b).

Contemporary nursing's political strategy in many states involves hooking the APN's concerns to expand scope of practice and prescribing authority to the "managed care" agenda, which is about money, not practice. Although the research on the cost-effectiveness of advanced practice nursing is still slim, it has been cleverly analyzed and combined with regulatory options by Barbara Safriet, an attorney, in a monograph that is often made part of public testimony (Safriet, 1992). Having this information compiled by an attorney who is not a nurse has the effect of making the data even more powerful because it does not seem self-serving.

CREATING THE AGENDA: A MINI CASE STUDY

The ANA's political agenda is and, since taking on collective bargaining, has been preserving and protecting nursing jobs. The ANA took a very unpopular stance to support Medicare very early on (Lewis, 1961; Marmor, 1973) because Medicare would bring access to care, which meant more nursing jobs. The implementation of the Prospective Payment System and diagnosis-related groups (DRGs) under Medicare in 1983 had been resisted by organized nursing in public testimony on the basis of predictions of nursing jobs lost (Cole, 1982; Curtis, 1983; Diers, 1992a). By 1986 or so, the effect of the payment system was being felt in hospitals that had cut registered nurse (RN) positions because decreased admissions were anticipated. RN vacancy rates (not jobs lost) rose. The American Hospital Association (AHA), stimulated by the American Organization of Nurse Executives

(AONE), did several "quick and dirty" surveys. The average community hospital RN vacancy rate rose from 4.4% in 1983 to 11.3% in December 1987 (AHA, 1988).

At the same time, the Division of Nursing of the Bureau of Health Manpower of the Health Services and Resources Administration in the U.S. Department of Health and Human Services, which collects data on nursing numbers and employment rates, was reporting that there was no shortage of nurses (Division of Nursing, 1984).

Using U.S. Department of Commerce statistics under a model that estimated population trends and requirements for nursing personnel across settings, the National League for Nursing (NLN) concluded that the supply of associate degree graduates would exceed demand in 2000 and that the supply of baccalaureate and master's prepared nurses would be under demand by about 0.5 million each (Maraldo & Solomon, 1987).

So already we have four different nursing agendas, producing four different sets of numbers.

The ANA's agenda is jobs: we need more nurses. AONE's is recruitment and manpower: more nurses. NLN's is education—the health of schools of nursing in the supply pipeline: more nurses. The agenda of the Division of Nursing, as part of the Executive branch of government, is to decrease federal expenses: less funding is needed because there are enough nurses.

The Secretary's Commission on the Nursing Shortage (1988) took testimony from all the players mentioned above, and from others who had done other kinds of analyses of requirements for nursing. Aiken and Mullinix (1987) took apart numbers in an economic analysis that showed that when nursing salaries began to approximate salaries of other women workers, nursing vacancies declined. They also showed that the salary compression in nursing—nurses employed for a long time did not make a compensatory amount over newly hired nurses— was another factor. Aiken and others (Fagin, 1982) revealed "oligopsony," an economics term

---

[8]Senator Inouye is proud to announce that he was assisted into the world by a midwife. He also credits nurses who cared for him when he lost an arm in World War II.

meaning that where there are only a few large employers (hospitals) and an adequate supply of employees (nurses), the employers effectively have a monopoly in the nursing market and can conspire, deliberately or not, to constrain nursing wages and salaries. A nurse unhappy with her lot could simply change jobs to a higher-paying one, and an employer unhappy with a nurse could find another one easily—if there are enough nurses.

These data were powerful enough, but what was even more powerful was information that, combined with the above, nailed down the problem: it wasn't the *supply* of nurses, it was the *demand*. That is, the payment system changed and the incentives for hospitals were to admit fewer "easy" patients and try to discharge the "harder" patients earlier. This meant that nurses were confronted with caring for patients whose stay in the hospital could consist entirely of "acute" days, which require more nursing (Thompson, 1988).

The conversion of the agenda from supply to demand is still not well understood by committees and special commissions, who do not take into consideration the changing nature of patients and care requirements in hospitals, outpatient settings, nursing homes, and home care spawned by changes in funding.

The nursing shortage data, flawed as they were, pushed hospitals even in rate-regulated states to raise salaries so that nursing staff could be hired and retained. But within 5 years, something happened, and now highly paid nurses were part of the cause of escalating health care costs and should be reengineered and downsized out in favor of lower-paid, unlicensed personnel.

Nobody had any data here, either. The agenda shifted, and the actors did, too, after the flame-out of the first Clinton Administration's health care proposals. Terrified by the possibility of managed competition, business coalitions and the insurance market put health care definitively into the private (as opposed to governmental) mode. This changed the political landscape and left everybody, including nursing, at the low end

of a very steep learning curve. Business (the private system) does not operate by the same rules of engagement as government, which nursing had just begun to figure out.

AGENDA SETTING: THE CONTINUING STORY

In the wake of redesign and reengineering and other euphemisms for cost cutting, organized nursing has turned to data gathering in an interesting new way. Nursing jobs are not particularly the public's agenda. To gain public support, nursing has made the safety of patients cared for in hospitals, by strangers, the public relations target. Nursing in the Northeast has particularly used this strategy to publicize the notion that every patient deserves a nurse (as opposed to an unlicensed caregiver). The Robert Wood Johnson Foundation Hospital in New Jersey has produced a particularly effective advertisement (see p. 199).

Judith Shindul-Rothschild and colleagues (1996) conducted a study for the *American Journal of Nursing* that highlights the effects of downsizing and other corporate restructuring efforts on nursing practice through a national survey of the opinions of nurses. The study received considerable media play because it feeds into both the media's interest in juicy health care error stories and the national concerns for layoffs and job losses in a recovering economy. These are "people" stories, which make for easy sound bites and quick public testimony.

On the other hand, the IOM's study, *Nursing Staff in Hospitals and Nursing Homes: Is It Adequate?* (Wunderlich, Sloan, & Davis, 1996) expresses "shock" at the lack of available data on hospital quality and calls for stepped-up research on quality outcomes and their link to nurse staffing. Yet a study by the Minnesota Nurses Association (MNA) of workplace injury/illness rates as a result of hospital downsizing, made available to the IOM, was not included in the final report. The IOM staff said that the data stood alone and were not corroborated by any

They're taking care of Mrs. Miller today.

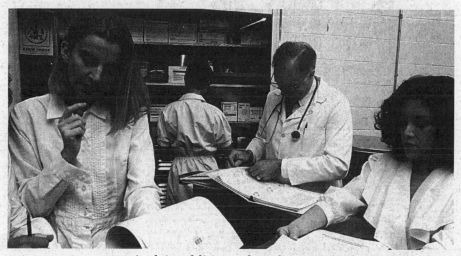

And, in addition to her physician,
one of the first people she'll see today and **every day** is a Registered Nurse.

You're hearing a lot these days about hospitals that have restructured, cutback staffing, or replaced registered nurses with unlicensed aides. Of course that concerns you. That's why you should know that at **Robert Wood Johnson University Hospital we have not reduced registered nurses at the bedside. In fact, our number of highly-trained nurses and medical professionals at each patient's bedside places us among the top tier of hospitals** throughout the country.

Delivering world-class patient care is always our first priority, and as our patient volume increased over the years, so has our staff of expert nurses. For our patients this means stellar care that is coordinated by a clinically elite team of physicians, nurses, pharmacists, and others that are recognized nationally for quality. **We're proud that our recognized quality care is there for you...from admission...to bedside...to discharge.**

Robert Wood Johnson University Hospital...
setting the standard for quality, value and service.
And, satisfying the most important standard there is...yours.

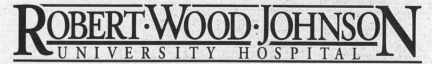

Core teaching hospital for UMDNJ-Robert Wood Johnson Medical School
Member of the University Health System of New Jersey
Hub hospital for the Robert Wood Johnson Health System

existing literature (Canavan, 1996). Because apparently no one had studied this issue before, of course there was no literature. MNA put its findings in the hands of the National Institute for Occupational Safety and Health, which made nursing work part of their research agenda (Wilburn, 1996). ANA has continued to push the issue of work-related injuries ("Growing physical workload . . . ," 1997), because its issue is nursing jobs. The IOM agenda, defined by Congress, which assigned IOM to this project and provided the funds, is to define the federal role in funding nursing education so that the supply of nurses is adequate for the health care needs of the nation (but only about 45% of U.S. health care dollars are public [government] funds). The subtext of the federal agenda, however, is to get the federal government out of the business of funding nursing altogether. Thus a finding that would seem to suggest that more rather than fewer nurses might be in order might conceivably not see the light of print.

RESEARCH AS POLITICAL: PRACTICE GUIDELINES AND AHCPR

The Agency for Health Care Policy and Research (AHCPR) is funded in part by a 1% "tax" on NIH research grants to support "evaluation" of the use of public monies for medical scientific research. The story of how this unusual provision came to be is itself an interesting commentary on policymaking[9] (Gray, 1992). AHCPR's portfolio has evolved over the years to include evaluation of health services, outcome studies, and the important work to pull together the existing science to support clinical practice guidelines under programs called PORTs (practice outcome research teams) (*Medical Care*, 1994, 1995). Multidisciplinary commit-

tees, which regularly include nurses in highly visible roles, review literature related to their assignment (e.g., pain, depression in primary care, cataract treatment) and develop publicly available guidelines in two forms, one for the consumer reader and one for health professionals. The proposed documents are peer reviewed and then published and widely distributed by the government. The process is rather straightforward, essentially nonpolitical, grinding hard academic work. But then it goes public.

One of the topics AHCPR picked was low back pain. The expert panel generated its report and subsequent guidelines, which said that 8 of 10 patients with acute back pain will recover in a month or so without therapy, that studies showed that surgery benefits only 1 in 100 patients, and that much diagnostic imaging was futile and unnecessary. Were the practice guidelines based on these findings to be implemented, there would be billions of dollars of savings and patients would be protected from unnecessary tests and ineffective treatment. The American Academy of Orthopaedic Surgeons endorsed the guidelines.

But the North American Spine Society, a group of surgeons, went up in smoke and got the attention of two Texas Republican representatives to Congress, who agitated to cut off AHCPR's funding entirely ("A spineless attack . . . ," 1996). A concerted lobbying effort by the Association for Health Services Research (AHSR), which, by the way, welcomes nurse members, eventually produced a compromise that took AHCPR out of the guideline business and into being "science partners" so that users can "develop their own high-quality, evidence-based guidelines" ("AHCPR drops guideline development," 1996). There was, of course, no requirement that anybody ever use the AHCPR guidelines, but clearly it would have been in the interest of payers, including Medicare and managed care insurers, to monitor the extent to which they were paying for evidence-based practices. AHCPR came close to losing its entire funding over this issue.

---

[9]The original name for the agency was Agency for Health Care Research and Policy, which produced an unfortunate acronym (see Gray, 1992).

MENACING THE MESSENGER[10]

Research isn't completed until it is peer reviewed and made available for public information and criticism. Recent reports have exposed the lengths to which special-interest groups or others who do not like the results of certain studies will go to prevent publication or use of the science. Deyo, Psaty, Simon, Wagner, and Omenn (1997) have collected their own and others' experiences. They show that the ox gored by the spine studies was the manufacturer of a pedicle screw sometimes used in spinal fusion. The manufacturer was being sued by patients alleging poor results from use of the device. Attorneys for the defendant subpoenaed documents from the original investigators, tying up their work for some time. Another pedicle screw manufacturer unsuccessfully sought a court injunction to prevent AHCPR from publishing its guidelines (Deyo et al., 1997).

Simon was caught in another controversy when research from his team questioned the value of immunodiagnostic tests often used to support disability and liability claims for chemical sensitivity (Deyo et al., 1997). The science was attacked by "parties whose financial interests depended on [the] testing: plaintiffs' attorneys, advocacy organizations for people with chemical sensitivity, . . . testing laboratories" (Deyo et al., p. 1177), and allegations of scientific misconduct were made to the federal Office of Research Integrity and the medical board in Washington State. Individual patients at Group Health Cooperative, where Dr. Simon worked, were "contacted and encouraged to attack his credibility" (p. 1177).

Psaty and his colleagues (Deyo et al., 1997) studied calcium channel blockers, diuretics, and beta-blocking agents and found that the short-acting calcium channel blockers were associated with an increased risk of myocardial infarction.

The media's handling of the story tended to play up the risk and downplay the science, and the manufacturers of the calcium channel blockers were bent out of shape. Pharmaceutical companies funded mass mailings to physicians from an "opinion leader" in hypertension management without identifying the source of funding for the mailing. The investigator's dean came down on him, too.

The April 16, 1997, issue of *JAMA* contains a fascinating report (Rennie, 1997) of a study that took 9 years to reach publication because it called into question the superior efficacy of Synthroid, a synthetic thyroid preparation (Dong et al., 1997). The study had been funded by the manufacturer of Synthroid, and several preparations other than this company's were tested. The investigators had submitted the manuscript to *JAMA,* with a cover letter to the effect that the sponsor of the research disagreed with the conclusions. While the results, which showed that all the preparations were essentially bioequivalent, were under review for possible publication, the manufacturer suddenly woke up to the fact that in the agreement to fund the research was a provision that the manufacturer had the right to approve any potential publications. The university counsel's office had not caught this provision, which is the kind of thing universities do not tolerate.

The manuscript was peer reviewed and eventually approved for publication, but it was abruptly withdrawn by the investigators when the manufacturer brought legal action against the university. At this time the company was being considered for acquisition by another pharmaceutical firm, and the comparative efficacy of its most important product was at issue. The company did its own reanalysis of data, reaching conclusions opposite to those of the original study, and published its findings in a new journal for which the company's investigator was an associate editor. The situation reached the notice of the *Wall Street Journal.* Suddenly an "inside" model situation converted to "outside."

The issue became a matter of public policy when the U.S. Food and Drug Administration,

[10]For an interesting update on a number of the instances discussed in this section, see "Intimidation of researchers by special-interest groups," a set of letters to the editor of the *New England Journal of Medicine* ("Intimidation of researchers," 1997).

led by Dr. David Kessler, entered and alleged that the company had mislabeled its product's efficacy, using the results of its own reanalysis, a violation of law. That apparently brought the company to the table with the university, and eventually the company agreed not to challenge publication of the original manuscript, which *JAMA* did in this issue (Dong et al., 1997). Several letters, including correspondence from the new owners and the original investigators, were also published in the same issue. "Thyroid Storm," *JAMA* called this sorry story.[11]

NURSING'S RESEARCH QUESTIONED

In nursing, we have not had to contend with this level of intimidation, but we have had our own experience with having research called into question or rejected when the conclusions offended conventional political wisdom.

Policy proposals, such as the late lamented Health Security Act to open reimbursement opportunities to APNs and perhaps even remove the grating barriers to practice that APNs have lived under, have made the questions we had hoped were already answered come back: Are NPs safe (unsupervised by physicians, of course)? Are they cost-effective? These are "internal" policy issues. There is as yet no public pressure to increase the freedom of choice of providers to include NPs or nurse-midwives.

When the Health Security Act provisions became known, both *JAMA* and *NEJM* weighed

in with editorial opinion and solicited commentary (Kassirir, 1994; DeAngelis, 1994), as did the American College of Physicians (1994), published in their own journal. *NEJM*'s editorial exposition was stimulated by a contribution from a nurse, Mary Mundinger, who has often provoked such response as a way to get nursing out there (Mundinger, 1994). In different words, the physician contributors[12] and the American College of Physicians asserted that the research results were as yet incomplete in regard to NPs, that the gold standard of the double-blind, randomized, controlled clinical trial (RCCT) had yet to be achieved, and that public policy therefore ought to wait a while until all the data were in. This response leapt lightly over the fact that it is not practically possible to do such an RCCT, which would have to involve randomly assigning exactly the same patients first to an NP and then to a physician and vice versa. This cannot be done because the first encounter would alter the second, and there is no way to "blind" either the clinicians or the patients. But simply declaring that the right study hasn't been done ignored more than 1000 research articles that have been summarized in federal documents (Office of Technology Assessment [OTA], 1988), analyzed in reviews (Brown & Grimes, 1995; Safriet, 1992), and used to argue for more federal funding to train NPs. It was amusing that the Burlington studies of NPs (Spitzer et al., 1974), which were allegedly RCCTs and always cited in this political context, were dredged up again when the faults of the method have been uncovered in subsequent critique (Diers & Molde, 1979). The original

---

[11]The curious reader might note that the Deyo article and the Rennie/Dong sequence were published by two different journals one day apart, April 16 and 17, 1997. Yet another example appears in the same issue of *NEJM*. Suzanne Fletcher (1997) describes her experience as part of the NIH Consensus Conference on breast-cancer screening, which had concluded that "the data available do not warrant a universal recommendation for mammography for all women in their forties" (p. 1181) and set off a firestorm of protest. Readers are urged to follow these arguments for themselves; they are very intricate as science, politics, and policy. By the time this chapter is published, there will be other examples as science and policy become more public.

---

[12]A phenomenon often used in the politics of public regulation where the issues are about nursing and (or versus) medicine occurs when the organized medical forces trot out "former nurses"—nurses who have become physicians—to testify to how dangerously uninformed/undertrained, and so forth, they have found nursing to be, now that they are doctors. Catherine DeAngelis (1994) began her professional life as a nurse. Unlike some others, she does not bash nursing but tries to bridge the policy gap between medicine and nursing. There is a policy dissertation in here somewhere for the right doctoral student.

author of the Burlington trials [sic] of the NP alleged that with time NPs might be discovered to be like thalidomide, introduced too soon with too little testing (Spitzer, 1984). Organized medicine's agenda here was to change the definition of the issue from freedom of choice to safety, which has always been code for economic opposition to advanced practice nursing (Safriet, 1992).

RESEARCH DESIGN FOR POLICY

It should be obvious by now that the quality of research may have little to do with its impact on policy. There are, however, some ways in which research can be made more useful and usable in policy decision making.

In the first place, research can be used to help define a problem, particularly to determine how big it is. The making of public policy is concerned with the "big picture"—the greatest good for the greatest number. Therefore studies that can document how widespread a problem is are likely to be more effective than single-site or single-state studies. The methodological concern here is sampling: how representative the data are of the larger problem.

Aggregating studies in the form of literature reviews or meta-analyses is the new hot research design for policy-related research (Conn & Armer, 1996; Grady & Schwartz, 1992; OTA, 1994). The intricacies of meta-analysis are beyond the scope of this chapter, but the advantage of meta-analysis or carefully constructed literature reviews is clear: small-sample but important studies can be made additive. AHCPR's PORT initiative has raised meta-analysis to an art form.

Pickiness about research design is not always relevant when the goal is to boil down a collection of disparate studies or other data to make a policy point. This is not at all the same as fudging the numbers. Politicians and policymakers are generally not entranced by arcane academic standards for methodologic technicalities. The OTA's (1988) gathering of NP literature, and Safriet's (1992) use of OTA and other studies, read, to the academic eye, as insufficiently critical of the studies cited. The Shindul-

Rothschild (1996) study sample consisted of readers of the *American Journal of Nursing* who chose to send in a tear-out questionnaire—not a representative sample. But to do an academic critique on either piece of work is surely beside the point of having this information gathered together by an unbiased critic, on the one hand, and an adroit use of a survey of nurses' experience on the other. Using a tight methodological critique would be like shooting ourselves in the foot.

Nursing's research support at the federal level has concentrated deliberately on personal health situations and services, to develop the science that underpins the professional practice and to distinguish research problems that are peculiarly related to nursing from more general health services delivery questions, which are funded by AHCPR. This distinction is necessary to protect the NINR's status within NIH, which was so difficult to achieve. NIH's mission is science, not service delivery, and nursing must fit. Many recognize that research directed more pointedly at policy issues, such as the effects of nursing on outcomes, cost-effectiveness, and substitutability, needs to be encouraged and supported (McCloskey et al., 1994).

Linda Aiken has provided many good examples of **large dataset** research for policy, including her linking of magnet hospitals to lower mortality rates, which conceptualized the nursing magnet in a way that made sense outside the field (Aiken, Smith, & Lake, 1994; Aiken, Sochalski, & Lake, 1997). For nursing, the trick is to conceptualize the variables in large datasets as *nursing* so that the results can be attributable to nursing. Length of stay and mortality are powerful variables from a policy point of view, and they can be linked to nursing given appropriate conceptualization and study design (Aiken et al., 1994; Diers & Potter, 1997). There are many variables, especially in standard, computerized hospital information systems, that can be taken as evidence of the effect of nursing (Pollack & Diers, 1994).

Florence Nightingale is justly credited with exquisite use of statistics to argue her points, and because in general nobody else had any data, she had the "first mover advantage." Nightingale was not above collecting and using her data to her own advantage (Thompson, 1990). Casting research in the best light to get the best attention to make the best policy point is the new test.

CONCLUSION

For research to be useful in policy, the policy agenda first ought to be clear. Elizabeth Hadley (1996), from her experience as an assistant attorney general, a lobbyist, and a staff member to one of the Health Security Act groups, writes about how the internal divisions within nursing compromise our policy strivings and make using data difficult.

No nursing journal has a circulation as large as that of *JAMA* or *NEJM*, nor the editorial courage of the editors of these two medical journals. There are scattered examples of using nursing journals for policy effect, but they are indeed scattered. And, like it or not, the official publication of nursing's largest professional organizations, the *American Journal of Nursing* for ANA and *Image* for Sigma Theta Tau, do not lend themselves to taking policy positions. ANA's policy agenda was discussed above. Sigma Theta Tau has no policy agenda.

Research is not something to be plugged in when a policy or political crisis rears up. Timing is everything. Nurses, as politicians, policymakers, and researchers, need to keep (or have access to those who keep) such close touch with what is happening in the policy and political environment that we can anticipate trends and design studies to speak to them. We need to have networks of information, now not difficult with Internet, MEDLINE, Nexus, Lexis, and all the other computer tools. We need to learn when anecdote is more powerful[13] than statistical significance and how to present our research to make a difference. We need to keep data on our own practices, especially advanced practice,

because there will—trust me—come a time when those data will turn a challenge around.

These, then, are the multiple and simultaneous strategies:

• Keep or find nursing data. Find and use the computerized information systems in the practice or the institution. Don't worry about whether the data are labeled as nursing. If you do the work, you own the information.

• Understand the agenda. Things are not always what they seem. Ask: "What is the problem here?" Or, "To what problem is this (reengineering, downsizing, policy change) a solution?" And follow up with: "How do you know? What are the data?"

• Shape the agenda. Believe (because it is true) that others do not necessarily know more than you do about the work, even if they are administrators or doctors. Know the players, teams, and organizations. What do *you* think ought to happen, and how can you get there? What's *right*? What's simple, cost-effective, or important? Then use information to support that because . . .

• Data are powerful, often more powerful than they deserve. But she or he who hath the data hath it all.

• Do good research. Nobody wants to do bad research, so what this is meant to signal is only that carefully designed and conducted research can stand on its own even in the face of methodological criticism, which will always come. If the research can have a policy hook—money, quality, equity—so much the better.

• Ride in on others' research. Read the research literature, mine it, distill it, use it to advantage even when it's not perfect.

• Recognize when anecdote is more powerful than large samples and multiple regression statistics. Learn how to write evocatively. Back up anecdote with numbers when you can. But true stories from true people can move mountains that no amount of data can. Don't be afraid to tell those stories. Nurses have millions of them.

• If you're a researcher and want to get your stuff out there, think about using the public relations (PR) people in your institution. Sorry about this, but researchers are often boring. PR

---

[13]Nursing has a good friend in Suzanne Gordon (1997), an investigative reporter who writes often, sensitively, and well about nursing as the work and as the economic and political reality.

people know how to convert boring information into powerful stories. Use them.

• Partner with nurses doing policy work. Every nurse who manages anything, including case managers, is doing policy-related work.

Finally, recognize that no amount of research will save us. Because research runs by the rules of science, it is rational, perhaps suprarational, according to those who would wish a less quantitative and more qualitative, human, and respectful notion of science. Politics, political science, and even policymaking have their own rules that are equally rational (Paltiel & Stinnett, 1996). Making research serve policy and political ends means learning the rules where research or science collides with values.

ACKNOWLEDGMENTS: I thank most sincerely (and in order of appearance) Donna Mahrenholz, RN, PhD, for help with finding obscure references; Sally S. Cohen, RN, PhD, for comments on an earlier draft; Sharon Eck, RN, MSN, doctoral candidate, for comments that shaped the final draft; and the editors for careful review.

REFERENCES

AHCPR drops guideline development. (1996, June). *HSR Reports,* p. 4 (Association for Health Services Research, 1130 Connecticut Ave. NW, Washington, DC 20036).

Aiken, L. H. (1983) Nursing's future: Public policies, private actions. *American Journal of Nursing, 83,* 1440–1444.

Aiken, L. H., & Mullinix, C. (1987). The nurse shortage: Myth or reality? *New England Journal of Medicine, 317*(10), 641–645.

Aiken, L. H., Smith, H. L., & Lake, E. T. (1994). Lower Medicare mortality among a set of hospitals known for good nursing care. *Medical Care, 32*(8), 771–778.

Aiken, L. H., Sochalski, J., & Lake, E. T. (1997). Studying outcomes of organizational change in health services. *Medical Care, 35*(Supplement), NS6–NS18.

American College of Physicians. (1994). Physician Assistants and Nurse Practitioners: Position Paper. *Annals of Internal Medicine, 121*(9), 714–716.

American Hospital Association. (1988). Draft report of the 1987 Hospital Nursing Demand Survey. Chicago: Author.

American Medical Association, Council on Scientific Affairs. (1992). Assault weapons as a public health hazard in the United States. *Journal of the American Medical Association, 267,* 3067–3070.

Blendon, R. J., Young, J. T., & Hemenway, D. (1996). The American public and the gun control debate. *Journal of the American Medical Association, 275*(22), 1719–1722.

Bonneyman, G. (1996). Stealth reform: Market-based Medicaid in Tennessee. *Health Affairs, 15*(2), 307–314.

Brown, S. A., & Grimes, D. E. (1995). A meta-analysis of nurse practitioners and nurse-midwives in primary care. *Nursing Research, 44*(6), 332–339.

Canavan, K. (1996, October). Minnesota study supports link between hospital downsizing and workplace injury/illness. *American Nurse,* p. 15.

Cobb, R., Ross, J. K., & Ross, J. H. (1976). Agenda building as a comparative political process. *The American Political Science Review, 70,* 125–138.

Cohen, S. S., Mason, D. J., Kovner, C., Leavitt, J. K., Pulcini, J., & Sochalski, J. (1996). Stages of nursing's political development: Where we've been and where we ought to go. *Nursing Outlook, 44*(12), 259–266.

Cole, E. (1982, November 22). Testimony before the House Subcommittee on Health and Environment of the Committee on Energy and Commerce. Washington, DC: U.S. Government Printing Office (Serial 97–183).

Commentary: Should there be a National Institute of Nursing Research? (1984). *Nursing Outlook, 32*(2), 119–122.

Conn, V. S., & Armer, J. M. (1996). Meta-analysis and public policy: Opportunity for nursing impact. *Nursing Outlook, 44*(12), 267–271.

Culliton, B. (1983). A nursing institute for NIH? *Science, 222,* 1310–1312.

Curtis, B. (1983, February 14). Testimony before the Subcommittee on Health of the House Ways and Means Committee. Washington, DC: U.S. Government Printing Office (Serial 98–6).

DeAngelis, C. (1994). Nurse practitioner redux. *Journal of the American Medical Association, 271*(11), 868–871.

Deliver, then depart. (1995, July 10). *Newsweek, 126*(2), 62.

Deyo, R. A., Psaty, B. M., Simon, G., Wagner, E. H., & Omenn, G. S. (1997). The messenger under attack: Intimidation of researchers by special-interest groups. *New England Journal of Medicine, 336*(16), 1176–1179.

Diers, D. (1992a). Diagnosis-related groups and the measurement of nursing. In L. H. Aiken (Ed.), *Charting nursing's future* (pp. 139–156). Philadelphia: Lippincott.

Diers, D. (1992b). Nurse-midwives and nurse anesthetists: The cutting edge in specialist practice. In L. H. Aiken (Ed.), *Charting nursing's future* (pp. 171–193). Philadelphia: Lippincott.

Diers, D., & Burst, H. V. (1983). Effectiveness of policy-related research: Nurse-midwifery as case study. *Image, 15*(3), 68–74.

Diers, D., & Molde, S. (1979). Some conceptual and methodological issues in nurse practitioner research. *Research in Nursing and Health, 2*(2), 73–84.

Diers, D., & Potter, J. (1997). Understanding the unmanageable nursing unit with case-mix data. *Journal of Nursing Administration, 27*(11), 27–32.

Division of Nursing, Bureau of Health Manpower, Health Research Services Administration, U.S. Department of Health and Human Services. (1984). The registered nurse population, findings from the national sample survey of registered nurses, November 1984. Washington, DC: Author.

Dong, B. J., Hauck, W. W., Gambertoglio, J. G., Gee, L., White, J. R., Bubp, J. L., & Greenspan, F. S. (1997). Bioequivalence of generic and brand-name levothyroxine products in the treatment of hypothyroidism. *Journal of the American Medical Association, 277*(15), 1205–1213.

Dumas, R. G., & Felton, G. (1984). Should there be a national institute for nursing? *Nursing Outlook, 32*(1), 28–33.

Editor's note (1997, April 3). *New England Journal of Medicine, 336*(14), 1034–1035.

Fagin, C. M. (1982). The national shortage of nurses: A nursing perspective. In L. H. Aiken (Ed.), *Nursing in the 1980s* (pp. 21–40). Philadelphia: Lippincott.

Fletcher, S. (1997). Whither scientific deliberation in health policy recommendations? Alice in the Wonderland of Breast-Cancer Screening. *New England Journal of Medicine, 336*(16), 1180–1183.

Glantz, S. A., Fox, B. J., & Lightwood, J. M. (1997). Tobacco litigation: Issues for public health and public policy. *Journal of the American Medical Association, 277*(9), 751–753.

Gold, M. (1997). Markets and public programs: Insights from Oregon and Tennessee. *Journal of Health Politics, Policy and Law, 22*(2), 633–666.

Gordon, S. (1997). *Life support: Three nurses on the front lines.* Boston: Little, Brown.

Grady, M. L., & Schwartz, H. A. (1992). Medical effectiveness research data methods. Rockville, MD: U.S. Department of Health and Human Services (Agency for Health Care Policy and Research).

Gray, B. H. (1992). The legislative battle over health services research. *Health Affairs, 11*(4), 38–66.

Grisham, J. (1996). *The Runaway Jury.* New York: Doubleday/Dell.

Growing physical workload threatens nurses' health. (1997). *American Journal of Nursing, 97*(4), 64–66.

Hadley, E. H. (1996). Nursing in the political and economic marketplace: Challenges for the 21st century. *Nursing Outlook, 44*(1), 6–10.

Hinshaw, A. S. (1988). The National Center for Nursing Research: Challenges and initiatives. *Nursing Outlook, 36*(2), 54–55.

Institute of Medicine. (1983). *Public policies and private actions.* Washington, DC: National Academy Press.

Intimidation of researchers by special interest group. (1997). *New England Journal of Medicine, 337*(18), 1314–1319.

Jacox, A. K. (1983). Significant questions about IOM's study of nursing. *Nursing Outlook, 31*(1), 28–33.

Jacox, A. K. (1985). Science and politics: The background and issues surrounding the controversial proposal for a National Institute of Nursing. *Nursing Outlook, 33*(2), 78–84.

Kassirer, J. (1994). What role for nurse practitioners in primary care? *New England Journal of Medicine, 330*(3), 204–205.

Kassirer, J. (1997). Practicing medicine without a license: The new intrusions of Congress. *New England Journal of Medicine, 336*(24), 1747.

Katz, A. (1997, April 8). Personal values get in way of bridging science, policy. *New Haven Register,* p. A6.

Kellerman, A. L. (1993). Obstacles to firearm and violence research. *Health Affairs, 12*(4), 142–153.

Koop, C. E., & Lundberg, G. B. (1992). Violence in America: A public health emergency—time to bite the bullet back. *Journal of the American Medical Association, 267*, 3075–3076.

Lewis, E. P. (1961). Pressure points. *American Journal of Nursing, 61*(6), 41.

Maraldo, P., & Solomon, S. (1987). Nursing's window of opportunity. *Image, 19*(2), 83–86.

Marmor, T. (1973). *The politics of Medicare.* Chicago: Aldine.

Maternity leave. (1996, February). *Harper's Magazine, 292*(1749), 14.

McCloskey, J. C., Maas, M., Huber, D. G., Kasparek, A., Specht, J., Ramler, C., et al. (1994). Nursing management innovations: A need for systematic evaluation. *Nursing Economic$. 12*(1), 35–44.

Medical Care (1994, Annual Supplement), *32*(7); (1995, Annual Supplement), *33*(4) [PORT updates].

Medical journal's article seriously flawed, NRA says. (1989, January). *American Rifleman,* 55–56.

Mirvis, D. M., Chang, C. F., Hall, C. J., Zaar, G. T., & Applegate, W. B. (1995). TennCare: Health system reform for Tennessee. *Journal of the American Medical Association, 274*(15), 1235–1241.

Morone, J. A. (1991). Framing political issues. *Journal of Health Policy, Politics and Law, 16*(2), 213–214.

Mundinger, M. (1994). Advanced-practice nursing: Good medicine for physicians? *New England Journal of Medicine, 330*(3), 211–214.

Normand, J., Vlahov, D., & Moses, L. (Eds.). (1995). *Preventing HIV transmission: The role of sterile needles and bleach.* Washington, DC: National Academy Press.

Office of Technology Assessment. (1988). *Nurse practitioners, physician assistants and certified nurse-midwives: A policy analysis.* Washington, DC: U.S. Government Printing Office.

Office of Technology Assessment. (1994, September). *Identifying health technologies that work: Searching for evidence.* Washington, DC: U.S. Government Printing Office.

Paltiel, A. D., & Stinnett, A. A. (1996). Making health policy decisions: Is human instinct rational? Is rational choice human? *Change, 9*(2), 34–39.

Pearson, L. (1997). Annual update on how each state stands on legislative issues affecting advanced nursing practice: A survey of legal authority, reimbursement status and prescriptive authority. *The Nurse Practitioner, 22*(1), 18–86.

Pollack, C., & Diers, D. (1994). Finding nursing management data. *Seminars in Nursing Management, 2*(2), 58–62.

Redman, E. (1973). *The dance of legislation.* New York: Simon & Schuster.

Rennie, D. (1997). Thyroid storm. *Journal of the American Medical Association, 277*(15), 1238–1243.

Safriet, B. (1992). Health care dollars and regulatory sense. *Yale Journal on Regulation, 9*(2), 417–488.

Secretary's Commission on the Nursing Shortage. (1988, December). *Final Report,* Vol. 1. U.S. Department of Health and Human Services. Washington, DC: Author.

Shindul-Rothschild, J., Berry, D., & Long-Middleton, E. (1996). Where have all the nurses gone? Final results of our patient care survey. *American Journal of Nursing, 96*(11), 25–39.

Sloan, J. H., Kellerman, A. L., Reay, D. T., Ferris, J. A., Koepsell, T., Rivara, F. P., Rice, C., Gray, L., LoGerfo, J., et al. (1988). Handgun regulations, crime, assault and homicide: A tale of two cities. *New England Journal of Medicine, 319*(19), 1256–1262.

Sloan, J. H., Rivara, F. P., Reay, D. T., Ferris, J. A., & Kellerman, A. L. (1990). Firearm regulations and rates of suicide: A comparison of two metropolitan areas. *New England Journal of Medicine, 322*(6) 369–373.

A spineless attack on the AHCPR. (1996). *Geriatrics, 51*(4), 9–10.

Spitzer, W. O. (1984). The nurse practitioner revisited: Slow death of a good idea. *New England Journal of Medicine, 310,* 1049–1051.

Spitzer, W. O., Sackett, D. L., Sibley, J. C., Roberts, R. S., Gent, M., Kergin, D. J., Hackett, B. C., & Olynich, A. (1974). The Burlington randomized trial of the nurse practitioner. *New England Journal of Medicine, 290,* 251–256.

Tanenbaum, S. J. (1996). Medical effectiveness in Canadian and U.S. health policy: The comparative politics of inferential ambiguity. *Health Services Research, 31*(5), 517–532.

Thompson, J. D. (1988). DRG prepayment: Its purpose and performance. *Bulletin of the New York Academy of Medicine, 64*(1), 25–51.

Thompson, J. D. (1990). Under hostile banners: Florence Nightingale and the relocation of St. Thomas' Hospital. Unpublished manuscript, Yale University Department of Epidemiology and Public Health, New Haven, CT.

Todd, J. S. (1991, May 3). Support for H.R. 7, the "Brady Handgun Violence Prevention Act." Letter to members of the U.S. House of Representatives. Available from the American Medical Association, Chicago.

Turning a new leaf: Liggett breaks ranks with "Big Tobacco" (1997, March 31). *Newsweek,* 50.

Varney, H. (1996). *Varney's midwifery* (3rd ed.). Boston: Jones & Bartlett.

White, D. L., & Hamel, P. K. (1986). National Center for Nursing Research: How it came to be. *Nursing Economic$, 4*(1), 19–22.

Wilburn, S. (1996, October). MNA study captures national attention. *American Nurse,* p. 15.

Wunderlich, G. S., Sloan, F. A., & Davis, C. K. (Eds.). (1996). *Nursing staff in hospitals and nursing homes: Is it adequate?* Washington, DC: National Academy Press.

Chapter *12*

THE ECONOMICS OF HEALTH CARE

SUZANNE MOORE, FRANKLIN N. LAUFER, AND MARY BETH CONROY

Many areas of public policy are characterized by a scarcity of the resources needed to achieve desired ends. As a consequence of such a scarcity of available resources, policy choices or decisions are required from among the potential alternative uses to which such limited resources can be devoted. Economic evaluation, specifically through such techniques as cost-benefit analysis and cost-effectiveness analysis, is useful for aiding policymakers in resource allocation decisions and has been applied in both the public and private sectors to evaluate issues pertaining to health and medical care. After a brief review of the place of health care in the market economy, this chapter provides an overview of economic evaluation techniques and their application to questions regarding health and medical care allocations.

THE DYNAMIC HEALTH CARE MARKET

In the United States, many policymakers profess that health care has been transformed into a market-driven system that has reduced rate increases for private purchasers and consumers. As recently as 1992, many contended that health care could never be treated as a commodity in the "market." The essence of a free market is that there is a buyer and a seller. The seller must compete for the buying power of the consumer. Competition constrains prices, and the market assumes that the consumer can evaluate the quality of the commodity, decide how much he wants or needs, and buy the best quality at the lowest price.

It is true that, in the past decade, consumers have become better educated about their health care needs and are making decisions based on value. We have seen the proliferation of health maintenance organizations and managed care products that were called "alternative delivery systems" in the 1980s and are now the norm. We have also seen the demise of hospital rate regulation (in 1997 only 1 state in 50 still regulated hospital rates), forcing hospitals to compete on price and quality and develop product lines that purchasers demand. There is no question that health care has evolved into a competitive market-driven system, but in an economic sense, does it or could it fit the economist's concept of the perfectly competitive economy?

Most believe that the properties of idealized economies involve large numbers of profit-maximizing firms and utility-maximizing consumers. The self-motivated behavior of these players leads to patterns of consumption and production that are efficient in the sense that it is impossible to make some person better off without making some other person worse off, a concept referred to as "Pareto efficient." Utility-maximizing behavior of consumers and the profit-maximizing behavior of firms distribute goods through the "invisible hand" in such a way that no one could be better off without making someone worse off. Economists do recognize many situations that violate the basic assumptions of the idealized competitive economy and thus interfere with efficiency in consumption or production, and these are called "market failures."

The traditional market failures are such things as public goods, natural monopolies, or instances where the consumer does not have adequate information. Market failures, as described, necessitate some form of regulation, often under the guise of public policy. The term *public goods* appears frequently in the economic literature. The blanket use of this term hides a uniqueness among a variety of public goods.

To qualify as a public good, a product must be nonrivalrous in consumption, nonexcludable in use, or both. A good is nonrivalrous in consumption when more than one person can derive benefits from a given level of supply at once. For example, a water filtration system is nonrivalrous because all citizens in the community enjoy the benefits without reducing the benefits to others. A good is nonexcludable if it is physically or legally impractical for one person to maintain exclusive control over its use. A third characteristic, congestibility, is useful in describing public goods. Congestibility means that the marginal social cost of consumption can increase beyond some level of consumption. In the example of the water filtration system, if the community reaches a certain population density, the filtration system may become ineffective.

The three characteristics, therefore, that determine whether in fact a good is considered a "public good" and can lead to Pareto inefficiency that results from market failure are nonrivalry in consumption, the extent of excludability or exclusiveness in control of its use, and the existence of congestion.

Keeping in mind the definition or characteristics of public goods, does health care qualify? If so, can it be forced into a market system, or will some degree of government intervention in the form of regulation always be necessary? In a market, the consumer is knowledgeable and able to decide how much of a product he needs or wants. Traditionally, the consumer has been at the mercy of the physician who is trained to decide the type and extent of health care needed. Even if a consumer becomes "informed," he cannot be expected to determine the extent of his "need." As Arnold Relman (1980) points out,

most consumers in health care are not "consumers" in the Adam Smith sense; medical insurance converts consumers into claimants who want medical care in spite of cost. It is sometimes difficult to define who the consumer is in the health care market. Is it the patient or the payer (the insurer or employer or government entity)? In a traditional market the consumer is also the payer. Because financial risk is spread among so many players in each health care transaction and because frequently the patient is bearing none of the financial risk but is the consumer of the product, health care is not and cannot be a truly competitive commodity.

ECONOMIC EVALUATION

Today's health care market is very much concerned about cost control. The rapidly increasing popularity of managed care over traditional indemnity insurance options leaves health care practitioners and advocates concerned about the assurance of high-quality, low-cost health care. It is important to ensure that limited resources are allocated on the basis of the maximum value and usage to the health care consumer. There are always implicit and necessary tradeoffs among the alternative uses of health care resources, programs, or both. Weinstein and Stasson (1977) described the need for a methodology to help health care providers make decisions on the distribution of finite resources. They describe a methodology that utilizes the best current information on both the efficacy of a medical practice and the cost. Cost-benefit analysis (CBA) and cost-effectiveness analysis (CEA) attempt to use existing information in an area of health care to develop criteria for allocating resources. In the 1960s, these economic decision tools that were common in the military became widely used in health care planning. There are other derivative forms of economic evaluation (e.g., modified CBA, qualitative CBA, economic impact analysis, risk analysis, cost minimization, and cost-utility analysis), but they are beyond the scope of this discussion, which is to provide the reader

Table 12-1 Examples of Areas Where Economic Evaluation is Applicable

AREA OF HEALTH CARE	AREAS FOR EVALUATION
Environmental health	Safe drinking water (Congress of the United States, 1995)
	OSHA standards (Bartel & Thomas, 1985)
	Food safety standards (Zeckhauser, 1985)
Health systems management	Purchasing versus leasing medical equipment
Hospital and nursing home administration	Neonatal intensive care units (Boyle, Torrance, Sinclair, & Harwood, 1983)
Health care financing	Long-term care treatment options for chronic disease and disability
	Home care versus long-term care (Cummings & Weaver, 1991)
	Inpatient care versus ambulatory (Churchill, Morgan, & Torrance, 1984)
	Cost to public payers (Medicare and Medicaid) of alternative models of health care delivery (Moore & Martelle-Conroy, 1996)
Injury control	Seatbelt laws (Nelson, Peterson, Chorba, Devine, & Sachs, 1993)
	Motorcycle helmet laws (Muller, 1980)
	Traffic safety—speed limits (Castle, 1976)
Mental health/mental retardation/ developmental disabilities	Inpatient versus outpatient models of care (Weisbrod, Test, & Stein, 1980)
	Medication options for the mentally ill
Public health/disease control/addictions	Vaccinations/immunizations (Lieu et al., 1994)
	Needle exchange programs (Kahn, 1993)
	Methadone maintenance programs
	Needlestick injury prevention (Laufer & Chiarello, 1994)
	Prenatal care options for the prevention of birth defects (Hargard & Carter, 1976)
Standards and surveillance	Nosocomial infection prevention programs (i.e., handwashing, air circulation ventilation systems)

with a sound understanding of the principles of economic evaluation.

Economic evaluation is useful in judging the effectiveness of a single program, multiple programs, or pilot programs. Economic evaluation may be used for regulatory purposes (i.e., a CBA or CEA may be required before a regulation is adopted or continued). An economic evaluation may be used to support the status quo or used as an argument for change.

As mentioned earlier, the role of economic evaluation in health care is crucial to the allocation of scarce health care dollars where the maximum value to the public good will be realized. Some of the areas where various

methods of economic evaluation may be used are listed in Table 12-1.

The economic analysis of health care is a complex, multifaceted judgment that must be made on an inclusive basis after the broad, full range of effects of an identified program or policy are analyzed. This may seem an intimidating ordeal, but once this broad view is broken down into easily understandable parts (i.e., a listing of all possible costs and benefits), an alternative that provides the greatest good at the lowest cost becomes apparent.

CBA is, in itself, a simple concept: costs are identified and then assigned a dollar value, benefits are identified and assigned a dollar value (undesirable benefits should be classified as costs), and then a net benefit is derived (the sum of the benefits minus the sum of the costs). It is important to remember that in a CBA everything is reduced to a dollar value—that is, both costs and benefits are quantified—and the decision on which program is efficient is based on the relationship of these quantified terms.

CEA differs from CBA in that effectiveness is presented in a nonquantified format. Costs between programs are compared on the basis of a single measure of effectiveness. In CEA the costs of a program or intervention are measured against nonquantified health outcomes. CEA is often chosen over CBA when it is deemed in poor taste or judgment to place a dollar value on a human life. A CEA is designed to determine the effectiveness of a health care program in achieving a nonquantified health outcome on the basis of the costs of the program in achieving the desired outcomes.

Economic evaluation of health care is a sensitive, highly important tool for public welfare. Whereas an analyst must always expect uncertainties in an analysis, areas of controversy or ambiguity must always be clearly defined and stated along with the analysis.

Cost-Benefit Analysis

CBA is the principal analytical framework used to evaluate, usually on an *ex ante* basis, decisions involving public expenditures. As a project evaluation technique, CBA was originally applied during the 1930s to analyze water resource projects and has been more widely used recently not only in the public sector for evaluating alternative uses of resources but also in the medical and health care policy sectors as well. CBA requires the systematic enumeration, from a societal perspective, of all benefits and costs that will accrue from the adoption of a particular project. With the use of monetary estimates of both costs and benefits, the decision rule on which all CBAs hinge is to select the alternative that produces the greatest net benefit (Nas, 1996; Stokey & Zeckhauser, 1978), that is,

the alternative that achieves the greatest level of economic efficiency. This section is intended to provide only a brief overview of the CBA approach, because several texts on CBA are accessible to the reader who wishes to obtain more in-depth treatment of any of the aspects of CBA discussed here (e.g., Mishan, 1988; Nas, 1996; Pearce, 1983), as well as to use as guides for applying CBA to medical and health care policy questions (Drummond, Stoddart, & Torrance, 1987; Gold, Siegel, Russell, & Weinstein, 1996; Warner & Luce, 1982). In addition, two health-related applications of CBA will be summarized.

ESTIMATING COSTS

CBA is used to evaluate alternative uses of resources in terms of the economic rather than the financial effects of the allocation decision. Resources are valued in terms of their *opportunity costs:* "If we use resources for project A, what alternative uses of those resources have been forgone?" An analyst examining the cost-benefit of an in-house workplace exercise program, for example, would need to consider not only the costs of exercise equipment to be purchased as a result of program implementation but also the cost of the space used to house the program and that portion of the cost of human resource personnel who may administer the exercise program, as there are alternative uses to which these resources could have been applied but which are forgone in favor of implementing the exercise program.

It is also important for CBA purposes that resources are valued at their incremental cost levels. In our example of the workplace exercise program, if a new program is contemplated, then the full cost of the resources (e.g., people, space, equipment) used to implement the program would be used for CBA purposes. However, if an expansion of an existing program is contemplated and additional resources will be required, a CBA of the expansion considers only the (incremental) costs of those additional resources and not those resources already consumed by the existing program.

A final consideration, and one that is particularly pertinent to evaluating clinical or public health–related interventions, is that resources generally should be valued at their costs rather than at their charges. Costs reflect the price of resources consumed to produce a service or product, as distinguished from the price actually charged consumers. For example, a patient or his or her insurer is charged $50 by a hospital for a specific laboratory test, but a CBA should consider only the actual cost to the hospital of performing that test. For more on this topic, see Finkler's (1982) discussion.

CATEGORIES AND VALUATION OF COSTS

Two categories of costs are used to value inputs (costs) and outcomes (benefits): direct costs and indirect or, more appropriately, productivity costs. Direct costs reflect the organization and provision of the intervention that may affect both current and future resource consumption; therefore, an appropriate time span over which resource use will be valued needs to be determined. Inputs such as health professionals' time, supplies and equipment, transportation, and capital and utility costs all reflect changes in the use of health-care and non-health-care resources and need to be included in a CBA. Costs borne by patients, their families, and other caregivers also need to be included. Analyses should also recognize the time spent by individuals who are volunteering or giving up time for which they would otherwise be paid to act as caregivers. Omitting such unpaid time biases the analysis in favor of programs that rely on donated or volunteered services over those which rely on purchased services (Drummond et al., 1987; Gold et al., 1996).

Productivity costs are intended to measure the value to society of lost productivity caused by changes in life expectancy and morbidity (Drummond et al., 1987; Gold et al., 1996). As an expression of the benefits of an intervention, these costs measure the lost productivity averted from implementing the intervention. Two approaches—the human capital approach and the willingness-to-pay approach—have been used to measure productivity costs. The human capital approach takes the perspective that "you're worth what you're paid" by valuing benefits of health care to an individual as his or her future flow of earnings that would otherwise be forgone because of death or ill health. In a cost-benefit evaluation of counseling, testing, referral, and partner notification services for persons infected with the human immunodeficiency virus (HIV), for example, Holtgrave, Valdiserri, Gerber, and Hinman (1993) valued program benefits for the prevention of HIV transmission to an individual as the sum of lifetime HIV treatment costs averted and that individual's expected future earnings.

The willingness-to-pay approach takes the perspective that "you're worth what you would pay" for an intervention. Through surveys or interviews, people are asked what they would be willing to pay either to obtain the benefits provided by the intervention or to avoid the costs of illness. For example, Thompson (1986) interviewed patients with rheumatoid arthritis to assess what percentage of their household monthly income they would be willing to pay on a regular basis for a complete (and hypothetical) cure for arthritis. The average respondent was willing to pay 22% of his or her household income for such a cure, a finding that did not vary with respondents' income. Although criticisms and limitations of both the human capital and willingness-to-pay approaches have been noted in the literature (see Johannesson & Jonsson [1991] and Robinson [1993], for example), consideration of these is beyond the scope of this review.

DISCOUNTING

An important aspect of an economic evaluation such as CBA is the recognition that future costs and benefits need to be discounted or presented in terms of their present value. However, discounting should not be confused with nor appear to be necessitated by inflation. Simply put, the reason that discounting is required is that people will value having a dollar in hand today rather than the promise of a dollar next year because having a dollar today presents opportunities for spending or investment. To use a simple example, if I am indifferent to receiving either $1.00 today or $1.05 next year, then that $1.05 received next year has a present value to me of $1.00. This implies that I have "discounted" my future earnings at a rate of 5%.

Productivity costs as benefits also need to be discounted so that they can be valued relative to the current dollars represented by the discounted stream of direct costs or expenditures. Short-term costs and benefits (i.e., those realized within 1 year) are usually not discounted.

Although discounting is recognized as an integral part of any economic evaluation, a critical issue is the rate at which discounting is done. Depending on the policy issue and the federal agency performing the CBA, rates range from as low as 2.1% up to 7% (Gold et al., 1996; Nas, 1996). For CEAs of health and clinical interventions, Gold et al. recommended that both 3% and 5% be used.

SENSITIVITY ANALYSIS

Many of the parameters in the analysis may have been estimated under uncertainty. That is, any specific parameter may take on a value within a certain range. After an initial base-case analysis is performed, in which the base values assumed for the variables are incorporated into the analysis, a sensitivity analysis is conducted to examine any effect on the results that may be caused under different assumed values for these parameters. For example, it is appropriate to perform a sensitivity analysis over a range of discount rates (usually over rates ranging from 0% to 8%, as recommended by Gold et al. [1996]), as well as over reasonable ranges of vaccination rates and protective efficacy, life expectancy, projected earnings, and any parameters, specific to the particular study, that have been estimated with uncertainty.

TWO EXAMPLES OF COST-BENEFIT ANALYSIS

The studies summarized in Case Examples 1 and 2 were chosen to demonstrate applications of CBA both to preventive services (immuniza-

tion) and to curative services (neonatal intensive care). Interested readers are encouraged to consult the published studies for more extended descriptions of the respective analyses.

CASE EXAMPLE 1 **Vaccination for *Haemophilus Influenzae* Type b Disease**

Infants infected with *Haemophilus influenzae* type b (Hib) disease may contract meningitis, pneumonia, septicemia, or some other Hib disease. Immunization, however, can prevent Hib infection, and Hussey, Lasser, and Reekie (1995) employed a general cost-benefit approach to measure prospectively the expected net benefit from a hypothetical Hib vaccination program for the metropolitan area of Cape Town, South Africa. Hussey et al. assumed a birth cohort of about 47,000, for which 310 of these unvaccinated infants would contract Hib disease. Under base assumptions for imperfect vaccine efficacy and coverage, the opportunity costs were calculated for about 221 cases averted.

The analysis accounted for both direct medical care costs and productivity costs for the Hib cases averted. Direct medical care costs included the hospitalization costs for treating unvaccinated infants across the Hib disease spectrum. Mortality and long-term morbidity, resulting in lost or reduced productivity through infants' lifetimes, were valued by using both the human capital and the willingness-to-pay approaches to determine the economic value of an individual life. (The latter approach combined projected subsistence costs during an individual's nonemployment years with lost earnings for an individual's employment years.) These categories of costs represented the economic benefits of implementing the vaccination program.

The costs of administering the vaccine and of care for any vaccinated infants having severe side effects, representing the incremental costs to be used in the analysis, were also estimated. Both costs and benefits were discounted to current (1992) levels. In 1992 U.S. dollars the total avoidable disease costs (mortality, hospitalization, and long-term morbidity costs) for the 221 cases of Hib disease averted were estimated to be about $3.5 million when the human capital approach was used and about $3.9 million when the willingness-to-pay approach was used. Vaccine administration costs for the birth cohort, including the costs of treating infants for severe side effects, were estimated to be $2.7 million. Benefits exceeded costs when both the human capital ($0.9 million) and the willingness-to-pay ($1.3 million) approaches were used; the benefit-to-cost ratios were calculated as 1.29 ($3.6 million/$2.7 million) with the human capital valuation of benefits and 1.44 ($3.9 million/$2.7 million) with the willingness-to-pay approach. Sensitivity analyses demonstrated the effects of varying the base assumptions, such as the value of life, the discount and economic growth rates, and the vaccination coverage rate. On the basis of the economic savings demonstrated by their analysis, Hussey et al. (1995) recommended implementation of a national vaccination program.

CASE EXAMPLE 2 Cost-Benefit of Neonatal Intensive Care for Very-Low-Birth-Weight Infants

An often-cited cost analysis is that performed by Boyle, Torrance, Sinclair, and Horwood (1983) to determine the cost-benefit of neonatal intensive care of very-low-birth-weight (<1500 g) infants. (Their cost-effectiveness analysis, examining the cost per life-year gained and the cost per quality-adjusted life-year gained, will be summarized in the next section.) Boyle et al. compared costs and outcomes of care before and after the introduction of a regional neonatal intensive care program in a portion of Ontario, Canada, performing separate analyses for infants weighing 1000 to 1499 g and those weighing 500 to 999 g.

Direct costs associated with neonatal intensive care were identified, including in-hospital and other follow-up medical care, ambulance transport, and physician charges (note: not costs). Direct costs also included the costs of other current or projected institutional care, special services, durable medical equipment, special education, and other miscellaneous items as determined according to parents with surviving low-birth-weight children. Forecasts of outcomes and lifetime costs, including life expectancy, future functioning, productivity as a percentage of normal productivity, and consumption of medical resources as a percentage of normal consumption, were provided by two developmental pediatricians. The analysis also used census data on individual income to determine earnings; regional data on health care costs; and published and unpublished studies for

yearly costs of parental care and subsistence of disabled children in the home.

Incremental costs and benefits were determined per live birth to three thresholds: to discharge from hospital, to age 15 years (projected), and to death (projected). Because expenditures for neonatal care result in benefits realized at a later date, a discount rate of 5% was applied to costs and earnings to value these future monetary effects at their present value. Net economic benefit was defined as the difference between the change in earnings per live birth less the change in costs per live birth. For both birth-weight groups, the increase in costs exceeded the increase in projected earnings: the net economic loss (expressed in 1978 U.S. dollars) was $2,280 for the 1000 to 1499 g class and $14,120 for the 500 to 999 g class. Sensitivity analyses, performed on the discount rate, life expectancy, and other parameters demonstrated that the net benefit was generally unaffected by changes in these parameters, excepting that the net benefit per live birth for the 1000 to 1499 g class was positive at discount rates lower than about 3.5%. More specific analyses were also performed for infants in 250 g subgroups within the two original birth-weight classes. Boyle et al. (1983) conclude with the relevant observation that programs may not meet the cost-benefit criterion of having benefits exceed costs but are justified by society on the basis of the positive benefits produced.

CBA is used to evaluate the economic efficiency of alternatives as an aid to decision making in many areas of public policy. Valuing both costs and benefits in monetary terms permits comparisons between alternatives across different policy areas (e.g., environmental programs can be compared with transportation programs). However, CBAs' dependence on an economic valuation of benefits—specifically the value of a human life—is often difficult and is viewed as controversial by many researchers and decision makers. This has hindered the application of CBA to medical and other health-related policy choices and is perhaps the main reason why cost-effectiveness has been increasingly relied on in health and medicine.

Cost-effectiveness Analysis

CEA is one form of economic analysis available to examine the costs and consequences of health care programs. CEA summarizes costs into one number and benefits into another and prescribes rules for making decisions based on the relationship between the two. CEA does not attempt to assign monetary values to health outcomes but expresses benefits in simpler, more descriptive terms such as years of life gained. A useful CEA must be comprehensive and broadly applicable. Usually the overall societal view in evaluating costs and effectiveness is taken; however, the objectives of the actual decision makers may vary considerably.

HOW TO CHOOSE A MEASURE OF EFFECTIVENESS

Measures used to indicate effectiveness should be outcome oriented. Process measures are often useful proxies for outcome measures when the latter are not available. Intermediate outcomes or process measures have the advantage of being more immediate and potentially more measurable. The disadvantage is that their relationship to the larger goal or to the program itself is often indirect or elusive (Weinstein, Graham, Siegel, & Fineberg, 1989).

One recent evaluation used CEA to measure the efficiency of inpatient rehabilitation for patients with traumatic brain injury. The functional recovery at the end of the rehabilitation stay was used as the effectiveness measure. That measure is only a step in the whole recovery process and yet is clearly linked to the end result (Moore, 1992).

The term *cost-effectiveness* is frequently misused. People often make statements asserting the cost-effectiveness of a procedure or treatment without providing or referring to relevant cost and outcome data. Doubiet, Weinstein, and McNeil (1986) listed the varying criteria used for determining cost-effectiveness. The first is that cost-effectiveness means cost saving. This criterion is unsatisfactory in medicine because many programs that do not save money but do provide a benefit at an "acceptable" cost would be eliminated. The second erroneous criterion is that cost-effective means merely effective; costs are not considered. The third criterion is that cost-effective means cost saving with an equal or better outcome. This is too stringent for medicine because it would eliminate approaches that reduce costs greatly but lead to a small decrease in effectiveness, which is unacceptable. The last and most acceptable criterion is that being cost-effective means having an additional benefit worth the additional cost. However, this criterion depends on the relative value one places on the health outcome and the monetary cost.

CEA can be used only to analyze economic problems with a marginal impact on the entire economic and social structure of society. For example, if malaria were to be eradicated, a major demographic impact would be felt throughout society, not only in the short run, but also for the next 20 to 30 years. Another disadvantage of CEA is that equity and distributional concerns are often avoided in an attempt to maximize economic growth by maximizing the return to society's investment (Dunlop, 1975).

MacIntyre (1977) contends that CEA and CBA treat the social world as predictable and calculable and ignore arbitrary factors. These tools presuppose a decision as to what is a cost and what is a benefit. The decision expresses the author's values and not necessarily societal values. Shepard and Thompson (1979) list several disadvantages of CEA. They contend that it rarely yields a single answer but that this is compensated for by the fact that assumptions are made explicitly and their effect on the results is made clear. They also allude to the practical difficulty of incorporating consumers' input and to the unquantifiable nature of human values. However, CEA, unlike CBA, does avoid the quantification of human values and human life. Graham and Vaupel (1981) describe the variation in the value of life from $217 million to $625 million, depending on which method the analysis incorporates. CEA avoids this difficult problem of money valuation, but unlike CBA it does not yield a single answer.

CEA has been used extensively in medicine to evaluate primary preventive programs as well as secondary and tertiary programs. CEA is responsible for eliminating universal smallpox vaccination once smallpox was eradicated from the world (Russell, 1986). Eddy (1981a, 1981b), using the best clinical information on the natural history, detection, and treatment of cervical cancer, found that administering Pap tests to adult women every 3 to 4 years would produce almost as much health benefit at less than a third of the cost. This CEA caused the American Cancer Association to change its recommendation concerning the frequency of Pap smears. Hypertension screening and treatment and lifestyle changes such as exercise and improved diet have been under economic scrutiny for several years, and the result has been major changes in health care delivery and funding (Russell, 1986). The cost-effectiveness of HIV prevention programs, including premarital screening, condom promotion in secondary schools, and the distribution of bleach among intravenous drug users, is currently being evaluated (Weinstein et al., 1989).

Weinstein and Stasson (1985) examined the cost-effectiveness of interventions to prevent and treat coronary artery disease. The interventions they evaluated were admission to a coronary care unit, the use of beta-blocking agents in postinfection patients, and the use of coronary artery bypass grafts. Albrect and Harasymiw (1979) used CEA in their evaluation of the rehabilitation of patients with focal cerebral injuries and spinal cord injuries in 10 centers. They found that the three factors responsible for the variability in cost-effectiveness were the center, the time from incident to rehabilitation, and age. Lehman et al. (1975) studied the cost-effectiveness of stroke rehabilitation. They found that, for the given life expectancy of a stroke patient, the cost of rehabilitation is more than compensated for by the savings from not placing some successfully rehabilitated patients in nursing homes. They contend that CEA stud-

ies should be done to demonstrate to politicians and policymakers that better support of rehabilitation through private insurance, or through state and federal agencies, actually reduces the overall cost to society of disability.

THE BASIS OF THE METHODOLOGY

Choosing the Correct Measure. The first step in choosing a measure is defining the objectives of the program. If one objective is the most salient, the analysis should be based on this dimension.

Look for a common measure that can be used to compare interventions or disparate programs (i.e., "cost per life-year gained").

Collecting Data on Effectiveness. The medical literature is the major source of the data necessary to evaluate and compare programs. The quality and relevance of the outcome data must be evaluated. Generally this is an epidemiological and biostatistical issue, and the appropriate sources should be consulted. If no good clinical evidence exists, one can proceed by making assumptions about the medical parameters or can design a study that will generate the effectiveness data required (Drummond et al., 1987). If one is making assumptions, *sensitivity analysis* of the economic results, in comparison with different assumptions, should be done.

COSTS

Inclusion of Indirect Costs. As one calculates costs, the question arises as to which costs should be considered. Should direct costs of an intervention (labor and materials) be considered, or should the indirect costs, such as lost wages of a relative who has turned care provider, be considered? When determining costs, the analyst must be aware of the methodology used by other economic analysts, which may be used as a comparison. Methodological consistency in a comparison of cost analyses is essential.

Should Effects Occurring in the Future Be Discounted? If the effects occur in a short period, discounting is not necessary. Though discounting makes sense in the context of resources where one would expect future generations to be wealthier, it may not make sense in the context of a health effect. However, leaving effects undiscounted while discounting costs can lead to inconsistencies.

TWO EXAMPLES OF COST-EFFECTIVENESS ANALYSIS

CASE EXAMPLE 1   Neonatal Intensive Care for Very-Low-Birth-Weight Infants

In addition to performing a CBA on neonatal intensive care for very-low-birth-weight infants, Boyle et al. (1983) performed CEAs evaluating the cost per life-year gained and the cost per quality-adjusted life-year (QALY) gained. Costs of neonatal intensive care were determined as described in the previous section. Additional life-years gained for the study subjects were projected by means of survey responses of parents of surviving infants and the expert opinion of developmental pediatricians. To assess QALYs gained, the authors developed a classification of health states to measure the health of survivors with respect to health problems and levels of physical, social, role, and emotional functioning. The social preferences for health states, characterized by various combinations of these health states, were determined by the results of a random survey of parents and schoolchildren who were asked to rate the utility (i.e., desirability and undesirability) of each of the possible health states relative to the reference states "healthy" and "dead," which are by convention usually assigned utility values of 1 and 0, respectively. The authors note how some parents also rated certain chronic dysfunctional states in children as worse than death, however, which resulted in utility values for health states ranging from 1 for normal health to −0.39 for these worse-than-death states. Life-years were adjusted for quality by these utility values so that, for example, a life-year in a health state judged to be 0.65 in utility would represent 0.65 QALYs.

The results of the analyses showed that the incremental cost of neonatal intensive care for the 1000 to 1499 g birth-weight class was $789 per life-year gained and $877 per QALY gained; for the 500 to 999 g birth-weight class, the cost was $6402 per life-year gained and $15,348 per QALY gained. (All values are in 1978 U.S. dollars.) By these results, as well as the results of their CBA, Boyle et al. (1983) concluded that "it was economically more feasible to provide intensive care for the relatively heavier infants" (p. 1334), a finding consistent over all sensitivity analyses conducted as part of the economic evaluations performed.

CASE EXAMPLE 2   Screening for Carotid Stenosis in Asymptomatic Men

A more recent CEA (Lee, Solomon, Heidenreich, Oehlert, & Garger, 1997) examined the cost-effectiveness of screening for carotid stenosis in asymptomatic 65-year-old men. Using published data from clinical trials, the costs and outcomes of screening were compared with no screening for carotid stenosis. Screening would be done with Doppler ultrasonography, followed by angiography for stenosis found to be 60% or greater. If angiography confirmed stenosis and was uneventful, carotid endarterectomy would be performed. The sequence of possible events and outcomes was modeled by means of decision analysis, beginning with the decision to screen through surgery and its potential outcomes and complications.

Charges were used as proxies for medical and other nonclinical treatment costs; productivity costs such as lost earnings, however, were omitted. Utility values were assigned to each health state (well health, after strokes of differing severities, after acute myocardial infarction, and death). The probabilities of the events and outcomes incorporated into the decision analysis and the future costs and utilities were estimated at a baseline value and at a plausible range for purposes of performing sensitivity analyses. A discount rate of 3% was applied to both future costs and future utilities, although the discount rate itself was not varied.

The results demonstrated that the marginal cost-effectiveness of the screening strategy over the no-screening strategy was $120,000 per QALY gained (in 1994 U.S. dollars). Only under certain implausible conditions, such as a 40% prevalence of carotid stenosis in this population rather than the 5% baseline prevalence assumed, would the cost per QALY gained decrease to $50,000 or less, a level at or below which interventions are generally considered acceptable from a cost-effectiveness perspective (Laupacis, Feeny, Detsky, & Tugwell, 1992). The authors also compared their results with previously published analyses of screening programs (hypertension) and curative interventions (coronary artery bypass graph surgery for left main artery disease) that have been demonstrated to be cost-effective. The authors conclude that screening for carotid stenosis is not cost-effective because the number of candidates found for surgery is low, and when a candidate is found, the modest absolute (5%) reduction in stroke rate achieved by surgery is realized at a substantial cost.

ECONOMIC EVALUATION AS PART OF THE POLICYMAKING PROCESS

The two techniques reviewed in this chapter—cost-benefit analysis and cost-effectiveness analysis—enable policymakers to evaluate alternative policy choices and make recommendations. CBA is considered a more comprehensive and theoretically sound economic evaluation technique than CEA. However, CBA has not been as widely used as CEA to evaluate medical and other health-related interventions. CBA requires valuing both costs and benefits, or outcomes, in monetary terms, and valuing outcomes (e.g., losses of productivity from morbidity and death) in dollars and cents has been considered complex and controversial by researchers and decision makers in the health policy arena. CEA, on the other hand, requires that outcomes be measured in natural units (e.g., number of people screened) or in quality-adjusted life-years gained. These outcome measures are considered to be more easily derived, contributing to the widespread application the CEA technique has enjoyed in health care evaluations.

Recent attention has been paid to the economic evaluation of prevention programs. Prevention programs may involve high expenditures for relatively little benefit. For example, Eddy (1990) estimated that annual rather than biennial screening for cervical cancer will cost all payers an additional $1 million per year of life gained. However, public values such as altruism or distributive justice or fairness cannot be expressed in monetary terms but may play a role in policymaking (Ubel, DeKay, Baron, & Asch, 1996). In addition, researchers have questioned how future benefits of preventive services are discounted. Prevention programs generate ex-

penditures today, but related beneficial health outcomes often are realized well into the future. As a result, high current and generally undiscounted costs are compared with far-off and heavily discounted health benefits or outcomes, thus creating unfavorable cost-effectiveness ratios. We do not discuss this issue further here but refer the interested reader to such sources as Ganiats (1997) and Phillips and Holtgrave (1997) for more detailed discussions of these and other related issues.

Examples of the application of CEA to the evaluation of preventive or screening programs, as well as curative or clinical interventions, have been presented here. Insurance carriers as third-party payers, whether public or private, often look to the results of CEA as input to coverage decisions (Neumann & Johannesson, 1994). Economic evaluations of new drugs and other medical technologies play an important part in determining whether such services will be covered as part of an insurance benefit package. Perhaps the most interesting and relevant application of CEA to the allocation of health care resources is the effort by the Oregon Health Services Commission to prioritize health services in order to ensure the affordability of and access to some minimum, or "basic," level of health care for its citizens. Because Oregon's prioritization project receives expanded treatment elsewhere in this book (see Unit II Case Study), we restrict ourselves here to the role of economic evaluation in this project.

PRIORITIZATION OF HEALTH SERVICES: THE OREGON EXPERIENCE[1]

The methodology adopted by the Oregon Health Services Commission for the prioritization of health services followed three steps. The first step was to rank a set of health service categories (e.g., care for acute fatal conditions,

---

[1]This description is based on portions of the Oregon Health Services Commission's 1991 report, *Prioritization of Health Services: A Report to the Governor and Legislature,* unless otherwise noted.

maternity care, preventive care for children, and comfort care). This ranking was done by the commission members but was based not only on their own judgments of importance but also on the social values and public priorities identified through a series of community meetings and public hearings. Condition/treatment pairs (e.g., acute myocardial infarction/medical therapy) were then created and subsequently categorized into these health service categories. By placing each condition/treatment pair within these ranked health service categories, an initial prioritization was accomplished.

The second step involved deriving the "net benefit" for each condition/treatment pair and combining this net benefit with cost information. Net benefit was intended to represent the extent to which an individual feels better or worse after being treated or not. A set of potential health states and symptoms, intermediate between perfect health and death, was determined for each condition/treatment pair, both with and without treatment, on the basis of literature review and by data provided by service providers. The Quality of Well-Being (QWB) Scale (Kaplan & Bush, 1982; Kaplan & Anderson, 1988) was selected to provide a health-related quality-of-life measure by which to quality-adjust expected health states. The survey used to assess QWB scores was modified and subsequently administered to a random sample of 1,001 people through a telephone survey. From the survey responses, numerical values were derived to represent the public's feelings about the desirability or utility of the intermediate health states and symptoms characterizing each condition/treatment pair. This QWB adjustment was then multiplied by the expected duration of the benefit of treatment, providing a measure of net benefit.

Charges for professional and hospital services were used to define costs; opportunity costs were not included. Net benefit was combined with cost data to provide a cost-effectiveness ratio. A simplified ratio can be expressed as follows:

$$\frac{\text{Cost}}{(\text{Net benefit}) \times (\text{Duration of benefit})}$$

This ratio was intended to compare the health benefits received in relation to the money spent for the different condition/treatment pairs being considered. The combination of ranked health services categories with the cost-effectiveness ranking within these categories provided an initial draft list of prioritized health services.

Preliminary ratios, expressed as dollars per year of healthy life gained, ranged from $1.46 to more than $300,000. For example, the cost-effectiveness ratio for antibiotic treatment of candidiasis was $1.66, compared with ratios of $52,243 for liver transplant for treatment of alcoholic cirrhosis or $129,658 for surgery for bursitis (Patrick & Erickson, 1993).

The third step in the process involved commission members' using a "reasonableness" test to adjust the objectively ranked health care services. Commissioners examined the placement of condition/treatment pairs on the list in terms of public health impact, cost and effectiveness of treatment, incidence of condition, and social cost. Services ranked in the top part of the list were those considered by the commission to be lifesaving, maternity care, and preventive services for children, followed by reproductive services, comfort care, preventive dental services, and preventive care for adults. Infertility services, preventive services considered less effective for adults (e.g., sigmoidoscopy for persons less than age 40 years), and treatment that results in minimal or no improvement in quality of life (e.g., surgical treatment for chronic pancreatitis) were ranked in the lower part of the list. As a result of the prioritization process, and other activities not described here, a prioritized listing of 709 health services was recommended to the Oregon state legislature for budgetary allocation decisions.

The Oregon state legislature establishes the budgetary constraint and the cutoff point below which no public funding is provided. In 1993 the funding provided by the legislature was sufficient for a benefit package consisting of treatment for the first 587 condition/treatment pairs. Subsequently, available funding for 1994 enabled the package to include the first 606 of the

744 health services on the list. (The listing is continually reviewed and revised by the Oregon Health Services Commission.) Effective in 1996, available funding enabled coverage of the first 581 services, and the funding level for 1997 covers the first 578 services.

CONCLUSION

This chapter provides the reader with an overview of economic evaluation as a policy-analysis tool for decision making in health care. Specifically, the techniques of cost-benefit analysis and cost-effectiveness have been reviewed here in brief. As exemplified by the Oregon prioritization process described above, perhaps the most important contribution that economic evaluation techniques make to the policymaking process is to provide a systematic approach to evaluating, from an economic perspective, the costs and benefits of alternative uses of resources. As such, economic evaluation should be considered an aid to decision making and not the sole source of information on which a decision is based. Applying economic evaluation to policy choices requires that values—whether monetary or desirability, such as in utility assessment for deriving quality-adjusted life-years—be made explicit and be presented in support of a policy recommendation. However, as Neumann and Johannesson (1994) have noted, economic evaluation is only one step: "Conducting cost-effectiveness analysis will not remove the need for difficult resource allocation decisions. But explicitly illuminating the trade-offs involved should help the process; thus, it represents a prudent step forward in public policy" (p. 212).

REFERENCES

Albrect, G., & Harasymiw, S. (1979). Evaluating rehabilitation outcome by cost function indicators. *Journal of Chronic Disease, 32,* 525–533.

Bartel, A., & Thomas, L. G. (1985). Direct and indirect effects of regulation: A new look at OSHAs impact. *Journal of Law and Economics, 28*(1), 1–25.

Boyle, M. H., Torrance, G. W., Sinclair, J. C., &

Horwood, S. P. (1983). Economic evaluation of neonatal intensive care of very low birth weight infants. *New England Journal of Medicine, 308*(22), 1330–1337.

Castle, G. (1976). The 55 MPH speed limit: A cost-benefit analysis. *Traffic Engineering, 46*(1), 11–14.

Churchill, D. N., Morgan, J., & Torrance, G. W. (1984, January-March). Quality of life in end-stage renal disease. *Peritoneal Dialysis Bulletin,* 20–23.

Congress of the United States, Congressional Budget Office. (1995, September). *The safe drinking water act: A case study of an unfunded federal mandate.* Washington, DC: Author.

Cummings, J., & Weaver, F. (1991). Cost-effectiveness of home care. *Clinics in Geriatric Medicine, 7*(4), 865–874.

Doubiet, P., Weinstein, M., & McNeil, B. (1986). Use and misuse of the term cost-effectiveness analysis in medicine. *New England Journal of Medicine, 314,* 253–255.

Drummond, M. F., Stoddart, G. L., & Torrance, G. W. (1987). *Methods for the economic evaluation of health care programs.* Oxford: Oxford University Press.

Dunlop, D. (1975). Benefit cost analysis: A review of its applicability in policy analysis for delivering health services. *Social Sciences and Medicine, 9,* 133–139.

Eddy, D. M. (1980). *Screening for cancer: Theory, analysis and design.* Englewood Cliffs, NJ: Prentice-Hall.

Eddy, D. M. (1981a, October). Appropriateness of cervical cancer screening. *Gynecologic Oncology, 12,* S168–187.

Eddy, D. M. (1981b). The economics of cancer prevention and detection: Getting more for less. *Cancer, 47,* 1200–1201.

Eddy, D. M. (1990). Screening for cervical cancer. *Annals of Internal Medicine, 113,* 214–226.

Finkler, S. A. (1982). The distinction between costs and charges. *Annals of Internal Medicine, 96,* 102–109.

Ganiats, T. G. (1997). Prevention, policy, and paradox: What is the value of future health? *American Journal of Preventive Medicine, 13*(1), 12–17.

Gold, M. R., Siegel, J. E., Russell, L. B., & Weinstein, M. C. (Eds.). (1996). *Cost-effectiveness in health and medicine.* Oxford: Oxford University Press.

Graham, J., & Vaupel, J. (1981). Value of life: What difference does it make? *Risk Analysis, 1,* 89–95.

Hargard, S., & Carter, F. A. (1976). Preventing the birth of infants with Down's syndrome: A cost-benefit analysis. *British Medical Journal, 1*(6012), 753–756.

Holtgrave, D. R., Valdiserri, R. O., Gerber, A. R., & Hinman, A. R. (1993). Human immunodeficiency virus counseling, testing, referral, and partner notification services: A cost-benefit analysis. *Archives of Internal Medicine, 153,* 1225–1230.

Hussey, G. D., Lasser, M. L., & Reekie, W. E. (1995). The costs and benefits of a vaccination programme for *Haemophilus influenzae* type B disease. *South African Medical Journal, 85,* 20–25.

Johannesson, M., & Jonsson, B. (1991). Economic evaluation in health care: Is there a role for cost-benefit analysis? *Health Policy, 17,* 1–23.

Kahn, J. B. (1993). How much does it cost to operate NEPs? In P. Lurie & A. L. Reingold (Eds.), *The public health impact of needle exchange programs in the United States and abroad.* San Francisco: Institute for Health Policy Studies, University of California, San Francisco.

Kaplan, R. M., & Anderson, J. P. (1988). A general health policy model: Update and applications. *Health Services Research, 23,* 203–235.

Kaplan, R. M., & Bush, J. W. (1982). Health-related quality of life measurement for evaluation research and policy analysis. *Health Psychology, 1,* 61–80.

Laufer, F. N., & Chiarello, L. A. (1994). Application of cost-effectiveness methodology to the consideration of needlestick-prevention technology *American Journal of Infection Control and Epidemiology, 22,* 75–82.

Laupacis, A., Feeny, D., Detsky, A., & Tugwell, P. X. (1992). How attractive does a new technology have to be to warrant adoption and utilization? *Canadian Medical Association Journal, 146,* 473–481.

Lee, T. T., Solomon, N. A., Heidenreich, P. A., Oehlert, J., & Garger, A. M. (1997). Cost-effectiveness of screening for carotid stenosis in asymptomatic persons. *Annals of Internal Medicine, 126,* 337–346.

Lehman, J. F., Delateur, B. J., Fowler, R. S., Warren, C. G., Arnhold, R., Schertzer, G., Hurka, R., Whitmore, J. J., Masock, A. J., & Chambers, K. H. (1975). "Stroke: Does rehabilitation affect outcome?" *Archives of Physical Medicine and Rehabilitation, 56,* 375–382.

Lieu, T. A., Cochi, S. L., Black, S. B., Halloran, E., Shinefield, H. R., Holmes, S. J., Wharton, M., & Washington, E. (1994). Cost-effectiveness of a routine varicella vaccination program for U.S. children. *JAMA, 271,* 375–381.

MacIntyre, A. (1977). Utilitarianism and cost benefit analysis: An essay on the relevance of moral philosophy to bureaucratic theory. *Values in the chemical power industry.* Chicago: Notre Dame Press.

Mishan, E. J. (1988). *Cost-benefit analysis: An informal introduction* (4th ed.). London: Unwin Hyman.

Moore, S. (1992). *The effectiveness and efficiency of inpatient brain injury rehabilitation: Factors that predict success.* Boston: Boston University, The University Professors Dissertation.

Moore, S., & Martelle-Conroy, M. B. (1996, April 9). *Alternative models of ensuring access to primary medical care in nursing facilities demonstration project.* Final Report to the Robert Wood Johnson Foundation.

Muller, A. (1980). Evaluation of the costs and benefits of motorcycle helmet laws. *American Journal of Public Health, 70*(6), 586–592.

Nas, T. F. (1996). *Cost-benefit analysis: Theory and application.* Thousand Oaks, CA: Sage.

Nelson, D. E., Peterson, T. D., Chorba, T. L., Devine, O. J., & Sacks, J. (1993). Cost savings associated with increased safety belt use in Iowa, 1987–1988. *Accident Analysis and Prevention, 25*(5), 521–528.

Neumann, P. J., & Johannesson, M. (1994). From principle to public policy: Using cost effectiveness. *Health Affairs,* Summer 1994, 206–214.

Oregon Health Services Commission. (1991). *Prioritization of health services: A report to the governor and the legislature.* Salem: Oregon Health Services Commission.

Patrick, D. L., & Erickson, P. (1993). *Health status and health policy: Allocating resources to health care.* New York: Oxford University Press.

Pearce, D. W. (1983). *Cost-benefit analysis.* New York: St. Martin's Press.

Phillips, K. A., & Holtgrave, D. R. (1997). Using cost-effectiveness/cost-benefit analysis to allocate health resources: A level playing field for prevention? *American Journal of Preventive Medicine, 13*(1), 18–25.

Relman, A. (1980, October 23). The new medical

industrial complex. *New England Journal of Medicine, 303*(7), 963.

Robinson, R. (1993). Cost-benefit analysis. *British Medical Journal, 307,* 924–926.

Russell, L. B. (1986). *Is prevention better than cure?* Washington, DC: Brookings Institute.

Shepard, D., & Thompson, M. (1979). First principles in cost-effectiveness analysis in health. *Public Health Reports, 94,* 535–543.

Stokey, E., & Zeckhauser, R. (1978). *A primer for policy analysis.* New York: Norton.

Thompson, M. S. (1986). Willingness to pay and accept risks to cure chronic disease. *American Journal of Public Health, 76,* 392–396.

Ubel, P. A., DeKay, M. L., Baron, J., & Asch, D. A. (1996). Cost-effectiveness analysis in a setting of budget constraints: Is it equitable? *New England Journal of Medicine, 334,* 1174–1177.

Warner, K. A., & Luce, B. R. (1982). *Cost-benefit and cost-effectiveness analysis in health care: Principles, practice, and potential.* Ann Arbor, MI: Health Administration Press.

Weinstein, M., & Stasson, W. (1977). Foundations of cost-effectiveness analysis for health and medical practices. *New England Journal of Medicine, 296,* 716–721.

Weinstein, M., & Stasson, W. (1985). Cost-effectiveness of interventions to prevent or treat coronary heart disease. *Annual Review of Public Health, 6,* 41–63.

Weinstein, M. C., Graham, J. D., Siegel, J. E., & Fineberg, H. V. (1989). Cost-effectiveness analysis of AIDS prevention programs: Concepts, complications and illustrations. In C. F. Turner, H. G. Miller, & L. E. Moses (Eds.), *AIDS sexual behavior and intravenous drug use.* Washington, DC: Commission on Behavioral and Social Sciences Education, National Research Council.

Weisbrod, B. A., Test, M., & Stein, L. I. (1980). Alternatives to mental hospital treatment. II. Economic benefit cost analysis. *Archives of General Psychiatry, 37,* 400–405.

Zeckhauser, R. (1985). Measuring risks and benefits of food safety decisions. *Vanderbilt Law Review, 38*(3), 529–569.

Chapter *13*

THE ROLE OF THE MEDIA IN INFLUENCING POLICY: Getting the Message Across

Diana J. Mason, Barbara Glickstein, and Catherine J. Dodd

When President Bill Clinton first took office in 1992, one of his primary domestic policy priorities was the guarantee of comprehensive health care coverage for every American. In September 1993, he released the Health Security Act to Congress and the public with the hope and anticipation that this would become landmark legislation. The nursing community was particularly supportive of this legislation because it recognized advanced practice nurses as important providers of primary care. Two curious characters, Harry and Louise, were to play a key role in dashing the hopes of the President, much of the nursing community, and others who saw the legislation as an important remedy for an ailing health care system.

Harry and Louise is the name of a series of television advertisements sponsored by the Health Insurance Association of America, which adamantly opposed the President's plan. Harry and Louise portrayed a couple discussing the bill with grave concern. They said: "Under the president's bill, we'll lose our right to chose our own physician" and "What happens if the plan runs out of money?" Although the advertisements were not the only reason for the demise of the Health Security Act, *Harry and Louise* effectively planted fear and negativity in the hearts and minds of many citizens within the span of 60 seconds (Annenberg Public Policy Center, 1995).

What many do not realize about the *Harry and Louise* commercials is that the target audience was not the public directly. Rather, it was policymakers and those who could influence how the public perceived the issue (i.e., journalists). The ads originally aired in Washington, D.C., Los Angeles, New York City, and Atlanta and were subsequently seen and reported on by journalists. In fact, the ads got more air time by becoming part of the journalists' news stories. Much of the American public who saw the ads did so through viewing them as part of the evening news (Annenberg Public Policy Center, 1995).

Harry and Louise is an example of media advocacy because it was a deliberate strategy to mobilize a public constituency around public policy. The media saturate this nation and much of the world with images that change people's opinions, shape their attitudes and beliefs, and transform their behavior (McAlister, 1991). The media shape the public's image of nursing and nurses, influence which public policies get developed, and affect the outcomes of political campaigns. The power of the media is recognized by all significant players in policy and political arenas. Competing to control the media and their message is common in today's political world. Woodruff (1995) contends that health care providers "are in an optimal position for promoting health public policy through the media" (p. 812). The public views nurses as credible, moral, and trustworthy. Though nursing organizations are increasingly sophisticated in their use of media to influence public opinion, individual nurses need to recognize the far-reaching influence of the media, how they can be used effectively, and for what purposes.

THE POWER OF THE MEDIA

Schmid, Pratt, and Howze (1995) argue that individual-focused interventions for changing health behaviors are limited in long-term effectiveness; rather, they maintain that community or aggregate-focused interventions hold the greatest promise for improving the health of communities. An example of aggregate-focused interventions is public policy such as U.S. sanitation laws, which had a dramatic effect on the health and quality of life for many people. The media provide a potentially powerful aggregate approach to influencing public policies that can promote health.

Certainly, media can be viewed as a political tool. Turow (1996) notes that "journalists now recognize that public discussions of medicine are necessarily political—i.e., they are ultimately about the exercise of social power" (p. 1240). The media's power arises from their ability to get a message or information to a large number of people or to key people (i.e., policymakers). Talk radio has proliferated during the past decade because of the way that it engages listeners. The Internet is increasingly taking center stage as a vehicle for sharing information and shaping public opinion. It provides uncensored access, speed, and a snowballing effect in which the message can take on a life of its own. Former Speaker of the House of Representatives Tom Foley found that his reelection defeat in 1994 was brought about by an Internet campaign against him launched by a few dissatisfied citizens. It quickly became an initiative to test the power of the Internet in defeating a political candidate.

Nurses are often keenly aware of how the media misrepresent them and their work. In many news articles, nurses may appear in the text and story without being identified. In the mid-1990s, organized nursing mounted a deliberate campaign to shape public opinion about the importance of what nurses contribute to health care. During this decade the cost-focused reengineering, restructuring, and downsizing of health care organizations led many to eliminate nursing positions and substitute unlicensed assistive personnel. In response to the American Nurses Association's campaign slogan "Every Patient Deserves a Nurse," the New York State Nurses Association invested several million dollars to launch a media campaign with the message "Every Patient Deserves an RN–a Real Nurse." Television, radio, and print ads appeared in targeted areas throughout the state, including the capital city, where policymakers and their staff would see the ads. When the campaign offered a "hospital evaluation kit" that people could use to evaluate the adequacy of nursing in their hospital, 75,000 people received the kits. Policymakers talked about the campaign, as did nurses' neighbors, friends, and family. The vignette following this chapter provides the details of this effective media campaign.

What the media do or do not cover is equally powerful in determining what issues are considered by policymakers. For example:

- The epidemic of acquired immunodeficiency syndrome is recognized as having been exacerbated by a lack of coverage by the media, who saw it as a problem limited to promiscuous gay men and to drug abusers (Shilts, 1987; see also the End Case Study by Ungvarski and Ballard).
- When the front page of an influential newspaper carries a headline and story about the use of nurse practitioners as primary care providers, the issue is "on the agenda" of policymakers and the public.
- Walt Bogdanich and his colleagues at *The Wall Street Journal* published a front-page article in February 1987 on the misreading of Pap smears by laboratory technicians that left

some women with a misdiagnosis. One year later, Congress passed the Clinical Laboratory Improvement Amendments, requiring minimum standards for laboratory operations and technician training (Otten, 1992).

Although the news media are instrumental in getting issues onto the agenda of policymakers, nonnews entertainment television programs can mobilize public constituencies around an issue. On the popular prime-time television program *Murphy Brown,* episodes that addressed Murphy's becoming a single mother stimulated Vice President Dan Quayle's comments about "family values." Although his comments were meant to criticize Murphy Brown, his response created media attention to the policies and support that are needed by single parents.

Public officials often first learn about an issue through the press. In fact, a bill can be wallowing in the mire of legislative bureaucracy with no hope of passage until media highlight the issue that the bill addresses. For instance, many states and local communities had considered policies to restrict teenagers' access to cigarettes, but it took a media exposé on the deliberate targeting of adolescents for smoking through the "Joe Camel" ads to get some of the legislation passed.

Media can also highlight the outcomes of a public policy. In 1989, New York State decided to try to reduce the mortality rate after cardiac bypass surgery by requiring all hospitals to report on the case mix, risk factors, and outcomes of this surgery. The state analyzed these data, developed a method of ranking hospitals on their mortality rates, and released these rankings to the public. The media responded with feature stories highlighting "the best" and "the worst," or which hospital outranked another in the same community. In addition, one newspaper won a court case requiring the state to release the ranked data by individual surgeon. Unfortunately, not all journalists knew statistics well enough to realize that some of the differences in rankings that they were highlighting were not statistically significant or clinically meaningful. As a result of such misinterpreta-

tions of the data, the state decided to educate journalists about the outcome initiative, interpretations of the data, and the need to emphasize what hospitals and surgeons were doing to improve the quality of care. Subsequent media coverage has highlighted the quality improvements that were made. Although the state once feared that the media coverage could undermine their effort to push for public reporting of medical outcomes, the program is now considered a model that will be replicated in other states and for other conditions or procedures (Chassin, Hannan, & DeBuono, 1996).

Media can also determine who gets elected to public office. When a candidate running for public office wakes up to a news report on the candidate's questionable financial dealings, the candidate worries, even if the story is unfounded. The image of the candidate in the minds of many can be tarnished forever. Similarly, the candidate's campaign manager and staff will read the letters to the editor of the newspaper to see which issues and positions are of concern to a community. They will also stage *media events.* These are a type of on-site press conference at a place that provides the visual images (for television and press photos) representative of an attention-getting problem that the candidate commits to address through policy initiatives. For example, the American Nurses Association announced its endorsement of the Clinton-Gore ticket in 1991 at a hospital in California in which patients, staff, and nurses from all over the state gathered to show support for the nomination. This event highlighted Clinton's commitment to health care and the support of nurses, a group that the public trusts.

With all this power vested in the media, one is justified in being concerned about who controls the media. This is becoming increasingly important as large corporations buy up networks of television or radio stations (Naureckas, 1995). Public media, such as National Public Radio and the television's Corporation for Public Broadcasting, are threatened with cutbacks from the federal government, raising concerns about whether there will be any media in the United

States that are not privately controlled. In recent years, public radio and television stations began providing more visible and lengthy acknowledgments of corporate contributions. Although the style of these notices differs from that of ads on commercial stations, their impact is noticeable and raises concerns about the corporations' influence on programming.

On another level, one can argue that individual journalists are equally responsible for their choice of issues to cover and how they are covered. Getting to know the nature and quality of particular journalists' work can help you to decide how much trust to place in their work. Do they frequently misrepresent issues? Are their stories sensationalized, overplayed, exaggerated? Or do they present all sides of an issue with accuracy and depth? Journalists rarely have the same depth of knowledge about a topic as insiders.

Fallows (1996) provides an informative critique of and challenge to the media in his book *Breaking the News*. He argues that the media have contributed to a public cynicism of politics and policymakers that has resulted in a largely uninvolved citizenry. This is due partially to journalists' having limited expertise on particular issues; as a result, they often cover the political dimensions of an issue (see also Turow, 1996).

In addition to the *Harry and Louise* commercials, the media influenced the demise of President Clinton's Health Security Act in other ways that demonstrate this point. Dorfman, Schauffler, Wilkerson, and Feinson (1996) reported that in-depth analysis and explanation of the issues and the legislation were scarce in local news coverage; the focus tended to be superficial coverage of the risks and costs of the legislation to specific stake holders. In fact, Naureckas and Jackson (1996) note that full debate of approaches to remedying an ailing health care system was not available to most citizens, because the single-payer alternative was rarely covered by the press. In an analysis of media coverage of the issue, the Annenberg Public Policy Center (1995) found that the press

concentrated on only a few of the alternative proposals for health care reform, focused their reporting on strategy rather than the pros and cons of proposals, magnified the impact of negative fear-based advertisements by focusing on them, and "had a tendency to filter both elections and policy debates through a set of cynical assumptions, including the notion that politicians act out of self-interest rather than a commitment to the public good" (p. iv).

Fallows' (1996) point is also illustrated in reporting on health-related research. It is not uncommon for journalists to report the findings of one study as definitive, without considering prior research and the limitations of the present study. For example, the media widely reported on a study that found daily intake of oat bran could lower blood cholesterol. After people incorporated oat bran into their diets (e.g., oat bran cereal, muffins, cookies, cakes, and bread) in large quantities, a subsequent study found that oat bran probably had little, if any, direct effect on cholesterol. Occurrences such as these threaten the public's faith in research, rather than in the media's reporting.

ANALYZING THE MEDIA

Although this chapter advocates that nurses more frequently and effectively use the media as a political tool, the first obligation that all nurses have is to be a knowledgeable consumer of media messages. Each nurse needs to be able to critically evaluate media messages.

What Is the Medium? The first step is to ask yourself where you get your information and news. Do you read a daily newspaper? What is its reputation? Is it known for its balanced coverage of health-related issues? Does it cover national as well as state and local issues? Is it a credible source of information about health issues and policies? What television and radio news–related programming do you regularly tune in to? These questions provide a basis for you to judge whether the information and news that you are getting is credible and representative of a broad sector of public opinion. On any particular issue of concern, you will want to sample various media presentations of the issue and evaluate their messages and effectiveness. Turow (1996) points out that nonnews television entertainment is particularly loaded with rhetoric that often stereotypes power relationships and may be more successful than the news in shaping people's images of the world:

> [H]ighly viewed TV presentations of medicine hold political significance that should be assessed alongside news. Like the rhetorical struggles in news about medicine, series such as *ER, Dr. Quinn, Medicine Woman, Diagnosis: Murder,* and *Chicago Hope* are ultimately about power. Every week, they act out ideas about the medical system's authority to define, prevent and treat illness. [p. 1249]

Such programming can shape people's expectations, beliefs, and opinions of medicine, nursing, and health care.

Who Is Sending the Message? Who is sponsoring the message and why? Part of understanding what the real message is about comes from knowing who is behind the message. You could interpret the real message behind the *Harry and Louise* commercials against President Clinton's health care reform legislation once you knew they were sponsored by the Health Insurance Association of America (HIAA). If the legislation had passed, the majority of insurance companies would have been locked out of the health care market. Instead, their success left them in control of health care in the United States.

What Is the Message and What Rhetoric Is Used? What is the ostensible message that is being delivered, and what is the real message? What rhetoric is used to get the real message across? For example, "family values" became important rhetoric during the Reagan Presidency. The President used the phrase regularly to convey a safer, saner society that supported the "traditional" values of the American family. Yet his presidency was remarkable in the extent to which it did not advocate public policies that supported families. Similarly, President George Bush picked up the rhetoric and subsequently vetoed the Family and Medical Leave Act, which eventually was adopted and remedied the reputation of the U.S. as the only industrialized country not to have such a leave.[1] Subsequently, other candidates—Republicans, Democrats, and independents alike—running for public office frequently have referred to their support of "family values" in their political advertisements. Is the message that the candidate will support family-friendly public policies, or is the message "I am the person who will keep government out of your lives" or "I will make you feel safe and secure—vote for me"?

Is the Message Effective? Does the message attract your attention? Does it appeal to your logic and to your emotions? Does it undermine the opposition's position?

Is the Message Accurate? Who is the reporter and what reputation does the reporter have? Is the reporter credible, with a reputation for accuracy and balanced coverage of an issue?

The box on p. 228 provides an exercise to analyze newspaper reporting critically.

RESPONDING TO MEDIA

One of the most important ways to influence public opinion is to respond to what is read or seen or heard in the media. The vignette at the end of this chapter describes the power and use of letters to the editor and of listener call-ins to talk radio programs. There are several other ways to respond to the media: writing an opinion editorial, mobilizing grassroots efforts

---

[1]One of the first acts of President Clinton's first term was to sign into law the Family and Medical Leave Act. Although it guaranteed employees leaves of absence for family health problems or emergencies, without fear of job loss, the United States remains one of only three industrialized nations not to have a *paid* leave.

HOW TO ANALYZE NEWSPAPER REPORTING

The following exercise on how to analyze a newspaper expands one that was developed by Douglas (1991) for Fairness and Accuracy in the Media (FAIR), a national media watch group that critically analyzes news reports to raise consciousness about, and to correct, bias and imbalance.

- Get a recent copy of two or more national newspapers. Find an issue of concern and compare the papers on their coverage of the issue.
- First, note where the article is placed. Is it on the front page? Is it buried amid advertisements in a small portion of one column in the last section of the paper? Why do you think it received front, or last, page coverage?
- Second, note who wrote the article. The reputation of journalists can give you a sense of what bias might appear in the reporting, whether the coverage is likely to be balanced, and whether this journalist is someone who is known for in-depth investigative reporting.
- Third, what are the sources of information that are reported in the article? Every time a government official (e.g., president, other administration official, congressional representative, or staff) says something, highlight the passage with a yellow marker. This includes "anonymous high-placed public officials" whose names and formal titles are not included. Every time the source is nongovernmental, highlight the passage with a pink marker. With a blue marker, note every time a woman or a person of color is mentioned or quoted. Now compare these passages. The ratio of yellow to pink to blue suggests what and who are routinely considered most important.
- For health reporting, note how often journalists quote or refer to nurses as opposed to physicians. How might the article be different if nurses were a primary source of information on the topic?
- What is the focus of the article? Does it present all sides of an issue? Is the coverage confined to the politics of an issue, rather than the content of the issue itself (Fallows, 1996)?
- Do any photographs included in the article reflect the issue and the people involved in it? If it is a story on some aspect of patient care, for example, does the photograph include and name nurses who are providing the care? Or are only the physicians shown and named?
- Who sits on the board of directors of a newspaper, and what interests do they represent? What is or is not being said in the editorials that might be directly or indirectly critical of these interests?

---

to boycott sponsors and call producers, being proactive, and saying thanks.

Writing an Opinion Editorial (Op Ed). Opinion pieces allow more in-depth response to current issues and provide a way to get an issue on the public's agenda. Though they are often solicited by the newspaper or magazine, particularly in large cities, local community papers are often eager to receive editorials that describe an important issue or problem, include a story that illustrates the impact of the problem, and suggest possible solutions to the problem.

Mobilizing Grassroots Efforts to Boycott Sponsors and Call Producers. For commercial media, disturbing programs and stories can be suppressed by threatening to boycott the sponsors who bought advertising time or space attached to the program, or by expressing concerns to the producers, editors, or station managers. A successful nursing grassroots effort arose from the airing of *Nightingales,* a prime-time television program that portrayed nurses as mindless sex objects. Nursing organizations contacted their members and asked them to write to the producers and sponsors of the program, noting that they would not buy the sponsor's products. When a sponsor knows that a group of more than 2 million people (with family, friends, and professional colleagues) doesn't like the program their ads are paying for, they'll think twice about continuing to sponsor such programs. *Nightingales* was withdrawn from the network before the season was over.

Being Proactive. Contacting producers can also be done proactively to ensure appropriate representation of nurses or an issue. A powerful example came in the 1960s with the airing of *Dr. Kildare* and *Ben Casey,* two television programs featuring smart, caring, "nice guy" physicians. The American Medical Association (AMA) actively encouraged the producers to present these images:

> In return for showing their organization's seal of approval at the end of each programme, AMA physicians demanded the right to read every script and make changes in the name of accuracy. To them, however, accuracy also meant a proper doctor's image. During the height of its power in the 1960s, the AMA Advisory Committee for Television and Motion Pictures tried to make sure that with few exceptions the physicians who moved through doctor shows were incarnations of intelligent, upright, all-caring experts. AMA physicians were even insistent about the cars their TV counterparts drove (not too expensive), the way they spoke to patients (a doctor could never sit on even the edge of a female patient's bed), and the mistakes they made (which had to be extremely rare). . . . [Later] Doctors' organizations expressed anger that the programmes were holding nurses and psychologists to the same status as MDs. [Turow, 1996, p. 1241]

Although the AMA's influence over television programming waned in the 1970s, physicians are frequently consulted on health-related entertainment programs. Nurses have also served as consultants, and sometimes they have volunteered their services to a producer.

Saying Thanks. One of the most important strategies that nurses can use to influence the media is to thank the journalist who did a fine job in covering an issue of importance on nursing and health care. This can be done in person or in writing. It goes a long way toward developing a relationship with the journalist that can be of help later when you have a story or an issue you would like covered.

INFLUENCING MEDIA: WHAT MEDIA?

Media are not simply television and radio. They include print and electronic media. Print media include newspapers, magazines, newsletters, and billboards (and similar public displays of a message). Although organizations' newsletters (e.g., newsletters of the American Cancer Society, Children Now, and the American Heart Association) are not commonly considered a form of media that influences policy, they are often accessible to nurses who can write columns that will both promote the visibility of the nurse as expert and influence readers' opinions about health policies.

These media differ in a variety of ways that are important to consider as you think about which media to use:

1. **The audience the media reach.** Different segments of the public gravitate to television for their news, rather than to newspapers.
2. **The depth of coverage of an issue** (which to a certain extent influences who uses a particular medium). Television relies on "sound bites," and the message must be crafted carefully to be effective; however, talk radio has become an increasingly popular vehicle to discuss current issues. Newspapers have learned that their survival is often dependent on in-depth coverage and analysis of issues, after a catchy headline.
3. **The extent to which the media are accessible** (again, influencing who may use the medium). For example, only those with access to computers can use the Internet, and one can listen to the radio but not watch television while driving or (sometimes) working.
4. **The cost.** The cost to mount a political campaign has increased dramatically over the years, as candidates have tried to reach larger audiences through television and radio advertisements.

These differences do not mean that one medium is better than the next, but they need to be considered when one is trying to influence an issue.

GETTING THE MESSAGE ACROSS

Considering the medium you want to reach requires careful planning. For example, to get television coverage, you must have a visual attraction. In the State of California, nurses staged a media event on a senior health issue by staging a "rock around the clock" marathon, with seniors in rocking chairs outside an insurance company. They got press on the event, which elicited some supportive letters to the editor, as well as some negative press from seniors who said that they were stereotyping elderly persons.

The following guidelines will help you shape your message and get it delivered to the right media:

1. **The Issue**
   a. What is the nature of the issue?
   b. What is the context of the issue (e.g., timing, history, and current political environment)?
   c. Who is or could be interested in this issue?
2. **The Message**
   a. What's the angle? What is news?
   b. Is there a sound bite that represents the issue in a catchy, memorable way?
   c. Can you create rhetoric that will represent core values of the target audience?
   d. How can you frame nursing's interests as the public's interests (e.g., as consumers, mothers, fathers, women, taxpayers, health professionals)?
3. **The Target Audience**
   a. Who is the target audience? Is it the public, policymakers, or journalists?
   b. If the public is the target audience, which segment(s) of the public?
   c. What medium (media) is appropriate for the target audience? Does this audience watch television? If so, are the members of this audience likely to watch a talk show or a news magazine show? Or do they read

newspapers, listen to radio, or surf the Internet? Or are they likely to do all of these?
4. **Access to the Media**
   a. What relationships do you have with reporters and producers? Have you called or written letters or thank you notes to particular journalists? Have you requested a meeting with the editorial board of the local community newspaper to discuss your issue and how the members of the board might think about reporting on it?
   b. How can you get the media's attention? Is there a "hot" issue you can connect your issue to? Is there a compelling human interest story? Do you have printed materials (including a press release) that will attract their attention within the first 3 seconds of viewing it? Are there photographs you can take in advance, and then send out with your press release? Can you digitalize the images and make them available on a web site for downloading onto a newspaper?
   c. Whom should you contact in the medium (media) of choice?
   d. Have you been getting prepared all along? Are you news conscious? Do you watch, listen, clip, and keep track of who covers what and how they cover it? What is the format of the program, and who is the journalist? What is the style of the program or journalist?
   e. Who are your spokespersons? Do they have the requisite expertise on the issue? Do they have a visual or voice presence appropriate for the medium? What is their personal connection to the issue, and do they have stories to tell? Have they been trained or rehearsed for the interview?
5. **The Interview**
   a. Who is in control? Remember, *you* want to be in control. Keep your agenda focused on the one, two, or (at most) three major points that you want to get across in the interview. What is your sound bite? Even if the interviewer asks a question that does not address *your* agenda, return the focus

of the interview to *your* agenda and to *your* sound bite with finesse and persistence.

b. Try to be an interesting guest. Come ready with rich, illustrative stories. Avoid yes or no answers to questions.

c. Remember that being interviewed is an anxiety-producing experience for many people—it's a normal reaction! Do some slow deep-breathing or relaxation exercise before the interview, but know that some nervousness can be energizing.

d. See the box at right for tips on the "Do's and Don'ts of Being a Good Radio Show Guest." Many of these points are similar for interviews on television and other media.

6. **Follow Up**

a. Write a letter of thanks to the producer or journalist afterward.

b. Provide feedback to the producer or journalist on the response that you have received to the interview or the program or coverage.

c. Continue to offer other ideas for stories on the same or related topics.

MEDIA ADVOCACY

Harnessing the media for your own purposes is an important strategy if you are seeking public support for health-promoting policies. Media advocacy is the strategic use of mass media to apply pressure to advance a social or public policy initiative (Jernigan & Wright, 1996; Wallack & Dorfman, 1996). It is a tool for policy change—a way of mobilizing constituencies and stake holders to support or oppose specific policy changes. It is a means of political action (DeJong, 1996).

Media advocacy differs from social marketing and public education approaches to public health. Table 13–1 delineates some of these differences. Media advocacy defines the primary problem as a power gap, as opposed to an information gap, and thus mobilization of groups of stakeholders is needed to be able to influence the process of developing public policies. Wallack and Dorfman (1996) use the example of

---

THE DO'S AND DON'TS OF BEING A GOOD RADIO SHOW GUEST

The key concept to grasp in talk radio is "talk." This is not lecturing, and it is not news. It is personal conversation between host and subject, and between listeners and guests.

Do

- Provide the host with the way you wish to be introduced. Include your professional and academic affiliation but evaluate whether you need clearance from your institution to include your affiliation with it.
- Be prepared. Know your information.
- Focus on the questions, listening attentively to the interviewer.
- Keep eye-to-eye contact with the interviewer.
- Be a storyteller. If you are a great storyteller, you've got it! The appeal of talk radio is the person-to-person conversation.
- Be enthusiastic.
- If you don't know the answer, say so. Offer to get back to the host and to follow up at a later date.
- Give information to the producer, and to the guests if appropriate, on how you can be contacted.
- Offer to be available in the future on the same topic or another topic that you can speak to.
- Have fun. It really is fun to do.

Don't

- Be late.
- Read from a paper. You can bring a reference sheet, but don't prepare a written statement; it doesn't work over the air because people tune out.
- Wrinkle paper or wear jangling jewelry.
- Give yes or no answers.

---

tobacco control to illustrate the focus of media advocacy. The dangers of smoking were well known, albeit not admitted by tobacco companies until 1997. During the past 25 years, public policies that attempted to limit smoking created "a shift in the acceptability of smoking" (p. 298). More recently, advocates have focused on the tobacco producers instead of the users. As Wallack and Dorfman summarized: "In tobacco con-

Table 13–1 Media Advocacy Versus Social Marketing/Public Education Approaches to Public Health

MEDIA ADVOCACY	SOCIAL MARKETING/ PUBLIC EDUCATION
Individual as advocate	Individual as audience
Advances healthy public policies	Develops health messages
Changes the environment	Changes the individual
Target is person with power to make change	Target is person with problem or at risk
Addresses the power gap	Addresses the information gap

Adapted from Wallack, L., & Dorfman, L. (1996). Media advocacy: A strategy for advancing policy and promoting health. *Health Education Quarterly, 23*(3), 297, Copyright © 1996 Sage Publications. Reprinted by permission of Sage Publications.

trol, as in other public health issues, the challenge we face is to change the environment, and media advocacy provides a tool to help us meet that challenge" (p. 298).

Mothers Against Drunk Driving (MADD) is another illustration of the potential of media advocacy. MADD developed a policy agenda aimed at preventing drunk driving. They developed a "Rating the States" program to bring public attention to what state governments were and were not doing to fight alcohol-impaired driving. After a national press conference just before Thanksgiving, the beginning of a period of high numbers of alcohol-related traffic accidents, MADD representatives held local press conferences with their state's officials and members of other advocacy groups to announce the state's rating. Local and national broadcast and print press coverage resulted in the exposure of an estimated 62.5 million people to the story. Subsequently, action was taken in at least eight states to begin to address the problem of drunk driving (Russell, Voas, DeJong, & Chaloupka, 1995).

Getting on the news media agenda is one of the functions of media advocacy (Wallack, 1994). With numerous competing potential stories, media advocacy employs strategies to frame an issue in a way that will attract media cover-

age. But *how* the message is presented is as important as simply getting the attention of the news media. The demise of the Health Security Act demonstrates this point. It got on the media's agenda, but the important messages were lost in the discussion of managed competition.

Getting on the agenda and then controlling the message require *framing.* Framing "defines the boundaries of public discussion about an issue" (Wallack & Dorfman, 1996, p. 299). *Framing for access* entails shaping the issue in a way that will attract media attention. It requires some element of controversy (albeit not over the accuracy of advocates' facts), conflict, injustice, or irony. The targeted medium or media will shape how the story is presented. For example, television requires compelling visual images. If a broad audience is to be reached, several media need to be targeted. It also helps to attach the issue to a local concern or event, anniversaries, or celebrities, or to "make news" by holding events that will attract the press, such as releasing research or in some other way being "newsworthy" (Jernigan & Wright, 1996).

Framing for content is more difficult than framing for access. Though a compelling individual story may gain access to the media, there is no guarantee that the reporter will focus on the public policy changes that are needed to address problems illustrated by the individual. Wallack and Dorfman (1996) note that this framing "involves the difficult process of 're-framing' away from the usual news formula" (p. 300). The authors suggest that this reframing can be accomplished by the following:

- Emphasizing the social dimensions of the problem and translating the individual's personal story into public issues
- Shifting the responsibility for the problem from the individual to the corporate executive or public official whose decisions can address the problem
- Presenting solutions as policy alternatives
- Making a practical appeal to support the solution
- Using compelling images
- Using authentic voices—people who have experience with the problem

- Using symbols that "resonate with the basic values of the audience" [p. 300]
- Anticipating the opposition and knowing all sides of the issue

Jernigan and Wright (1996) argue that media advocacy is most effective when it is "linked to a strong organizing base and a long-term strategic vision" (p. 314). In addition, it is enhanced by a long-term strategy that incorporates continually setting up future efforts. For example, highlighting the way that one group in a community is negatively affected by an issue can lead to that group's lending its support to the next media advocacy strategy around the issue. Training and designating spokespersons are important to controlling the message.

Increasingly, computer-based electronic communication systems, including specific networks (e.g., SCARNet, an electronic communication network that has been used by advocates in the alcohol control movement to plan strategy jointly and rapidly) and the Internet, are being used by media advocates.

CONCLUSION

The media in our society are tremendously powerful and may be the single most influential force on public policy. They are diverse—including everything from network television and Hollywood movies to your local *Pennysaver* and your hospital newsletter. They may contain information and points of view that strive to be fair and balanced, as well as opinions with the singular goal to change your mind or get your money. Nurses, like all members of our society, have a big stake in what gets reported and how an issue is treated. Nurses, both individuals and groups, can influence public policy by supporting candidates that support nurses, by writing letters to journalists and congresspersons, and by simply responding to media messages, from whatever source, both positively and negatively. You can make a difference in public policy and the future of nursing and health care in this country.

REFERENCES

Annenberg Public Policy Center of the University of Pennsylvania. (1995). *Media in the middle: Fairness and accuracy in the 1994 health care reform debate.* Philadelphia: Author.

Chassin, M. R., Hannan, E. L., & DeBuono, B. A. (1996). Benefits and hazards of reporting medical outcomes publicly. *New England Journal of Medicine, 334*(6), 394–398.

DeJong, W. (1996). MADD Massachusetts versus Senator Burke: A media advocacy case study. *Health Education Quarterly, 23*(3), 318–329.

Dorfman, L., Schauffler, H. H., Wilkerson, J., & Feinson, J. (1996). Local television news coverage of President Clinton's introduction of the Health Security Act. *Journal of the American Medical Association, 275*(15), 1201–1205.

Douglas, S. J. (1991). Reading the news in more than black and white. *EXTRA!, 4*(7), 1, 6.

Fallows, J. (1996). *Breaking the news: How the media undermine American society.* New York: Vintage Books.

Jernigan, D. H., & Wright, P. A. (1996). Media advocacy: Lessons from community experiences. *Journal of Public Health Policy, 18,* 306–329.

McAlister, A. L. (1991). Population behavior change: A theory-based approach. *Journal of Public Health Policy, 12,* 345–361.

Naureckas, J. (1995). Corporate ownership matters: The case of NBC. *EXTRA!, November/December,* 13.

Naureckas, J., & Jackson, J. (1996). *The FAIR reader: An EXTRA! review of press and politics in the '90s.* Boulder, CO: Westview Press.

Otten, A. L. (1992). The influence of the mass media on health policy. *Health Affairs, Winter,* 111–118.

Russell, A., Voas, R. B., DeJong, W., & Chaloupka, M. (1995). MADD rates the states: Advocacy event to advance the agenda against alcohol-impaired driving. *Public Health Reports, 110*(3), 240–245.

Schmid, T. L., Pratt, M., & Howze, E. (1995). Policy as intervention: Environmental and policy approaches to the prevention of cardiovascular disease. *American Journal of Public Health, 85*(9), 1207–1211.

Shilts, R. (1987). *And the band played on.* New York: St. Martin's Press.

Turow, J. (1996). Television entertainment and the U.S. health care debate. *Lancet, 347,* 1240–1243.

Wallack, L. (1994). Media advocacy: A strategy for empowering people and communities. *Journal of Public Health Policy, 15,* 420–436.

Wallack, L., & Dorfman, L. (1996). Media advocacy: A strategy for advancing policy and promoting health. *Health Education Quarterly, 23*(3), 293–317.

Woodruff, K. (1995). Media strategies for community health advocacy. *Primary Care, 22*(4), 805–815.

VIGNETTE

Free Media Coverage: Using Letters (Messages) to the Editor

Catherine J. Dodd

In 1987 after Congresswoman Nancy Pelosi was elected to the U.S. House of Representatives, I was asked to join her staff because of the effective role I played in coordinating a "Nurses for Pelosi" effort within her campaign. I quickly learned many lessons in working for a member of Congress. One of my first assignments was to rotate through the early morning "letter to the editor" clipping and faxing job in the office. This meant leaving the house by 5 AM to purchase the first issue of the morning paper at an all-night newsstand and arrive at the San Francisco Congressional Office by 5:30 AM to read, clip, and fax back to Washington, D.C., the editorial page with the letters to the editor so that they would be on Congresswoman Pelosi's desk by 9 AM. Why? Because newspaper subscribers tend to be homeowners, and homeowners vote in every election.

Letters to the editor reflect what voters are thinking about local issues. The editor of the editorial page usually does not publish a letter until more than one letter on the same issue has been received, so published letters reflect the views of lots of voters. A catchy, well-written letter to the editor that is published has much more political weight than a personal lobbying letter on an issue. (So if you are going to write just one letter, write the letter to the editor; better, though, to write your lobbying letter, as well!)

This in no way means that Congresswoman Pelosi concerned herself only with homeowners/newspaper subscribers. She was fortunate enough to represent a district that is overwhelmingly Democrat, so her reelection was certain. She is an advocate for voters and those unable to vote—children and the many noncitizens who live in San Francisco. She still listens to and is concerned about what the voters think.

Today, in campaigns for ballot initiatives as well as candidates, press staff are orchestrating letters-to-the-editor campaigns to show "voter support" of candidates and issues. For statewide issues and candidates, only six different letters are needed. Six basic letters are drafted and faxed to six volunteer letter submitters in the geographic area of every major daily in the state. The letter submitters put the text of the letter on their personal letterhead and fax the same letter to the same paper to which five other people are faxing their letters. The same plan works on local issues as well. Major papers like to demonstrate the breadth of their circulation, so they frequently publish letters received from nearby cities and suburbs. Editors of the editorial page want to be viewed as fair, so they will attempt to balance the gender of letter authors. This gives women an excellent chance of being published, because women do not write as much or as often as men.

In my graduate class on health policy and politics at San Francisco State University, nursing students are offered extra credit for every letter to the editor they write. In 1994, California voters passed Proposition 187, a mean-spirited, anti-immigrant initiative that, among other things, denied prenatal and emergency care to undocumented persons. After the election and just before Thanksgiving, a student who had immigrated from Russia with her family wrote a letter to the editor about how our country's first immigrants would not be celebrating Thanksgiving, they would be hiding from immigration officials had Proposition 187 been the law of the land at that time. It was published with headlines on Thanksgiving day and was the subject of several days' worth of subsequent letters supporting the provision of prenatal care and education to undocumented people. Those four points of extra credit had a lasting effect. Other students report the therapeutic effect of writing a letter on something you feel angry or passionate about and knowing that, if published, it will reach the eyes of tens of thousands of readers.

A similar strategy can be used for radio talk shows, which reach hundreds of thousands of people at one time. (General commercial radio audiences, as opposed to public radio listeners, cannot be categorized as perennial "always" voters.) Radio talk shows can be used to educate the public about new treatment modalities, changes in the quality of care, dangerous patient care situations, or any number of issues that nurses are concerned about. Having a group or "radio response squad" of well-prepared registered nurses listening to a talk show and prepared to call in on an issue or during an "open" session can be an effective advertising tool. Callers should be cautioned to write down the three points they want to make and practice them on a friend. If they get to the producer and are asked what their position is, they should be neutral and have a question they want to pose. (If there has just been an on-air caller who expressed your position, the producer will not air another caller with the same position.) Once on the air, callers should make their point and say, "I will stay on the air for your response," being prepared to defend their statements. "Taking a response" off the air allows the host or talk show guest to have the last word.

Regardless of the medium, if you are advocating for the public (as opposed to advocating for nursing's professional interests), always identify yourself as a registered nurse. The public trusts and values nurses, and your message will carry more clout.

VIGNETTE
Every Patient Deserves a Nurse
Judy Sheridan-Gonzalez and Marva Wade

Nothing prepared registered nurses (RNs) for the full-scale assault launched against our existence by the controlling forces in the health care industry in the 1990s. It was only in the 1980s that the surge in unionization and aggressive labor tactics by RNs, the critical nursing shortages, the rise in technology, the increased acuity of hospitalized patients, and the sophistication and demands of certain consumer groups created an insatiable thirst for RNs in the United States. Nursing school enrollments swelled, salaries skyrocketed, and versatile and innovative RNs started treading newground. Some became advanced practice nurses, whereas many others simply began to assert control over, and to formally define, our bedside practice. Those were heady days.

With all the talk about health care reform after President Clinton's election, it seemed logical that we would have a place in the sun. We looked with enthusiasm toward the creation of the new health care system. We knew that we were the critical link in the holistic pathways that seemed to be emerging as society presumably wanted to embrace a wellness model of health care. As health care consumed more and more of the gross domestic product, policymakers and big providers, as well as insurers and other players, began to look toward different models of care. Keeping people healthy, preventing illness and injury, working with communities to take control over their health—all these things—began to look attractive in the middle of all the cost-cutting hysteria. We knew that RNs would be essential in promoting, planning, and implementing these newer types of care models that we naively believed would be adopted. Nursing school waiting lists lengthened while new jobs opened up.

The rapidity with which the for-profit groups and other parasites moved in and took control over the direction of health care policy in this nation, as well as the hearts and minds of the population, was astounding. In its search for the middle ground (and the least common denominator) the Democratic Party isolated the single-payer sector of its health care reform "movement" and catered, instead, to the managed care pundits. The Clinton plan, as presented to the American public, became a hodge-podge of plans that was so ill defined, redefined, and complicated that no one could enthusiastically describe it, let alone support it. Meanwhile the Health Insurance Associations of America moved in with the *Harry and Louise* commercials, playing on everyone's worst fears and confusion and defeating any hopes of systemic change. Thus the 30-odd million uninsured became 40-odd million, and the rest of us became slaves to profit motives in health care—the worst of both worlds.

How, in the face of the nation's desire to reduce health care inflation, can insurance companies, managed care corporations, health-related supply, equipment, and research companies, and the for-profit provider/manager/financing systems corporations turn over such huge profits? *They demand cuts* in services and in the work force. Suddenly, RN salaries, which began to reach a level that could comfortably sustain a family, became a liability. Expensive consultants were hired by health facilities to look at "the way we do business." "What do these nurses do?" they wondered, that some (cheap) trained technicians could not do easily

enough? The factory model of health care provision began to be more attractive to hospital administrators looking to save dollars. What nurses did, who we were, and what patients needed was questioned: "What *exactly* do you do, and how long does it take?" And most important, "Who else can do it?"

The Rise of the "Nurse Extender"

No one had a problem with nurses' extending ourselves, literally and figuratively, as long as we weren't putting in for overtime and were being dismally underpaid. Hospital administrators began looking frantically for alternatives as salaries climbed, fringe benefits improved, and passivity receded (it is rumored that more RNs took their lunch breaks in the 1980s than in any other decade!). Some sought out licensed practical nurses (LPNs) or vocational nurses (who, previously, had been systematically eliminated in many parts of the country). Others, with the aid of business-minded and "customer focused" consultants and efficiency experts, transformed the concept of the "nursing assistant" into "nursing replacement."

Similar attempts by the American Medical Association several years ago, with its introduction of the registered care technician, were soundly defeated by organized nursing and their political allies. This new attempt at replacing RNs was more insidious, more vague, and made to sound like an improvement. "Oh, let's have these folks help you out so you can focus on the truly professional aspects of your job" was the guiding mantra. We were sent to classes. Patients and staff were "customers." We needed to be multiskilled and cross-trained. We were one big close-knit family of "associates" ("employees" was too polarizing) in imminent danger of being anachronized by our competitors if we couldn't produce the best buy for the rising managed care aristocrats. Nursing salaries, as well as our desire to promote "unrealistic (high-quality) care models," were seen as major obstacles in the fiscal viability of acute care facilities. This was the ideology that we faced as the reorganization of the work force translated into a radically altered professional-to-nonprofessional staff mix.

Every Patient Deserves an RN

In June 1994, in response to issues of understaffing and replacement, the American Nurses Association (ANA) launched its "Every Patient Deserves a Nurse" campaign. With pamphlets and press releases, ANA hoped to publicize the potential hazards inherent in certain hospital restructuring plans. Local state nurses associations were encouraged to embellish the campaign. The New York State Nurses Association (NYSNA) took this charge seriously, launching its "Every Patient Deserves an RN" campaign soon afterward. Stickers, bumper stickers, buttons, and postcards were distributed to nurses and nonnurses, exhorting, "Every Patient Deserves an RN—Not an Imitation." The postcards were collected for future use for the benefit of state legislators and basically consisted of two distinct messages. One, by registered nurses, described the negative implications of "downskilling" and replacement. The other, on behalf of the lay public, extolled the virtues of having RNs at the bedside and insisted that this practice continue.

However, it wasn't until NYSNA's annual convention, in October 1994, that the campaign got the kick it needed. Many hospital-based staff nurses were buzzing with fears, confusion, and horror stories while facing layoffs for the first time in years. The use of unlicensed assistive personnel (UAPs) had increased dramatically. We were killing ourselves to meet patient care needs: skipping breaks, leaving late, bringing paperwork home, and generally working at a frenzied pace. Patients were not only being denied "extra touches," they were missing out on real care essentials. Problems were being missed. Complications related to inadequate nursing care were on the rise. Mistakes were being made. Registered nurses were spending less time with patients and more time monitoring "assistants" and engaging in reimbursement-related paperwork.

There seemed to be a concerted effort to force older (senior, better-paid, but also most experienced) nurses out by means of increased disciplinary actions for minor errors and illness, and demanding a breakneck pace that some nurses just couldn't keep up with. People returning one day past a maternity leave were told their jobs were filled or, more often, eliminated. Nurses who voiced their concerns were isolated and ostracized by administrators. On May 23, 1994, the Supreme Court overturned a critical Ohio National Labor Relations Board decision. It ruled that several LPNs who protested what they believed were unsafe conditions for patients at their nursing home were not protected by the National Labor Relations Act and were therefore justifiably terminated. It vaguely and ambiguously implied that they functioned as supervisors (by virtue of directing other employees) and rejected the argument that the employer could possibly *not* have the clients' best interests at heart! This had a chilling effect on whistle-blowing and concerted activity on the part of all licensed nurses. Patients and nurses were suffering, and NYSNA was exhorted to "do something."

These were the conditions that prompted us to draft a resolution directing NYSNA to (1) launch an aggressive media campaign to alert the public, (2) forge coalitions with other health professionals, providers, workers, and consumers—locally and nationally, and (3) increase organizational support for nurses on the front lines. Many staff nurses who never got up to the microphones at conventions in the past delivered emotional appeals to the organization to pass the resolution. There was some discord among several educators and administrators who believed that we were premature in proposing such a drastic resolution and inaccurate in describing conditions so dramatically. Adequate research linking quality care, patient outcome, and professional nursing care had not been completed. How could we pass a resolution based on anecdotal evidence alone? The last word on the subject was provided by a staff nurse who confided in the voting body that this was her first time speaking to an issue at a convention. She urged passage of the resolution, stating that conditions were extremely serious, that she was the next nurse on the "chopping block" at her institution, and that she might not be around next year if we did not respond immediately and forcefully to the crisis facing nursing practice and patient care. The resolution passed.

Ask for a Real Nurse: Ask for an RN

NYSNA proceeded to build a multimedia advertising campaign with an eventual budget of nearly $1.4 million over 1995 and 1996. Our specific goals were as follows:

- To alert the public about unlicensed workers' being substituted for RNs in New York hospitals
- To associate high-quality patient care with care delivered by RNs
- To encourage consumers to ask questions about their care and to "ask for an RN"

The campaign, built around the slogan "Ask for a Real Nurse—Ask for an RN," consisted of a television commercial aired in the New York City (NYC) metropolitan area for 22 weeks, radio commercials aired in seven New York cities (including greater NYC), newspaper ads in five cities, a magazine ad, ads in NYC bus shelters located near large hospitals, subway ads, commuter railroad ads, billboards in NYC and near the New York State Legislature in Albany, and an informational postcard sent to all consumers who called the toll-free number featured in the television and print ads.

Within a 12-week period, we received 15,000 calls to our toll-free number. We received scores of calls from reporters asking for more information on the replacement of RNs, followed by press coverage, including mentions in a national magazine, in out-of-state and out-of-the-country newspapers, and by columnists and editorial writers. The television ad was aired in its entirety on ABC's *Nightline* program (May 9, 1996) dealing with the RN replacement issue. Nurses across the state reported being asked by

patients, "Are you a real nurse?" There was also more than anecdotal evidence that the public began to link the term "real nurse" with "RN." We began to see hospitals and agencies advertising their services with headings like, "You'll be cared for by real nurses (i.e., RNs) here." A National Public Radio broadcast said that hospitals were substituting technicians for "real nurses." At legislative hearings and speak-outs, thousands of postcards previously collected from nurses and consumers demanding care by RNs were distributed. Legislators commented on our advertisements and couldn't miss our colorful bumper stickers (yellow on purple).

Analysis of the Response to the Campaign

The "Ask for a Real Nurse—Ask for an RN" media campaign succeeded in igniting concern among the general public. Our challenge as an organization would be to sustain and strengthen that concern and to broaden the concept into a form that might promote concrete action. One of our goals was to dramatize the potential dangers of "de-skilling" (which was actually occurring across the country and across the industry) and to put firmly on the public's agenda their need to assert their rights for quality health care. It was a form of coalition building (through the use of mass media) that we had not engaged in extensively as an organization in the past. Our hope was to enhance the grassroots work around coalition building that had been occurring and accelerating in the recent period. Moreover, recognizing the power of the media, we wanted to launch our campaign and define the situation *before* the wealthier forces (who were replacing nurses with UAPs, kicking patients out of hospitals, and denying care) attempted to twist the public's perception or confuse the issues.

What proved to be difficult (and remains so) was describing to the public the totality of our role in the provision of health care. Patients who had experienced skilled nursing care at first hand, or who were able to understand our contribution to their well-being, understood.

Nothing in our society—the inaccurate portrayal of nurses in history books, in the popular media, or in the news media—nothing except for direct experience, prepared the average citizen to understand who we were and what we did. Unfortunately, we couldn't synthesize it into a 20-second sound bite, either.

The response to the campaign was overwhelmingly positive. We discovered that consumers respect nurses in general and were pleased that someone was looking out for them. However, a few RNs reacted negatively to the campaign, anxious that they were being placed under a microscope. In the face of tremendous cutbacks in staff, they believed that they were being held to even higher standards. When a patient demands an RN, what is she supposed to do if she can't get to that patient? The campaign had nothing in place to fill the gaps created by patient expectations and demands and by severely short-staffed nursing units. In addition, attention was focused on cases of mediocrity on the part of some RNs. This is the dilemma faced by many of us in service-oriented or professional fields, who know of colleagues who are not up to par. We are hard-pressed to defend certain behaviors. Deficiencies become even more glaring when the profession is under attack, even though this is the exception rather than the rule.

Some LPNs raised concerns about the phrase "Ask for a Real Nurse—Ask for an RN." What did it say about LPNs? In addition, some skilled and valuable technicians, functioning within legal parameters, believed that their contribution to patient care was minimized by the campaign. These problems reflect the downside of advertising. How do you explain the history and implications of "de-skilling" in half a minute? Our organization responded to all letters of concern, explaining the restrictions of expensive advertising. All members of the health care team are valuable. Illegal and harmful replacement of higher-skilled individuals by others puts *everyone* in jeopardy. This is evidenced by the concerns of various UAPs who said that they are being assigned to tasks they don't feel qualified

to do and by the concerns of consumers who described incidents and accidents as a result of the absence of RNs.

Significantly, the campaign placed RNs squarely on the health care diagram. We entered the public's vocabulary as an entity, as people who knew what to do, who wanted to continue to look out for patients and deliver care, and who were facing obstacles in attempting to do so. NYSNA became more established as a voice for organized nursing and as a force in the health care debate. Nurses, who were initially intimidated out of wearing their "Every Patient Deserves an RN" buttons to work, put them back on as a statement of pride and of defiance, and as an outstretched arm to patients—as allies. The name NYSNA started to look familiar in different spheres. This not only supported the work of our political action committee but created a context for nurses who raised issues in our communities and workplaces. There's something especially magical about television in our society, and we had to chuckle to ourselves whenever patients approached, inquiring whether or not we were their RNs.

Most important, the campaign laid the groundwork for deflating the myth of "reengineering" as a corporate means of improving quality. Ads that followed (often around labor disputes in NYSNA-represented institutions) were able to build on previous campaign ads in exposing hospital cost-cutting measures that jeopardized patients. Ads placed by the councils of nurse practitioners at Mount Sinai and Columbia-Presbyterian medical centers in New York City evoked much public sympathy. Our concerns about our jobs and our practice were beginning to be seen as linked to the well-being of patients and their families.

NYSNA's Campaign Continues—Getting the Word Out

Despite the flaws in collecting and reporting accurate data, recent studies indicate that "as RN staffing increases there is a statistically significant decrease" in several selected adverse patient outcomes (*Report*, NYSNA, April 1997).

As more and more studies link patient outcomes to RN staffing, NYSNA will continue to publicize these results. Our latest media campaign (started in early 1997) includes television and radio ads aired in several big cities, and newspaper and magazine ads from *The New York Times* to *TV Guide.* Included in our informational strategy are compact "hospital evaluation kits," sent to all those who call any of the 800 numbers in the ads and distributed in various other settings. These portable cardlike foldouts contain information about downsizing and replacement and describe the importance of RNs and nursing care. They contain a list of phone numbers of all area hospitals and a guide as to what questions patients should ask before selecting a hospital or other health care organization, particularly regarding their access to RNs. Though the message of the campaign still uses the same slogan ("Ask for a Real Nurse . . ."), it has been expanded to offer consumers a more complex view of the RN's role. NYSNA's two paid lobbyists have made a point of making sure that every legislator has a kit for himself or herself. NYSNA members and friends are leaving a kit in legislators' offices whenever they make a visit, not only to promote the campaign, but also as a way of introducing themselves as nurses and voters.

These strategies are having a measurable effect. By the end of 1997, we had distributed 75,000 kits. We are increasingly consulted and sought out for our input on issues where nursing and health care are concerned, by legal officials and by the media. Nursing and NYSNA have moved to the forefront, identified as leaders in the battle for consumer safety. We have delivered testimony after testimony at public hearings. Our credibility as spokespersons for the profession has been enhanced. We have strengthened our relationships with consumer advocacy and community groups, as well as with other unions. We take every opportunity to broaden our influence very seriously, and we are more diligent in developing positions on various issues. Perhaps one of the most telling measures of our success in awakening the public has been manifested by a sudden increase in ads by hospitals, health plans, and physician groups describing how *their* facilities have prided themselves on the number of RNs caring for patients! A recent full-page ad in *The New York Times* by an NYC metropolitan-area hospital described how the first and last people whom patients see in that facility are RNs. In placing these ads, these facilities are actually augmenting *our* own advertising campaign at no cost to us! (See reprinted advertisement on p. 199.)

Our ultimate success will depend on several factors:

- How well we can form and sustain community-labor coalitions around the concept of health care as a right, not a privilege
- How effectively we can continue communicating to the public, by advertising, letters to the editor, television appearances, interviews, public hearings, and word of mouth, *what nurses do* and why we are as essential *as we are* to any health care system
- How well we can link our struggle to defend nursing practice and ensure quality care to a superior health care policy, such as a national health system (single payer)
- How we can support each other in our workplaces (and outside) to function on a day-to-day basis and to generate the communal courage to take a stand on critical issues
- How we can win over the hearts and minds of our own nurses about the need to find a unified agenda and a unified voice to salvage the science and art of nursing—to take back our practice

Chapter *14*

ETHICAL ISSUES: Politics, Power, and Policy

MILA ANN AROSKAR

Nurses are confronted with ethical challenges wherever they practice in the turbulent world of health care. Responding to ethical questions and problems always requires a reasoned approach and often requires political action and policy work in health care organizations and in the wider community. Ethical issues such as requests for assisted suicide (also known as assisted dying), access to an adequate level of competent health care, evolving managed care arrangements and hospital restructuring that create worries about patient care and treatment, emerging infectious diseases, and proposed cuts in Medicare and Medicaid influence nursing care at the bedside, influence policy in health care organizations, and influence public policy. Public policy development then influences policy development in organizations and decision making at the bedside directly or indirectly. This chapter explores the ethical terrain of nursing's political and policy activities in organizations and the wider society—important and underexplored areas of nursing activity.

ETHICAL ISSUES IN NURSING: NEED FOR POLITICAL ACTION

Nursing's Agenda for Health Care Reform (American Nurses Association, 1992) articulated important goals of ensuring universal access to needed health care and promotion of health. One key to meeting these goals is the active participation of nurses in political and policy activities at organizational and societal levels of the health care enterprise. The last item in the American Nurses Association (ANA) *Code for Nurses* (1976, 1985) states that nurses collaborate with other health professionals and citizens in promoting community and national efforts to meet the health needs of the public. The code uses the language of obligation to emphasize the importance of nurses' participation in promoting equitable access to nursing and health care for all people. Participation in political and policy-making processes is, indeed, an ethical obligation for nurses, as both citizens and professionals. Nurses must be sensitive to the fact that such participation may create ethical conflicts and struggles similar to those in clinical care but with fewer formal structures such as institutional ethics committees or identified consultants for assistance. Nurses often turn to respected colleagues for assistance with their ethical struggles when other identified resources do not exist.

The financing and delivery of health care are key policy issues in the United States. Ways to ensure access and rights to health care in evolving health care structures and to ensure assistance in dying continue to be debated. Many managed care arrangements are still to be proved as effective and ethically supportable responses to escalation of health care costs and provision of quality care. End-of-life care and decision making are receiving more public attention than ever before. As essential providers of care, nurses are and should be playing key roles in these national debates that influence individual and organizational decision making. Without nursing services and values of caring and respect for persons, health *care* systems cannot long survive. The nursing profession advocates for humane values of nurturing and caring for individuals and populations who are vulnerable and suffering: the terminally ill, the elderly, the chronically mentally ill, and children in poverty. Nursing's values will be reflected in evolving health care systems only if nurses and their professional organizations actively participate in politics as an obligation of public and professional ethics and if nurses insist on participating in organizational and public policy development at every level—from the hospital, nursing home, and home care agency to government programs and research policies.

Fifty years ago, nursing leader Katharine Densford spoke to the need for political action by nurses, as have many other leaders since. In the book *Ethics for Modern Nurses* (Densford & Everett, 1946), she wrote, "All professional people, including nurses, should plunge into the midst of politics" (p. 241). Starting in the 1920s a proposed code of ethics for nurses emphasized that their role as citizens is a primary obligation (Fowler, 1984). Over the years, however, this emphasis has weakened; in the latest formulation of the *Code for Nurses,* citizenship is not mentioned explicitly as an ethical obligation. At the same time, the bioethics community has rediscovered citizenship as a way of analyzing and responding to issues in health care that combines respect for personal autonomy and concerns of individual and social justice.

Nursing cannot meet its goals in isolation from politics, power, and health policy formulation (Abdellah, 1991). In other words, nurses cannot divorce their roles as professionals from their roles as citizens, nor can they separate their interests in the well-being of individuals from their interests in the collective well-being of society. It is part of nurses' professional practice and social mandate to work for the individual patient's good and the public good. It is no less than an ethical obligation, and all the

more essential in the context of our complex and turbulent society and the demands that society makes on nursing and health care delivery systems.

Unequal or closed access to health care; homelessness; epidemics such as adolescent pregnancy, substance abuse, family and workplace violence, and sexually transmitted diseases; stresses related to growing ethnic diversity and unstable international relations—all these are part of the rapidly changing social context in which nursing must fulfill its individual and collective obligations. Meeting individual, family, or even community client health care needs is not enough to meet the social mandate of professional practice. In summary, as members of the moral community of nursing who possess specialized knowledge and expertise and commitment to values of caring and health, nurses must work toward both individual and public good in collaboration with others (Aroskar, 1995).

LINKS BETWEEN ETHICS AND POLITICS

Many people, including nurses and politicians, may consider ethics and politics separate, almost diametrically opposed realms of human thought and behavior. Whereas politics is the essence of "the public life," many consider ethics a private matter, concerned with an individual's own definition of what constitutes good conduct. This, however, is a limited concept. Ethics is a philosophical discipline that systematically studies what our conduct ought to be in relation to ourselves, others, and the environment and how to justify what is right or good. Ethics addresses the whole of life, and that includes our ethical obligations as individuals, professionals, and citizens.

The practice of politics often carries negative connotations because of the actions of some politicians and a moral ambivalence toward the exercise of power. Indeed, I suspect that most "politicians" would not identify themselves as taking part in activities that are clearly ethical in nature. But if we look at politics more closely, we can see that it consists of a rich array of concepts that do not necessarily carry negative overtones: politics as a science dealing with the regulation and control of people in society, the work of government and legislators, or any human activity concerned with the advancement of the interests of society or any group within society. The term *politics* can also refer to relations between leaders and nonleaders in society or within groups such as a patient care unit or a professional nursing organization ("Webster's third, . . ." 1986).

Other formulations of what is political more clearly point to the overlap with ethics (Aroskar, 1987). Politics can be seen as the practice of public ethics, as in pursuit of the public's welfare; as a branch of ethics concerned with the state as a whole rather than with individuals; as a division of moral philosophy dealing with ethical relations and duties of government or other social organizations such as health care institutions; or as the totality of the complex and usually conflicting interrelations among persons living in society. These formulations highlight one common area of ethics and politics: the often occurring conflict of individual needs and interests with those of a group or community. Examples include individuals infected with human immunodeficiency virus (HIV) who refuse to notify their sexual partners or to use safe sex practices, dying patients who ask nurses to help them die, and nurses with "inside" knowledge about a political candidate's conflict of interest that could affect the candidate's ability to legislate equitable health policy.

Aristotle (1976) discussed both ethics and politics as concerned with what is good and what is just conduct. He claimed that politics is the supreme practical science and is even more honorable than medicine. For Aristotle, politics was practical action in accordance with goodness, the content of ethics. Politics and ethics, then, far from being unrelated domains of human activity, are closely intertwined in our personal and professional lives as nurses.

In nursing, there are obvious situations in which ethical, political, and power aspects intertwine in organizational and public domains. For example, a nurse has to decide whether to blow the whistle on a physician who uses inadequate hand-washing technique on a bone marrow transplant unit or to remain silent. Nurses participate in ethics committees where power issues are an implicit part of the dynamics in discussion and recommendations for action. A professional nursing organization has to make decisions about the use of limited resources for economic and general welfare activities in competition with programs for membership development and education. Nursing organizations make decisions about support for political candidates and consider potential consequences of such actions as part of the decision-making process. Professional nursing organizations also have to decide whether and how they will participate as members of the national and international nursing communities in such critical areas as the protection of nurses' human rights. For example, nurses in some war-torn countries have been tortured and killed for providing care to wounded citizens. The American Nurses Association has taken a strong position against such blatant violations of human rights, thus standing courageously for humane values in countries where these values are negated by those in power. All these situations illustrate the intertwining of ethics, politics, and power in different ways that affect individual and public good.

ETHICAL ISSUES AND ANALYSIS IN NURSING

Similar to ethical issues that arise in clinical practice, the ethical issues of politics and policy-making are concerned with decisions about the following:

- Our conduct with each other
- Whether our conduct is right or good
- Identification of our duties and obligations
- What we ought to do when ethical values conflict with each other or with other values, such as economic or cultural values

Ethical values are reflected in ethical principles. The ethical principles that have received the most attention in the bioethics literature during the past two decades are respect for individual autonomy, nonmaleficence (avoiding or preventing harm), beneficence (providing benefits to others), and justice as equity and fairness. Truth telling and fidelity to patients are additional ethical principles of significance to nursing found in the *Code for Nurses.*

In politics and policymaking, ethical issues and concerns occur at every level—in the workplace, the community, health care delivery systems, professional organizations, and government. Many current health care problems cut across all four areas of decision making. Consider the many value conflicts and issues concerning HIV infection and the acquired immunodeficiency syndrome (AIDS): development of policies for HIV testing; issues of protecting patient confidentiality; informed decision making and consent regarding treatment; protection of individuals and communities from a lethal communicable disease; allocation of limited financial and social resources to prevention, treatment, and research; and the impact of AIDS on nursing care needs around the world. Individually and collectively, nurses can contribute sensitivity, clinical expertise, and advocacy for the vulnerable to the policy decisions that these issues require. The ethical conflicts that arise in such organizational and public policymaking require explicit attention and the development of legally, economically, socially, *and* ethically supportable responses.

Other health care policy issues that require nursing's perspective, ethical values, and active leadership include public policy that moves Medicaid patients into managed care delivery structures, restructuring and downsizing of hospital nursing staff which create situations that jeopardize patient safety, and inadequate planning for continuity of patient care. Each of these issues involves groups of people at risk, including patients and nurses, and demands explicit consideration of such ethical values as respect for individuals, avoiding harm, providing benefits, truth telling, fairness, responsibility, accountability, and personal and professional integrity. Each issue also involves decision-making activities and environments in which power and political dynamics often present compelling practical constraints.

Ethical reflection requires use of a moral reasoning process by nurses individually and in group dialog to work through difficult issues systematically in clinical and other organizational settings:

1. Determine that the problem in question is primarily ethical rather than, for instance, a legal or communications problem. Defining the problem guides one's response and therefore one's decisions and actions.
2. Specify the ethical and value conflicts in the situation and identify those who have a stake in these conflicts.
3. Consider alternative actions to resolve the situation.
4. Determine whether these alternatives are congruent with ethical principles and values.
5. Identify any practical constraints (e.g., legal, economic).
6. Choose a course of action and carry it out.
7. Evaluate the effects and what has been learned that will inform responses to similar situations in the future.

Using such a moral reasoning process will immediately force nurses to confront the moral complexities of the environment in which they attempt to deliver care. The realities of today's health care system in the United States—intense cost-containment efforts that seem to overwhelm other goals, use of sophisticated technologies with the potential for both torturing people and saving lives, the lack of access to health care for millions (many of them children) in the world's wealthiest nation—challenge nurses with ethical dilemmas in direct patient care activities and in organizational and public policymaking activities that are often dominated by economic and power issues.

In practice, these and other troublesome realities of evolving health care systems and policymaking bodies often boil down to questions about the allocation of finite resources, about which society must make some difficult decisions. Society's resources are not only financial and economic. Access to an adequate level of needed health care, availability of nursing time for patient care, professional expertise, affordable housing, and opportunities for education and employment are also societal resources, and they are in limited supply. Kalisch and Kalisch (1982) assert that "the basic definition of politics is the authoritative allocation of resources" (p. 31). Clearly the ethical problems that nurses face have a political dimension, and political and policymaking participation often creates ethical struggles for nurses who see themselves primarily as advocates for their individual patients. Nurses use formal mechanisms such as their professional organizations and dialog with colleagues to decide how to respond to ethical struggles.

A FRAMEWORK FOR ETHICAL ANALYSIS IN POLICY DEVELOPMENT AND EVALUATION

In an article on social change and intervention, sociologists Warwick and Kelman (1976) have provided the components for a framework that nurses can use to identify and evaluate the ethical dimensions of existing and proposed institutional and public policies:

1. **What are the goals of the proposed or existing policy?** What values are maximized or minimized when we consider, for example, prospective reimbursement or managed care systems that have cost containment as a major goal? Are economic values maximized at the expense of humane and ethical values, such as respect for persons, which incorporates respect for autonomy and respect for persons as interconnected members of the human community, and universal access to needed health care?

2. **What is the definition of the target of change in forming a specific policy: that is, who or what is supposed to change?** Are patients, clinicians, administrators, payers, or organizations being asked or forced to change? How are they involved in the process of setting goals and in policy development or revision in clinical or business areas that affect care and treatment directly or indirectly?

3. **What means are chosen to develop, implement, and change policy?** Are they coercive means that negate respect for individual autonomy and simply use raw power to achieve

results, or are they facilitative means that encompass respect for individuals and considerations of fairness? For example, smoking policies in the workplace raise questions about the means used to implement them. Should workers who are addicted to nicotine be forced into treatment programs, with compliance linked to salary incentives? Should there be surveillance of smokers even when they are not in the workplace, thus jeopardizing individual privacy? Use of such coercive means runs counter to our deeply held societal values of individual liberty and freedom of choice, even though we are not free to do things that harm others.

4. **What direct and indirect consequences of existing or proposed policy can be identified?** What are the economic, psychological, and emotional costs (and benefits) as issues of fairness and justice? How are people affected, directly and indirectly, by a proposed health policy and its costs? What is its potential impact on the welfare of the most vulnerable when the most advantaged individuals or groups, such as chief executive officers of large corporations, will clearly benefit?

This framework can be used when one is considering the ethical adequacy of proposed policies for women's health care services and research at the federal level, in hospitals and clinics, and in managed care systems. Areas in women's health for which funding priorities must be established include breast health services and treatment of breast cancer, prevention of cardiovascular diseases and HIV infection, development of safe drugs and medical devices, and any occupational and environmental health issues that primarily affect women. Using the framework for ethical analysis, policymakers would address the goals of proposed and existing policies for women's health; how women at risk participate in the development of policy goals and plans for implementation; the representativeness of the women who participate; and the means recommended to implement policy. Policymakers would also discuss the direct and indirect consequences of policy from an ethical perspective as well as legal, economic, and social perspectives. All the policies that may be developed in women's health care will be influenced by the allocation of societal resources, rationing, and other cost-containment efforts. Nurses, as essential health care providers, must participate actively in these policy debates and decisions, as they have in efforts to pass patient protection legislation in evolving managed care arrangements, the assisted suicide debate, and advocacy for the health of women and children.

Public policy goals for women's health care might be developed to provide health benefits for the greatest number of women. On the face of it, this seems to be an ethically justifiable way to proceed, but, in fact, such a utilitarian policy might ignore consequences to the most vulnerable and sickest women, who are smaller in number. Conflicts might arise among women with no known health problems, those who are infected with HIV, and the poor elderly with multiple chronic health problems. How are the interests and values of these different groups represented and heard in the policy development process? Some policymakers might opt to allocate more resources to preventive activities than to research or treatment. Will the health of an already advantaged group of women be improved at the expense of a less advantaged group? What are the means recommended for implementation of policies such as providing funds for existing services, using noncoercive incentives for healthy lifestyles, or invoking penalties for failure to comply with treatment recommendations? What are the consequences for traditional nursing values of individual patient advocacy and access to an adequate level of needed health care for all women? What are the consequences of proposed policies in the area of women's health programs in the allocation of finite societal resources to health needs of infants, children, and men? These questions suggest additional areas that must be addressed from an ethical perspective to arrive at comprehensive and reasoned policies in women's health care that are ethically supportable.

The explicit consideration of ethical aspects in policy development does not automatically mean that there will be ethical consensus about a single policy or set of policies; reasonable people may still disagree after much debate and careful ethical analysis. Reasoned ethical analysis, however, would result in the summary rejection of policies that trample on respect for the most vulnerable individuals. At a minimum, decision makers could clarify the ethical trade-offs in proposed and existing policies, whether in health care institutions or public policy, and could make the difficult required choices in an ethically sensitive way. At best, the most vulnerable individuals and groups would clearly benefit from policy development and evaluation that incorporated ethical principles and values. Nurses are logically the participants to draw explicit attention to principles and values of the nursing profession that are at stake or in conflict in political and policy debates. This requires courage in the face of an often overwhelming emphasis on economic consequences and values and consideration of the consequences to oneself in identifying ethical aspects of decision making and policy development. Nurses should not have to be moral heroes or heroines to protect and promote the health of all.

ETHICAL PRINCIPLES, VIRTUES, AND POLITICAL BEHAVIOR

Ethical principles and virtues are integral aspects of our moral lives as nurses. Virtues refer to certain dispositions or character traits, such as integrity, trustworthiness, respectfulness, honesty, courage, and kindness. They are evidenced by behaviors and are expressive of ethical principles, such as truthfulness, respect for persons, and beneficence. Virtues and ethical "bottom lines" of nurses are tested not only in clinical situations but also in participation in political arenas and policy development. As noted earlier, such participation often brings with it ethical struggles that differ from those in patient care. For instance, some legislators and politicians view lying and deception as an accepted part of doing business. Philosopher Hannah Arendt (1969, p. 4) warns us that "truthfulness has never been counted among the political virtues, and lies have always been regarded as justifiable tools in political dealings." This is a different and threatening reality that jeopardizes assumptions that the social fabric of the community and our daily lives depends on truthful communication.

Nurses who participate in political circles at local, state, or national levels may be faced with the uncomfortable realization that behaviors commonly practiced in that context challenge their own personal and professional integrity. It is critical to be aware of this challenge and of the potential moral costs of participation in political activities that are essential to furthering nursing's health care goals. But it is also important to understand that nonparticipation poses costs as well, particularly the absence of nursing's voice and values in the development of institutional and public policy. We must recognize the paradox that in many instances what is ethical and what is politically expedient in the day-to-day practice of politics and public policy development will be painfully incongruent and will create moral turmoil.

A first step in dealing with a situation that creates moral turmoil is to recognize the incongruity and what is at stake for one's own integrity. Discussing the situation with trusted colleagues or friends will help to identify the personal and professional values that are challenged in the situation and potentially generate decisions and actions that take the tradeoffs into account in an ethically supportable way. Such deliberation may also end in an individual's withdrawal from such activities or summoning the courage to confront them directly. It is important to anticipate the possible consequences of each option for action. One test is to consider the options in terms of whether you would be willing to publicize them on the nightly television news. Ethical reflection and discernment will rule out options such as participation in a deliberate cover-up of information that is critical to the public's health and welfare, even though that information is detrimental to interests of powerful corporations such as tobacco companies that are influential in financing political campaigns. Undoubtedly, nurses who participate in political activities have opportunities to check their own ethical barometers for integrity and honesty.

CONCLUSION

Nurses, individually and collectively, have an ethical obligation to participate in political activities and policy development to achieve nursing's goals for the health of individuals and the public, recognizing that ethical conflict comes with the territory. Expansion of nursing's political activities on behalf of the public good is particularly critical because the focus for the past few decades in nursing, medicine, and society has been on sickness care for individuals. We are increasingly aware that the health of individuals is profoundly interdependent with the health and well-being of families and communities locally, nationally, and globally. Violence, emerging communicable diseases, long-term physical and mental illness, and the health of the environment are powerful examples that illustrate this reality.

The concept of the nurse as citizen is critical when one is considering the choices involved in the ethical obligation to work with others to achieve nursing and health care goals. There are costs and benefits to individual nurses and the profession both in choosing to participate and in choosing not to participate in the political/power aspects of decision making in organizations and the wider society and in the ethical struggles that may ensue. Individual nurses and the profession must balance the costs and benefits and clarify what values are nonnegotiable when they participate in traditionally defined political activities and the development of professional, institutional, and public policies. This discussion has not yet occurred broadly in the nursing community. Consideration of the ethical dimensions of one's political activities as a nurse in organizations and in society can occur in informal discussions with trusted colleagues, in professional workshops that focus on a variety of nursing topics, and increasingly in health care organizations that are developing system-wide ethics plans in response to identified need and accreditation requirements.

Nursing's voice and participation are critical to the health of our society, particularly the health of the most vulnerable, as many individual nurses and professional nursing organizations already recognize. Advocacy by nurses, individually and collectively, for patient protection legislation and advocacy for health care reform at federal and state levels are just two examples. Indifference to political activities and participation is unacceptable, given nursing's social mandate to care. Recognition of the ethical problems and struggles that occur in political participation and reflective support for nurse participants are obligations for all members of the moral community of nursing.

REFERENCES

Abdellah, F. (1991). *Nursing's role in the future.* Indianapolis, IN: Sigma Theta Tau International Center Nursing Press.

American Nurses Association. (1976, 1985). *Code for nurses with interpretive statements.* Kansas City, MO: Author.

American Nurses Association. (1992). *Nursing's agenda for health care reform.* Washington, DC: American Nurses Publishing.

Arendt, H. (1969). *Crises of the republic.* New York: Harcourt Brace Jovanovich.

Aristotle. (1976). *Ethics* (Radice, R. [Ed.], Rev. ed.). New York: Penguin Classics.

Aroskar, M. A. (1987). The interface of ethics and politics in nursing. *Nursing Outlook, 35*(6), 268–272.

Aroskar, M. A. (1995). Envisioning nursing as a moral community. *Nursing Outlook, 43*(3), 134–138.

Densford, J. J., & Everett, M. S. (1946). *Ethics for modern nurses.* Philadelphia: W. B. Saunders.

Fowler, M. D. M. (1984). *Ethics and nursing, 1983–1984: The ideal of service, the reality of history.* Unpublished doctoral dissertation, University of Southern California.

Kalisch, B. J., & Kalisch, P. A. (1982). *Politics of nursing.* Philadelphia: J. B. Lippincott.

Warwick, D. P., & Kelman, H. C. (1976). Ethical issues in social intervention. In W. G. Bennis, K. D. Benne, R. Chinn, & K. E. Corey (Eds.), *Planning of change* (3rd ed., pp. 470–496). New York: Holt, Rinehart & Winston.

Webster's third new international dictionary. (1986). Springfield, MA: Merriam-Webster.

UNIT II CASE STUDY

Rationing Health Care: The Oregon Story

Cecelia Capuzzi

In 1805, Lewis and Clark blazed across the country and reached the Pacific Ocean, traveling through the territory that is now Oregon. They have since been followed by hundreds of thousands of people who have migrated to the Northwest, bringing with them a culture of progressiveness and independence. This pioneering spirit is reflected in the state's political system. Oregonians pride themselves on having a legislature composed of ordinary citizens who meet every 2 years to enact the will of the people; often it is referred to as a "user friendly" legislature. State legislators are accessible to the public, and average citizens frequently testify at legislative hearings on bills of interest. In this political climate, the Oregon Health Plan was created in 1989.

RATIONING OF HEALTH CARE: AN IMPLICIT POLICY

Before the enactment of the Oregon Health Plan, the Oregon legislature made its funding decisions biennially, trying to match available dollars with citizen needs. Frequently the decisions about the funding of health care resulted in some citizens' becoming uninsured; health care rationing occurred implicitly. There were no explicit rules to determine how this allocation process would occur, nor were the consequences of these actions openly acknowledged as being rationing (Capuzzi, 1994).

Several events that occurred during the 1980s caused the issue of access to health care to be recognized and adopted as a major legislative initiative. In the mid-1980s, the state's economy was improving and Oregon increased its spending on health care, but 350,000 Oregonians (16%) less than 65 years of age still did not have health insurance (Oregon Health Services Commission, 1991). In addition, certain health indicators were declining; for example, for the first time in 10 years, the state's "inadequate prenatal care rate" (the number of births to women who had fewer than five prenatal care visits or had no prenatal care until the last trimester of pregnancy) was increasing (Oregon Health Division, 1987).

Not all of the uninsured were jobless; in fact, 65% of those without health insurance were employed either part time or full time, or were dependents of employed individuals (Joint Legislative Committee on Health Care, 1990). As health care costs in the United States continued to escalate, employers' insurance costs increased 18% to 30% (Governor's Commission on Health Care, 1988), and many small companies dropped health insurance benefits for their employees. Additionally, an increasing number of individuals were unable to obtain affordable health insurance because they had a preexisting health condition.

In 1987 the issue finally came to a head. The state's Medicaid program was experiencing financial problems, and the Oregon legislature was considering more than $48 million in social program needs but had only $21 million in the budget (Kitzhaber, 1991). Its solution was to discontinue funding for 30 organ transplants, totaling approximately $800,000, and to use the monies to extend health care to approximately 3,000 other Oregonians who lacked health insurance (Kitzhaber, 1990). This policy was attacked by the media when it featured a young boy with leukemia whose family was unable to pay for a bone marrow transplant; he subsequently died. Rationing had become a reality.

RATIONING OF HEALTH CARE: AN EXPLICIT POLICY

THE BEGINNING OF CHANGE: ISSUE RECOGNITION AND ADOPTION

THE OREGON HEALTH PLAN. In January 1989, when the sixty-fifth session of the Oregon Assembly opened, I began a legislative internship and was working with a nonprofit advocacy group. I spent the first 6 weeks familiarizing myself with the political and legislative processes while attempting to keep abreast of current events. Six weeks later, I sat in a large room on the Willamette University campus adjacent to the state capitol, listening to a presentation of a pilot project report on prioritizing health services. After the presentation, Senate President John Kitzhaber unveiled his plan for decreasing the number of uninsured Oregonians before an audience that included key state leaders, as well as health lobbyists and the media. We knew that the issue of access to health care had been adopted by this legislature and that this legislation would be a major priority during the 1989 session.

Senator Kitzhaber's plan to increase access to health care consisted of three pieces of legislation. The first bill, SB 27, expanded Medicaid to include all individuals whose income was below the federal poverty level. The second bill, SB 935, created a health insurance pool and offered tax credits to small-business employers so that they would provide health insurance to their employees and their dependents. The third bill, SB 534, created a high-risk insurance pool for those who were unable to obtain health insurance (Capuzzi & Garland, 1991).

SB 27, the most controversial of the three bills, proposed the development of a list of health service priorities by an 11-member commission; critics called this "rationing health care." After it was determined which services would be offered, this package would constitute the basic health care package offered by Medicaid, the small business insurance pool, and the high-risk insurance pool. Moreover, leaders envisioned that this package would eventually govern the required insured health services offered by all insurance plans in the state. SB 27 required that the basic health services be provided by managed care systems when feasible.

ISSUES OF CONCERN TO NURSES. A core group of nurses were particularly interested in this legislation: staff and members of the state nurses association, nurses involved with other advocacy groups, faculty from the Oregon Health Sciences University School of Nursing, and me. After study and discussion of the proposed legislation, we concluded that although the plan benefited the majority of citizens in the state, we still had several concerns.

Our first concern was the proposed composition of the Oregon Health Services Commission (HSC). SB 27 mandated that the commission have 11 members: 5 physicians, 1 public health nurse, 1 social services worker, and 4 consumers. We thought that fewer physicians were needed if changes in the health care system were to occur; we looked for an emphasis not on medical treatment but on health promotion and disease prevention.

Our second concern was related to the first one. Although the language of the bill and accompanying speeches by Senator Kitzhaber and his aides discussed the changes needed in the health care system, most of their examples were related to the delivery of medical care.

Finally, we questioned whether the requirement for prepaid managed care services would preclude or limit consumer access to services provided by nurses and other nonphysician providers, because the original bill did not contain language to ensure that all health care providers would be eligible to participate in a managed care system and receive reimbursement.

POLITICAL STRATEGIES USED BY OREGON NURSES. We used numerous political strategies to ensure that nurses' input and concerns were heard before implementation of the legislation. The first strategy was to gain access to the political arenas where the policy was being formulated: the senate president's office, committee hearings, work sessions, and interest group meetings. Because many of us had been politically involved in preceding years with other health care issues, it was not difficult to gain access to these policy arenas.

After SB 27 was referred to the House Human Resources Committee, there were six additional hearings. At least one member of the core nurses' group was present at all hearings to monitor amendments, hear the arguments for and against the bill, identify which groups were supporting the bill, assess committee members' views, and talk with others who were following the bill. We also monitored the SB 935 and SB 534 hearings.

We met frequently with staff in the senate president's office and with staff of select legislative committees to monitor the progress of the bills. Besides giving us access to information, our presence promoted our reputation as knowledgeable health professionals who were actively concerned with the issues involving consumer access to health care.

A second political strategy was to present testimony. We testified at the legislative hearings and presented our concerns, provided expert knowledge about the difficulties our patients had in gaining access to health care services, and lobbied for comprehensive health services. We emphasized that health care is broader than medical care, that health promotion and illness prevention should be included, and that the language of the bills should reflect these principles. We presented data about the effectiveness of nurses' providing certain types of health care services and asked that the language of the bill not be limited to physician providers. And we urged that more nurses be appointed to the HSC, particularly if the intent of the legislation was to look at cost-effective

health care services that nurses can and do provide.

Marketing was a third strategy we used. These activities were often the same as those involved in gaining access and lobbying. For example, we met with key policymakers and provided information about the nursing profession, nurses' roles in the health care system, and the cost-effectiveness of health and nursing care delivered by nurses. We invited key players to meetings such as the state nurses association's annual conference, where the senate president was invited to speak on SB 27 and answer questions.

We believed that all nurses needed to be informed about the legislation and initiated several measures: each of us reported regularly to our organizations, wrote articles for newsletters, and made presentations to groups of nurses around the state.

A fourth political strategy we effectively used was networking. We were members of our professional organizations but also of other advocacy groups. An advantage of belonging to such groups was the opportunity to interact with other health professionals who shared our interest in the legislation. We explained our concerns, and our fellow health professionals became our advocates; we in turn listened to their concerns and often supported issues of importance to them. At times, coalitions were formed. One example relates to our first concern, that of nursing representation on the HSC. One advocacy group we had discussed our views with lobbied for additional nurses on the commission. Later, this group thought the legislation lacked enough cost-control measures and sought our support for subsequent legislation. The networks we developed also provided us with a means to obtain pertinent information before it appeared in the media, thus giving us extra time to plan and respond, as well as to squelch rumors.

The final strategy was mobilization of other nurs/es. Through our informal networks, we identified other nurses who could monitor the legislation, testify at hearings, and lobby their local legislators. At times, we provided nursing colleagues with the tools necessary to participate: one-page summaries of the key issues, guidelines for the preparation of testimony, information about upcoming hearing dates and times, and names of legislators to lobby on various issues.

These political strategies helped Oregon nurses to be successful in alleviating two of our concerns. The language in SB 27 was amended to use the term *health care* rather than *medical care,* and language was added that prohibited managed care systems from excluding the services offered by nurses or other nonphysician providers. In addition, the strategies we employed added to those used by other groups to ensure passage of the legislation. Nurses' expert testimony about patients' needs helped to convince policymakers that the legislation would benefit health care consumers and influenced the final shape of the health care plan.

After testifying on this concern, we stopped lobbying for an additional nurse commissioner and began to plan new strategies for achieving this goal after enactment of SB 27. At the end of the 1989 legislative session, the Oregon House of Representatives and the Senate passed the three bills, and the governor signed the legislation into law.

POLICY IMPLEMENTATION

The implementation of SB 27 had three stages: priority setting, budget setting, and implementation (Capuzzi & Garland, 1991). Each stage involved different primary actors and different political arenas.

PRIORITY SETTING STAGE. The HSC was responsible for developing the ranked list of health services. The legislation specified that the HSC obtain input from public hearings, community meetings, advocates, and health care providers including nurses. The legislature emphasized that the values of Oregonians be considered when the ranked list of health services was developed. Additionally, the ranked list needed to include provider services and supplies, outpatient services, inpatient hospital services, and health-promotion and disease-prevention services. After the HSC developed the ranked list of condition/treatment pairs, actuaries attached a cost to each item. This list, with the specified costs, was forwarded to the 1991 Oregon legislature.

BUDGET SETTING STAGE. The primary actors for setting the budget were the Oregon legislators. Using the ranked list of condition/treatment pairs with actuarial costs, the legislature determined how far down the list could services be funded for the Medicaid program. By law, the legislature could not change the order of the list. If they wanted to fund more conditions/treatments, the legislature had to allocate additional monies. Thus the allocation process was explicit.

IMPLEMENTATION STAGE. Again the actors and the arena changed, this time to the Oregon Medical Assistance Program (OMAP). OMAP first sought a waiver from the federal Health Care Financing Administration (HCFA) because the Medicaid funding portion of the Oregon Health Plan was at variance with that allowed by current HCFA rules. The first area of variance was with the services provided. By using the ranked list of conditions/treatments, Medicaid was not providing some services mandated by federal guidelines. The other area of variance concerned the populations to be served. Medicaid would include *all* individuals who fell below the federal poverty level; this group included single adults who were excluded in the federal regulations. In 1994, Oregon received the waiver for a 5-year period and the Medicaid portion of the Oregon Health Plan began.

During this third phase, OMAP also established the criteria for providers and insurance companies to offer health care to groups of Medicaid clients under managed care contracts.

Whereas, in the past, individual health care providers treated Medicaid patients and then billed directly for reimbursement on the basis of a fee-for-service model, now health providers had to be part of a managed care plan and payment was based on a capitated system.

Implementation of the other two bills that composed the Oregon Health Plan, SB 534 and SB 935, occurred within Oregon's insurance division.

ISSUES OF CONCERN TO NURSES. During these policy implementation stages, there were old and new concerns. First, at the priority-setting stage, we wanted to know who would be appointed to the nurse, physician, and consumer positions of the HSC. Second, we continued to be concerned about the emphasis on medical care rather than health care, despite the amendments that had been made to SB 27. Third, we believed that the outcome of the health services ranking process might restrict nursing practice. Our new concerns included getting input into the priority-setting process, measuring health values, securing consumer input, and ensuring the welfare of health care consumers.

During the budget-setting stage in the 1991 legislature, the main issue was the legislative appropriation for Medicaid. We wanted to ensure that there were sufficient monies to fund what we considered to be the minimum needed services. During the Medicaid implementation stage, we again were concerned that the restructuring of the health care system for Medicaid clients not limit their access to health care nor limit their access to nursing services.

POLITICAL STRATEGIES USED BY OREGON NURSES. We continued to use the same political strategies that were employed before the Oregon Health Plan was enacted. We needed to maintain access to the political and policy arenas, although these arenas had changed. Again, our previous involvement gave us ready access. At the beginning of the priority-setting stage, I was asked to join the Oregon Health Decision's

advisory committee that was charged by the HSC to assess community values about health care. Other nurses who were involved earlier also were asked to join. The Oregon Nurses Association (ONA) selected a member to represent them at the HSC's meetings; she also assisted with the Oregon Health Decision's community values assessment. It was the participation of many nurses that ensured consumer involvement in the priority process.

Nurses attended the HSC meetings. During some meetings, we were asked for information and were encouraged to participate. We also attended the public hearings and the community values meetings. Our presence allowed us to obtain information, monitor the process, and demonstrate our concern. The organizations to which we belonged submitted nominations for the nurse, physician, and consumer positions on the HSC, which proved to be a valuable strategy: two of our nominees, one physician and one consumer, were selected. We introduced ourselves to each newly appointed commissioner and worked closely with the nurse commissioner.

We continued to use lobbying strategies, testifying at the public hearings and participating in the community values meetings. We discussed the points that had been made at previous legislative hearings: (1) the need for reimbursable, preventive, and health promotion services, (2) the importance of case management, (3) the need to consider health services broadly so as to include such things as transportation and child care, and (4) the need to provide cost-effective services that health professionals other than physicians can offer. We cited case examples to illustrate our points: the effectiveness of diabetes education in preventing complications and hospitalizations, the story of one mother's need for transportation to the prenatal care clinic from a rural area, and the success of case management for a pregnant teenager who later had a full-term, normal-weight infant.

The marketing strategy was continued in order to make the commissioners aware of our expertise and value as a resource. In three specific instances, this proved to be valuable. One type of data the HSC collected was the judgment of health providers about the outcome and effectiveness of treatments for specific conditions. The ONA assisted by having nurse practitioners complete the questionnaires.

In another instance, the commission struggled over the meaning of *case management.* Was it an advocacy or a gatekeeping activity? Since we had some very definite ideas about this, the ONA Cabinet for Health Policy invited three commissioners to a meeting at which the American Nurses Association's *Nursing Case Management* document (Task Force on Case Management, 1988) was presented to them. Additionally, we proposed a definition of case management and urged the commissioners to adopt it. Our ability to provide expert information constituted an important source of power.

The public hearings and the community values meetings made it clear that consumers viewed health promotion and prevention services as a high priority (see Box below). However, the inclusion of those specific services were missing because the standard list of medical service codes focused only on treatment-of-illness services and did not have codes for preventive services. A group of individuals, including the nurse commissioner and me, formed a task force. We reviewed various documents and recommended the adoption of *Guide to Clinical Preventive Services* (Report of the U.S. Preventive Services Task Force, 1989), a document with recommended frequency of preventive services based on research that was not limited to illness codes. The HSC incorporated this list of preventive services into the priority list and created service codes.

We also continued to network with other nurses and health professionals around the state. Members of one group actively involved in health care reform asked us to join them. Their group included a variety of health care professionals, and our involvement with this multidisciplinary group allowed us to present a nursing perspective.

Finally, we continued to mobilize other nurses by keeping them informed and providing the necessary tools for their involvement. I was chairperson of the Oregon Health Sciences University School of Nursing's External Affairs Committee, and we arranged a series of forums

---

RANK ORDER OF COMMUNITY VALUES BY FREQUENCY OF DISCUSSION AT COMMUNITY MEETINGS

1.	Prevention	Very high (all meetings)
2.	Quality of life	Very high
3.	Cost-effectiveness	High (more than three fourths of the meetings)
4.	Ability to function	Moderately high (three fourths of the meetings)
5.	Equity	Moderately high
6.	Effectiveness of treatment	Medium high (more than half of the meetings)
7.	Benefits many	Medium (half of the meetings)
8.	Mental health and chemical dependence	Medium
9.	Personal choice	Medium low (fewer than half of the meetings)
10.	Community compassion	Medium low
11.	Impact on society	Medium low
12.	Length of life	Medium low
13.	Personal responsibility	Medium low

for nursing faculty. At the first forum, we reviewed the state's access-to-health-care problems and the intent of the Oregon Health Plan. At the second forum, we invited one of the commissioners, and after providing an update on the commission's progress, she asked for information on case management. Two faculty members testified at the next commission hearing, and another volunteered to collect data on rural health nursing.

Once again, nurses served as a valuable resource to the commission. When the final ranked list of condition/treatment pairs was presented on February 20, 1991, we were satisfied that our major concerns had been addressed. There was an appropriate emphasis on prevention, and the condition/treatment list considered a broad spectrum of health services. Moreover, the outcome of the health services ranking process had not restricted nursing practice.

Lobbying was the primary strategy used during the budget-setting stage. Nurses testified about what they considered to be a basic package of services that should be available to each Oregon citizen and what the consequences of lower funding would be. We added our voice to that of others, and by the end of the 1991 legislative session, $35 million in new resources had been appropriated, funding the list through line 587, or 83% of the services on the list of priorities.

During the implementation phase of the Oregon Health Plan, we supported OMAP's efforts to obtain the HCFA waiver by writing letters of support. We also reviewed the information presented by groups and individuals that were critical of this plan and responded with our own written evaluations. Frequently, we found that these groups were misinformed about the Oregon Health Plan, and we provided accurate information. We also communicated with the American Nurses Association, which had become interested in what was occurring in Oregon.

While OMAP was initiating the criteria for providers and insurance companies under managed care contracts, we reviewed drafts of OMAP's proposals, raised questions, and offered suggestions. One major issue was how health professionals in the public health system would be part of this new managed care system. In the past, many Medicaid patients were served by local public health clinics and public health nurses. These patients were either seen at no cost or the local health departments billed Medicaid. Because OMAP was proposing that all managed care systems eligible to be reimbursed for Medicaid patients needed to provide both inpatient and ambulatory care, the effect on public health was significant. Public health nurses were active in advising OMAP on this issue. Today the issue of the integration of public health services and the Oregon Health Plan continues, and nurses are active on governmental task forces and in professional organizations dealing with this subject.

CONTINUING POLICY DEVELOPMENT

THE OREGON HEALTH PLAN TODAY. It has been 8 years since the enactment of the Oregon Health Plan; two subsequent legislative sessions have occurred since the ranked list of condition/ treatment services was funded. During the 1991 session, three additional bills were passed that became part of the Oregon Health Plan. This legislation expanded the scope of the plan to include the aged, blind, and disabled populations receiving Medicaid (SB 44); initiated additional small-business health insurance reforms (HB 1076); and created the Health Resources Commission (HRC) to examine alternatives to a certificate-of-need process (HB 1077). Two years later the mandate to the HRC was revised to focus on health care cost-containment, with specific emphasis on technology assessments to guide health care policy and spending (Oregon Legislative Administration Committee, 1993).

During the 1993 and 1995 legislative sessions, additional bills were passed to "fine tune" the Oregon Health Plan. In 1993, SB 5535 created the Office of the Health Plan Administrator, which is responsible for overseeing the entire Oregon Health Plan (Oregon Legislative Administration Committee, 1993). Another bill, SB 5530, directed the director of human resources to seek federal waivers (1) so that a prioritized list of mental health and chemical dependency services could be integrated into the medical services list and (2) so that senior citizens, blind and disabled persons, and foster children also would be included in the new plan for providing care to Medicaid clients. This bill also delayed for 2 years the date when both small and large businesses were required to provide health insurance for their employees. HB 3582, also enacted in 1993, connected the public health services to the Oregon Health Plan (Oregon Legislative Administration Committee, 1993).

SB 935, the employer mandate, was never implemented. After this bill was enacted, it was determined that this mandate conflicted with the Employee Retirement Income Security Act (ERISA), a federal law that prohibits states from enacting laws or regulations relating to employee benefits. The state applied for a federal waiver, but it was not granted and the legislation lapsed in 1996 (Conviser, 1997).

Some outcome data on the Oregon Health Plan is beginning to emerge. The number of uninsured persons has dropped to 11% in 1996; the number of children less than age 18 years without health insurance has dropped from 21% in 1990 to 8% in 1996. Additionally, more than 9,000 Oregonians who were unable to obtain health insurance because of a preexisting condition now have coverage through the high-risk insurance pool, and more than 54,000 uninsured small-business employees and their dependents now have health insurance in the private market through the state's Insurance Pool Governing Board. The majority of persons participating in the Medicaid program in 1996 indicated satisfaction with access (88%) and health care services (84%) and consider their health to be good to excellent (76%) (Oregon Health Plan Administrator's Office, April 1997). Select health indicators also are improving. The percentage of expectant mothers receiving adequate prenatal care has risen to 79%, and the infant mortality rate has dropped to 7.1 per 1,000 live births (Oregon Health Plan Administrator's Office, March 1997).

ISSUES OF CONCERN TO NURSES. The issues of concern to nurses were the same as at the earlier stages of the policy process. We continued to monitor the access and quality of health services to all Oregonians and ensure that the climate in which nurses practice is optimal.

POLITICAL STRATEGIES USED BY OREGON NURSES. Oregon nurses continued to use the same political strategies that were adopted when the Oregon Health Plan was first conceptualized. We have access to many political arenas, and we actively participate in the ongoing development and expansion of the Oregon Health Plan. Nurses were involved in the HSC's work to develop a prioritized list of mental health and chemical dependency services; the chair of this subcommittee was the nurse commissioner. Nurses also have been appointed to subsequent policy-making groups such as the Oregon Health Council. I spent 1 year on sabbatical with the Oregon Office of Health Policy as a research analyst on a Robert Wood Johnson grant that furthered the state's health reform plans. We continue to critique new proposals and testify on issues where we have expert knowledge. We are assessing the emerging outcome information regarding clients in the Oregon Health Plan. We also continue to inform other nurses about emerging issues.

The national debate triggered by this legislation has abated*; likewise, health care reform at the national level has stalled. It is at the state

---

*For more information about the critique of the Oregon Health Plan, a select reference list is provided at the end of this case study.

level that experiments in improving health care are occurring (Capuzzi, 1997). It is at this level that nurses need to be actively involved.

LESSONS LEARNED

Many of the nurses who were involved in the development and implementation of the Oregon Health Plan had expertise in the policy arena. They had prior experience in dealing with other issues and were knowledgeable about the use of effective political strategies and the creation of health policy. Although the Oregon story reinforces what is written in the literature, this experience produced some additional lessons.

EARLY INVOLVEMENT

Involvement in the policy process begins early in the game and continues after legislation is enacted. Most authors discuss the implementation of policy (e.g., lobbying, testifying), but they do not emphasize the importance of being involved during the issue recognition and adoption stages. Early involvement allowed us a voice in shaping the issue and setting the agenda; entry at a later point allows only for working on what already has been created. We were able to shape the Oregon plan so that it included prevention, case management, and a broad array of services that are often ignored. Moreover, being involved early facilitated our entry into other policy arenas as the project proceeded. Volunteering to do some of the tedious work and attending all meetings had a payoff. In several instances, we were able to ensure that key points were preserved in the plan because we had taken notes and had attended all the meetings. Enactment of the legislation was just the beginning of change; the process of implementation needs to be monitored to ensure the desired outcomes. Additionally, as new related legislation in health care reform is proposed and enacted, these policies need to be critically evaluated and monitored.

EXPERTISE AS A SOURCE OF POWER

Nurses' expert knowledge to shape health care reform is a valuable source of power. Furthermore, when nurses are willing to contribute their expert knowledge, they are seen as a priceless resource. For example, after we had offered to provide information in one area, the HSC came back for assistance with other problems. Health care reform must be dealt with in all states—and the need for many to lend their expertise is great.

ADVOCACY AND COALITIONS

Involvement in both advocacy groups and coalitions of health professionals is vital. The nursing profession stresses the importance of nurses' involvement with their own organizations, and this has merit, but nurses must collaborate more with other health professionals and with public advocacy groups if they are to influence the development of creative and effective policies needed to respond to the health care crises that face our country.

OPPORTUNITIES TO ACHIEVE GOALS

There is often more than one opportunity to achieve a specific goal. We found that if we did not get a desired change the first time, we could plan a new strategy and prevail another time. We advocate compromise, but we also urge nurses to consider ways to achieve the ideal outcome before deciding to compromise.

A LONG-TERM ENDEAVOR

Political and policy involvement is a long-term endeavor. Again, all books on politics and policy except this one do not convey this fact, even though common sense would lead to this conclusion. Books discuss the policy process, implying that there is an end point. We have learned that this is not accurate. Although one aspect of the issue may be solved, new, related issues emerge; new twists and turns occur. Policymaking is truly incremental and ongoing. Nurses need to be prepared to be involved for the long term, especially if significant changes are to occur. But long-term involvement does produce effective results, and that is rewarding.

References

Capuzzi, C. (1994). The Oregon model of decision making and its implications for nursing practice. In J. McCloskey & H. K. Grace (Eds.), *Current issues in nursing* (4th ed., pp. 711–717). St. Louis: Mosby.

Capuzzi, C. (1997). Toward a comprehensive health care system: Example of a statewide system. In J. McCloskey & H. K. Grace (Eds.), *Current issues in nursing,* (5th ed., pp. 434–438). St. Louis: Mosby.

Capuzzi, C., & Garland, M. (1991). The Oregon plan: Increasing access to health care. *Nursing Outlook, 38*(6), 260–26J, 286.

Conviser, R. (1997). A brief history of the Oregon health plan and its features [On-line]. Available: www.das.state.or.us/ohpa.

Governor's Commission on Health Care. (1988). *Report to Governor Neil Goldschmidt on improving access to health care to all Oregonians.* Salem: Oregon Office of Health Policy.

Hasnain, R., & Garland, M. (1990). *Health care in common: Report of the Oregon Health Decisions community meetings process.* Portland: Oregon Health Decisions.

Joint Legislative Committee on Health Care. (1990). *The Oregon health standard.* Salem: Oregon Legislature.

Kitzhaber, J. (1990, June 12). *Presentation to the Catholic Health Association,* Washington, DC.

Kitzhaber, J. (1991). A healthier approach to health care. *Issues in Science and Technology 7*(2), 59–65.

Oregon Health Division. (1987). *Oregon vital statistics, 1986.* Salem: Oregon Department of Human Resources.

Oregon Health Plan Administrator's Office. (1997, March). *Health, health insurance and children in Oregon: A summary of findings from the 1996 Oregon population survey.* Salem: Author.

Oregon Health Plan Administrator's Office. (1997, April). *Effects of the Oregon health plan: A summary report.* Salem: Author.

Oregon Health Services Commission. (1991). *Prioritization of services: A report to the governor and legislature.* Salem: Author.

Oregon Legislative Administration Committee. (1993, September). *1993 summary of major legislation, Oregon Legislative Assembly.* Salem: Author.

Oregon Legislative Administration Committee. (1995, October). *1995 summary of major legislation, Oregon Legislative Assembly.* Salem: Author.

Report of the U.S. Preventive Services Task Force. (1989). *Guide to clinical preventive services: An assessment of the effectiveness of 169 interventions.* Baltimore: Williams & Wilkins.

Task Force on Case Management. (1988). *Nursing case management.* Kansas City, MO: American Nurses Association.

References on the Critique of the Oregon Health Plan

Budette, P. P. (1991). Medicaid rationing in Oregon: Political wolf in a philosopher's sheepskin. *Health Matrix, 1,* 205–225.

Callahan, D. (1991a). Commentary, ethics and priority setting in Oregon. *Health Affairs, 10*(2), 78–87.

Callahan, D. (1991b). The Oregon initiative: Ethics and priority setting. *Health Matrix, 1,* 157–170.

Daniels, N. (1991). Is the Oregon rationing plan fair? *Journal of American Medical Association, 265*(17), 2232–2235.

Fox, D. (1991). Rationing care in Oregon: The new accountability. *Health Affairs, 10*(2), 7–27.

Kelly, K. (Ed.). (1994, March). Health care rationing, dilemma and paradox. *Series on Nursing Administration, 6.*

Strosberg, M. A., Wiener, J. M., & Baker, R., with Fein, I. A. (1992). *Rationing America's medical care: The Oregon plan and beyond.* Washington, DC: The Brookings Institution.

Unit *III*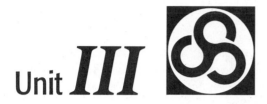

POLICY AND POLITICS IN THE WORKPLACE

Unit III

explores policy and politics in the workplace. Although the emphasis is on the hospital environment, the principles and issues discussed are relevant to all settings where nurses work.

The unit begins with a discussion of contemporary issues in the workplace. The chapter explores the reconfigurations of health care delivery systems brought about by the need to reduce costs, shift to an emphasis on primary care, and enhance continuity of care. The challenges that these reconfigurations and other societal changes pose for nurses are discussed. One response to these challenges has been the proliferation of nurses in case management roles. The vignette that follows this opening chapter examines the policies and political nuances that have accompanied this phenomenon.

Change is everywhere in health care. Nurses who are skillful at creating and sustaining change in the workplace will have opportunities to move their vision for better care. Chapter 16 outlines strategies for effective change in the workplace, and Chapter 17 elaborates on the necessity for communication and collaboration in the process of change in the workplace.

Chapter 18 explores the issues that are confronting advanced practice nurses and staff nurses as they try to provide comprehensive, high-quality care to patients and their families. It also examines the strategies that are being used to ensure the future of all nurses in clinical practice. The vignette that follows this chapter describes strategies—some successful, others yet to be—that one state's organization for nurse practitioners has been using to ensure the viability of these providers.

The controversy of collective bargaining continues within the profession. Chapter 19 examines this controversy, as well as the history, policy issues, and politics of collective bargaining. It includes a description of "whistle blower" legislation that has been proposed to protect nurses who speak out about poor, unsafe, or mismanaged care. The vignette that accompanies this chapter presents one nurse's courageous story of blowing the whistle on fraudulent activities that left a vulnerable population of prisoners without adequate health care.

Nursing research is increasingly important to demonstrating nursing's contributions to health care and to ensuring that interventions and approaches to care are producing desired outcomes. Though many would view this endeavor as an apolitical one, the authors of Chapter 20 discuss the political dimensions of nursing research and its conduct.

This unit ends with an inspiring case study that illustrates the importance of values for changing structures and policies in the workplace and for the development of political strategies. This case study is important reading for any nurse who is involved in workplace change. It provides hope for the future of health care and demonstrates the vision and leadership that nurses can provide in turbulent times of change.

Chapter *15*

CONTEMPORARY ISSUES IN THE WORKPLACE: A Glimpse Over the Horizon into the New Age of Health Care

TIM PORTER-O'GRADY

The past two decades have brought major social, cultural, and technological transformation to the lives of everyone on the global stage (Barnet & Cavanagh, 1994). The growth of the computer chip as the basic unit of communication, productivity, and information management has altered the world's social and political structures. In an instant, deals can be struck, information generated, relationships established, money moved, products planned and produced, and communication facilitated at any moment from anywhere in the world (Negroponte, 1995). These dramatic developments are not simply changing what we do, they are transforming who we are.

Innovation has become the definitive word in constructing social and business institutions. No longer can organizations operate as independent units outside the context of their relationship to other components of the social system. No longer can systems fail to recognize the need for balanced stewardship of scarce resources. No more can the cost associated with services be carelessly ignored or stretched beyond the ability of the social and economic systems to recover them (Bennis & Mische, 1995).

In the past, health services were provided in a way that essentially ignored the financial constraints related to their use. Choice and selection of methods and modalities were frequently undertaken without consideration of either their long-term viability or their short-term cost. When access to and growth of health services was the driving force for health care leadership, there was no overt reason to make choices based on "lean" availability of resources. There was always a "fat" supply of resources available for a growing system. Inevitably, the "fat" supply of dollars was bound to dry up, as it has, driving health professionals and leadership to make "lean" choices. Unfortunately, experience has not left administrators and providers with the necessary insight and skills to undertake substantive and meaningful change (Henderson, 1996).

It is into this atmosphere of increasing access to innovative and viable technology, and of shrinking resources, that the health professional is tossed today. These times have arrived without much enthusiasm or readiness for them. Consequently the decisions being made in response to the changing times appear inadequate. Nurses, alongside their colleagues in medicine and allied health, may be both mystified and overwhelmed by the radical nature of both the shifting social and economic equation and the system leaders' responses to it. As a result, a significant sense of loss has all but crippled many health care providers. Challenges and conflict have emerged in all areas of the system at a level of intensity rarely experienced in the recent past (Freeman, 1994).

For many, the system has suffered a loss of meaning under the dramatic changes of the recent past. The sacred values attached to patient care now seem to be inexcusably "thrown to the wind." It seems as if the health care system has lost its core and is now reeling schizophrenically in response to the multiple and sometimes conflicting demands of its many customers (Coile, 1994).

The ability to discern short-term shifts from more sustainable changes allows organizations and health professionals to respond favorably to the demand for change. Connecting the current health care shifts with those under way in other forums places these changes in a firmer context and reveals their actual meaning. Additionally, current developments in health care have created substantive changes in the service arena, affecting what nurses do and how they do it. Nursing must consider the meaning imbedded in the following health care developments:

- Mergers and acquisitions are creating more complex organizational arrangements, challenging nurses to establish new cultural and service relationships with new players and partners. Configuration of such systems are directed to positioning the organization in a way that ensures broadest access to essential services across the continuum of care within specific population categories (managed lives).
- Newer managed-care models demand different allocation of service and call for providers to recognize the different configuration of both payment and service provision. Providers are required to be more intimately involved in planning service structures within the new context instead of grieving the need for newer models of health care.
- Cost controls and new service configurations require a different mix of workers in the service setting. This shift can create a threat to current roles and service expectations. Providers must diligently ensure that such provider changes result in quality outcomes.

At first view, these changes appear threatening to the work integrity of the nurse. Nurses often feel that the dismantling of "hard won," high-quality patient care merely in the interest of cost containment and constraining resource availability is completely unacceptable. It is disheartening to know that the focus of health care service is changing when the personal evidence available to nurses suggests that the patient in the bed still has a set of needs and demands that must be met, regardless of the degree of shift toward outpatient care. The immediate challenge currently confronting health professionals, especially nurses, is looking past machinations and reactions to the present demand for change and taking a futuristic view on the notion of sustainable change.

SUBSCRIBER-BASED APPROACHES TO HEALTH CARE

In the past model of health care, individuals would approach their illnesses incrementally and in an event-based way. The individual would become sick, see a physician, require intervention, obtain that intervention, get well, and return to his or her previous way of life. For the most part, the health care service provided could be defined as event based and intervention driven. Indeed, rather than a health care model, the system has been operating predominantly on a sickness care model.

All health care services were constructed to support this particular flow of activities, including provider roles, which were built on a set of distinct and differentiated responsibilities: physicians diagnose and intervene, nurses provide care and therapeutic activities, technologists test and assess, and therapists intervene and advise. All the payment structures were set up essentially to respond to this specific dynamic.

The problem is that this dynamic is expensive. As a result, health care costs have spiraled at some 14% to 16% a year for the past 30 years.

The health care system has been operating at a growth rate that is 10% higher than the growth rate of any other industry (Goldsmith, Goran, & Nackel, 1995). Over the years, there were no cost constraints, no indications that cost levels would be reduced, and no control over growth. Furthermore, the predominant model of health care delivery embraced the most expensive and cost-intensive technological advances in order to make diagnoses and render treatment.

Health care costs simply have risen beyond the ability of a social and political system to sustain it. Employers, third-party payers, and governments have all initiated some attempt to control the dollars they use for provision of health care services. As a result, critical decisions about controlling and distributing resources, including mechanisms for stewardship of the funds, have changed the character of services, the structure of activities, and the relationship between the health system and those who pay for health care. These decisions, however, have not always been wise or judicious, resulting in approaches that compromise service, reduce quality, and put the consumer at an increasing level of personal risk (Clare, Sargent, Moxley, & Forthman, 1995).

It is out of this set of conditions that managed care has emerged. The managed care approach manages services and costs over the term of the consumer's relationship with the service organization. Managed care requires the careful enumeration and adjudication of the services provided within a specified cost framework for all who might use it (Coile, 1997). As managed care has matured, the various components of the managed care approach have resulted essentially in a change in the focus, as well as the design, of health care with regard to how it is provided and how it is paid for. For the first time in the history of the United States, the past decade of health service has been more devoted to the need to control costs than to the provision of health care services.

Subscriber-based service means aggregating populations and billing them under one payment structure. Those who represent large groupings of patients negotiate directly with providers to determine the service expectations and the costs that might attend those services. Therefore one of the unique characteristics of the emerging managed care environment is the aggregation of populations together for the purpose of negotiating both the character and the cost of service for that population at one time in advance of the service. To varying degrees and at varying levels, this model is unfolding as the predominant model for the health care delivery system in the United States.

Subscriber-based health care has changed the relationship of the health care professional to the service that is provided. It requires health care professionals to understand the needs and characteristics of the population, geographic and economic considerations, service mix, and other factors that converge to create a service system that fits as tightly as possible to the target population. Institutions are moving through a number of stages on the way to population-based service. From patient-focused care strategies to product lines, these efforts are simply the first stage of reallocating structure and resources. Ultimately provider-based and institutional models of service will shift to create population-driven models like centers of excellence, patient and service pathways, and point-of-service designs that align structure and service for a better fit with the demands of specified populations.

Though nurses may view change (product lines, integration, interdisciplinary practices) as an interruption to the smooth functioning of the established health care system, each of these stages enumerates processes that demand a shift in perspective and practice and serve as the foundation for subsequent changes.

FIXING THE PRICE OF SERVICE IN ADVANCE

Advanced pricing is emerging as the prevailing model for addressing the cost of health care and obtaining control. The ultimate demand of the changing pricing structure in a subscriber-based approach is to achieve some level of value. The best possible care and the highest level of intervention are no longer the goals of health service. More serious and studied delineations such as the best cost/benefit ratio, the most effective service for the price, and the most efficient ways of delivering work while balancing cost and quality are all numerators of today's focus on value across the health care system.

The primary concern in advanced pricing is to make sure that a clear delineation of dollars is established at the outset of service delivery so that the financial parameters are clear to all players. This rather finite, clear, and fixed notion of the relationship between inputs and outputs is a relatively new notion for health care providers in the United States. For the first time in health care, advanced pricing defines specific, clear, and identifiable parameters under which the resource provider must operate in offering clinical care to the defined subscriber population.

Nurses and nursing as a discipline must recognize that the fundamental change to a subscriber-based, advanced-pricing system alters the very characteristics of the relationship among providers and between providers and those they serve. The structures of the health care organization must give not only evidence of fiscal responsibility but also evidence of a "tightness of fit" between the services that are provided and the price that is paid for them. Though nurses and other professionals have always been aware of certain budgetary considerations to choices that are made, there has never been an overwhelming demand that those considerations be a part of every choice regarding what actions or activities will be undertaken in providing service to consumers. This led to a habit of "best choice" practices by nurses. No judgment or action, no plan or activity, no function or process can be undertaken without first identifying both its cost and its benefit in relation to the outcomes of service. These two factors, cost and service integration, form the driving force for service-delivery considerations in delineating health care in any part of the system. As a result, this has led to a demand for a skill-set shift for nurses from "best choice" to "wise choice" practices, which include conditions of value in nurse decision making.

BUILDING THE CONTINUUM OF CARE

Perhaps the most significant and least obvious development in the unfolding models of health care service is the slow emergence of the focus on a continuum of services across the subscriber base. The establishment of the new cost and service parameters and the recognition of a managed care approach in subscriber-based structuring have led to a deeper understanding of the need for a composite, continuously linked set of services. For a measurable effect on both the cost and the quality of service to specific populations, there is a growing understanding of what is required to create the right conditions:

1. *A comprehensive linkage of providers across the continuum of service.* Buyers of services and those who represent subscribers are increasingly aware of the cost of incrementally negotiating services from a wide variety of groups. There is an increasing demand for a linkage of services across the continuum of care, with the ability to negotiate with key players representing all the service elements under one umbrella.
2. *A stable subscriber base.* High subscriber turnover results in high per-unit costs. To reduce costs, the health care system must be able to have a long-term, abiding relationship with the subscriber and become involved in life span decisions affecting health status and health behaviors.
3. *Early intervention.* Early subscriber assessment and intervention reduce the intensity of service, the risk to the individual subscriber, and the cost of services provided to that individual over the long term.
4. *Team-based approaches and integrated-service structures.* In a changing system, it is interdependence that is defining the charac-

ter of health service. It is neither effective nor sustainable for individual services to operate as though they are independent of each other. Therefore protocols, critical paths, clinical pathways, best practices, care maps, and other devices used for integrating the activities of various disciplines around specific populations are the methods of preference for delineating the character and content of service in a managed care environment (Zander, 1995).

5. *Subscriber-specific and population-based health care.* Providers must be highly mobile, moving health care services to where subscribers are and fitting those services directly and "tightly" to the population served.

The new framework for health care is unfolding with relatively clear parameters. What is required of nurses is to articulate the value, meaning, and application of their roles. This is perhaps both the greatest opportunity and the greatest challenge for nurses and the profession within the next decade.

QUALITY AND THE NEW ACCREDITATION

There are three elements to creating sustainable value: cost, quality, and labor. One cannot alter any one of these variables without directly affecting the other two. In health care there has been a dramatic focus on price for the past two decades. In many ways this emphasis has operated at the expense of quality at a number of different levels, from the quality of service to the competence of the provider. Now, and for the next decade, there will be a growing emphasis on the issue of quality and the impact of change on the outcomes of service.

As hospitals become health systems and create integrated-service structures, newer methods and processes of accreditation and quality assessment emerge. The Joint Commission on the Accreditation of Healthcare Organizations, the National Committee on Quality Assurance, the Community Health Accreditation Program, and a host of other groups are becoming

the moderators of quality for a dramatically altered health care system. State agencies and federal bodies are becoming more aware of the power of outcomes, rather than the importance of functional processes, and are expanding their use of outcome measures within their regulatory activities, including licensing.

The changing focus of accreditation and evaluation will have a powerful impact on the practice of nursing. The main thrust of these changes consists of the following:

- Less focus on process-oriented factors and more emphasis on outcome-driven activities
- Increasing demand for and assessment of clinical relationships among providers, rather than review of individual nonaligned clinical activity
- Identification of the critical elements of care services that have the most sustainable impact on the health of the consumer and the quality of care services
- More emphasis on linked, comprehensive services and the determination of their collective impact on patient care and the consumer by accrediting agencies
- Development of comparative standards of measure by reviewing bodies, making it possible for buyers and consumers to compare the performance of health systems against each other through use of a template that incorporates community, regional, and national standards
- Use of computer technology to advance more specific performance standards and to measure them more consistently

There is growing competition between the various quality measurement and accreditation agencies to be viable and relevant to the future of health care services. Because the technology for quality measurement is improving every day and the standards of measure are being continually refined, it is essential for nurses to be both aware of and involved in the entire process associated with quality determination and measurement across the continuum of care.

POLICY AND PLANNING CONSIDERATIONS FOR NURSING

The policy considerations of these changes are considerable. Clearly, for nursing, there are many implications that become the foundation of defining the requisites and focus of nursing practice in the future. All nurses have a stake in decisions that affect institutional or system changes in patient care delivery, in resource allocations, and in service design. Nurses should play an active role in the dialog, design, implementation, and evaluation of clinical care models and their changes at any level of a cost-constrained service system. Some of the more critical considerations are enumerated below:

1. Subscriber-based approaches require that the population served be identified and understood as fully as possible. The demographic, service, and demand requirements of the population will provide the foundation for determining the service needs of that population.
2. Service evaluation and the quality improvement processes will continue to be built on a protocol, critical-path, best practices, or care-continuum framework. Clinical pathways, consumer relationships, performance evaluation, and outcome validation will need to be clear, to be well articulated, and to result in the achievement of clinical expectations, as well as to address contemporary issues in the workplace and in the arena of consumer health.
3. Because costs continually influence choices that are made in patient-care services, there is a risk that nursing values, roles, and applications will be lost in the process. The movement to interdisciplinary care models, alternative care providers, and unlicensed assistive personnel will require that nurses be increasingly clear and specific about the service risks, the cost, and the delineation, accountability, and articulation of roles and functions in a way that best benefits the population served.
4. The role of case management in managing the continuum of services in an early engagement system will require a growth in nursing roles in managing subscriber populations across the life continuum. There is an expanding need for nurses in primary care roles directed at assessing, planning, evaluating, teaching, and referring subscribers across the continuum of care. In expanding the skill base in such practices, a new standard is established for the basic preparation of the nurse.
5. There is a need to develop a standard set of best nursing practices that are grounded in cost-benefit methodologies. Tying nursing care into costing and pricing strategies directly (rather than indirectly, as has been the case in bed-based costing) will strengthen the value of nursing in light of specific services and defined populations. One of the major activities of the profession during the next decade will be identifying this price-service relationship.
6. Nursing practice can no longer be identified in isolation from its relationship to the practice of other disciplines around defined populations. Nurses must provide leadership in gathering the requisite disciplines together in a composite activity of patient care planning. Therefore the central activity of nursing during the next decade is building essential relationships between and among the disciplines, creating necessary partnerships, and together designing, implementing, and evaluating the different models, approaches, protocols, and processes of health service delivery.
7. Nurses must establish a more comprehensive database that more clearly indicates the value and the return on investment of nursing services in the system. All activities related to value determination, and to tying rewards and benefits to the measures of value, will strengthen and reaffirm the contribution of nursing to delivery of health care services.
8. There is a need to focus and design nursing curricula in a way that builds on core

competencies in a variety of applications and settings across the continuum of care for basic nursing practice.

9. There will be a growing demand for high-level professional education, specifically for associate degree–prepared nurses, to operate in interdependent settings. These nurses will continue to require carefully moderated and supervised settings where their technical application will be the primary framework for their service delivery. Reallocation of large sums of public dollars for education to baccalaureate and advanced nursing education will be a major policy reorientation.

10. Increasingly, a critical element of nursing practice are those activities that affect the formation of direction, structure, and legislation or other policies having an impact on health care delivery. It is of growing importance for every nurse to know that decisions in the legislative arena have as many implications for practice as decisions in the practice environment have. All nurses have a political obligation to articulate the issues and to be advocates for their practice and their profession.

Each of these areas has significant policy implications in the academic, service, and political settings and at the local, systems, regional, and national levels. The national level of nursing leadership is obligated to establish standards, guidelines, and a framework for dialog that can guide the thought and action of nurses in the local and regional health systems where planning activities unfold. Nursing and health care administration has an ethical and moral obligation to ensure that nursing is involved in all issues related to governance, patient care planning, service delivery, protocol development, and outcome evaluation. No sustainable patient care delivery program can be outlined in a meaningful way without the involvement, investment, and engagement of the nursing discipline. Failure in this endeavor would compromise the viability and the safety of the approach to the consumer and would increase both the amount of time required and the energy necessary to readdress inadequate design and structure when it becomes evident that an approach is nonsustainable.

Consequently, nursing will need to be considerably assertive in this decade in clarifying its role, valuing its contribution, and affirming its obligation to advocate for subscribers receiving health care in any number of arrangements. Rather than wait for an invitation to the policy table, nurses should initiate the establishment of patient-care policies, structural models, cost parameters, and service-based frameworks.

TRANSITIONS IN NURSING LEADERSHIP

With many of the recent shifts in health care, it has appeared as though nursing leadership has been sidelined and diminished in its contribution to the health system. Many nurse executives have seen their positions eliminated in the process of integrating the health care organization. Though it is correct to assume that some of this movement is unnecessary or even illegitimate, most of it is not. Many of the most effective nurse executives have actually moved into more significant and powerful positions in the integration processes, with more nurses becoming chief executive officers and chief operating officers than at any time in recent nursing history. The ability to influence political and economic power in these roles is of far greater value to the patient and the profession than the myriad roles that have been eliminated were ever able to achieve.

The role of nursing leadership is no longer focused on protecting or advancing the role of the nurse in a vertically articulated organization. Instead, it is to position the nurse critically at the point of service along the emerging integrated continuum of services. As health care becomes more population driven and subscriber based, the critical location for leadership will not be in the bureaucratic compartments of an antiquated organizational framework. Rather, leadership will be grounded in the clinical processes and relationships necessary to meet the comprehensive needs of defined populations across the continuum of care in a system driven more by the need to preserve health than by the need to treat illness.

The nursing leader of the future is presiding over a system whose journey is away from expensive, highly intensive, late-stage health care to less costly, minimally invasive, early-engagement health service in a managed environment. Indeed, the nursing leader of today should be leading this journey, and in many successful emerging health care systems she or he is doing so. Power in the new environment is not in the vertical location and control one has within a departmental structure but, instead, is located in the horizontal relationships one creates to sustain multifocal and transprovider interfaces in an integrated environment.

There are a number of new expectations for nursing leaders in the emerging health care environment:

- Positioning nurses in key coordinating positions at the point of service, directed to coordinating, integrating, and facilitating the provider partnerships around patient and population processes along the service continuum
- Creating and managing integrated service environments
- Creating structures that merge all providers around patient and service pathways
- Building effective teams
- Facilitating nursing partnerships with physicians
- Constructing better models of comprehensive service delivery across the life span that reflect a subscriber-based system and focus on health processes rather than sickness interventions

THE END OF THE JOB AGE

As we move out of the industrial age into the new sociotechnical age, shifts occur in the context of work. The job, a creation of the industrial age, clearly no longer has imbedded in it the same characteristics that once gave it form (Bridges, 1994a). Most jobs are specifically

defined, functionally focused, and fixed in their location. As work becomes more flexible and decentralized, the ability of the individual to shift more quickly into new activities, functions, roles, and opportunities is the current requisite for success. The measure of work efficacy in today's emerging workplace is no longer simply functional proficiency but a tightness of fit between the skills of the individual and the demands of the workplace for those skills.

Both the kinds of skills required to manage in a decentralized, continuum-based, noninstitutional model of health care and the ability to move fluidly from one locus of service to another are especially traumatic for the nursing profession. Though nurses have traditionally been available to all areas of health care, they have been notably identified with a specific function and activity in a given unit or department. As those activities become more linked and integrated across the continuum of care, they are less position or site specific. This creates a demand for nurses to look more at the flexibility of their activities and functions in a variety of settings and less at expertise and proficiency in any one locus or setting and service (Cummings & O'Malley, 1993).

In the next decade, fewer than half the beds that were available in 1980 in the United States will be used. The focus on case management, primary care, nonhospital intervention, and outpatient services is changing the locus of control from the bedside to the home, business, community, plant, school, and other places where the focus is on prevention and early intervention. Historically, between 60% and 70% of nurses have traditionally practiced in bed-related service environments. With beds being reduced by 50% during the next decade, clearly a large number of nurses (about one third of the profession) will need to move to other settings and service arrangements if they are to thrive.

This shift in both service characteristics and locus also represents a shift in the focus on the relationship between clinical process and definitive outcomes. Increasingly, in a cost-constrained world, the tight control of resources requires considerable emphasis on "deliverables" and value. Therefore a much stronger emphasis on the relationship between activities and results creates increasing pressure on professionals to give evidence of the value of their activities and functions in light of the outcomes that they either influence or directly achieve (Allred et al., 1995). Unfortunately, there are few aggregated data that suggest any clear relationship between nursing activities and sustainable results. Though there is a growing body of data in relation to process and outcome in nursing, there is little research examining sustainable results directly related to nursing action alone. The data that do exist are not broad based nor well defined in conjunction with other activities associated with achieving clinical outcomes and improving the circumstances and health of those served (Fagin, 1990).

As the focus moves from jobs to positions, roles, and relationships, critical elements must emerge which ensure that the needs of both the consumer and the professional are equally addressed. When the needs of either the provider or the consumer are lost in the process of change, service suffers, its ability to be sustained is compromised, and the quality of the service is significantly reduced. In addressing the issues related to the changing workplace, nurses must focus on the following:

- Developing policies related to the critical role of the nurse in the continuum of care, universal standards of care based on validated protocols, community expectations for the delivery of health service, protocols for ensuring the "tightness of fit" between service structures and the specific needs of defined populations, and the relationship of nurses' roles within the interdisciplinary team format
- Ensuring the portability of tenure, remuneration, benefits, and position as nurses move fluidly across a variety of service settings within a health care system
- Clarifying the core functional expectation of nursing roles in facilitating team process, patient activities, continuum-based planning, and the movement of patients across the service settings

- Verifying and ensuring the role of nursing in providing leadership in the planning, development, and implementation of innovative initiatives for the delivery of health care across the system's service continuum

A TIME OF CHANGE FOR UNIONS

In this era of reorganization and retooling of the workplace, collective bargaining units are facing great obstacles and challenges. What was once clear in a growth-oriented, expanding health care marketplace is no longer true in a constraining, efficiency-obsessed health system. The ability to negotiate is severely compromised, and the foundations for advancement through the collective bargaining process are brutally challenged. In many instances today, nurses are forced to negotiate simply to keep their jobs.

Many of the strategies used by unions in the collective bargaining process no longer achieve the results once expected of them. While unions are touting the value they have and the role they play on behalf of employees, they cannot protect the worker from the vagaries of necessary changes and the essential retooling of the health care system. All of the downsizing, role reconfiguration, and cost-managing activities are central to the organization's effort to reconfigure itself for a changing health care environment.

Therefore it is imperative that unions expand their role with and for nurses. They must begin the shift to a different frame of reference if they are to be sustained. The percentage of collective bargaining agreements will not grow substantially over the long term unless there is a tighter fit between the functions and purpose of the union and the values of the nurse. Furthermore, the union must be more cognizant of the realities affecting the future of health care and the health system's response to those changes. Following are some of the shifts necessary to ensure that health care unions thrive:

- A union agenda more specifically aligned with that of the localities. One of the most significant complaints of union membership is the sublimation of the local needs to those of the larger union priorities.

- Financial elements of the union contract that include performance measures and some connection of salaries to productivity and the financial status of the health care organization.
- The realization that the character of health care for the foreseeable future is grounded in building partnerships at all levels of the system. The union, too, must build partnerships and be a stake holder in the viability of the organization.
- Union recognition that negotiating for one group has direct implications for the relationships with other groups. The organization cannot simply negotiate compartmental and segmented elements of a relationship with one party at the expense of its relationships with other members of the system.
- The establishment of multiunion negotiating. Where possible, unions will need to join with other unions in the organization to bargain conjointly so that the time and resources of all the parties are not fragmented and stretched. Establishing some common frameworks around which to negotiate creates efficiency and builds consensus around issues.
- Evolutionary thought regarding the relationship of the worker to the health care system. Increasingly the worker is a stake holder in the emergence of the system. Systems are communities requiring a different set of relationships than institutional and industrial models have had in the past. Unions must see themselves as members in the process of creating the future and become co-creators of models and processes that better fit what health care is becoming.
- Flexible definitions of worker roles and environments. Workers in the future work environment will need to have mobile skill sets and to be able to move fluidly through a number of different arenas of service in the system. The notion of finite roles and fixed settings for work is simply nonsustainable.
- Judgment about work conditions and circumstances based on better data processes. Anecdotal stories of horror, lack of safety, and inadequate service are emotionally compelling but are not the foundations on which to build an economic and social contract.

Neither unions nor health care organizations can act as though the conditions and circumstances influencing their relationship haven't changed. The old industrial-age adversarial model is no longer a sustainable format for their relationship in the emerging health system. Both groups must alter approaches and methods to create a more equitable relationship and a more even table at which to negotiate. Both must extend to the other the information and data that underpin the reality to which each is responding. Both must know they are stake holders of the future and that decisions cannot be made which hold the future hostage to an inadequate view and recidivistic processes.

THE NEED FOR COORDINATED AND INTEGRATED NURSING PRACTICE

One of the emerging problems in the health care system is the location of well-prepared, quality providers both in the management of subscribers and in primary-service provision in an early-engagement delivery system. The focus of early engagement requires more emphasis on early assessment and intervention before high-intensity, high-cost, high-intervention needs arise. Increasingly, primary care and the services related to it become of vital importance. If the goal is to keep costs low and generate a healthier subscriber population, a great deal of emphasis on the appropriate location, use, and preparation of primary care providers and managers of the continuum of care is vital.

Certainly, physicians will play a major role in the processes associated with primary care. The medical establishment is working quickly and diligently to expand the number of primary care practitioners available to the emerging managed care market place. However, what will be needed in the new managed care environment will be less medical attention and more health service. The script for the emerging market over the long term is early engagement, delay of onset of symptoms, and personal accountability for health, development, education, and prevention. All these issues, though an important foundation for medical practice, are really broader health-based issues that require a different education from that traditionally and currently being taught in medical schools, even in the arena of primary care.

Fortunately for the health care system, the curriculum, framework, scope, and perspective for preparing the future nurse are health driven and broad based. The nurse in the emerging managed-care environment must now exhibit skills that relate to and integrate well with the skills of many other providers. The integration of the expectations, behavior, insights, and breadth of education of the future nurse will need to incorporate skill sets that include relationships, communication, critical thinking, group dynamics, and team processes.

Though specialization will still have some value, most specialization in a managed care environment will follow the requisites of clinical paths that represent the population's rather than the provider's delineation of services (Cronenwett, 1995). Instead of using diagnostic models to discern service requirements, population- or health-based models will be employed. For example, instead of obstetrics and gynecology as practice delineation, women's health is emerging as the predominant practice delineation. Nurse providers in women's health will require a broad-based preparation and understanding of women's issues across the life span. Structural organization of services may emerge around such delineations as adult health, family health, women's health, the health of children, gerontology, behavioral health, and community health. All provide the legitimate, conceptual, contextual, and content framework for advanced nursing practice in the near future. The following are specific and immediate concerns around changing nursing practice roles that will need to be addressed in the next decade.

- A radical retooling of the educational institutions to prepare an adequate number of nurses with broad-based preparation to as-

sume care roles in rural, urban, systems, community, and acute care settings will be necessary in the short term.

- Partnership currently defines the character of interdisciplinary relationships in the health care workplace. Partnership requires a share in both the demands and the rewards of service provision. Therefore nurses should develop collaborative relationships with physicians and other disciplines in a way in which they share the obligation, benefits, and rewards of the practice. Nurses should be treated no differently, in terms of remuneration, benefits, and other rewards, from physicians and other interdependent professionals.

- Competition in the health care system will continue; however, the competition will be more broad based—that is, between health systems rather than between practitioners or hospitals. The competition between systems will be based on the evidence they provide with regard to the efficacy, efficiency, quality, and value of health care across a number of measurable variables documented by the national quality databases of the Health Employer Data Information Set, the National Committee on Quality Assurance, and others. In this way the buyer, consumer, or subscriber can make more useful, informed choices with regard to those health systems that better meet the needs and interests of the consumer. Nursing's value and competence must be tied to outcome expectations if that value is to be measured and translated into sustainable, consumer-based outcomes.

- Regulation of licensure at the state level has been a historic mandate in the United States; however, differentiation between requirements in one state and another is certainly diminishing, if not disappearing. In the next decade, serious efforts at creating a national standard of practice and national criteria for licensure will make mobility within the health system easier, the standardization of expectations clearer, and the measurement of competence more consistent across the nation.

- There will be increasing caution with regard to the preparation and use of unlicensed assistive personnel (UAPs) in the health care delivery system. There is already ample evidence to suggest that UAPs do not necessarily ensure the viability, quality, and effectiveness of care delivery. Therefore each health system will give more careful consideration to the role and number of UAPs, as well as to the expectations of their relationships with others. During the next decade it will become clearer that there is limited value for this minimally skilled worker in a more complex, distributive, judgment-based health care system. Unlicensed and unregulated workers will be primarily relegated to functional tasks and iterative activities under the direct planning, control, and supervision of licensed nurses. There will not be an uncontrolled proliferation of unregulated workers to the extent that most nurses today fear. The obligation for clear policy and functional, skill-based determinations regarding the role of the unregulated worker will be an important obligation of the nurse at every level of the health care system. This obligation is a subset of the role of patient advocacy as it recognizes the consumer's right to expect nursing advocacy for the appropriate, effective, yet efficient level of service (which includes UAPs) aligned with the best possible achievable outcomes within the prevailing cost framework.
- Granting credentials and privileges to nurses will be made easier by the demand for their role within health systems. Depending on the strength and assertiveness of nursing within health systems, advanced practice nurses will be privileged. Increasingly, the law will make it possible for those disciplines not historically credentialed by medicine to be credentialed in more broad-based health systems. There is already evidence that chiropractors, holistic health practitioners, and acupuncturists, as well as advanced practice nurses, are obtaining privileges in continuum-based and full-service health systems.

- Policy structures and hospitals and health systems will be necessarily more broad based. The formation of unilateral, discipline-specific, departmental, and compartmentalized policy is being replaced by policy that is inclusive, horizontal in its delineation, and effective at addressing needs across the system.

It can be anticipated that the preparation and the use of nurses will unfold within these contextual frameworks. As we move to pathways of health service for population groups, we will increasingly need nurses in the workplace, because 70% to 90% of those working-aged adults paying for health care are employed. Increasingly the control of employees' early diagnostic and preventive care will become an important part of the service delivery structure and the continuum of care. Therefore nurses must also have skills in occupational, social, and family dynamics in a host of care settings, including the workplace. This is no less true with the underserved, the aged, and those with behavioral and social adjustment problems. All will require some level of early intervention and engagement to prevent later high-intensity, high-cost, high-intervention, and high-risk service. A percentage of the population will require, from time to time, the high-cost, high-intensity, high-intervention services. Nurses with basic preparation, as well as advanced practice nurses, will be required in these settings as well. Indeed, a growing arena for nursing practice will be the acute care environment. These nurses will provide both case management and high-tech care.

CONCLUSION

Clearly there are a number of policy and practice issues emerging in every place in the health care system. The greatest challenge for nursing at this point in the transition is to get past issues that relate to mourning necessary losses of a style of practice that is forever gone. They must now respond to a call for a new context and character for practice that is more mobile, fluid, and integrated with the activities of a team. Many of the institutional constructs that defined nurses' work are now gone or are going quickly. Nursing cannot be constrained by perceptions of its role, its relationship, functions, and activities that are firmly grounded in the old delivery structures. Nurses now must respond to the conditions and circumstance of this shift in reality in a way that advances their work and the outcomes of that work.

The reality is that we are constructing a new health care system. The journey on the way to transforming the system will be noisy, painful, uncertain, questionable, and certainly challenging. The requirement of the profession and of every professional will be to engage in the process of dialog and negotiation, of strategizing and planning, and of designing and implementing new prototypes, models, frameworks, and processes associated with creating a new cost-efficient, effective, early-cycle, primary-care, health-based delivery system. The movement from a predominantly sickness, late-cycle system to a health-based system will not be easy.

Issues of cost control, efficient structuring, valid outcomes, and value delineation will create a context that increases the stakes and variables adding to the complexity of change. However, it is the work of the time. Nurses have always exhibited the ability not only to confront the issues but also to generate creative strategies in response to them. Nurses are both efficient and effective in generating a higher level of health care and a better health service structure for the community they serve.

The fact that there is confusion, discord, lack of clarity, poor judgment, broad-based latitude, and good structures and bad simply creates the conditions within which the profession must unfold its work. The challenge of the time is to look past the issues of transition toward the process of transformation. While the task is challenging, it is necessary to read the signposts of the journey well, to design the prototypes and experimental responses to the demand for change carefully, to evaluate judiciously, and to make what changes are sustainable and appro-

priate to advance the health of society. This remains the fundamental mission of nursing and the obligation of its work in fulfillment of its social mandate.

REFERENCES

Allred, C., Arford, P., Michel, Y., Dring, R., Carter, V., & Veitch, J. (1995). A cost-effective analysis of acute care case management outcomes. *Nursing Economics, 13*(3), 129–136.

Baker, S., & Armstrong, L. (1996, September 30). The new factory worker. *Business Week,* 59–68.

Barnet, R., & Cavanagh, J. (1994). *Global dreams: Imperial corporations and the New World Order.* New York: Simon & Schuster.

Bennis, W., & Mische, M. (1995). *The 21st century organization: Reinventing through reengineering.* San Diego: Pfeiffer.

Bridges, W. (1994a). The end of the job. *Fortune, 130*(6), 62–74.

Bridges, W. (1994b). *Job shift.* New York: Addison-Wesley.

Brown, M. (1995). The economic era: Now to the real change. *Health Care Management Review, 19*(4), 73–82.

Carlson, L. K. (1994). From garden peas to global brains. *Healthcare Forum Journal, 37*(3), 24–28.

Clare, M., Sargent, D., Moxley, R., & Forthman, T. (1995). Reducing health care delivery cost using clinical paths: A case study on improving hospital profitability. *Journal of Health Care Finance, 21*(3), 48–59.

Coile, R. (1994). Transformation of American healthcare in the post reform era. *Healthcare Executive, 9*(4), 8–12.

Coile, R. (1997). *Five stages of managed care.* Chicago: Health Administration Press.

Cronenwett, L. (1995). Molding the future of advanced practice nursing. *Nursing Outlook, 43*(3), 112–118.

Cummings, S., & O'Malley, J. (1993). Designing outcome models for patient focused care. *Seminars for Nurse Managers, 1*(1), 16–21.

DeWoody, S., & Price, J. (1994). A systems approach to multidimensional critical paths. *Nursing Management, 25*(11), 47–51.

Fagin, C. (1990). Nursing's value proves itself. *American Journal of Nursing, 90*(10), 17–30.

Freeman, R. (1994). *Working under different rules.* New York: Russell Sage Foundation.

Goldsmith, J., Goran, M., & Nackel, J. (1995). Managed care comes of age. *Health Care Forum Journal, 38*(5), 14–25.

Hammer, M. (1996). *Beyond reengineering.* New York: Harper Collins.

Henderson, H. (1996). *Building a win-win world.* San Francisco: Berrett-Koehler.

Hitt, M., Keats, B., Harback, H., & Nixon, R. (1995). Rightsizing: Building and maintaining strategic leadership and long-term competitiveness. *Organizational Dynamics, 23*(2), 18–32.

Leider, R., & Shapiro, D. (1995). *Repacking your bags.* San Francisco: Berrett-Koehler.

Negroponte, N. (1995). *Being digital.* New York: Knopf.

Porter-O'Grady, T., & Krueger-Wilson, C. (1995). *The leadership revolution in healthcare: Altering systems, changing behavior.* Gaithersburg, MD: Aspen.

Slocum, J., McGill, M., & Lei, D. (1995). The new learning strategy: Anytime, anything, anywhere. *Organizational Dynamics, 23*(2), 33–48.

Zander, K. (1995). *Managing outcomes through collaborative care: Care mapping and case management.* Chicago: American Hospital.

VIGNETTE
The Politics of Case Management
Toni G. Cesta

My career in case management began in 1988, when I became involved in the first study funded by the United Hospital Fund of New York (UHF) to look at nursing care delivery and its relationship to length of hospital stay. The UHF is a philanthropic organization in New York City that supports health care research in various forms. This project, called "The Nursing Initiatives Program," was the first nursing research that the UHF had funded. Five New York City hospitals were selected as research sites. I was hired by Long Island Jewish Medical Center to direct its study.

The study had several goals, including reduction in length of stay and improvement in nursing and staff satisfaction through the introduction of new and different ways of delivering care. As I began to implement the study on the first pilot units, little did I know that I was designing and implementing a case management model. In essence, this meant that specified nurses, whom we were then calling "patient care managers," were removed from direct patient care to coordinate the care process for their patients, with an eye to speeding up the care process and reducing length of stay. Satisfaction scores for patients and staff were also tracked for the 2 years of the study (Ake et al., 1990).

In New York City in 1988, this was radical thinking. With very little managed care penetration in the area and barely an understanding of the prospective payment system, the notion of length-of-stay reductions was "cutting edge." Yet there were some physicians who believed that practice guidelines (critical paths) were the right way to go and were interested in supporting the study. We were able to get several clinical groups together, with physician participants, and develop these radical new tools for cost and length-of-stay management.

Unfortunately, the resistance to change in the organization came not so much from the physicians as it did from the administration. One administrator told me that the critical paths would increase length of stay. He believed this to be true because if the path called for a 5-day length of stay and the patient was ready to go home after 4 days, then the nurse would keep the patient the extra day. During these years, it was hard to get length-of-stay data because they were considered confidential. Case management had not yet taken the firm foothold it would take during the next few years.

The study was a success. The length of stay went down, and patient and staff satisfaction scores improved on most of the units. This type of successful pilot study of case management is needed to propel the model forward. Each successful research study, demonstration project, or pilot gives additional data that support the need for case management and demonstrate that it truly does work. Since 1988, I have directed the implementation of case management in four hospitals in New York City and consulted with many others across the country. I have seen at first hand the power of this model when implemented correctly. I have made mistakes and learned from them. And I have influenced others in their thoughts regarding case management, a care delivery model that I believe is essential for our present and future health care systems.

The Historical Development of Case Management

Case management, despite its popularity today, is not new to health care. It has been around for more than 50 years and began as a community model within the fields of psychiatry and social work. In the 1930s, case management was adopted and used by public health nurses. Case management was first introduced into acute care settings in 1985 in response to the prospective payment system. In the 1990s, case management is viewed as a care delivery model that can support the management of quality patient care in fiscally responsible ways (Cesta, Tahan, & Fink, 1997).

In the 1970s, several demonstration projects, funded by the federal government, studied the effects of case management on long-term patient populations. These initial demonstration projects offered comprehensive case management services to Medicare, Medicaid, and some patients under private reimbursement. Populations such as the mentally ill and the elderly were targeted for case management that provided services across the continuum and included nursing, social work, medical care, physical and occupational therapy, and nutrition services (Cohen & Cesta, 1994).

It became clear in the late 1970s and early 1980s that these case management approaches were effective in coordinating services for complex groups of patients. In the 1980s the federal government began its first significant attempt at controlling health care costs. It was apparent that health care costs were out of control and that much of this cost was associated with misuse or overuse of resources. It was further recognized that much of this waste was occurring in hospital settings (Cohen & Cesta, 1997). The demonstration projects of the 1970s had shown that patients could be effectively managed in alternative care settings outside the acute care environment, and that they could do very well. Acute care settings had become extremely narcissistic, believing that only they could provide quality patient care. But the world of health care was changing, and hospitals were no longer the center of the health care universe. This fundamental change in thinking was a painful one for many health care providers, and one that many still struggle with today.

Prospective Payment

During several years in the early 1980s a prospective payment system for hospital care reimbursement was developed to control the cost of health care and the use of resources. The diagnosis-related groups (DRGs) were created to categorize "like type" patients into groupings that would determine hospital reimbursement. The industry abruptly moved from a "fee for service" reimbursement to a fixed-sum reimbursement. The candy jar's lid was sealed. Health care providers could no longer bill and be paid for each and every thing they did, or for each service they provided, essentially without question. DRGs meant fixed sums of reimbursement based on the category into which the patient was placed after discharge. This *wake-up call* to health care providers meant that they had to control their own expenditures because the dollars flowing in were now finite and fixed.

The prospective payment system, mandated

for all Medicare patients, was eventually adopted by many states for Medicaid patients. Some states adopted it for other payers as well. This system, using the DRGs as the foundation, was designed as a mechanism to control both cost and length of stay in the hospital. The premise was that if hospitals were paid fixed amounts for various case types, they would be forced to control their expenditures. Unfortunately, one critical concept was overlooked. Though this system controlled dollars paid to hospitals, it did not do the same for physicians, particularly those caring for medical patients. For these physicians, reduced length of stay and reduced admissions translated to reduced income. Many physicians were resistant to adopting any conceptual model that would affect their income, and they hid behind threats that "quality" would be affected in negative ways. Terms such as "discharge them quicker but sicker" became mantras for those opposing any controls on spending. Even though the literature abounded with documentation of waste and overuse in the industry, many physicians resisted altering their practice. And because, in the final analysis, physicians ultimately control costs, the prospective payment system was essentially and finally a failure.

Managed Care

It was during this period that the managed care organizations began to take a firmer foothold in the industry, negotiating extremely competitive insurance rates. Managed care proliferated in this dysfunctional health care system. And though the prospective payment system had little impact on physician income, a managed care system meant heavy income cuts, either in the form of negotiated discounted rates or capitated risk contracts. To survive, physicians formed alliances such as physician groups and independent practice associations (IPAs), with the goal of pooling resources, managing costs, and maintaining profits.

Hospital-Based Case Management

In 1985, case management was introduced into hospitals as a care delivery system for controlling cost and length of stay under both the prospective payment and the managed care reimbursement systems (Cohen & Cesta, 1997). It became apparent that the means of delivering care in acute care settings had to change dramatically if organizations were going to survive. Though case management was initially slow to gain popularity, a direct relationship can be seen between the amount of managed care penetration in a geographic area and the degree to which case management is being used as a delivery system. The initial case management models were introduced in direct response to prospective payment, but it quickly became evident that there was a relationship between case management and managed care. Today, organizations are more likely to view case management as a system to respond to managed care; thus the perceived need for this type of delivery system has grown.

Change is Still a Dirty Word

I am often asked where I find the greatest difficulties and barriers in implementing case management in hospitals and community organizations. Even though we now deal with a shrinking hospital-based health care system and with tremendous layoffs and downsizing, nurses, physicians, social workers, and administrators are still reluctant to change the status quo. This is mind boggling. Even after layoffs have occurred, there are still those incumbents who do not understand what has happened or why it has happened.

The greatest resistance to change comes from two factions. The first are the staff nurses. Many staff nurses continue to function in a political void. They may have a limited understanding of what is going on in health care in the broad sense, and they therefore are incapable of translating these broader issues to their daily experience where they work. If they have not stayed abreast of current events and the professional literature, "selling them" on case management takes months and years. This resistance comes from a failure to understand the reasons that changes need to take place and what they will mean to our profession with time. Some nurses do not understand that the ability to demonstrate skills that no other profession has, such as those of the nurse case manager, makes us marketable and indispensable.

The other shortsighted and highly resistant group is the physicians. Though a small minority accept case management because they see it as a means to an end, a greater number almost seem to blame the very vehicle that can help them. I believe that this resistance is completely driven by financial considerations. In markets such as New York, where managed care penetration is around 30%, physicians still believe that tremendous financial gains can be made by inappropriately admitting patients, extending the length of stay, and using vast amounts of resources. They choose not to acknowledge that these are the very behaviors and attitudes that have brought managed care to our doorstep. Not until the financial rewards have completely dissipated will the vast majority of physicians support case management as a strategy for survival.

In today's health care environment, the best way to win the support of any group is through education. It has been my experience that nurses educated to the current issues in health care are much more supportive of the changes that take place in organizations with the introduction of case management. I conduct on site educational programs that include topics such as health care reimbursement systems, the role of the case manager, and outcomes management. The more educated the nurses are, *and the more educated all the disciplines are,* the more supportive they will be.

A Case Manager Is a Case Manager Is a Case Manager

Confusion continues to surround case management and the role of the case manager. In managed care organizations, the utilization functions of the insurance company are conducted by an employee of the managed care organization, using the title of case manager. This role is typically one of utilization review conducted by the insurer. Length of stay, resource utilization, and discharge planning benefits are distributed or denied on the basis of these reviews. Because this function is a financial one, some physicians and administrators are confused when case management is introduced into a care delivery setting outside the insurance company. Many have had experience with the case manager in the insurance company and are not familiar with the clinical functions of a case manager in a care delivery setting, where the role is more clinical and less financial.

Time and resources are needed to educate the physicians and other care providers to clinical case management and the various types of case managers, and to assist them in understanding that in the care delivery setting the case manager has functions above and beyond those of utilization review. Today's case managers are found in all care delivery settings across the continuum, including acute care, community care, and subacute, long-term, and home care. They perform clinical functions including assessment, planning, monitoring of outcomes, negotiation of benefits with third-party payers, discharge planning, and patient education, just to name a few.

The history of case management in the social work profession adds another level of confusion. Social workers have traditionally used the title of case worker or case manager, but today's case manager's functions are distinct from those original roles from the 1940s through the 1970s. Two things have happened concurrently. The first has been the questioning of the social worker's place in the acute care setting. With shorter lengths of stay and rising acuity levels, social workers have been less able to develop therapeutic relationships with patients and families. Many had taken over discharge planning functions during the past two decades. When the social worker has had to pass the baton to a nurse to answer the third-party payer's clinical questions or to make the most appropriate clinical discharge plan, time has been wasted, length of stay has been extended, or insurance denials have occurred. Discharge planning now includes high-tech clinical services in the home, and clinical assessment skills are critical to the process. For these reasons, discharge planning has been moving under the umbrella of case management functions and has caused social workers to feel anxious and fearful of their job security and their place in the future health care system. Though social workers can have beginning relationships with patients and families while they are in the hospital, the bulk of their work in the future will take place in community outpatient settings.

Designing Case Management Models

In the hospital setting, case management can be designed in a number of different ways. When an organization decides to implement a case management model, design issues must be agreed on. These include some fundamental and basic questions:

- Who will be the case manager?
- What role functions will the case manager assume?
- How will other departments be affected by the creation of a new role?
- Will a case management department be necessary?
- What other jobs/positions in the organization can be eliminated with the introduction of this new role?
- To whom will the case managers report?

Clearly, these design questions may represent serious restructuring issues for an organization considering development of a comprehensive case management model.

Though it seems logical to assume that a care delivery system would be designed to meet the needs of the patients and the organization in the most effective way, this has not always been the case. Internal political battles rage around case management's place in the organization and its functions and scope of responsibility.

Case management departments have been restructured under many different departments, including operations, nursing, quality assurance, medicine, social work, and finance. Typically, once an organization has decided to implement case management, many departments may vie for case management to come under their

jurisdiction. Though these decisions should clearly be based on the case management department's design, goals, and staffing, in reality there may be other driving forces. These are generally political.

Implementation of a comprehensive case management model will result in the integration of previously disconnected departments. This may cause tremendous *turf battles* for the administrative incumbents who are trying to protect their departments. Ultimately the decisions driving design and accountability may be based on the political strength of an administrator or department.

For example, it may be more appropriate to place the case managers under operations or under nursing. The vice president of operations may have less political strength than the physician leadership, and the case managers may ultimately find themselves reporting to a physician, although this design may not be the best for the organization.

Successful Case Management

The key to a successful case management model lies in the organization's ability to put aside politics and, as objectively as possible, to create a design that meets the organization's current and future needs. The ability to put logic ahead of politics may be so subjective that outside consultants may be necessary. External consultants can be directed by the organization in a particular way, or they can be given free reign to design the model. If given free reign, they will have no political allegiance or agendas and may be best prepared to make the most objective decisions for the organization. If the model is designed solely around political agendas, it may not be designed for success.

In the final analysis, effective case management models must incorporate design elements that meet the goals of the organization. The case managers must be clinically competent and must assume enough role functions to be effective. If their function is redundant, the model will be too expensive to operate and the outcomes and goals will not be achieved. In other words, clear delineation of the case manager's job functions and responsibilities must be teased out from those of others already in the organization. These others may include social workers, utilization review nurses, and discharge planners.

Education must be an emphasized step in the implementation process. Educational programs should be geared toward physicians, nurses, social workers, administrators, and all support departments. A lack of education will make the change process much more difficult and potentially less successful.

Summary

We have finally begun to see case management move toward being viewed as a specialty area with a unique set of skills and a specialized knowledge base. This recognition is taking place in professional organizations such as the American Nurses Association and in academia. Universities and colleges are acknowledging the need to introduce case management concepts and related issues into undergraduate and graduate programs. Topics such as health care reimbursement systems, quality care measures, and continuous quality improvement are being added to curricula. This formalization of case management as a specialty will fully legitimate it and, it is hoped, finally have it fully accepted by our profession. After all, how can we expect other disciplines to accept case management when our own profession still struggles to define and recognize it?

If politics is indeed defined as "influencing the allocation of scarce resources," then the role of the case manager may be considered first and foremost a political one. Case managers balance health care resources with the clinical needs of their patients—resources that are generally dictated by a third-party payer. Case managers must balance dwindling health care dollars against the patient's needs, the physician's plan, and the available resources, and they make these kinds of decisions every day.

Developing and implementing a new case management delivery system takes courage and commitment on the part of the organization, the leadership, and the care providers. In today's increasingly complex health care system, how can we expect anything less?

References

Ake, J. M., Bowar-Ferres, S., Cesta, T., Gould, D., Greenfield, J., Hayes, P., Maislin, G., & Mezey, M. (1990). The nursing initiative program: Practice-based models for care in hospitals. In I. E. Goertzen (Ed.), *Differentiating nursing practice into the twenty-first century.* Kansas City, MO: American Academy of Nursing.

Cesta, T. G., Tahan, H., & Fink, L. (1997). *The case manager's survival guide: Winning strategies for clinical practice.* St. Louis: Mosby.

Cohen, E., & Cesta, T. (1994). Case management in the acute care setting: A model for health care reform. *Journal of Case Management, 3*(3), 110–116, 128.

Cohen, E., & Cesta, T. (1997). *Nursing case management. From concept to evaluation* (2nd ed.). St. Louis: Mosby.

Chapter *16*

STRATEGIES FOR CHANGE IN THE WORKPLACE

KARREN KOWALSKI

Because change is a continuous, evolving process, human beings accept change when it is gradual and doesn't create too much discomfort. Resistance occurs when change is excessively rapid, is radical in nature, or requires significant alterations in individual behaviors (Senge, 1990). For example, moving an office may be a nuisance but is not the end of the world in terms of change. Switching from a typewriter to a computer requires a different set of skills and thought processes. It is an opportunity for the person to "look inadequate or inept" and can be threatening; thus resistance sets in.

Convincing someone, whether it's a secretary or a nursing-school faculty member, to make a major change can involve the highest level of political skills. Politics is merely a set of tools that focus on persuasion, the effective use of power, the analysis of problems or obstacles, and the creation of effective teams. These political tools are all used to accomplish goals within organizations. When stated in this way, the use of skills and tools has a positive connotation. Yet politics in the workplace is often seen in a negative way. One point of view includes utilizing power and influence to acquire something by competing with others (O'Malley, Cummings, & King, 1996). This competitiveness can be set up in a win-lose format so that the person using the best politics wins and everyone else loses. In fact, politics is much like power, in that it can be perceived in a negative context. Because power is defined as the ability to do or act, it is a neutral

concept. The critical issue becomes how politics and power are used. Either can be used for good or used in a selfish or an egotistical way for the aggrandizement of personal means and goals.

When we are looking at what has an impact on the politics of an organization, the external forces can be knowledge of competitors, strategies and approaches, demographics of patients, rate of change related to health care, and how the institution is viewed by the community. The internal forces that have an impact on the politics of change include being able to identify where the power is and the decision making occurs. Is decision making formal or informal? What are the needs of the individuals who influence the decision-making process? With whom do you build coalitions? Who is sympathetic to your plans or ideas? Is it realistic to believe that some resources can be shared? Is the timing appropriate? Consider the following example:

In the process of creating a new program, one nurse executive was asked by the perinatal physicians to create an expanded or advanced clinical practice role that would support them in increasing the volume of high-risk patients. Considerable resources were to be expended on education and preparation. The nurse executive was concerned that these new nurse practitioners be accepted on a broad basis within the specialty area, rather than seen as minions of one particular physician. She explored the needs of the remaining physicians to see whether she could construct the role in such a way that the remaining physicians would have need of the services. To this end, these nurses were trained to scrub in the operating room for emergency procedures, specifically cesarean sections, and were made available to the general obstetricians. The physicians could do surgery at night without calling their partners in to assist. This saved time and money. The physicians discovered that the nurses were competent, able to assist them, and extremely knowledgeable about specific procedures as well as reproductive anatomy and physiology. With a positive experience in the surgical suite, the physicians began to use the nurse practitioners to care for other patients in the facility. Within 3 to 6 months, not only were the advanced practice nurses scrubbing for cesarean sections, they were also monitoring patients in labor, doing various procedures such as biophysical profiles, and providing assessments of patients to physicians when they were in their offices.

The role of advanced practice nurses has been immensely successful because the nurse administrator paid attention to the needs of the physicians and the skills of the nurses and created a useful role for both physicians and their patients. She also focused on the nursing perspective through emphasis on both the curriculum and practice of the role of traditional clinical nurse specialists. She developed a broad perspective, looked for ways to build coalitions of support, justified the financial impact, and compromised with competing interests.

- She persuaded administration to give her 6 to 12 months to get the obstetricians/gynecologists (OB/GYN) to support the new role (they were initially resistant—they wanted residents).
- She identified where the power was (the perinatologists and then the OB/GYNs) and sought to obtain support and build coalitions, first with one group and then with the second group.
- She identified the obstacles (resistance on the part of the OB/GYNs) and developed strategies (help in the middle of the night, which saved them time and money) to overcome the obstacles.

- She developed a team of nursing administrators, perinatologists, staff nurses, and students who were all focused on the same goals—developing the new critical care nurse practitioner role.
- She involved allied health professionals (e.g., social workers and respiratory therapists) so that they were included and enrolled in this significant change.
- She was conscious of timing. There was no need to force issues or acceptance of the role by the OB/GYNs. No conflict was created. She merely made a service available and waited for physician need to accomplish the goal.

POLITICAL STRATEGIES FOR INFLUENCING THE HEALTH CARE ORGANIZATION

Influencing health care organizations will ensure the survival and focus of nursing for the next century—more nurses have learned the skills and tools to be able to exercise such influence. Frequently we see nurses moving into senior administrative positions that are responsible, not just for nursing, but for much of the operation of the organization.

Identify Decision Makers

One of the most important political skills is to identify who makes the decisions in the organization and where the organization's power lies: who controls the resources, which includes the allocation of time, money, personnel, and space. For example, if there is a major special project such as preparation for the Joint Commission on Accreditation of Healthcare Organizations (JCAHO), how much time, money, and personnel are dedicated to the project? How is the assessment made regarding the extent of the project, the number of people needed to accomplish whatever goals have been identified, and the amount of time to be devoted to preparation for the JCAHO review (people who would otherwise be providing care for patients)? It is also important to identify who will support the nursing perspective on how the project should move forward and what the advantages are for administration, physicians, and others to support it.

Another important aspect of identifying where the decisions are made is clearly identifying your own personal strengths. To a great extent, influence or power comes from *competence.* When you are competent, you are perceived to be knowledgeable, reliable, creative, and able to solve problems. Competence includes self-acknowledgment of your competence: having the confidence to know that you can do whatever needs to be done. It is also knowing that if your ideas or perspective do not win the day, there is always another opportunity, another day.

Develop a Plan

When one is proposing a project or significant change, it must be clearly thought out and presented with the use of the format and style acceptable to the institution. It may be a business proforma, which each institution seems to do differently. It may be an oral presentation with only basic tables of information. It may be a discussion or lunch with the most influential member of the executive committee or a member of the board of directors. It is most important to discover how these ideas or projects are presented and to honor the format, at least in the beginning.

Identify Financial Resources

If an idea or project requires financial support, and few do not, it is pivotal to be creative about where such funding might be obtained. Financial support could be available through philanthropic entities, grants, or cost savings from other areas or investments. It is important to demonstrate that you have thought through the financing. Have some ideas about how the project could be cost effective or cost neutral.

Manage Conflict

When strong passions and commitment exist and resources are limited, conflict and adversarial positions can result. The nurse who facilitates conflict resolution also furthers the cause of the profession, enhances a reputation for competence, is a team player, and furthers the mission of the institution. It is valuable to learn and practice conflict management skills (Northway, 1996). (See also Chapter 9: Conflict, Politics, and Policy.)

Common Mission and Goals

It is helpful to connect the proposed projects to the espoused mission and goals of the organization (Mason & Leavitt, 1995). For example, utilizing the patient and family as central to the mission of the organization often unites opposing points of view. Physicians want the best possible care for their patients, and this goal can be used to move to common ground when there are differences in perspectives that create some animosity. Everyone wants to generate enough income to remain financially viable. This common ground can also be used to shift people from immovable positions.

Timing

The timing of discussions and requests for various special projects is critically important. For example, nursing is most apt to receive additional resources to improve charting in preparation for JCAHO visits. Money to support a perinatal nurse practitioner program came from a need to maintain the high-risk perinatal service when OB/GYN residents were withdrawn from the institution. Be flexible enough to take advantage of such situations. On the other hand, an example of poor timing is asking for additional staff when redesigning and downsizing are the major focus of the organization.

Communication

Effective politics requires effective communication skills, much like those used to persuade a staff nurse to work an extra shift or to persuade an unwilling postoperative patient to turn and cough. Such communication tools include speaking effectively, listening actively, eliminating blame and judgment, creating compassionate relationships, and writing clearly.

SPEAKING EFFECTIVELY

Traditional research (Wallechinsky, Wallace, & Wallace, 1971) indicates that public speaking is the number one fear expressed by the majority of Americans (death is number seven). Many people believe that they are unable to speak effectively, and some people demonstrate that they cannot speak effectively. Because speaking effectively is key to communication, it is valuable to devote time and energy to learning this skill. Being a powerful presenter is like many other aspects of life and politics: it is a "learned" skill. Such skills increase the likelihood that nurses can accomplish their goals and objectives.

LISTENING ACTIVELY

Active listening means that the listener is completely focused on the speaker. It means listening for the essence of the conversation so that the listener can actually repeat, back to the speaker, the speaker's intended meaning. It also means being 100% present, absorbing words, posture, tone of voice, and all the clues accompanying the message, so that the intent of the communication can be understood. This activity requires a very high level of concentration and eliminates the option of developing a defensive response or argument in a listener's head while the speaker is talking. Examples of active listening include conveying interest, helping to clarify problems, pulling out key ideas, responding to people's feelings, and summarizing specific points of both agreement and disagreement.

ELIMINATING BLAME AND JUDGMENT

The most effective speakers and communicators are those who refrain in both public and private conversation from blaming others for the issues and problems in the organization. They avoid judgment and gossip about who is being ineffective. Both of these activities involve making someone else wrong, which allows the speaker to be right. We all have an intense desire to be right. Being right gives us a sense of control over our environment. However, it also builds walls and prohibits us from learning about other human beings and their ideas—learning that can have immense value in accomplishing goals and solving problems.

CREATING COMPASSIONATE RELATIONSHIPS

One of the ways to avoid blame and judgment is to think compassionately about the individual with whom one disagrees. Strive to understand the other person's struggles. At the core of most disagreement is pain and fear. For example, it is easier to be compassionate about physicians who are upset if we focus on the pain and fear that create their response. Understanding the pain and fear allows us to have more compassion for where that person is and what it is that he or she is attempting to accomplish. It decreases blame and judgment and supports each of us to solve problems rather than to be angry and defensive.

WRITING CLEARLY

The use of basic writing tools is also a learned behavior. Remedial writing is available in colleges across the United States. The ability to write clearly is easily acquired.

Use of these five skills enables the nurse to influence various groups within an institution and to influence the distribution and utilization of resources. Effective use of these skills generates respect for nurses.

Attitude

Attitude is paramount to one's success in political negotiations, both in the workplace and in life. Attitude is a way of thinking, acting, or feeling toward a situation or person. It is the outward manifestation of our core beliefs. There is considerable research about the importance of one's attitude (Brown, Cron, & Leigh, 1993; Cooper, 1979). In business, the one who is most successful is the one with the best attitude. Although research varies in this area, there is general consensus that approximately 20% of success can be attributed to aptitude, which includes information, intelligence, and skills; 80% of success is attributed to attitude. It is the dominating factor that separates top producers in the business world from mediocre producers.

The most successful people have a "can do" attitude. They believe there isn't anything they can't organize or accomplish. All the changes in the health care system and the constraints placed on available resources could easily impact people's attitudes in a negative way. Stress, anxiety, frustration, anger, and resistance—all are negative emotions and are common responses to intense pressure in health care. Such negative attitudes and emotions contribute to the impression that "I can't accomplish whatever needs to be done." One of the most important deterrents to a positive "can do" attitude is fear and self-doubt.

A negative attitude is highly contagious. It not only impacts individual performance but prohibits people from building liaisons and cooperative ventures to solve problems. One nurse executive is fond of talking about the glass being half full or half empty. Those people who consistently see the glass as half full focus on opportunities: "I can." They feel empowered, and they have fun. Those who see the glass as half empty often focus on all the things that aren't working, who is to blame, and why they are powerless to take action. Who would you rather spend time with?

INTERDISCIPLINARY COLLABORATION VERSUS COMPETITION FOR SCARCE RESOURCES

Collaboration hinges on relating to coworkers, including physicians, administrators, and allied health workers. One of the key aspects of getting things accomplished, politically, is

developing strong relationships. Experienced nurses know that they are much more apt to succeed in creating a change in patient-care delivery if they collaborate with the doctors, administrators, or allied professionals who must concur with the changes.

The most critical relationship in a health care institution is the relationship between nursing and medicine. Is it collegial, or is it adversarial? Collegial relationships obviously create more opportunities to accomplish goals than do adversarial relationships. Yet nursing is often in an adversarial relationship with medicine. There are reasons for the adversarial relationships, not the least of which are power struggles, differences in education, differences in focus or emphasis, and competition for scarce resources.

In the evolution of adversarial relationships, some people feel excluded. The concept of "in-ness and out-ness" can have far-reaching ramifications. Most of us want to be valued and recognized within our institution. We want to be known and understood. Within the leadership group, most people want to be at the core of decision making, power, and influence. In other words, they want to be in the "in group." Research has demonstrated that those who feel "in" cooperate more, work harder and more effectively, and bring enthusiasm to the institution (Weisburg, 1988). The more people feel as though they are respected and have access to information and resources, the more they contribute. The more "out" people feel, the more they withdraw, work alone, daydream, and engage in self-defeating behaviors. Conflict between groups results when individuals feel they are "out" and are striving to be "in." These folks are more apt to use negative behaviors. Thus adversarial relationships are created that can lead to schism and divisiveness, prohibiting groups from accomplishing goals.

Constructive relationships are good for goal attainment, which is paramount in the delivery of patient care. The Pew-Fetzer Task Force issued a monograph entitled *Health Professions Education and Relationship-centered Care* (Tresolini, 1994). They describe relationships as the core of patient healing. They identify the relationship between the practitioner and the patient as the essence of the care that is given. This relationship is vitally important to both parties because it is the medium of exchange for information, feelings, and concern. It is a major factor in the success of therapeutic interventions and an essential aspect of patient satisfaction. The task force identifies this relationship as the most therapeutic aspect of the health care encounter. When these relationships disintegrate, litigation ensues.

The task force not only identifies the relationship between the patient and the provider as key to the therapeutic intervention; it also discusses the major impact of the relationships between providers and the influence they have on the healing process of the patient. The relationship between providers requires teamwork, shared values, mutual learning and sharing of expertise, and support for others to learn and develop. The ideal relationship supports setting aside issues such as hierarchy, privilege, and "specialism."

The task force encourages health care practitioners in their personal growth in the following four areas:

- Self-awareness
- Continuing self-growth
- Developing and maintaining relationships with patients
- Communicating clearly and effectively

These areas of self-growth apply not just to individuals as patient-care providers but to anyone who wishes to be politically astute. It is critical for individuals who want to motivate change and successfully accomplish goals to be self-aware and have an ongoing interest in their own self-growth. This includes expanding both a knowledge base and interpersonal skills, which facilitate the development and maintenance of relationships with peers and others in the system. The task force believes that practitioners, as human beings, are the most relevant factor in the quality of care provided and especially in the quality of the relationships that are established. Self-respect and respect for patients and other

care providers are essential. It may not even be important to be a charismatic communicator if one's intention, purpose, compassion, and respect for others is clearly identifiable and modeled.

An example of nurses' working on both their own personal growth and collaboration is the following case study:

Recently a team of neonatologists and neonatal nurses experienced a breakdown of communications with a subspecialty group of cardiologists. The cardiac specialists were excellent clinicians and significantly increased the patient volume for the hospital. They had worked extensively with the pediatric internists, were comfortable with these relationships, and wanted all their patients to go to the pediatric intensive care unit. Incorporating the cardiologists into the neonatal team proved to be an exercise in frustration. There were clinical disagreements and interpersonal conflicts. The interpersonal interactions disintegrated to the point where they could best be described as mutual distrust, lack of cooperation, and conflict over control of the patients. It would have been easy for all parties to throw up their hands and say: "Enough, get these guys out of here. We're done." This kind of response would have been in direct conflict with the philosophy of the institution, which promoted patient- and family-centered care and healing. There was also a strong emphasis by leadership for staff to have meaningful work relationships among interdisciplinary team members. The members of the unit's leadership bided their time while being supportive to the cardiologists. When negative incidents occurred, the nurses resisted blaming anyone and focused on the best care for neonates. They did problem solving with staff and physicians. Because the nurses were so calm and evenhanded, the physicians were willing to be more reasonable. The nurses continued in a calm way to make points for both quality patient care and problem solving.

The neonatalogists and the cardiologists both shared the goal of the best possible care for babies. From this perspective, the team members decided that they would make additional efforts to enroll the specialists. The nurses waited for an appropriate time, when the cardiologists' need for help and service was high. The nurses succeeded in getting everybody together in the same room, and both groups of medical professionals were able to identify areas of mutual respect. Both groups were willing to listen to each other's concerns. Care guidelines and areas of responsibility were identified, ideas on how to improve communication were discussed, and a plan based on patient needs and the corresponding agreements was implemented.

Relationships improved dramatically. Are there still issues that come up between the specialists and the neonatal group? Of course. But a concerted effort to rise above conflict was demonstrated, and it has been successful in shifting how the team members relate to one another.

INTERFACING WITH CONSULTANTS

Most institutions, when faced with cost containment, downsizing, reduction of staff, and staff resistance, seek to accomplish these changes through the use of consultants. Most often, consultants come in to tell the caregivers how to institute changes. Given the stress that downsizing produces, it would be natural for staff to be negative toward consultants. Negative attitudes, hostility, or open conflict may provide short-term gratification but in the long-term may prove excruciatingly painful when the consequences of the negative behavior occur. Consequently, it works best if nursing personnel and nursing leaders are positive about the opportunities to make changes and to create a more cost-effective, patient-focused system. Know up front that the nursing personnel budget is usually more than 60% of the hospital budget. Of course, consultants will look first at cutting positions.

Stay current with the literature. Offer suggestions based on what has been researched and found effective. Keep track of what has worked in other parts of the country, as well as what hasn't worked. Bring as much data and information to discussions as possible. Administrators like data and "facts." These can help make a case and create options. Be willing to give up some things that are relatively painless so that the most important items, such as bedside caregivers, can be retained. In negotiations, always have a Plan B and a Plan C just in case Plan A is rejected. It is important to speak up respectfully. Don't go quietly into the night. It works best to be proactive, using powers of persuasion and political knowledge of the organization to influence consultants on behalf of nursing and patients. This is accomplished primarily by being cooperative and providing data and information needed by the consultants while asking many questions about how the consultants see things. At the same time, maintain a positive attitude and convey clearly, in writing and verbally, what the nursing perspective is and any creative ideas for solving problems.

When consultants come into institutions to tell caregivers how to institute changes, it is easy to see the consultants as threatening. Units close and staff members are laid off, downsized, or encouraged to take "early retirement." Staff members feel out of control in such situations. A psychiatric nurse colleague is fond of saying that human beings want two things out of life: to have control over their environment and to create meaning in their lives. When major change such as downsizing occurs, staff members feel uncertain and believe they have lost control over their lives. With these radical changes, some people question the meaning of their work because the finances appear to take precedence over the quality of care for patients. Staff members become fearful, and the quality of the work environment deteriorates.

CREATING AND MAINTAINING A SUPPORTIVE WORK ENVIRONMENT

A supportive, high-quality work environment makes a world of difference in accomplishing goals. It provides a positive environment for learning (Senge, 1990) and helps to create mutual trust and respect. Such an environment begins with a vision—usually of a better work world. One nurse executive said she wanted to create a healing place for patients and families as well as for staff. That would translate into a place where all are treated with mutual respect while blaming and making others wrong are minimized (Kowalski, Burton, & Rehwaldt, 1997).

In support of such a creation, guidelines or agreements about how people will relate to one another help staff to accomplish the goal of a positive work environment. One example (see Box) was compiled by Marie Manthey (1992). When guidelines are written and shared, it is much easier to hold people accountable for behavior that deviates from the agreements. Some institutions are now incorporating evaluations of these behaviors into performance appraisals.

Because how we treat each other is key to our political goals, to our ability to influence others in the organization, and to our maturation as professionals, it is appropriate to evaluate these behaviors. In some settings, staff have been counseled to find other employment because they were unable or unwilling to control behaviors that violated the agreements. Though this approach has not been common, it will become so in the next century because of the vital importance of effective teams.

A negative or unsupportive work environment is hazardous to physical well-being; thus nurses will be considering the environment when making job decisions. The positive, creative, flexible staff will be drawn to a supportive environment.

Regardless of how unsupportive a work environment seems to be, nurses have choices. Even though they sometimes feel out of control and powerless, they have options. The dualism of our society leads us to believe that the choices are A or B, black or white, yes or no, go or stay. However, there are always multiple choices. The number of choices is limited only by our own creativity. We can take an active part in how the workplace is redesigned; we can change jobs within the workplace; we can move on to case management or quality assurance; or we can acquire additional education and skills (i.e., advanced practice roles in nursing). And if the situation seems impossible, we can go after another job or start an entrepreneurial venture.

COMMITMENT TO MY CO-WORKERS

As your co-worker, with a shared goal of providing excellent nursing care to our patients, I commit to the following:

- I will accept responsibility for establishing and maintaining healthy interpersonal relationships with you and every member of this staff. I will talk to you promptly if I am having a problem with you. The only time I will discuss it with another person is when I need advice or help in deciding how to communicate to you appropriately.
- I will establish and maintain a relationship of functional trust with you and every member of this staff. My relationships with each of you will be equally respectful, regardless of job titles or levels of educational preparation.
- I will not engage in the "3 B's" (bickering, backbiting, and blaming) and will ask you not to as well.
- I will not complain about another team member, and ask you not to as well. If I hear you doing so, I will ask you to talk to that person.
- I will accept you as you are today, forgiving past problems, and ask you to do the same with me.
- I will be committed to find solutions to problems, rather than complaining about them or blaming someone for them, and ask you to do the same.
- I will affirm your contribution to quality patient care.
- I will remember that neither of us is perfect, and that human errors are opportunities, not for shame or guilt, but for forgiveness and growth.

Written by Marie Manthey, reprinted by permission of Creative HealthCare Management, 614 East Grant Street, Minneapolis, MN 55404.

There are always choices. In politics, there is always the next election. In health care, there are new administrations and new opportunities!

Change and politics are a constant in the workplace. But each of us chooses how we respond to the workplace, how we effect change, how we use skills and tools, and how we create, build, and exercise political influence in the organization.

REFERENCES

Bridges, W. (1991). *Transitions: Making sense of life's changes.* Reading, MA: Addison-Wesley.

Brown, S. P., Cron, W. L., & Leigh, T. W. (1993). Do feelings of success mediate sales performance–work attitude relationships? *Journal of the Academy of Marketing Science, 21*(2), 91–100.

Cooper, M. R. (1979). Changing employee values: Deepening discontent? *Harvard Business Review, 57*(1), 117–125.

Kowalski, K. E., Burton, L., & Rehwaldt, M. (1997). Revisioning, re-educating, re-generating and re-committing: Nursing in the 21st century. *Nursing Outlook, 45*(5), 220–223.

Manthey, M. (1992). *Commitment to my coworkers.* Minneapolis, MN: Creative Nursing Management.

Mason, D. J., & Leavitt, J. K. (1995). The revolution: What's your readiness quotient? *American Journal of Nursing, 95*(6), 50–54.

Mason, D. J., Talbot, S. W., & Leavitt, J. K. (Eds.). (1993). *Policy and politics for nurses: Action and change in the workplace* (2nd ed.). Philadelphia: W. B. Saunders.

Northway, R. (1996). Leading to politics. *Nursing Management, 3*(7), 12–13.

O'Malley, J., Cummings, S., & King, C. S. (1996). The politics of advanced practice. *Nursing Administration Quarterly, 20*(3), 62–72.

Senge, P. M. (1990). *The fifth discipline: The art and practice of the learning organization.* New York: Bantam Doubleday Dell Publishing Group.

Tresolini, C. P., & The Pew-Fetzer Task Force. (1994). *Health professions education and relationship-centered care* (Rep. No. 415-476-8181). San Francisco: The Pew Foundation.

Wallechinsky, D., Wallace, I., & Wallace, A. (1971). *The book of lists.* New York: Bantam.

Weisburg, M. (1988). *Team work: Building productive relationships.* In W. B. Reddy & K. Jamison (Eds.), *Team building blueprints for productivity and satisfaction* (pp. 62–71). Alexandria, VA: National Institute for Applied Behavioral Sciences; San Diego, CA: University Associates.

Chapter *17*

COMMUNICATING AND COLLABORATING FOR CHANGE IN THE WORKPLACE

ANNA MARIE BUTRIE AND HANK NOWOHOLNIK

As the health care system evolves, the rate and magnitude of change will increase and the landscape will be filled with failed change efforts. As the environment continues to heat up and the number of players escalates, the opportunities for managing change effectively will become more apparent. The need to do so will become more critical.

The effective management of major, multiple, and constant organizational change is the specific competency that will determine the extent to which organizations will survive, much less thrive in the future. To keep pace with and successfully lead all these health care changes, nurse leaders must become comfortable with the ever-changing health care environment. This is often difficult because human beings are extremely control oriented. We feel the most competent, confident, and comfortable when we believe that we have some level of control in our lives. This control assures us that our expectations for what is and what will happen are being met. Change disrupts those expectations and often results in feelings of anxiety, fear, conflict, and stress. Even if we see the change as a positive one, these emotions will surface as we

Reprinted from *Journal for Healthcare Quality, 18*(5), 9–11,30, with permission of the National Association for Healthcare Quality, 4700 W. Lake Avenue, Glenview, IL 60025-1485. Copyright © 1996 National Association for Healthcare Quality.

experience and learn new behaviors and as we learn to adjust to new expectations in our environment (Ernst & Young, 1996). Consequently the effective nurse leader needs to expect change to occur, anticipate the change, and then manage the disruption associated with it in the organization. This requires that nurse leaders manage the entire situation, including the short- and long-term implications of the change (e.g., implementation of new technology).

BARRIERS TO AND ENABLERS OF ORGANIZATIONAL CHANGE

Major organizational change initiatives do not have a particularly good track record of successful implementation. Though some efforts have succeeded wonderfully, others have spelled failure from the very beginning and throughout the process, mainly because of poor implementation practices rather than because of pursuing the wrong solution.

In our experience, failed major change efforts in organizations occur because of the lack of appropriate action on two fronts:

1. Dealing with the fear, at all levels in the organization, that surfaces when any major change effort occurs
2. Generating and maintaining the necessary commitment of executive and key stake holders to sustain the process until successful implementation

Fear: An Ingredient of Major Organizational Change

By definition, fear is present in every change initiative, at every level. This is true for both personal change efforts and organization-wide efforts. It is a natural and necessary human response to all unknowns. It keeps us alive and keeps us going. Deming noted in his 14 points that, to achieve change (Total Quality Management [TQM]), one must "drive out fear" from the organization (Walton, 1985). This statement by itself is misleading. To remove all fear is likely impossible and certainly impractical. In fact, it is fear that motivates change far more often than anything else does. Tony Robbins (1986), nationally recognized personal performance guru, states that everything we do is motivated by either fear or pleasure and that, of the two, fear is the more powerful. If we think about everything that we or our organizations have done, we will realize that fear has often been the principal motivator: fear of lost opportunity, fear of failure, fear of success, fear of being ignored, fear of being found out. Yet, in major change efforts, we sometimes fail to recognize or appreciate the fear that is present and to act in accordance with it.

Executive Commitment: A Determinant of Success

The presence or lack of strong executive commitment to the major change initiative is an important determinant of whether the effort will succeed. Only the executives have the power to legitimate and drive the change through successful implementation. Senior management's decision to begin a major change does not necessarily mean there is sufficient commitment to sustain the initiative. The senior management's resolve must be strong enough to overcome the fear that surfaces during the initiative.

Fear of reprisals, fear of the physicians, and fear of loss of power or status are common. These fears sometimes result in an inability to take the hard stand, to make the hard decisions, or to take the necessary steps. We sometimes forget that change is a long process, and, as such, commitment levels must be built, sustained, and strengthened throughout the life of the process. Anticipating fear and resistance and managing them, while building and maintaining strong commitment by executives and others throughout the process, are key to successful implementation. Doing those things is what is called "change management," the use of which is critical for the success of any major change effort.

As attempts are made to manage each change effort, it is important to remember that change is a process, not an event. Regardless of the merits of the individual change effort, it is unlikely that implementation of the change will be successful just because "it is a good idea," "it is the right thing to do," or even if "the CEO wants it." Many variables within the organization need to be orchestrated and managed to implement major organizational change. The extent to which these variables are present and effective in the organization enables successful change; the extent to which they are missing or ineffective creates barriers to successful change. These variables include the following:

- Communication
- Consequence management
- Education
- Management of resistance
- Development of change agent skills
- Organizational alignment

Besides managing events that occur up to and on the actual day of implementation, other things such as individual personalities, the corporate culture, and resource constraints must be addressed. Senior management, including nurse leaders, must take ownership for leading the organization, managing the individuals, and focusing the resources to ensure that change will occur successfully. These senior executives must recognize that their organizations are composed of complex dynamics. One change, no matter how small, will have a ripple effect on the multiple systems within the organization. Nurse leaders must anticipate the effect that the change will have on the organization and must orchestrate the appropriate steps to ensure successful implementation.

INCREASING THE CHANCE OF SUCCESS

Successful major change initiatives require the management of multiple implementation issues within the organization for the duration of the effort, and often beyond. Because of limited resources (time, money, people), it may be necessary to prioritize these issues. In our experience, the highest priority should be given to the following activities:

- Building and sustaining executive and key stake holder commitment
- Communicating
- Anticipating and dealing with resistance

The following provides some further discussion of these implementation issues.

Building and Sustaining Executive and Key Stake Holder Commitment

For successful change to occur at all levels of the organization, the change mandate must come from the top. However, it is important to remember that the demonstration of commitment from senior management is more than just the communication of the vision and the decision to implement. It also includes the issuance of directives, the use of consequence management when necessary, and "walking the talk" both publicly and privately. Senior management must take responsibility for the successful implementation of the change. Senior management can delegate implementation tasks to others, but it cannot delegate responsibility for the success of the effort or for the necessary changes needed to be made by the executives themselves.

Communicating

It is important to recognize not only the commitment level needed but also the types of communication necessary to build that commitment. One can never overcommunicate the vision, goals, objectives, and status of any major change effort. For large-scale efforts, it is critical to develop a comprehensive communication plan. The communication plan should address who in the organization needs to receive information, what message should be sent, how often it should be sent, and when it should be delivered. All effective modes of communication that currently exist should be used, including newsletters, rounds, and meetings. In addition, new modes of communication should be explored, including videos, posters, presentations, and a change-specific newsletter. The frequency of updates to the various constituencies should also be determined. It is imperative that the communication modes provide for both upward and downward communications. This will allow senior management to identify resistance early and throughout the process, so plans can be developed to address effectively the identified resistance issues.

When one is developing communication messages, it is important to recognize that communication is not the same as "education." Some organizations assume that sufficient communications are provided regarding the change initiative when employees are being educated. Although an educational session provides a wonderful opportunity to communicate bidirectionally, communication occurs when a message is delivered and received, whereas education exists when knowledge or skills are transferred. Although related, the two are separate and should be used differently.

Who provides the communication and education varies with the message that needs to be delivered and the skills that need to be transferred. It is important to have the change message communicated by the key sponsor, whereas education should be provided by the technical expert. The amount of time and the cost that should be attributed to the communication and education effort vary by the amount of change that will result in the organization. The larger the groups affected by the change effort (both directly and indirectly), and the more roles that are affected by the change, the greater the amount of communication and education needed to implement the change successfully.

Anticipating and Dealing With Resistance

Resistance can best be described as the push back, or the drag on any effort to change or move from the current state. Regardless of how well you communicate the vision, goals, and objectives of the change initiative, resistance will occur. Regardless of whether the changes are perceived as positive or negative it cannot be avoided. Resistance is not necessarily a sign that something is wrong but, rather, an indication of the amount of disruption that people are feeling during the state of transition.

Let's look at this issue in another way. Imagine a large box, and that our job is to move that large box some great distance. On the basis of our previous experience, we know that moving the box will cause resistance. In physics, we call that resistance friction. The friction that is caused depends on the size of the box, the box's weight and composition, the distance to be traveled, the condition of the surface to be moved across, and so forth. To overcome this resistance and successfully move this box may require many more steps than just getting behind the box and pushing. For example, some or all steps we could take include the following:

- We may prepare the surfaces of the box or the surface to be moved across.
- We may get more people to help us move the box.
- We may remove some of the obstacles in our path.
- We may employ some sort of pulley system to aid our efforts.

The resistance to any major change effort must be anticipated and managed. The strength and reasons for the resistance must be determined, and actions must be developed to address the resistance, drive new behaviors, and avoid backsliding. The following are key levers to define and reinforce needed behaviors (Ernst & Young, 1996):

- Clear communication of the vision, the business imperative, and the status of the effort
- Identification and clarification of desired roles and behaviors
- Development of education and training programs to enable staff to learn these new behaviors and skills
- Identification of performance measures and reward systems to reinforce and encourage these required behaviors
- Development of compensation systems to further encourage the appropriate behaviors and actions
- Demonstration of leadership behaviors to support the major change
- Development of an organizational structure to support these new work behaviors

These actions help the organization to realign itself in such a way that desired changes are reinforced by the organizational, human resource, and management systems in place. In addition, behaviors previously sought or accepted but no longer desired in the new organization are discouraged and no longer reinforced or rewarded.

As an example, in a reengineered patient registration process, registrars are responsible for the collection and verification of demographic and insurance information and for registering the patient on admission. New behaviors that may be sought could include accuracy and timeliness of the capture of patient demographic and financial information, and the timeliness of greeting the patient and following through. The effectiveness of the new process could be ensured by supporting and encouraging actions that could include measuring and monitoring the registrar's performance on the basis of new criteria such as payment denials. Compensation and reward would be based on this performance.

For further reinforcement of these new behaviors, the organizational structure may be realigned to reflect the new process. For example, the registrar could report organizationally through the service line division, where performance will be evaluated on the basis of new indicators.

CONCLUSION

A successfully implemented major organizational change requires that the change process be managed effectively. Seeking the right solution is a necessary but insufficient element in today's health care environment. Not only does the solution need to be right, but it must also be successfully implemented. Some of the following issues should be considered for high priority when major organizational change is implemented: building and sustaining commitment, communicating effectively, and managing resistance.

If these issues are addressed and a transition plan is developed to manage the people, process, and technological objectives of your organizational change effort, your level of success is likely to improve. Without the use of these "change management" techniques, your level of success will most assuredly be lower.

REFERENCES

Ernst & Young, National Office. (1996). *Business change implementation framework.* Cleveland: Author.

Robbins, A. (1986). *Unlimited power.* New York: Ballantine Books.

Walton, M. (1985). *The Deming management method.* New York: Dodd, Mead.

Chapter *18*

ENSURING THE FUTURE OF NURSES IN CLINICAL PRACTICE: Issues and Strategies for Staff Nurses and Advanced Practice Nurses

BEVERLY L. MALONE AND DAVID KEEPNEWS

Nurses today face challenges as never before as we seek to continue what we have always done—provide the best, highest-quality care to all patients and populations. Changes in practice, in the organizational and financial contexts of health care delivery, and in the political and policy arenas all demand not only that nurses remain flexible and adaptable but that we identify and hold fast to the core values that define our profession—and that we find the best ways to effect those values.

The impact of these changes on nurses and on nursing practice—both the short-term effects and the potential long-range implications—are innumerable. What do these changes mean for nurses? What are the prospects for nursing's continued role in the health care delivery system? What strategies will be needed to ensure that role?

NURSING AS A CLINICAL DISCIPLINE

In its essence, nursing is a clinical discipline. As a profession, and as a discipline, nursing is concerned with the health of individuals, families, and communities—with identifying what interventions are needed to maintain or to restore health or to ensure comfort and optimal functioning and then carrying out those interventions. This identity and these functions are what all of nursing has in common. Although nurses play a broad spectrum of roles in health care delivery, this clinical core of nursing practice is what unites every type and variety of nursing role and specialty.

To be sure, a great many nurses have applied their nursing education and experience, with great creativity and a continued commitment to patient care, to a myriad of roles. For example, nurses serve as policymakers, attorneys, lobbyists, political activists, and public officials and, in those roles, have continued to serve their profession and the cause of safe, quality health care services. These roles build on their incumbents' clinical background, which enriches their abilities to serve in those roles. But they do not negate or alter nursing's basic identity as a clinical profession.

That identity has been forged since Florence Nightingale's time and has been redefined, expanded, and refined into a consistent and proud tradition of providing an increasingly broad range of preventive, restorative, and therapeutic health services to individuals, families, and communities in all settings. The broad-based education that nurses possess, their ability to serve in a wide variety of roles, along with their organizational placement within health care agencies and institutions, has thus far meant that nurses' central role in health care delivery appears assured.

Nursing's continued centrality as a clinical discipline is challenged and shaped by the same factors that are altering the health care delivery system as a whole.

A common complaint from nurses in health care institutions—staff nurses and managers alike—is the increasing role of nonclinical personnel in making administrative decisions. Many health care institutions, following the lead of other businesses, have eliminated much of their "middle management" level. This has often meant that the nurse managers responsible for administering hospital clinical services have been eliminated and replaced by nonclinical managers with graduate-level business or health administration preparation. The diminished nursing presence in hospital governance often means that the clinical impact of day-to-day budgetary, staffing, and other administrative decisions may not be taken into account. Many hospitals have shifted the "traditional" director-of-nursing position to add other patient care areas and, often, nonclinical operational areas. Some have "decentralized" their organizational structures in such a way that there is no identifiable "head" of the nursing department. Many have eliminated mid-level nursing management positions, often replacing them with managers who possess no clinical background or professional affiliation. To some extent, these moves mirror attempts to reduce nursing's clinical role at the bedside. They contribute to a decrease in nursing departments' cohesive identity within hospitals and other institutions and systems. The support for the clinical and career development of the registered nurse (RN) becomes lessened. This lack of a clear commitment to RN careers affects the RN's ability to meet the challenges of a changing, technologically evolving system of delivering valued health care services.

Indeed, nursing's position within the health care system is changing, in large part because of the economic and business changes that have overtaken the system as a whole. Whereas, under fee-for-service arrangements, the length and intensity of inpatient services had a direct and positive correlation with hospital income (i.e., the more services delivered, the larger the hospital's charges), under capitated systems of payment this is no longer the case. Rather than representing a source of revenue (through delivery of more intense hospital services), RNs appear to many institutions to represent a cost only.

That perceived change in relationship to hospital cost and revenues has, in part, led to changing patterns in utilization of RNs. As health care institutions seek to reduce costs, their operating budgets, of which labor is a significant component, make an obvious target. RNs are among the most highly paid hospital employees, as well as among the most numerous. Thus hospitals have, in many instances, decreased their use of RNs while increasing their utilization of unlicensed assistive personnel and other ancillary workers. At the same time, because of both capitation and technological advances, patients are being hospitalized for shorter periods (or circumventing hospitalization altogether by receiving treatment on an outpatient basis), which means that the hospitalized patient population is, in general, more acutely ill and in need of more intensive services than before, including quicker patient education and other preparation for discharge.

Though there appear to be wide variations, regional and otherwise, in nurse staffing patterns, for a great many RNs these changes in staffing patterns, coupled with growing patient acuity, have made for more stressful and significantly more difficult work. Old assumptions about safe staffing levels no longer hold as hospitals experiment with a variety of reengineering and patient care redesign schemes. Unfortunately, these experiments are often undertaken with little or no data to suggest their safety or efficacy. RNs, challenged with continuing their professional and ethical duties to provide and ensure safe, compassionate care to the patients under their charge, report increasing difficulty in ensuring safe, let alone quality, patient care.

Endemic to many patient care redesign initiatives is an effort to move RNs away from the bedside into roles as managers or coordinators of care provided by ancillary personnel. Of course, the nurse's role in coordinating and overseeing care is nothing new; what is new is an effort to remove the centrality of the nurse's role in providing direct care. An appreciation of nursing's clinical role must include a recognition of some of the functions that nurses perform beyond direct-care tasks: for instance, assessment of patient care needs, planning and evaluation of care; discharge planning, patient teaching, and oversight of ancillary personnel. Many nurses, however, aptly question the feasibility of performing these functions in isolation from the role of direct caregiver.

CHALLENGES TO ADVANCED PRACTICE REGISTERED NURSES

Increasingly, advanced practice registered nurses (APRNs) face challenges to their clinical roles as well. For one, APRNs continue to encounter many of the same barriers that have limited them for decades: limitations on insurance reimbursement, artificial restrictions on scope of practice, limited prescription-writing authority, difficulty in gaining admitting privileges, and other factors that impede their ability to practice to the full extent of their preparation and abilities. Nursing has achieved some hard-won successes in eliminating many of the restrictions on APRN practice during the past several years. The most recent and most prominent example is discussed later in this chapter: the passage of legislation in 1997 to provide Medicare coverage of nurse practitioner (NP) and clinical nurse specialist (CNS) services regardless of geographic setting. Since 1989, federal law has also required state Medicaid programs to cover the services of certified family NPs and certified pediatric NPs. At the state level, impressive victories have been won in the area of scope of practice, including prescription-writing authority.

However, even these important victories are to some extent threatened by other changes in the health care system. As increasing numbers of state Medicaid programs move into managed care arrangements, often using a primary care case management, or "gatekeeper," approach, many APRNs find themselves shut out from these critical primary care roles. This threatens their ability to provide services for Medicaid patients. Similarly, many private insurers that have moved to utilize preferred provider arrangements or other systems that require patients to receive services from a panel of approved practitioners (or that provide significant financial incentives to do so) have excluded APRNs from their provider panels (Mason, Cohen, O'Donnell, Baxter, & Chase, 1997). As more businesses have moved to provide services by means of "self-insured" plans, they have also freed themselves from state-imposed mandates (including, where applicable, requirements to cover APRN services) because of the federal Employee Retirement Income and Security Act (ERISA), which preempts state regulation of such plans.

Another challenge to the APRN role has come with an increasing emphasis on the training and production of primary care physicians: after a decades-long period during which physician specialists and subspecialists found more prestigious and lucrative careers than their generalist colleagues, more and more physicians have adopted the primary care role, encouraged by opportunities under managed care and by some conscious efforts to attract physician trainees into primary care residency programs. For those who have viewed APRNs in primary care provider roles as physician "substitutes," this shift has raised the question as to whether APRNs are necessary. Predictions of a physician surplus have suggested to some observers that the need for nonphysician practitioners may be sharply reduced.

Whether such predictions are realized or not depends on a number of factors, including whether significant numbers of physician specialists are able and willing to be retrained or redeployed as primary care practitioners. It also depends in part on society's interest in expanding access to primary care services for currently uninsured populations—an interest that was expressed in legislative health care reform initiatives in the earlier part of this decade but that has currently faded from national focus since the failure of those efforts and the increased role of the "market" in determining health care priorities.

There is little question that a variety of health systems, including managed care plans, have utilized APRNs successfully in providing both primary care and specialty services. Under the impact of short-term competition between systems and plans, however, some may seek to alter the role of the APRNs whom they utilize: for instance, some plans may seek to capitalize on consumer concerns about health care choice and quality by limiting the role of APRNs and promising consumers that they will receive services from a "real doctor."

One recent development in the opposite direction is worth noting. In February 1997, Columbia-Presbyterian Medical Center in New York City entered into an agreement with Oxford Health Plans, a large managed care organization, under which Oxford's subscribers who receive treatment at Columbia-Presbyterian may, at the patient's option, be seen either by a physician or by an NP who will serve as the primary care provider and whose services will be reimbursed at the same level as a physician's services (Winslow, 1994). The announcement of this pilot project drew a great deal of attention, including prominent media coverage and predictable criticism from organized medicine (Freudenheim, 1997; Jacobs, 1997). This project will potentially offer much useful data about the utilization and cost-effectiveness of the APRN and about patient satisfaction with these services. The APRN in this model is not presented as a physician competitor but as a different provider who emphasizes prevention of disease and promotion of health.

ROLE OF THE CLINICAL NURSE SPECIALIST

As nursing moves forward in establishing APRNs' authority to provide primary and specialty care services, it will also need to reexamine how the role of the CNS can continue to develop and to thrive. The CNS plays a variety of roles, from providing patient care services to serving as a clinical expert, consultant, and support to other nursing staff in hospital, ambulatory, and other clinical settings. Some CNSs fear that an emphasis on the APRN as a provider of "medical" services undercuts the CNS role as a clinical nursing expert. Indeed, CNSs have struggled for the visibility and public understanding of their role that NPs have to a large extent achieved. Many schools of nursing have expanded their NP programs or created new ones while CNS programs have been reduced or closed. At the same time, CNSs in several states have been successful in winning legislation that provides recognition of the CNS as a category of APRN or, at the very least, provides title protection—that is, sets legal standards as to who can be called a CNS. Nursing will need to continue to work to ensure that the CNS role—and changes in that role—are understood, that the CNS role as an APRN is appreciated, and that CNSs are empowered to apply their clinical nursing expertise to the provision of high-quality nursing services in all patient care settings.

DIVERSITY IN NURSING

Another challenge to the continued clinical role is in the increasingly diverse populations that require health care services from RNs. These nurses are, in their great majority, white; the populations for whom they care are increasingly African American, Latino, and Asian. Nurses face the challenge of obtaining and maintaining the skills and values to provide culturally competent, sensitive care. This also means that it is necessary for nursing to take seriously the need to increase recruitment of ethnic minorities into the profession and to make the nursing population begin to mirror the diversity of the American people, for whose care they are responsible. This will mean acknowledging and addressing the financial and other barriers that may disproportionately affect ethnic minorities' access to higher education.

OPPORTUNITIES

Along with the challenges to nursing's role outlined above come many opportunities for nursing, not only to defend its clinical role in the emerging health care system, but to expand it. Some of the expanding roles for nurses that emphasize clinical skills and judgment can already be seen in the increasing use of nurses as case managers in a variety of settings—a role that utilizes the clinical knowledge and the relationship-building, assessment, and care-coordination skills that are central to nursing. Some managed care companies are making greater use of RNs as liaisons between the plan and members of the provider panel. An increasing utilization of home health agencies offers the potential for new opportunities and roles for nurses in providing and coordinating care in the home. This care coordination skill of nurses provides the evolving health care system with the realistic possibility of seamless care between the hospital and the community. It is nursing's gift to health care that foretells the possibility of a technologically merged system based on a partnership between the individual, family, community, health care entities, and providers (including nurses), with the nurse orchestrating the overall coordination of the various services.

The need for nurses in the evolving health care delivery system, however, goes beyond what might be indicated in the "help wanted" section of today's newspaper. During this period of rapid change and of the current ascendancy of "market" forces in the health care system, the demand for RNs is likely to fluctuate for some time to come. To be sure, the not-so-old days in which new graduates could name their pick of jobs and shifts is no longer with us. Predictions and forecasts of the future need for nurses vary wildly—from the Pew Commission's 1995 prediction of a 200,000 to 300,000 surplus of RNs

(Pew Health Professions Commission, 1995), to predictions in California and elsewhere of a possible impending shortage (Sechrist, Lewis, & the California Strategic Planning Committee for Nursing, 1996).

Demand figures, however, even when consistent, tell only one part of the story. Draconian, "quick fix" cost-cutting measures that involve reductions of professional staff will, in many instances, yield to more sophisticated approaches to maintaining an efficient and effective operation.

What can nursing do to meet the challenges to its clinical role and to maximize its opportunities? Recent experience suggests some strategies, as illustrated in the following case examples.

CASE EXAMPLE **APRN Reimbursement Under Medicare**

The passage of Medicare reimbursement for NPs and CNSs in 1997 is a tremendously important example. It points to a number of the attributes that nursing needs to champion in order to meet with success: unity, grassroots activism, and most of all, persistence. On August 5, 1997, President Clinton signed Public Law 105-33—the Balanced Budget Act—into law. Though that comprehensive bill gained widespread public attention for its bipartisan support and for the fact that it included a balanced budget, for nursing the legislation was truly historic because of Section 4511 of that bill, which provided for coverage of NP and CNS services under Medicare Part B, effective January 1, 1998. The bill defines "physicians' services" (the principal service provided under Medicare Part B) to include services provided by an NP or CNS "which would be physicians' services if furnished by a physician," which the NP or CNS is legally authorized to perform.[1] In other words, if the service is within the NP's or CNS's scope of practice and a physician could be reimbursed for providing it, an NP or CNS can be paid for providing it.[2]

Medicare coverage for APRN services had been a central priority for nursing for more than 8 years.

---

[1] Social Security Act, Section 1861(s)(2)(K)(ii).
[2] The bill also, for the first time in federal law or regulation, provides a definition of the CNS: an RN who "holds a master's degree in a defined clinical area of nursing from an accredited educational institution" [Social Security Act, Section 1861(aa)(5)(B)].

Some initial steps toward this goal had been won in previous years. In 1989, Congress extended Medicare coverage to the services of NPs provided to patients in nursing homes. (As noted above, in that year it also mandated state Medicaid coverage of family NP and pediatric NP services.) In 1990, it added the services of NPs and CNSs in rural areas. These were tremendous advances, but nursing increasingly chafed at the limitations it placed on APRNs' ability to serve Medicare beneficiaries. "Rural areas," for instance, were very narrowly defined to include areas that were not within Metropolitan Statistical Area (MSA) counties—which, in practice, excluded some areas that were, in fact, "rural" by most standards and definitely underserved, but that were in the same county as part of an urban area. This situation was frustrating and grew even worse with census changes that reduced the number of non-MSA counties. These census changes also meant that NPs and CNSs in formerly non-MSA counties, who sometimes had built up practices and a steady clientele of previously unserved Medicare patients, were suddenly removed as Medicare providers.

Other problems continued to come up as well. In most urban settings, payment for NP and CNS services was sharply limited to so-called "incident to" coverage, under which services furnished by a physician's employee can be covered, subject to extreme restrictions—such as ongoing physician supervision and even requiring the physical presence of the physician when services are provided. Continued expansion of NP and CNS practice to new settings, and the increasing recognition of the ability of NPs and CNSs to provide services as independent practitioners, made the "incident to" restrictions increasingly problematic. In some settings, such as emergency departments and outpatient hospital clinics, lack of Medicare reimbursement became an economic concern for hospital administrators, often placing the employment of NPs and CNSs in these settings at risk. Clearly, winning NP and CNS reimbursement under Medicare, though long a top priority for nursing, was becoming imperative.

Efforts to secure Medicare Part B coverage for APRNs, regardless of geographic area, continued to gain ground, often coming up just short of success. Reimbursement was included in President Clinton's Health Security Act, as well as in most other comprehensive health care reform proposals in the 103rd Congress, none of which ultimately passed. Reimbursement for APRNs also passed in the 1996 Congressional budget bill, which was vetoed (for entirely separate reasons) during that year's famous budget impasse. The President's 1997 budget proposal included Medicare reimbursement for NPs and CNSs, and NP/CNS reimbursement continued to garner strong bipartisan Congressional support in 1997, thanks to successful mobilization of grassroots support, including through the N-STAT program of the American Nurses Association (ANA). Complementing ANA's activities was the support of nursing specialty organizations, including NP organizations and the American Psychiatric Nurses Association—the latter having a strong interest in Medicare reimbursement for advanced practice psychiatric nurses, including psychiatric–mental health CNSs and NPs. Unity, grassroots support, and more than 8 years of tireless persistence finally paid off on August 5, 1997, when the President signed the budget bill and Medicare coverage for NPs and CNSs became law.

Legislative victories are critical, but so is the successful implementation of those victories. People sometimes make the mistake of thinking that the effort is over once a bill is signed into law. But the process by which that law is implemented by government administrative agencies, often referred to as the regulatory process, is key. In the case of NP and CNS reimbursement, nursing is hopeful for a successful implementation process because the Administration has been in strong support of this measure and because of nursing's willingness to continue to put resources into the implementation phase of this bill. Moreover, the "step by step" victory in the area of reimbursement in which Medicare coverage was won first in nursing homes, then in rural areas, and now in all areas—has meant that the Health Care Financing Administration (HCFA), the federal agency that administers the Medicare program, is already familiar with NPs and CNSs as Medicare providers and has experience with NP and CNS issues to help guide it.

Nursing's victory in winning Medicare reimbursement for NPs and CNSs will also mean that the profession has to pay even closer attention to many of the bigger, broader issues surrounding reimbursement that have been of concern to physicians and other Medicare providers for years. These include billing issues; fraud, abuse, and other legal issues; the Medicare fee schedule (including the payment amounts for different kinds of services and procedures); and the coding of different services and procedures, including their listing and description in the *Current Procedural Terminology* (CPT) code book. Nursing has already been participating for some time in the processes by which provider organizations influence changes in coding and valuation. Nursing is represented in an advisory capacity to the CPT editorial panel, through which the American Medical Association (AMA) determines new billing codes each year. In addition, nursing works with the AMA's Relative Value Unit Update Committee, through which new values are proposed to HCFA for Medicare billing codes—a process that has a major impact on how certain procedures and services are valued by Medicare and thus on the levels at which they are paid.

The biggest challenge that nursing now faces is to demonstrate what NPs and CNSs really can do for their patients, now that Medicare beneficiaries have access to their services.

CASE EXAMPLE Safety and Quality

Another area in which nursing has made important strides in meeting its challenges and maximizing its opportunities is the issue of safety and quality of patient care services. Some of the problems related to health care quality, and the factors related to those problems, were explored earlier in this chapter.

It cannot be assumed that health care will face only a continually downward spiral of quality or that progressively fewer nurses will be utilized in health care settings. A variety of different influences and factors will continue to affect staffing and quality. There is already evidence that public concern is growing and may have an impact on administrators' and payers' actions. Focus groups convened by the American Hospital Association in 1996 revealed widespread consumer concern with decreasing quality of care in hospitals (American Hospital Association & Picker Institute, 1997) and indicated consumers' recognition of the key role that RNs play in safeguarding patient safety and giving quality care. Concern with the impact of managed care and cost cutting on consumer safety helped move President Clinton to appoint an advisory commission on consumer protection and quality in the health care industry, to address consumer and patient safety issues and to develop a consumer bill of rights. As another sign that nursing's role as guardian of patient health and safety is widely recognized, one of the authors of this chapter (B.M.) was appointed by the President to membership in this historic commission. In fact, of the 32 members of the commission, three are nurses: in addition to the ANA president, Dr. Mary Wakefield and Ms. Marta Prado were also named to the commission.

A critical component of nursing's efforts on behalf of quality and safety has been to demonstrate nursing's indispensable role in patient care. Public campaigns, such as ANA's "Every Patient Deserves a Nurse" campaign, and parallel efforts by state nurses associations in New York, Massachusetts, and many other states, are one strategy. Providing patients with tips for a safe, quality hospital experience that includes ascertaining that the provider at the bedside is an RN is an essential strategy for facilitating public support and awareness of quality issues.

Another strategy is reflected in ANA's work on nursing quality indicators. ANA has pioneered efforts to define and quantify outcomes and process indicators that will link patient care outcomes to nurse staffing levels and mix (American Nurses Association, 1995, 1996a, 1996b). Research efforts such as these can enable the profession to demonstrate the correlation between nurse staffing and positive patient outcomes—including financial outcomes. Currently, research efforts focus on acute care settings, but efforts are under way to launch similar efforts for community-based care. Nursing researchers have a critical role to play in the future of the nursing profession as they have the opportunity to document outcomes demonstrated in measurable ways that nursing makes a significant difference.

Nursing's efforts to address quality issues in health care, of course, cannot be successful as a "go it alone" strategy. It is more critical than ever to build alliances of all sorts with others who are concerned about quality issues—seniors, consumer groups, voluntary health organizations, advocacy groups for individuals with specific diseases (e.g., acquired immunodeficiency syndrome, breast cancer), traditional labor unions, and others. And we need to recognize and credit others' efforts to address these issues as well. These efforts come from a variety of sources. The Institute of Medicine, for instance, has an ongoing initiative to address quality issues in health care. As noted previously, the Clinton Administration has made efforts to address quality, including the appointment of an expert commission. Standard-setting organizations, including the National Committee for Quality Assurance, the Joint Commission on Accreditation of Healthcare Organizations, and others, have set specific guidelines by which managed care organizations should be assessed and granted (or not granted) accreditation. The Foundation for Accountability (FACCT) has started its work by developing guidelines for treatment, by managed care organizations, of specific conditions. One of the authors of this chapter (B.M.) also was appointed to the Health Plans and Professionals Committee of FACCT. As a committee member, Malone and other representatives from various health care organizations will help guide the organization in the selection and evaluation of performance measures, their implementation, and the use of performance data by health care organizations. FACCT's specific goals are to endorse a series of health system performance measures, advocate widespread adoption of those measures by existing oversight and consumer organizations, and promote consumers' use of the data obtained from these measures to help make better informed health care decisions ("Malone appointed . . .," 1997).

Nursing has involved itself in a wide range of efforts to address quality problems in health care. Many quality initiatives have focused primarily on managed care practices such as limits on care, lack of choice of providers, and lack of appeal rights. Efforts to "score" managed care plans often have centered on measures such as the time patients spend in the waiting room to see a practitioner, the time needed to book an appointment, and other aspects of plan administration. Though these factors are important, nursing has taken a leadership role in pointing out that a real examination of the quality of care provided under a health plan has to look at the care delivered to patients, whether provided directly by the plan or under contract with practitioners and institutional providers such as hospitals. How do the hospitals that provide care to a health plan's subscribers rate in terms of staffing and patient outcomes? This is a matter of accountability not just for the hospital but also for the health plan that contracts with it to provide care to its subscribers.

This concept of "shared accountability" encourages the open reporting and sharing of data not just at the plan level but also at the institutional level. ANA has spearheaded efforts to require public disclosure of staffing and patient outcome data, and ANA-supported federal legislation, the Patient Safety Act, would make such disclosure part of federal law by requiring it in order for a health care facility to participate (or to continue to participate) in the Medicare program. That Act would also provide protection for "whistle blowers" among hospital employees and would require federal oversight of the health and safety implications of any proposed health care merger or acquisition.

STRATEGIES

How can nursing best confront the challenges to its continued strength as a clinical discipline? How can we best take advantage of the opportunities before us? Step 1 has to be the continued building of strong professional associations at the national and state levels. The profession needs a source of leadership, a base of strength, and a foundation for analysis of challenges and opportunities and for strategic decision making to move the profession forward. Almost 500,000 nurses belong to some type of professional nursing organization. This leaves approximately 1.7 million without any professional involvement or connection. Membership, the collective power of organizations, is a primary strategy for shaping the development of a new, sensitive, patient-partnership health care system. The professional association provides the framework for the profession's collective strength, leadership, and growth. ANA and the state nurses associations (SNAs) are that framework for the profession as a whole. A strong ANA and strong SNAs provide the basis for strong, collegial alliances with other nursing organizations as well. A wide variety of nursing organizations reflect the diversity, specialization, and multiplicity of roles embraced by the profession. To ensure that this variety is associated with strength rather than fragmentation, all nursing organizations need to work as closely as possible and to draw on their common interests and needs.

Beyond alliances within the nursing profession, nursing also needs to build coalitions with other provider groups and, particularly, with consumer organizations. Because of common challenges and common interests, it is possible to work together with organizations that may have some differences from nursing in other areas.

A key part of nursing's strategy is to confront the current challenges by exerting vigorous legislative activity at the state and federal levels. This means working to introduce legislation that moves our goals forward. It also means supporting efforts initiated by others that fit within our goals, such as efforts to ensure expanded access to primary care services and to shape legislation.

Nursing is working on a number of other fronts, as well, to address both challenges and opportunities that face it. At the state level, SNAs continue to work to eliminate barriers to nursing practice. In addition, nursing is identifying new opportunities for the profession—new clinical roles, emerging settings, "growth" areas for professional nursing (e.g., home health care, expanded school health care, and subacute care). This also means pushing to make additional education and training available so that nurses can survive in a changing health care environment and take advantage of these new clinical opportunities as they develop.

One critical avenue for collective strength and power for the nursing profession is through collective bargaining. This has been a powerful weapon, not only to improve wages and benefits for nurses, but also for nurses to address, on a collective basis, the professional issues that confront them where they work. Collective bargaining has given many nurses the chance to negotiate contract language that addresses staffing issues and the use of unlicensed personnel, as well as broader issues, such as ensuring staff nurse input into clinical decision making and protecting nurses' ability and right to advocate for their patients and to engage in professional development activities.

One strategy that cannot be overlooked but is often minimized is the need for nurses to be in policy- and decision-making positions—which is one means of shaping the to-be-determined health care system, instead of merely reacting to continual changes in the system. Nurses must be visible in the media, on hospital and managed care boards, on city councils, in state legislatures and in Congress, as well as in committees and activities at the facility level, including collective bargaining activities. Using the collaborative strength of our organizational power, nurses must be the identifiable advocate for quality performance in the powerful role of traditional "keeper" of quality.

Nurses must achieve optimal power bases through partnering with patients. From this foundation will come the development of other partnerships moving across bridges of collaboration and focusing on the primary mission of meeting the health care needs of the nation.

These challenges demand an immeasurable commitment of time, energy, and resources. Nurses must learn to deploy their energy strategically, building in opportunities to rest, revitalize, and refocus, not only as individuals with family responsibilities, but also as professionals with the responsibility for developing a patient-sensitive system of caring that will not be dominated by cost.

CONCLUSION

There is no way to foretell exactly what the future of nursing's clinical role will be in 5, 10, or 50 years. Some predict the demise of nursing in the face of continued cost-cutting efforts and health care's current "business" focus, but such predictions have been heard before at various junctures in the history of our profession. We believe that, to paraphrase Mark Twain, reports of nursing's death have been greatly exaggerated. But this is not an excuse for complacency. *The future is inventable, not inevitable.* To ensure the best possible future for our profession and the best possible care for our patients, nurses must work today to build a strong professional association, to articulate nursing's messages to policymakers and to consumers, to operate with the greatest possible degree of internal unity based on a common commitment to nursing and patients, and to identify and work closely with our allies, and when necessary with our foes, to advance the cause of safe, high-quality patient care.

ACKNOWLEDGMENT: We thank Linda L. Minich for her research assistance and support in preparing this manuscript.

REFERENCES

American Hospital Association & Picker Institute. (1997, Summer). Eye on patients. *Journal of Health Care Financing, 23*(4), 2–11.

American Nurses Association. (1995). *Nursing care report card for acute care.* Washington, DC: Author.

American Nurses Association. (1996a). *Nursing quality indicators: Definitions and implications.* Washington, DC: Author.

American Nurses Association. (1996b). *Nursing quality indicators: Guide for implementation.* Washington, DC: Author.

American Nurses Association. (1997). *Position statement on privatization and for-profit conversion.* Washington, DC: Author.

Freudenheim, M. (1997, September 30). As nurses take on primary care, physicians are sounding alarm. *New York Times,* p. A11.

Jacobs, J. (1997, March 3). Primary care nurse. *American Medical News, 40*(9), 3.

Malone appointed to national foundation committee. (1997, July). *The American Nurse 29*(4), 3.

Mason, D., Cohen, S. S., O'Donnell, J., Baxter, K., & Chase, A. (1997). Managed care organizations' arrangements with nurse practitioners. *Nursing Economic$, 15*(6), 306–314.

Pew Health Professions Commission. (1995). *Critical challenges: Revitalizing the health professions for the twenty-first century.* San Francisco: Center for the Health Professions.

Sechrist, K. R., Lewis, E. M., & the California Strategic Planning Committee for Nursing. (1996). *Planning for California's nursing work force: Final Report of the Nursing Work Force and Education Forecasting Initiative.* Sacramento, CA: Author.

Winslow, R. (1994, February 7). Nurses to take doctor duties, Oxford says. *Wall Street Journal,* A3:4.

VIGNETTE
Ensuring the Future of Nurse Practitioners in Clinical Practice
Andrea Berne and Elaine Gelman

Ensuring the future of nurse practitioners (NPs) requires a multipronged strategy to influence policies in both the public and private sectors. The New York State Coalition of Nurse Practitioners (NYSCONP) has been developing and refining this strategy to advance NPs' practice in this state. The strategy includes working on legislation, negotiating with managed care organizations, and building coalitions.

Scope of Practice

The 1973 Nurse Practice Act (NPA) in the State of New York was historic in its definition of nursing as an independent profession that diagnoses and treats "human responses to actual and potential health problems." Although the New York State Nurses Association (NYSNA) held that this covered the work of NPs who were diagnosing and treating *illness and disease,* the need to amend the practice act became apparent as NPs in the state began to be charged with practicing medicine without a license.

In 1988, after a long and arduous battle, the NPA was amended to allow NPs to diagnose and treat illness and to prescribe in collaboration with a qualified physician. Most of this work was done by NYSCONP because the need was urgent and support from other groups was not forthcoming. The opposition of the Medical Society of the State of New York and NYSNA made NYSCONP's task even more difficult. Although a small group of NPs was able to overcome this opposition, NYSCONP was not as fortunate as NPs in other states who had the support of their state nurses associations and were able to get legislation passed quickly. NYSNA was opposed to any incremental change in the NPA that was directed at a particular group of nurses and any change that would be perceived as limiting the autonomy of nursing. As a result, the amendment includes language that was insisted on by the medical society but that we initially opposed. NYSCONP preferred no reference to physicians in the NPA, but because "supervision" by physicians had been proposed, we settled for "collaboration."

Though the 1988 amendment to the NPA authorized NP practice, it could not change the limitations imposed on our practice by previously written health-related legislation that never recognized NPs. NYSCONP responded by securing sponsorship for a "practice area" bill, which would remove several of these barriers to NP practice because it would authorize NPs to:

- Perform routine blood and urine testing without having to be licensed as a clinical laboratory. If this bill is approved, it would add NPs to the list of health care providers (doctors, osteopaths, dentists, and podiatrists) who can operate their own laboratories solely as an adjunct to the treatment of their own patients.
- Be medical inspectors in school.
- Prescribe or order home health aide services and personal care services.
- Certify that persons practicing nail specialty, natural hair styling, aesthetics, and cosmetology are free from infectious diseases by signing the certificate required by general business law.
- Perform the routine biennial medical inspection of bus drivers.

As of 1997, this bill had the support of the chair of the health committees in both houses of the New York State legislature.

NYSCONP also has bills in both houses that would allow doctors and NPs to form professional service corporations and permit NPs to perform Workers Compensation physicals and complete the examination report. Clearly the organization is pursuing the legislative route to changes when that is the most appropriate way to proceed. Because this route can be long and sometimes difficult, we attempt to use regulations to change policies when possible.

Direct Reimbursement

Barriers to practice for NPs in New York State are essentially the same as elsewhere in the country. By far the greatest obstacle to overcome has been the lack of direct reimbursement for NP services. NYSCONP has been dealing with this issue for many years.

The same year that the NPA was amended (1989), the New York State Medicaid program included NPs as providers receiving direct reimbursement. The attempt to achieve the same goal through other public and commercial insurers has met with limited success. Physicians are receiving reimbursement for services that NPs are providing. Because there is no mechanism in place for the NP to bill for his or her service, the claim form is submitted under the collaborating physician's signature. For several years, NYSCONP has had a direct-reimbursement bill before the legislature, proposing that this fraudulent activity be eliminated by reimbursing the NP directly. Arguments against passage include concerns that mandating reimbursement for a new category of provider would increase access to care and therefore would increase costs.

To support our position on direct reimbursement, NYSCONP commissioned a study to determine whether or not health care costs increased in states where NPs received direct reimbursement (Blevin, 1996). This study showed that in no instance were health care costs increased, and in most cases, health care costs have declined. The study was distributed to the legislators, and visits were made to the leaders of the health and insurance committees in each house to explain the study. Nevertheless, we have been unable to get legislators to pass the bill. Thus NYSCONP turned its efforts toward negotiating with commercial insurers on an individual basis.

In November 1995, NYSCONP communicated with Dr. Robert Jacobs, the medical affairs director of the Oxford Health Plans in New York City. When presented with the issues of concern to NPs, Dr. Jacobs and his colleagues were interested and sympathetic. We discussed the benefits to Oxford of the use of NPs as competent, cost-effective primary care providers (PCPs). After an hour of give and take, we came away with a commitment on the part of Oxford to explore the credentialing of nurse practitioners as PCPs. The credentialing process moved forward during the next several months with positive feedback. Following NYSCONP's efforts, a large New York City university began negotiating for a select group of its NPs to be credentialed by Oxford. An agreement to credential a group of this university's NPs was made, and the university made news of their unique relationship public. As a result of media attention, the Oxford physician providers were outraged. They insisted that no further credentialing of NPs be made even though only four NPs from the university had been credentialed as PCPs. Because 96% of Oxford providers are physicians, the administrators of the Oxford Health Plan were compelled to pay attention to their demands. NYSCONP will continue to bring pressure on the Oxford Health Plan in an effort to reverse the decision. Fortunately, there are other managed care organizations in New York State that have included NPs as PCPs in their plans (Mason, Cohen, O'Donnell, Baxter, & Chase, 1997). NYSCONP will increase its efforts to expand that list. We have an effort under way to solicit support for our position from our collaborating physicians and our patients. We believe that the health maintenance organizations will respond to that approach.

Coalition Building

After 1989, NYSCONP worked to expand membership awareness of the need for NPs to become politically active. Through a bimonthly newsletter and the continued active participation of the leadership of the organization, we were able to establish a statewide legislative committee. Each of the 20 chapters of NYSCONP has appointed a legislative representative who is responsive to the needs of the state legislative committee. Visits to the representatives in their home offices is a top priority. One outcome of this effort was the introduction of an organized "Lobby Day" at the State Capitol. Our work in this area is enhanced by the addition of a professional lobbyist to the NYSCONP staff. As membership in NYSCONP continued to grow to more than 2,100, the need to reexamine our

mission became apparent. In 1994 a representative group of NYSCONP officers and members met in a weekend retreat to formulate a mission statement and to review and revise the goals of the organization. The number one goal was to build relationships with other organizations and strengthen professional nursing's position in the health care system.

NYSCONP's first successful attempt at coalition building was gaining the support of physiotherapists (PTs), occupational therapists (OTs), and pharmacists to remove specific barriers to NP practice. The practice laws for OTs and PTs mandated that they accept referrals for their services from physicians only, and dispensing medication (samples, or small quantities of a drug) was the province of pharmacists only (and of physicians under special circumstances). By 1993, NYSCONP had secured the right of NPs to dispense medications (under the same rules as physicians) and gained authorization for OTs and PTs to accept referrals from NPs.

NYSCONP has been working on this goal on many fronts:

- We continue to meet with the Medical Society of the State of New York and NYSNA to discuss the changing health care delivery system and how we can work together to improve it.
- We maintain regular conversations among all advanced practice nursing leaders and NYSNA through participation in NYSNA's Nursing Organization Liaison Forum. This group of nursing leaders, representing specialty and ethnic nursing organizations, meets regularly and maintains contact between meetings by conference calls. The needs of each of these groups are discussed, and an attempt is made by all the groups to meet those needs. The Nursing Organization Liaison Forum could provide a powerful political tool for the profession.
- We have been working with physician's assistants interested in coalition building, and we participate actively in an annual conference where NPs and physician's assistants share issues of concern to both professions.

- In June 1996, NYSCONP held a 1-day seminar entitled "Building Bridges." This workshop was an attempt to bring together midwives, nurse anesthetists, CNSs, and NPs. The purpose was to create a better understanding of the ways in which we could work together to achieve our goals. The hope was that one of the other advanced practice groups would follow NYSCONP's lead and host a similar conference in 1997.
- The Ad Hoc Coalition of the New York State Professions was established to provide information on activities related to governance of the professions. This is the arena in which NYSCONP is able to monitor, along with the 37 other professional organizations, the regulation of professional practice. For example, in 1997 the governor of New York proposed legislation to transfer the activities of the Office of the Professions from the New York State Education Department to the Department of the State. This could put the regulation and governance of the professions in the hands of politicians and remove the professional from this role. A letter of opposition signed by this ad hoc committee has been sent to the legislature.

- On the national level, coalition building by NYSCONP took the form of participation in the establishment of the American College of Nurse Practitioners, a national organization devoted to advancing NP practice and accomplishing national and regional goals for all NPs. A grassroots movement to support financially an independent lobbyist to achieve passage of legislation for direct Medicare reimbursement to NPs arose during the annual meeting. The legislation was successfully passed in 1997.

Today, as a result of strong coalition building, advanced practice nurses in New York State are taking the lead in establishing the nursing profession's future in the health care delivery system.

References

Blevin, S. A. (1996). *New York State Coalition of Nurse Practitioners ask: Let the market in.* Albany: New York State Coalition of Nurse Practitioners.

Mason, D., Cohen, S. S., O'Donnell, J., Baxter, K., & Chase, A. (1997). Managed care organizations' arrangements with nurse practitioners. *Nursing Economic$, 15*(6), 306–314.

Chapter *19*

COLLECTIVE ACTION IN THE WORKPLACE

Mary E. Foley

The health care climate of the late 1990s is one in which care is delivered, or withheld, in an atmosphere dominated by financial high stakes and mergers of health care facilities into large corporations. Hospital mergers, closures, and acquisitions have transpired at dizzying rates. Serious staffing cuts have occurred nationally, and quality nursing care is jeopardized. Adequate staffing, quality of care, health and safety in the workplace, job security, and retaining an effective voice in the changing systems demand collective action. It is imperative that nurses be aware of the tools available to initiate collective action in the workplace.

Hospitals and other health care organizations do not want nurses to organize. Just as in other industries, managers do not want nonmanagerial personnel overseeing and participating in management issues. If collective bargaining is seen as a power struggle between union and management, and in many cases that is how it is defined and played out, the opposing parties are indeed seen as rivals, manipulating each other in an effort to improve and advance their respective positions. One definition of collective bargaining in the health care sector describes the broadly defined bargaining objectives (Stern, 1982, p. 11):

1. To protect the economic position and personal welfare of the worker
2. To protect the union's integrity as an ongoing institution
3. To recognize the outer limits imposed on collective bargaining outcomes by the economic conditions of the industry and the employer and by the climate of opinion

Collective action can range from shared governance to union representation, and many variations exist within those definitions. This chapter is not meant to be a primer on achieving or administering any specific strategy; it is meant to serve as an overview and to stimulate an interest in further exploration. Each setting will be different, depending in part on the administrative structure and more so on the beliefs and style of the chief administrative staff. Those factors can change with time, and strategies should be evaluated on a regular basis.

The chapter will also discuss collective bargaining for nurses from a policy perspective. Collective bargaining is a highly political and complicated legal process, and many guidelines govern the conduct of bargaining. Laws vary between the public and private sectors. In the public sector, laws may differ among states, and the federal system has its own regulations. Please refer to the wide range of other resources available for specific details.

CONTROL OF PRACTICE

Specific objectives that professional nurses identify as essential for control of their practice include the following:

- To improve the practice of professional nurses and all nursing personnel
- To recommend ways and means to improve care

- To make recommendations to the hospital management—for example, when a critical nurse staffing shortage exists
- To identify and recommend elimination of hazards in the workplace

Mechanisms to address practice issues within the institution derive from the nurse councils, practice committees, and other practice bodies that are established and empowered by either a governance model or a contract.

At the heart of each model is the interaction between the group and the leadership. Group problem solving is possible in any structure that encourages participation and that has a leadership that accepts the outcome of the participation. Committees are an example of group participation. Committees can be given a specific task to collect data, analyze it, and make recommendations. A committee can be representative and can involve individuals with specialized knowledge and direct interest. The downfall may be a prolonged process and a compromise that fails to address the problem at hand and may not really satisfy any of the participants.

Nurse Committees

Nurse committees, assisted by experts in nursing, can advocate against dangerous nurse reductions. New patient-care models must undergo careful analysis. When the nurse practice committee and management collaboratively design and implement a practice model, both nurses and the public will be better served. When layoffs are necessary, such as in true downsizing, every effort should be made to ensure safe care. The talents and expertise of nurses affected by the changes should be addressed by facilitating nurses' transition to new areas of practice. The nurse practice committee can assist in enforcing standards and competencies in the new arenas and can participate in designing and overseeing transitional learning opportunities for displaced nurses.

Magnet Hospitals

The early work by the American Academy of Nursing on the topic of magnet hospitals (American Academy of Nursing, 1983) describes professional practice environments that utilize a combination of staff involvement in unit and hospital decision making that influences practice. The managers and staff work as a team, and the sense of empowerment within both entities is measurable.

Shared Governance

Shared governance is defined as an arrangement of nurses (staff and managers) that attempts to emphasize principles of participatory management in areas related to the governance and practice of nursing. Also labeled self-governance, participatory decision making, staff bylaws, and decentralized nursing services, these efforts attempt to involve practitioners in the control of their practice. Shared governance is defined as a professional practice model that is an accountability-based governance system for professional workers (Porter O'Grady, 1987). The model works when nursing managers and practitioners engage in an atmosphere of joint ownership based on trust and not limited by structures that restrict true professional involvement. Although shared governance requires some structure, it is decision based and is constructed from the center of the workplace rather than from a hierarchy. Authority rests in specified processes, not in identified individuals. For the model to succeed, every nurse in the organization must believe in it. Nursing staff should be elected participants, not hand-picked favorites. Leadership of the committees may be rotated between managers and staff to be more equitable. It is not recommended that individual nursing units attempt to initiate the model unless the entire setting is committed, because this can lead to unit elitism and lack of interface within nursing. In some settings, once the nursing department adopts the rules or bylaws that govern them, these rules are approved by the hospital trustees as the operating rules of the nursing department. The model can also include a management decision-making forum for issues that support practice, such as finances and interdepartmental conflicts.

In reality, there are some serious limitations to shared governance models when they are tried in actual practice. Some shared governance models make no effort to conceal the fact that, in spite of the appearance of participation, a unilateral managerial decision-making authority remains in the institution. Such a practice negates the intent of the "shared" principle and only further distances management from nurses. Other warnings arise when the shared governance model is used to bypass or conflict with an already existing structure that has participation as a component, such as a collective bargaining agreement. Shared governance *can* exist in a unionized or nonunionized setting. Care must be taken to delineate clearly those topics that can be handled by the shared governance mechanisms and that would be subject to collective bargaining. Committee members could be identified by the union, much as it selects a practice committee representing all units. Another caution with collective bargaining is the legal precedent set in the academic setting, in which faculty members became so involved in the governance structure offered by the shared governance model that they were found to be ineligible for representation for collective bargaining because their roles were indistinguishable from those of managers (*Yeshiva*, 1980). And perhaps the greatest risk comes from lack of sustained commitment—the wisdom, courage, and patience of the managers and the staff may not survive the ups and downs of implementation.

Work Assignments

Registering an objection to a work assignment is considered an important professional obligation of nurses. Institutions provide an internal mechanism, known as an incident report or notification report, to communicate unexpected events or to document a problem; however, these forms are protected as proprietary property of the institution, and access to those data is restricted. Nurses have used a form called an "assignment despite objection" or "assignment under protest" while completing the assignment (or a nurse can risk charges of abandonment; see specific state practice acts for details). The forms are usually filed because of concerns over inadequate staff, poorly prepared staff, high patient acuity, and unsafe practice situations. The practice committee and nursing administration can then review the circumstances leading to the protest. If there is a pattern, a long-term solution can be developed. This strategy is not unique to the unionized setting and could be successful in any setting in which the channels of communication are supportive of joint problem identification and resolution. The union environment ensures a more formal follow-up.

Whistle Blower Protection

Professionals who speak out about working conditions, especially about issues of patient care, may not be protected from action by their employer. Holding a professional license may necessitate that you act as an advocate, but it will not ensure employment protection if what you say is unpopular with the employer. That protection, known as whistle blower protection, is not currently widespread but is gaining in popularity as a part of the next health reform agenda. The American Nurses Association (ANA) has promoted the Patient Safety Act, a bill to give consumers access to nurse-related data and to protect health care workers from retribution if they speak out about quality of care or working conditions.

New Models of Labor-Management Relations

There is some optimism that new models of labor-management relations will evolve in the next century. Studies were undertaken under the auspices of the U.S. Department of Labor, and in

1994 a report was issued by the Commission on the Future of Worker-Management Relations (U.S. Department of Labor, 1994). Underlying the report was a theme of employee participation and problem solving that could enhance workplace productivity.

Another nurse-specific example of new relationships is the work being done under the provisions of the U.S. Department of Labor Transitional Workforce Stability Provisions (U.S. Department of Labor, 1995). More than $200 million dollars was appropriated for retraining and other worker adjustments to assist health care workers affected by the transition to a restructured health care delivery system. The Michigan Nurses Association, a member of the ANA, participated in a 3-year grant funded by the Department of Labor to assist acute care nurses in making transitions to other settings.

CONTROL OF PRACTICE THROUGH COLLECTIVE BARGAINING

Collective bargaining agreements for nurses have traditionally been used as a means to equalize the power between management and nurses. Nurses have used contracts as a form of collective action to improve working conditions, hence improving care. Generically, unions in the health care setting stimulate better hospital management by fostering formal, central, and consistent personnel policies with better lines of communication, and they lead to improvements in the workplace so that recruitment and retention become easier (Juris & Maxey, 1981).

Should Nurses Organize?

In most commonly accepted definitions of a profession, the members of a profession have attained expertise after a specialized education. Society then grants the professional a measure of autonomy in her or his work in recognition of the expertise and the value of their service to the larger community. Autonomy permits professionals to make independent judgments and

decisions and to have special client-provider relationships, such as have been traditional in law and medicine.

Nursing has struggled with a modified definition of a profession. The work arrangements traditional to nursing have historically been as an employed professional—first by hospitals, nursing homes, and other health agencies, and now by health systems. Even though nursing meets many of the other criteria of a profession (education, expertise, a value recognized by society, and *some* autonomy in judgment), the role of nurses as employees has compromised the client-provider relationship. Hospitals have been organized as bureaucratic structures and have relied on hierarchical boundaries that are not congruent with the notion of a professional practice. Conflict arises when professionals believe that their professional autonomy and clinical judgment are challenged, and as a result, care is compromised. Medicine is now facing similar conflicts, with fewer physicians in private practice and managed care plans forcing clinical decisions that erode professional autonomy. Cost containment, productivity measurements, and issues of resource utilization are the stressors that stimulate interest by health professionals in collective action. In fact, physicians are beginning to use collective action, including collective bargaining, to reestablish professional authority, a remedy that is actually sanctioned by the American Medical Association (Jaklevic, 1997).

Nursing has used collective bargaining to its benefit, achieving professional goals and protecting and promoting public interest through lobbying efforts and political action. All other forms of collective action have a serious limitation! They work only when every party agrees they should. When neither party is bound to comply with the agreements, and no oversight exists to force compliance, the relationship can fail. An expectation that there would be benevolence in an industry that wasn't and isn't benevolent may answer why nurses have been willing to be organized for purposes of collective bargaining. Nurses who support collective bargaining view it as a way to control practice by a redistribution of power within the structure of a health care organization.

A study conducted by a Kansas City employee and labor relations consulting firm set out to ascertain why hospital employees and nurses join unions and how union organizers garner their support. The study was intended for use by hospital managers to define strategies to avoid outside representation for professional nurses. Their conclusion is self-explanatory:

> A myth widely subscribed to by hospital management is that big powerful unions organize professional nurses. In fact, unions do not organize nurses; professional nurses organize themselves. They do this because administrators and nursing supervisors fail to recognize and address nurses' individual and collective needs. [Stickler & Velghe, 1980, p. 14]

Another study, this one from the University of California, Berkeley, found that nurses who engage in collective bargaining do so because they believe it is the only solution to a management-employee power struggle. The authors concluded that nurses decide to unionize out of their "inability to communicate with management and their perception of authoritarian behavior on the part of management" (Parlette, O'Reilly, & Bloom 1980, p. 16). The age of this study by no means diminishes its importance or accuracy, because nurses of the 1990s who are selecting collective bargaining representatives are doing so in the face of great struggles over patient-care issues with managers who appear to have lost sight of the purpose of health services.

Nursing has been unable to come to closure on the debate about whether professional nurses should organize for collective bargaining. On one side of the debate are those who want nursing to be a profession that uses its prestige to ensure recognition. On the other side are those who view nursing as a professional or occupational group that can and should use collective action, in this case collective bargaining, to secure recognition. Virginia Cleland (1981), a legendary professor of nursing admin-

istration, stated, "The power bestowed upon the nursing profession should derive not from the hospital administrator's benevolence, but rather from the public's view of the value of services provided by the practitioner" (p. 17). Ada Jacox (1980), another esteemed nursing professor, criticized nursing departments that fail to acknowledge nurses as professionals and suggested that collective bargaining may be a way for nurses to achieve collective professional responsibility.

Hospitals have undergone extensive restructuring and reengineering in the 1990s, in part to survive but mostly to improve the profit margin. Despite record profits, 69% of hospital administrators reported plans to reduce operating costs as a "high priority" and 38% of 700 hospitals surveyed in 1994 reported plans to reduce the work force. Nursing personnel have been the targets of those cuts, with 27% of these hospitals planning to reduce the number of nurses or replace them (Burda, 1994). The ANA commissioned a survey in 1994 and confirmed that layoffs of registered nurses (RNs) were widespread, with more than 68% of the 1,800 national respondents reporting cuts at their institutions in the previous year. More than 53% of the respondents stated that RNs were taking care of more patients than before (Himali, 1995a). Hospitals are using labor costs as major factors in making employment and staffing decisions. The RN wages, higher than those of ancillary personnel, are not viewed in relation to RNs' contributions toward enhancing patient care but as a target for cost reduction (Buerhaus, 1995).

In place of the RN, some institutions have been aggressively cross-training hospital employees so that direct-care nursing previously done by RNs can be shifted to lower-paid employees. The result is a sharp reduction in the ratio of RNs to patients, accompanied by a cut in total employee positions (Hospitals, 1993). This development, called "patient-focused care," was documented in the 1994 ANA layoff survey, and in a 1996 survey (Shindul-Rothschild, 1996) in which RNs reported that their institutions were increasingly using unlicensed workers, some of whom have only 2 to 6 weeks of training, to provide direct patient care.

Nurse health and safety have been directly affected by the introduction of the restructured workplace. The combination of reduced staff, higher acuity, and pressure for increased productivity has led to an increase in nurse and other health worker injuries. These findings were documented by analysis of employer-provided data from 97 health care facilities for the years 1990 through 1994. The Minnesota Nurses Association has concluded the first phase of the study, and it confirmed what had previously been only anecdotal. The rise in patient acuity and the concurrent staffing changes caused a near doubling of RN workplace injuries (Himali, 1995b). It is important for representatives to make the connection between practice trends and health and safety issues. Health and safety issues are potential organizing issues and appropriate subjects of bargaining.

History of Collective Bargaining in Nursing

Nurses in the early 1900s were frustrated by their working conditions, and receiving little support from the established nursing organizations, a few thousand joined trade unions for assistance. In the 1940s, nurses in California, Ohio, and Pennsylvania were assisted in their workplaces by the state nurses associations (SNAs) of the ANA. In 1946, after considerable urging by the leaders of the states representing nurses, the ANA unanimously adopted a national economic security program. It was ANA's intent to encourage constituent members to act as the exclusive agents for nurses in the important fields of economic security and collective bargaining.

Other unions organized nurses, with more than 20 expressing an intent to solicit nurses in 1974. The competition has become more intense as the stakes get higher. The decline in traditional union membership in the United States, 14.5% of the workforce in 1996 from almost 25% in the 1970s, has made the nursing population an attractive new membership category.

Unions such as the Meatpackers, Paperhangers, United Food and Commercial Workers, Longshoremen, Teamsters, American Federation of Teachers, United Mine Workers, Service Employees International Union (SEIU), and Association of Federal, State, County and Municipal Employees (all members of the American Federation of Labor–Congress of Industrial Organizations [AFL-CIO]) have competed for nurse membership among themselves and with the SNAs.

Some nurses have chosen to be organized in independent unions, unaffiliated with either an AFL-CIO union or an SNA. One well-known independent union is the Committee for the Recognition of Nursing Achievement, at Stanford University in Palo Alto, California. Formed in 1964, this union has had a successful history of working closely with nursing administration to advance nursing standards and nurse recognition. Independent unions are at risk of raiding by other unions because of the difficulty and cost of providing the complex and expensive services of representation.

Who Represents Nurses (and Why Does That Matter)?

Who the bargaining representative is does make a difference to nurses. It is certainly going to have an effect on the public's perception of the profession. It can also determine who has the political clout in issues of legislation and regulation. Nurses who are considering a collective bargaining agent must do some values clarification. The underlying question must be addressed: Do nurses have identity *primarily* as nurses or as workers? The SNA collective bargaining agreements have historically focused on nursing practice issues, and their contracts are replete with references to the professional standards, the code of ethics, and professional practice committees that give nurses a voice, and a vehicle, to address patient care concerns. Indeed, trade unions do offer the appearance of bountiful resources and "strength" that derive from history and size. Their expertise has been in attaining wage and benefit packages and, in some cases, advocating for health and safety issues. In actuality, nurse unions, or units, which are subsumed within larger union structures, compete for resources, time, and attention to the patient-care issues that nurses consider important. Nurses find themselves trying to explain complex practice concerns to nonnurse labor staff, many of whom have voiced disdain for the professional issues that nurses are concerned about. Nowhere in the AFL-CIO leadership structure are nurses visible. As a result, the trade unions position nursing and patient-care advocacy as a minor plank.

The October 1995 election of John Sweeney (previously head of SEIU) as president of the AFL-CIO has ensured that competition for nurses by the trade unions will increase. SEIU represents more health care workers than any other union and, under Sweeney's leadership, was the only major union to grow in size during nationwide union membership losses.

For the first time, the AFL-CIO unions combined represent more registered nurses than those affiliated with the ANA. At this time, no single union within the AFL-CIO structure is larger than ANA, but organizing new units and "raiding" (see definition in the following section, "Electing the Agent") existing units are on the rise nationally. One of the historical debates within ANA is whether its multipurpose membership and mission make it stronger or weaker as a collective bargaining agent.

Within the ANA structure, the conflict, and the pressure to conform to traditional union methods, were played out in 1995. The California Nurses Association (CNA) voted to disaffiliate from ANA, severing a 98-year relationship with its national professional organization and becoming the first state affiliate actually to leave ANA. This vote removed all CNA member linkage to ANA. CNA had a growing relationship with SEIU and the United Mine Workers, which led to closer alignment with the politics and strategies of traditional trade unions. While remaining an independent union at this time, it continues to talk of nationwide nurse representation and a potential relationship with other

unions. CNA publicly described the need to splinter from ANA as a philosophical difference between ANA's and CNA's approaches to promoting nursing practice in the current shifting environment. In 1997 CNA represented fewer than 20,000 nurses, or about 7.5% of the RNs in the state (a decline from 26,000 nurses in the early 1990s, or 10% of the state nurse population).

THE COLLECTIVE BARGAINING PROCESS

Electing the Agent

When nurses decide to elect a collective bargaining representative, they are guaranteed legal protection, as all workers in the private sector are, as provided by the National Labor Relations Act (NLRA). The employer is also ensured some protection, especially protection against disruption of the workplace during the organizing or election process. Once the nurses/employees start a campaign for representation and 30% of the eligible nurses have signed cards signaling their interest in a representative, the employer is prohibited from engaging in certain activities that would constitute unfair labor practices:

- It may not fire the organizers in a retaliatory manner for their union activity.
- It is prohibited from interfering with, restraining, or coercing employees who choose to organize, form, join, or assist labor organization.
- It cannot refuse to allow dissemination of union information in the workplace.
- It cannot ignore a request for a vote of the workers for representation by the union as a collective bargaining agent.

After the campaign a vote is conducted under the guidance of the National Labor Relations Board (NLRB). Other unions may enter the race at this time. A vote of 50% of those voting, plus one (a simple majority), is required to select the agent.

Raids and Decertifications

Nurses represented by a bargaining agent have the right to drop or change (decertify) that agent by a similar campaign of signatures (30%) of the affected members, followed by a vote, again requiring 50% plus one. This is an increasingly common event, particularly fueled by competition between trade unions and nursing unions, and among trade unions themselves. When another union tries to decertify an existing union, the campaign is called a "raid," and raids are one of the easiest ways to recruit new members, making it more and more attractive. It is easier and cheaper to recruit a bargaining unit that is already organized than to recruit unorganized nurses (remember, nurses generally do not get organized from the outside; they organize themselves!). Competing unions often make exaggerated promises, and the larger trade unions have resources to use on raids. Critical questions must be asked: Are the promises delivered on? Are the services of the new bargaining agent better? And are the nurses better represented?

Recognition Appeals

An employer may choose to bargain in good faith on matters concerning employee working conditions by voluntarily recognizing the bargaining agent in lieu of awaiting the outcome of an election. This may occur if the support for one union is evident and a strong majority exists. More commonly, the employer will appeal employee requests for representation to the NLRB. The purpose of the appeal may be based on a technical distinction or definition, but the premise behind the appeal is the desire of the employer to prevent union representation in the workplace.

During an appeal, arguments about why, by whom, or how nurses will be represented are made before the NLRB. The net effect of the appeal may not change the outcome of the process, but it does come at a high price to the unions and the nurses in staff time, resources, and often loss of focus and momentum.

Insulation

Early challenges to nursing unions arose when the hospitals challenged whether the state nurses association was properly structured to be a labor union. In question was the membership of the SNAs: all RNs could belong to the association. Because managers could belong to the SNA, it was necessary to provide a real and substantial "insulation" of the collective bargaining program of the SNA from any potential managerial influence. This protection is required by the NLRB and prevents employers from interference, domination, or discrimination in an employee's pursuit of a representative for collective bargaining. In spite of a precedent-setting case in 1979, some hospitals appealed the SNA structure, and a series of cases in the 1980s ensued. Eventually the issue was resolved successfully for the SNAs and the nurses.

Unit Determination

Another example of challenges to nursing unions is the appeals on the issue of unit determination. When the NLRA and the subsequent 1974 amendments covering health care employees were adopted, Congress intended simultaneously to limit the number of individual bargaining units that an employer or industry would have to recognize and bargain with, and yet still allow for distinctions among employees that may have unique issues or circumstances. Nurses have historically been organized into all-RN bargaining units because they were believed to have a unique "community of interest" in the way they worked within the health care system.

In 1984 a dramatic change in nurse unit determination occurred when the NLRB ruled in a case involving St. Francis Hospital, in St. Paul, Minnesota, that the nurses were no longer eligible for a distinct, all-RN bargaining unit and, instead, would have to be included in what was called an all-professional unit. A professional unit could include respiratory therapists, social workers, physical therapists, librarians, pharmacists, medical clergy, the architect, and the business officer. This determination wreaked havoc with organizing, and it coincided with the beginning of the last great national nursing shortage in the late 1980s. That shortage led to serious nurse staffing problems and working conditions that were deplorable and unsafe. As the conditions worsened in hospitals, nurses all over the country were requesting organizing assistance. Despite the demand, there were very few successful elections from 1984 to 1991, mostly because of the NLRB ruling on all-professional units. First, it was difficult to organize and achieve a satisfactory election outcome among such a diverse group of health care employees. Second, though it might be possible to stimulate enough interest among employees to warrant representation, election of a single bargaining agent to represent the diverse needs of so many work classifications would be almost impossible.

The ANA and other unions representing nurses for collective bargaining decided to challenge the NLRB's decision. The major opponent in the challenge was the American Hospital Association, which worked strenuously to keep the determination in favor of the all-professional unit. After a successful ruling by the NLRB, affirming the rights of RNs to be organized in all-RN units, the American Hospital Association challenged that ruling in a federal court and an injunction was issued. Realizing that this issue stood in the way of nurses' being represented for collective bargaining as they tried to improve working conditions to protect patient care, the ANA and the NLRB appealed the case to the U.S. Supreme Court. In May 1991 the Supreme Court confirmed that the NLRB had ruled properly and reinstated all-RN bargaining units.

RN as Supervisor

A more recent employer-initiated legal strategy challenged the nursing profession and the future protection of nurses by the NLRA. In a shocking decision in May 1994, the U.S. Supreme Court ruled that any nurse who "directs other employees" is to be classified as working for the employer and could be fired for protesting job conditions or questioning management decisions that put the quality of patient care at risk, and therefore the nurse could be denied the protection of the NLRA. Nurses inevitably supervise a wide range of ancillary personnel, such as assistants, clerks, and, in the case of RNs, the licensed practical/vocational nurse. This ruling overturned a 20-year precedent of the NLRB that a nurse is *not* a supervisor when acting in the best interest of the patient in seeing that the work of aides is done properly. Historically the direction or assignment of others has been viewed as incidental to the treatment of patients and as exercised in the interest of the patient, not the employer. This ruling was a staggering setback for all nurses as they advocate for patient safety and quality in a climate of downsizing and restructuring. It is threatening to all unions, who strongly protest the "supervisory" label for nurses, because nurses would not be eligible for collective bargaining if this decision is upheld (*NLRB v. Health Care & Retirement Corp. of America*, 1994).

Because of the 1994 decision and the subsequent confusion it has created, the Supreme Court instructed the NLRB to reconsider its definition of "supervisory" as it pertains to nurses and to be consistent in the use of that term throughout all industries, therefore not treating nurses, or the health care industry, with any distinction. Employers have used this legal discrepancy and unsettled issue to delay or avoid bargaining with nurses. The *Providence Hospital* case (1996) started in 1994 when Providence Hospital, in Anchorage, Alaska, refused to recognize the newly elected bargaining representative, the Alaska Nurses Association, claiming that the charge nurses included in the proposed bargaining unit were, in fact, supervisors and were doing the work of the employer. The NLRB did not agree, the hospital appealed, and the matter was litigated in Alaska in July 1997. The ruling was favorable to nursing, and by all indications no appeals are anticipated. Not only the issue of bargaining-unit eligibility was at stake, but also the bigger issue of professional advocacy—being able, and expected, to speak out about patient care and related working conditions was in jeopardy and was legally upheld as a professional duty.

JOB SECURITY OR PROFESSIONAL/ CAREER SECURITY?

The economic environment in the health care industry, coupled with rapidly advancing technological breakthroughs, and a renewed interest in primary and preventive care has dramatically shifted health care away from the in-patient hospital setting.

New organizing will be difficult in light of smaller acute care settings and widely dispersed outpatient and home-employee groups. The new arrangements present an organizing dilemma to all representatives as resources and needs are spread further, the interests of the nurses are more diverse, and the numbers who can be organized in each campaign are smaller. Another formidable barrier to new organizing is the size and financial power of large, nationwide corporate systems, some of which have deep-seated and well-funded opposition to union activity.

These new paradigms have challenged nurses and their representatives to modify bargaining strategies and turn attention to issues of reductions in force and the transfer of nurses to alternative settings. The union that promises job security in the hospital setting and claims it can stop all these trends is setting itself up for failure. More seriously, however, some unions are misleading the nurses and are leaving large numbers of nurses unprepared for their future roles in health care. The ANA, through its affiliated members, has committed significant time and resources to maintaining the essential role of the RN in the acute care setting through bargaining agreements and workplace advocacy while simultaneously helping nurses prepare for the changing settings and roles.

Nurses of the future, if they are to survive the present, need professional advocacy and expertise. Professional representation involves much more than protest and requires a mature and balanced vision of nursing and health care. The ANA is facing major decisions on the future direction it will take to ensure nurses the best representation. Some advocate affiliation of ANA with AFL-CIO. Though not a new question, the present environment, competition for scarce resources, and competition for nurse members will force a new debate in the state and national arenas.

REFERENCES

American Academy of Nursing. (1983). *Magnet hospitals: Attraction and retention of professional nurses.* Washington, DC: American Nurses Association.

Buerhaus, P. (1995). Economics and reform: Forces affecting nurse staffing. *Nursing Policy Forum, 1*(2) 8–14.

Burda, D. (1994). A profit by any other name would still give hospitals the fits. *Modern Healthcare, 24,* 115–136.

Cleland, V. (1981). Taft-Hartley amended: Implications for nursing—the professional model. *Journal of Nursing Administration, 11,* 17.

Himali, U. (1995a). ANA sounds alarm about unsafe staffing levels. *American Nurse, 27,* 2.

Himali, U. (1995b). An unsafe equation: Fewer RNs = more workplace injuries. *American Nurse, 27,* 5.

Jacox, A. (1980). Collective action: The basis for professionalism. *Supervisor Nurse, 11,* 22.

Jaklevic, M. (1997). Doctors and unions. *Modern Healthcare, 27*(40), 99–106.

Juris, K., & Maxey, C. (1981). The impact of hospital unionism. *Modern Healthcare, 11,* 36.

Lutz, S. (1994). Let's make a deal: Health care mergers, acquisitions take place at a dizzying pace. *Modern Healthcare, 24,* 47–50.

NLRB v. Health Care & Retirement Corp. of America, 114 Supreme Court 1778 (1994).

Olson, M. (1977). *The logic of collective action.* Cambridge, MA: Harvard University Press.

Parlette, G. N., O'Reilly, C. A., & Bloom, J. R. (1980). The nurse and the union. *Hospital Forum, 23,* 14.

Porter O'Grady, T. (1987). Shared governance and new organizational models. *Nursing Economic$, 5*(6), 281–287.

Providence Hospital, 320 NLRB No. 49 (1996).

Shindul-Rothschild, J. (1996). Where have all the nurses gone? Final results of the AJN patient care survey. *American Journal of Nursing, 96*(11), 25–39.

Stern, E. (1982). Collective bargaining: A means of conflict resolution. *Nursing Administration, 6,* 9.

Stickler, F. B., & Velghe, J. C. (1980). Why nurses join unions. *Hospital Forum, 23,* 14.

Sullivan, E., & Decker, P. (1988). *Effective management in nursing.* Menlo Park, CA: Addison-Wesley.

U.S. Department of Labor. (1994, May). Health care workforce transition. Washington, DC: Author.

Yeshiva, supra, 103 LRRM at 2553 (1980).

VIGNETTE
Blowing the Whistle
Terri Havill

"Ideas Shine" glowed the posting from the ministry of attorney general. "Join our partnership initiative to find ways of delivering services to the public more effectively and efficiently," encouraged the unusual yellow bulletin.

Nervous excitement filled my chest as I read about a means of communicating to bureaucrats/officials in our capital city of Victoria. Intuitively I knew that this offer allowed me a way to address a taboo subject of the health care unit at my workplace.

In 1991 I was hired as a Nurse II–assistant head nurse at Vancouver Pretrial Services Center (VPSC), British Columbia. My previous experience as a "detox" nurse helped me in the transition to correctional nursing in a maximum security prison. VPSC is a remand facility that houses 220-plus prisoners. A remand institution is for accused persons awaiting trial. Remanded prisoners may be jailed because of serious charges that are not eligible for bail, or they may be remanded because of a history of failing to appear in court, or they may not be able to arrange bail payment.

People are often perplexed by the role of a jail nurse. Repeatedly I am asked with genuine interest, "Well, what do you do?" Unfortunately, the majority of prisoners are not the fit-weightlifter type who just want to eat three squares a day, exercise, and write home to mom. The majority of VPSC prisoners are substance abusers with a high incidence of infectious disease. As well, we care for the mentally disordered offenders who may be addicted and or infectious. The average length of stay is 9 days, with around 20 prisoners admitted or released daily. For many prisoners the first week in jail is a time to stabilize their health by undergoing detoxification, receiving wound care, receiving medication as directed by a medical doctor, improving nutrition and hygiene, and, of course, resting a tired body and spirit.

Pretrial staff frequently lament over the revolving door of the regular petty criminal. He may be underweight and wounded from fixing heroin or cocaine, or both, or he may be disoriented and injured from drinking rice wine—and he is back. He might have been released two months previously at 170 pounds, with skin intact. Now he is an irritable 135 pounds, with an abscess on the right forearm. Here we go again, meeting the needs of the regular inmate.

British Columbia's provincial correctional centers offer nursing, medical, psychological, psychiatric, and dental services in their health care facilities. On admission to a prison, an inmate is seen by an admissions nurse and a psychology intern. The nurse and intern may refer the inmate to the physician, dentist, psychologist, or "tower" nurse. The tower nurse is responsible for the ongoing care of the prisoner after he is admitted and transferred to one of the 12 living units in the six-story tower.

The psychology intern refers the troubled prisoner to the psychologist. One in ten inmates is noted as at high risk of suicidal or unpredictable, violent behavior. All inmates on the high-risk list are followed by a psychologist. The psychologist also cares for the inmate who has received a lengthy sentence, has experienced the recent death of a loved one, or is mentally unstable. To obtain sleeping medication, an inmate must see the psychologist and have sedation recommended. Some self-referrals to the psychologist are made in an attempt to acquire sleep aid.

Currently our physicians see 8 to 12 prisoners in a session ($3\frac{1}{2}$ hours). Inmates may be referred by a health care team member or may self-refer. All inmates' health complaints are screened by the nurse. Prisoners are placed on the health clinic list by the nurses according to priority medical needs.

On the outside, VPSC seemed to meet the five principles of the Canada Health Act: comprehensive, universal, accessible, portable, and publicly administered. Controversy arose when I questioned the quality and administration of prisoner health care. Rather than comprehensive care, prisoners received cursory care. Meanwhile the taxpayer paid for services that were routinely not given. Rapid care for prisoners by physicians and psychologists was a chronic problem ignored by management.

In February 1996, I wrote to the medical director of corrections for British Columbia, informing her of the quick care given to prisoners at VPSC by the two physicians and two psychologists. I described how data from 15 medical clinics, randomly reviewed, revealed an average of nine inmates seen at 5 minutes each. One physician saw 11 inmates for 3 minutes each on average per session, whereas the other physician saw seven inmates for 7 minutes each on average per session. I wrote: "If the institution does not require the professionals to prorate for partial sessions, as per contract, it allows one

to become accustomed to bonus remuneration. It can set up a keenness to do sessions quickly to maximize on the remuneration." I went on to describe the psychologists' practice of seeing an average of seven inmates for $5\frac{1}{2}$ minutes each and billing for $3\frac{1}{2}$ hours. In this same letter, I wrote, "It is important that partial sessions be prorated to ensure maximum availability of care can be provided." The medical director of corrections did not stop the clinicians' billing practice or effect positive change in service.

How does one address a significant concern of substandard care with creative billing done by professionals with historic impunity? Very carefully.

What did management have to gain by not enforcing the clinicians' contractual agreement regarding sessional psychological or medical services? They were able to maintain rapport and the window dressing of service being delivered. Bureaucrats said, "We don't want to create any unnecessary waves" and "This is a sensitive issue," as they procrastinated addressing my concerns. No one wanted to stick his neck out.

I was inspired by the British Columbia Nurses Union (BCNU) journal *Update*, which told the story of a nurse who blew the whistle on rural physicians using the hospital emergency department to see their regular patients. This increased the workload for the rural emergency nurses and enabled the physician to bill the province more for expensive emergency department service that could have been performed in the private-practice office at approximately half the cost. Judy Nowak, RN, decreased the workload for emergency department nurses and decreased billings from rural physicians province-wide by exposing this pattern of practice. She kept her job at Nakusp Hospital. I thought that if she could do this, maybe I could help bring change to VPSC.

Through the provincial government's Employee Recognition Program (Ideas Shine), I put forward two ideas to provide better prisoner care while saving money. I suggested that the psychiatrist be paid by the hour rather than per prisoner, which would save money and limit the incentive to see patients quickly for financial reward. Also I noted that the physicians and psychologists should prorate their incomplete sessions according to the contract. I recommended that the physician be available 7 days a week for 2 hours instead of 3½ hours for 6 days a week. This would provide daily service while lowering costs. Initially I thought 2 hours was appropriate because the average session was less than 1½ hours.

My ideas were supported in principle by the medical director of corrections. However, the evaluation of the ideas was shelved by local management. After 10 months I filed a Freedom of Information request for a year's worth of clinicians' billings and the health clinic documents completed by the correctional officer that showed the time doctors spent with each inmate. This document included the time the doctor arrived and departed, and the time the prisoner was in the office with the doctor. This health clinic record was concrete evidence of rapid care. One medical doctor's and one psychologist's visits with prisoners were less than 6 minutes on average. The other doctor and psychologist saw fewer prisoners but spent 3 minutes more per visit on average. Four clinicians each overbilled the equivalent of at least one welfare check for a family of four per month. Though the government was quick to crack down on welfare fraud, it ignored this problem, which could be systemic to other provincial institutions.

In August 1996, as directed by our shop steward, all available regular nurses and two auxiliary nurses completed professional responsibility forms (PRFs) on unsafe workloads at VPSC. This is a master collective agreement tool used in problem solving: nursing practice conditions, safety of patients and nurses, and workload. Our PRF's were given to local management. In my lengthy documentation (19 pages) I described how I was unable to meet the standards of the Registered Nurses Association

of British Columbia because of an unsafe workload and unsafe inmate/front-line nurse ratios in the tower: 220 inmates to one tower nurse, 24 hours a day. I included two pages on mismanagement of health care funds. I reported that funds were available to provide safe and effective nursing care by transferring the over-billed portion of the clinicians' sessions to nursing services.

The PRFs were also ignored, and a union group grievance for unsafe workload was completed in September 1996. We won this group grievance 10 days before arbitration, October 20, 1997. On October 4, 1996, I went to the ombudsman of British Columbia's office to make a formal complaint of unfair government practice at VPSC. The ombudsman's office agreed to investigate the management and the clinicians. I was informed by the ombudsman's investigator for the attorney general that "the ombudsman's office keep their cards close to their chest." A report is still forthcoming. I am unsure what action the ombudsman made to initiate change, but I believe the contact and investigation were part of the process of positive change. In November 1996 the BCNU wrote to the ministry of health about the overbilling at VPSC and outlined concerns regarding rapid care. This letter was also distributed as a news release. By December 20, 1996, the province newspaper wrote: "Doctor overbilling alleged. Physicians at pre-trial services centre are accused of spending less time examining people than had been reported."

Entering the doors of VPSC became harder for me. Lines were drawn and sides were taken. Instead of changing the practice of rapid service, the local management and accused clinicians decided to shoot the messenger. A letter was sent by the clinicians to management indicating that a more serious issue than the public allegations was that "one person" had "created an atmosphere which is incompatible with good patient care" and that they did not trust me to process their written orders. They offered their resignation for February 15, 1997, if the problem with the one person wasn't resolved.

January 1997 I met with the attorney general's auditors. I was informed by the auditors that the staff consensus was that the doctors were providing less than 1½ hours of care. The auditors treated me gently and respectfully. The Freedom of Information request made in February 1997 for the completed audit is expected to be released February 1998. A copy of the auditors' conclusion was given to me in September 1997.

The conclusion by the Internal Audit Branch is as follows: "We have concluded that the session hours billed by the physicians do not accurately reflect the actual time worked and on average, only 1.5 hours is spent at the centre, per session." "The issues surrounding contracted psychological services are virtually identical to those identified in our earlier report which addressed the allegation of over-billing for physician services within V.P.S.C." One physician used to come into the health care unit wearing his snowboard boots. He would visit with 15 prisoners and review 15 other prisoner's files in less than an hour and a half, leaving ample time for night skiing on Vancouver's local ski hills.

A full review of the centre's operation was ordered by Inspections and Standards for Corrections, British Columbia. This cultural audit was performed by retired chief coroner Mr. Vince Cain, in December 1996 and January 1997. I spent 4 hours with him in the capacity of nurse advocate. He was supportive and ethical.

Mr. Cain's report described how VPSC was being run in a "culture of fear and favoritism." "I am confident in concluding repercussions do exist, fear of repercussions does exist, and favoritism based on some knowns and unknowns likewise exist." I appreciate his noted opinion, "Use of administrative force emanates from personalities which are immature and insecure." He reported how medical and psychology care "was demonstrated to be in the vein of 'mill like assembly care.' Time spent with inmate patients by either physician appears minimal . . . The health care workers are stressed, the space [is] crowded; the inmates presenting a variety of ills, more help is needed in the area." When the government released Mr. Cain's report, all four senior management were transferred.

A review of the health care unit was recommended by Mr. Cain. Unfortunately, this was completed by old management despite Mr. Cain's warning that "the system must be honest, factual and objective if it is to have any integrity. I submit it is deficient in that respect at this centre." The operational review of the unit failed its mandate to assess the nurses' workload problems. The president of the BCNU, Ivory Warner, rejected the operational review of workload at VPSC. She wrote to Corrections' management: "While the review clearly recognizes there is a severe workload problem affecting nurses at the unit, it merely scratches the surface in documenting the problem, and then goes on to engage in the very type of personal scapegoating and harassment which was condemned in the report that gave rise to this 'review.'"

I spent many a late night deciding what was actually going to make a difference. I visualized myself playing chess with an antagonist and thought of strategies to use to checkmate management and the clinicians' king. It got to be a dirty game, and I was frightened. I thought a good defense is a strong offense. Although I had enlisted the support of the Registered Nurses Association of British Columbia, the BCNU, the John Howard Society (a prisoner advocacy group), and the ombudsman, as well as Mr. Vince Cain, still poor practice issues remained. I had communicated the issues from my immediate supervisor to ministerial assistants. One area I feared to tread was to speak to media, although I knew it was my trump card. Truth is the best defense. In early April 1997, my colleague Robert Ulm, RN, and I spoke to a health reporter with the province newspaper. A two-page feature came out April 25, 1997.

Headlines were "Jailhouse Nurse Calls Care Level Dangerous" and "Whistle Blower Pays the Price." This article described the workload problems and the issues leading to my whistle blowing.

Robert Ulm and I were not disciplined for speaking to media, even though we had signed an oath of confidentiality, because we had exhausted all avenues to elicit the necessary changes for safe care with appropriate costs.

The two psychologists offered their resignations after the newspaper article. A third psychologist resigned even though he was not audited. However, he was aware that Dr. Tana Dineen, the "Ralph Nader of the psychology industry," was questioning the old management on the quality of psychological services at VPSC. In the fall of 1996, I heard Dr. Dineen on our public radio station denounce her profession as entrepreneurs building their industry exponentially and exploiting the public safety net. I phoned her and told her about my workplace problems and how it related to her book, *Manufacturing Victims: The Psychology Industry.* Dr. Dineen did her own Freedom of Information requests on VPSC's psychology services. Her phone call to local management in February 1997 was followed by a third psychologist's resignation within a week. Both physicians had resigned before the news release. Their locum, or subcontracted physician, remained. He had never billed the province directly for his services; however, his subcontracted services were not prorated by the previous physician contractors, either.

Proudly, I can say that health care has improved significantly at VPSC as a result of my communications to the Employee Recognition Program, Mr. Vincent Cain, and the BCNU. Conclusions made by auditors Mr. Dan Peck and Ms. Sunny Matheson indicate that the medical and psychology services were less than $1\frac{1}{2}$ hours of a $3\frac{1}{2}$ hour session. Presently direct services from medical and psychology clinicians are approximately 3 to $3\frac{1}{2}$ hours of service. This represents a 100% increase in direct service and 100%-plus increase in the quality of care given to prisoners. Taxpayers have saved $90,948 annually from the previous unquantified and overused indirect service costs. We have reduced the number of psychologists from three to two for less cost and yet more noticeable and effective service.

I am thankful that there were avenues available to me to address my concerns on previous health care services at VPSC. Regretfully, it took significant personal effort and time to solve the taboo problems with health care services and health care management. People ask me, if I had it to do all over again, would I? I respond that indeed I would do it all again, and faster. The 1-year delay in responding to my concerns was unacceptable. These problems should have been rectified without the need for media to pressure for investigation.

The Code of Ethics for Registered Nurses and the Standards for Nursing Practice in British Columbia entitled me to speak up and advocate changes in the system (see Boxes for examples). These guidelines are what I based my nursing actions on in meeting the challenge of creating better health care delivery.

STANDARDS FOR NURSING PRACTICE IN BRITISH COLUMBIA

Standard 3   Provision of a Service to the Public: Provides nursing services, coordinates activities and collaborates with others in providing health care services.
- Participates in and encourages quality management.

Standard 4   Code of Ethics: Adheres to the ethical standards of the nursing profession.
- Expresses a philosophy of nursing that is congruent with the Canadian Charter of Freedoms.
- Reports unsafe practice or professional misconduct to appropriate person or body.
- Acts as an advocate to protect and promote a client's right to autonomy, respect, privacy, dignity and access to information.

CODE OF ETHICS FOR REGISTERED NURSES

Dignity: Nurses value and advocate the dignity and self-respect of human beings.

- Nurses relate to all persons receiving care as persons worthy of respect and endeavor in all their actions to preserve and demonstrate respect for each individual.
- Nurses exhibit sensitivity to the client's needs values and choices. Nursing care is designed to accommodate the biological, psychological, social, cultural and spiritual needs of the clients. Nurses do not exploit clients' vulnerabilities for their own interests or gains, whether this be sexual, emotional, social, political, or financial.

Fairness: Nurses apply and promote principles of equity and fairness to assist clients in receiving unbiased treatment and a share of health services and resources proportionate to their needs.

- Nurses promote appropriate and ethical care at the institutional/agency and community levels to the extent possible, in the development of policies and procedures designed to make the best use of available resources and current knowledge and research.

Practice environments conducive to safe, competent, and ethical care: Nurses advocate practice environments that have the organizational and human support systems, and the resource allocations, necessary for safe, competent and ethical nursing care.

- Nurses collaborate with nursing colleagues and other members of the health team to advocate health care environments that are conducive to ethical practice and to the health and well-being of clients and others in the setting. They do this in ways that are consistent with the professional role and responsibilities.
- Nurses practice ethically by striving for the best care achievable in the circumstances. They also make the effort, individually or in partnership with others, to improve practice environments by advocating on behalf of their clients as possible.

Postscript

As of Spring 1998, Terri Havill's efforts have resulted in the following:

1. Psychologists and physicians are paid only on a prorated basis by time.
2. With new management in place and after media coverage of the understaffing, the staffing was doubled.
3. The provincial premier and other officials are considering the creation of whistle blower protection legislation.
4. Terri received an award from the Employee Recognition Program for the savings that resulted from her whistle blowing; however, she is contesting the award because it underestimated the amount of savings that resulted from her exposure of the fraudulent billing practice.
5. Terri was nominated for the Nurse Advocate Award from the Registered Nurses Association of British Columbia.

Chapter *20*

THE POLITICS OF NURSING RESEARCH

DOROTHY BROOTEN, LINDA P. BROWN, AND SUSAN M. MIOVECH

Research is removed from politics–it is pure and almost holy. — Dorothy Brooten (1984)

Not Hardly!! — The authors (1997)

For the naive or for perhaps a very few basic scientists who are able to isolate themselves from the outside world, research may appear to be devoid of political influence. For other researchers, however, especially those whose work involves patients, providers, and health care delivery systems, politics is an ever-present part of the work. It influences all aspects of research, from the choice of a topic through the dissemination of the study results.

CHOICE OF A RESEARCH TOPIC

Most researchers consider a number of factors when choosing a research topic: the importance or significance of the study, its scope, and the cost and potential yield of the work. The political gain or loss associated with choosing a certain topic is also apparent. The choice of topic holds potential political ramifications for the researcher's professional career, the institution in which the researcher works, the researcher's professional group and the funding for the research, in addition to the broader societal implications.

Professional Career

In some ways, the selection of a topic is a personal statement. The choice may express the researcher's personality characteristics and style. Some conservative individuals consistently choose relatively safe studies over which they have maximum control. Risk takers and renegades cannot avoid choosing topics that challenge the status quo and conventional wisdom, placing them in the spotlight or isolating them from the mainstream of colleagues and support. And there are those ethereal individuals whose lofty thoughts, often enjoyed in isolation, generate additional theories. Some researchers prefer to study a narrow area in depth, whereas others superficially study the globe. In each case, the choice of topic reflects the researcher's values and the societal context and dictates, to some extent, collegial research and professional group associations.

The politics (influence) of choice of a research topic should be obvious. You should be able to envision the influence of the topic that has been chosen. From a personal standpoint, will the research increase your personal and professional contacts, improve professional or personal networking with key individuals or groups, or lead to further studies? When starting a program of research, especially in a time of scarce resources, ask yourself:

- Why is this topic important to me, to my organization, and to society?
- What will be the potential yield for me as an individual and researcher?
- Is the work a potential career enhancer?
- Is this the best research area I can choose to study?
- Who else is interested in the topic, and why?

Institutional Influence

The choice of a research topic can be a fit or a misfit within your work setting. If its focus is in keeping with the mission and goals of the organization, the research may promote the institution's image, improve the delivery of its service, or reduce the costs of providing that service. Research focused in these directions can be expected to be supported in some way or at least not be blocked. Research topics at odds with institutional philosophy, mission, or priorities are not likely to be facilitated and may not even begin because of institutional disapproval.

As an example, you cannot expect a Catholic institution to provide support for work on the most effective abortifacients. Other examples may be less obvious. A study to discharge low-birth-weight infants earlier than routine may have several scenarios, depending on the institution. If the payer mix of low-birth-weight infants is such that a longer hospitalization is revenue generating for the institution, the proposed research is not likely to receive much support. Alternatively, if the hospital's costs of providing care to this group exceed the charges for which it can be reimbursed, the institution is likely to support the work.

In considering the potential institutional influence on a research topic, determine how it might improve care or teaching and, if it does, for how many patients or students. How might it decrease costs or solve major nursing or health care problems within the organization? Perhaps the study will improve the institution's image or improve relationships among disciplines or between institutional and community groups.

Influence on the Professional Group

The choice of a research topic also holds potential import for your professional group. Will the study accomplish the following:

- Improve health care?
- Improve the profession's image with the public or with policymakers?
- Add to nursing's knowledge base?

- Provide data on the cost-effectiveness of nursing services?
- Help increase future funding for nursing?
- Fit with regional or national funding or health care priorities?

Alternatively, the choice of a research topic can have a divisive effect on a professional group. For example, studies that pit one discipline or level of nursing against another usually generate much energy that might be better focused on ways to improve patient care.

Funding

Securing funding for research raises a host of political issues:

- Will you need funding to conduct the study?
- Given the topic you have chosen to pursue, what is a likely funding source, and what are the politics involved in securing funding from that organization?
- If you receive funding, what will be the political fallout in the institution in which you work and with other staff?
- What are the political ramifications of receiving one or another level of indirect cost recovery on the grant?
- Will you, as the investigator, receive any of the indirect cost recovery or, perhaps, will your division or department?

Even if your study can be conducted without funding, you may experience pressure to have it funded anyway. The reason may be to secure extra money for the institution or division or to use the funded research to improve the organization's image or establish investigators' funding track record. Conducting funded pilot work may also be necessary to establish credibility in order to receive larger full-scale funding.

Usually the next political issue is where to apply for funding for the work. Federal funding, such as that from the National Institutes of Health (NIH), carries substantially greater indirect cost recovery than do most private sources. It may be 55% or greater. Thus a grant of

$100,000 submitted by an institution that has negotiated an indirect cost recovery of 55% actually costs the granting agency $155,000. The $55,000 indirect cost is for the institution's maintenance of its libraries, research space and research facilities, and so forth. Although the indirect cost recovery on federal grants is continuously under review, federally funded grants still carry much higher indirect cost recovery than do privately funded grants, which are generally around 10%.

Some institutions and schools are reluctant to allow investigators to seek private research funding because of the small indirect cost recovery. They claim that the cost of providing the research space and support that the investigators need far exceeds the indirect cost recovery provided by the grant.

If private funding is needed, the next step may be to investigate the unpublished priorities and politics of the funding agency. This is usually done through informal networking and contacts, a political exercise of its own. The research topic may not be fundable from a political standpoint. The work of Dr. Ann Burgess and Dr. Lynda Holmstrom during the 1970s is illustrative. In 1972 little scholarly research existed on the problems of rape victims and providing counseling services to them—but none of the agencies to which they submitted grant proposals stepped forward with funding. One agency, a foundation supporting research in women's studies, told them that their proposal was very well written but the agency could not become involved in their topic. Burgess and Holmstrom went ahead with the project but without funding, fitting the research in between full teaching loads. Within a year, they interviewed 146 rape victims at all hours of the day, conducted weekly follow-up interviews, and attended the rapists' trials. The study was completed and published widely. Today Dr. Burgess is an acknowledged national leader in the area of research on rape, violence, and victimization, and she continues to conduct research in these areas. Obtaining funding for this line of investigation is easier now than it was in 1972.

More recently, the dean of social sciences at the University of Chicago was notified that researchers at his institution had been awarded more than $1 million in federal funding to study the social patterns that govern the choice of sexual partners among adults. Several weeks later, he was informed that the funding had been delayed indefinitely because NIH grant officials were unwilling to submit the proposal request for review to the parent agency, the U.S. Department of Health and Human Services. A few years previously, the same team of researchers, at the request of the federal government, had designed a major national survey of sexual behavior to provide data needed by public health officials to understand the spread of acquired immunodeficiency syndrome (AIDS) and other sexually transmitted diseases. The House Appropriations Committee killed funding for the program some months later, citing its controversial aspects (Suplee, 1991). Congressional interests and influence have a clear and direct effect on the direction of and financial support for research.

The current increase in managed care is also affecting research funding, especially clinical research. Academic medical centers for many years have supported clinical research from the income generated through medical faculty practices. In addition, some clinical research costs (e.g., tests, medications) were underwritten as patient care costs. Managed care organizations have refused to pay such research-related costs and are forcing academic medical centers to compete in the marketplace with lower costs for providing patient care. This situation has the potential to reduce both revenue for medical clinical research and the time physicians have to conduct clinical research. Physicians are being forced to increase clinical practice time to maintain the same income level as before the incursion of managed care (Mechanic & Dobson, 1996).

The same managed care incursion may favor nursing research for several reasons. First, far less research conducted by nurses has been subsidized through clinical practice and patient care costs. Second, managed care organizations are interested in and supportive of research with findings that can be applied immediately to patient care. They are far less interested in basic research with findings that will benefit patients in future decades. Because patients enrolled in managed care plans generally remain in the plan for an average of 2 years, managed care executives are interested in findings that provide a market edge and that can be used before enrollees change plans. Third, administrators of managed care plans are interested in research that prevents illness and minimizes disability, a strength of nursing research (Brooten, 1997).

The funding of research also involves personality factors. Not all researchers approach the issue of funding in the same way. Several character types are discernible. The "research purist" is heavily invested in a line of research—so invested that she will not change areas, no matter what, including the unavailability of funds to conduct the work. The work may thus never really flourish. The "research prostitute," on the other hand, has no particular line of research but will propose to conduct any type of research, so long as the funding is potentially available, and in the long run develops no program of research. The "research realist" is invested in a program of research but is also cognizant of the reality of needing the funds to conduct the work. The realist generally seeks several potential funding sources and can skew a proposal to coincide with the organization's funding priorities, providing that the integrity of the research can be maintained. Some organizations that support research even have the equivalent of a "research pimp." Unlike a developmental model, in which a senior researcher gathers junior colleagues and works with them to develop their research skills and thus their independence, a research pimp creates a dependence model. The research pimp writes the proposals for junior colleagues rather than with them. The end result, if the proposals are funded, is a short-term increase in the organization's research funding. Unfortunately, the junior colleagues are not prepared to conduct

research or to prepare the subsequent follow-up study proposal. They become increasingly dependent on the research pimp for the next proposal and for maintaining the status that often accompanies funded researchers. Ultimately the organization will suffer, as will science, because the research pimp can oversee only a limited number of people unprepared to conduct what should be their own independent work. Unfortunately, the organization may reward the research pimp well, and those who become ever more dependent on him will do the same. This method may be viewed as the only viable solution for producing grant applications, particularly for non-research-intensive institutions, but it is shortsighted in regard to the long-term development of the organization. Though this situation is hardly pure and holy, it certainly is filled with the politics of research.

THE CONDUCT OF RESEARCH

There are as many political considerations associated with the actual conduct of a research project as there are with selection of a research topic. Choice of research team members and the role each plays in the project, selection of the site of data collection, and the politics within the home institution where the project originates represent significant potential sources of conflict.

Selection of the Research Team

Who is included on the research team and who is excluded can be a political hot potato. Careful selection of members of the research team—coinvestigators, project directors, specialty personnel (e.g., economists, statisticians, clinical specialists), and research assistants—is critical. In some institutions, the chief executive officer or department head may not support an individual's being included on a research team. This may be due to a personal dislike or fear of the person or a wish to dismiss him in the future. Success on a study, even as a team member, might make future termination more difficult.

A major concern of principal investigators is putting together a team of people who can work effectively as a collective (Clemen-Stone, Atwood, Barkauskas, & Dumas, 1988). This can be problematic from the start. In one study examining caffeine intake during pregnancy, a physician refused to participate as a coinvestigator if the obstetrical nursing clinical director was a member of the research team. Apparently, these two individuals had a long-standing history of problems with each other. Avoid such problems by investigating relationships among potential team members ahead of time.

Besides compatibility, choose research team members for their essential knowledge and skills, resources, and influence. For example, in clinical studies, access to patient populations is essential. Physicians often act as gatekeepers, sometimes blocking access to the patient group under investigation unless they are involved in the project. In one of our studies, which examined the most effective nonpharmacologic methods for treating breast engorgement in nonlactating women, a key physician in the obstetrical department would not grant access to inpatient postpartum women because "there is a pill to treat this problem." On further investigation it became clear that he felt bypassed because he had not been consulted on the research proposal before it was funded. Ego problems of this sort are not uncommon.

When physicians serve as coinvestigators, there are often benefits of access to subjects, increased subject safety, and opportunities for nurse-physician collaboration. Additionally, collaborative relationships with members of other disciplines promote a positive image of nurses as rigorous researchers and valued colleagues (Naylor, Brooten, Brown, & Borucki, 1991). Benefits to physicians and members of other disciplines from involvement in nurse-led research include money, involvement in funded research, publication, and presentations.

Research that requires nursing staff participation can be facilitated if key members of the staff are involved as coinvestigators, project directors, or research assistants. If the staff members are not compensated or do not see the value of their involvement, the result can be devastating. Feelings of frustration and outright resistance can occur when staff members believe that their time is being consumed by research tasks not clearly linked with patient care or their job responsibilities. They may also resent the fact that patients' available time is being used to meet research requirements.

Staff nurses who are involved in developing research protocols generally have a clearer understanding of why a certain protocol is necessary and provide extremely valuable information concerning practical day-to-day aspects of conducting the research within their institutions. The specific role that nurses play as members of the research team is determined by a variety of factors, among them, available time, job requirements, interest, research preparation, and institutional support for these activities. Potential benefits can accrue to individuals involved in the project, too: tuition subsidy, coauthor status on any publications, the opportunity to present the research, participation in additional research, and participation in a mentoring relationship with senior researchers. The potential career advantages for staff members is apparent in one example involving a funded pilot study on factors affecting milk volume in mothers delivering low-birth-weight infants (Brown, Hollingsworth, & Armstrong, 1990–1991). A staff nurse was the study research assistant at the data collection site. She was able to document her participation in the study in her application to a doctoral program; receive tuition reimbursement for two doctoral courses plus a small stipend; present one paper and two posters on the study; be listed as second author on one publication (Brown, Spatz, Hollingsworth, & Armstrong, 1992); and gain research skills that were helpful to her during her doctoral program. On completion of her terminal degree, she became a coinvestigator on a study funded by the National Institute of Nursing Research, NIH (Brown et al., 1995–2000).

Selection of the Site for Data Collection

Numerous factors affect selection of the site for data collection: the number of available subjects, the number of other studies being conducted at the site, pragmatic concerns such as travel to and from the site, established connections at the potential site, and the feeling of cooperation, or lack thereof, with key people. The political considerations are significant, as the following example shows.

Several years ago, a nursing colleague who had received major NIH funding for a study on elderly persons found herself embroiled in a fight to maintain access to adequate numbers of subjects. A physician, who had a smaller amount of private funding, wanted to begin his study with the same subject population and informed the nurse researcher that she could "have" the subjects he would not be using. The nursing research review committee for the hospital had reviewed and approved her study several months previously; the physician had never bothered to submit his study to the committee. Citing overlap with an ongoing study previously approved, the committee denied the physician access to subjects at the site. Though this was a "gutsy call" by the group, they were backed up by long-standing procedures at the institution. Situations such as this demonstrate the need to follow established institutional review guidelines, monitor the site continually for potential difficulties, and maintain a line of communication and good relationships with key individuals based at the data collection site. This ongoing communication is particularly important in today's climate of institutional reorganization, restructuring, and partnering.

In some situations the political game employed at the site is simply one of perceived raw power and control, or perhaps naiveté. In a study involving children with AIDS, a nurse researcher was denied access to a data collection site (one of two in the city) unless she named a physician as principal investigator. The study was her idea, and she had already developed the proposal. She chose to gain access to the other site and was successful; however, her subject numbers could have doubled if she had been permitted entry into both institutions.

In another example a nurse researcher had been conducting a pilot study on caffeine and pregnancy for more than a year. She invited a toxicologist to be a coinvestigator after the study had been developed and funded. His laboratory ran the analyses of serum and salivary caffeine. His was the only laboratory doing these analyses in the city, but there was no reduction in the price of the analyses, even though he was named as a coinvestigator. When the head of his department wanted to know what studies would be submitted for major funding within the next year in the department, the toxicologist telephoned the nurse principal investigator. He indicated that the information was needed by his department head and that, if a major study would be submitted from the pilot, it would come from his department, not from the nursing school. His department, he informed her, needed the indirect cost recovery. Not being sure whether he was naive or simply attempting a power move, the nurse researcher was firm: if major funding was sought as a result of the pilot, the application would indeed originate from the nursing school. She pointed out that she had come to him with a study already developed and funded; she had graciously asked him to join the work, and he was providing no reduction in the cost of the analyses; and the nursing school also needed indirect cost recovery from its researchers. She concluded by saying that she hoped that her position was clear and that she had addressed his concerns because she would prefer not to end their work together but would have to do so if she was forced to send her samples to another laboratory. He not only grasped the message but gained a new perspective on nurses.

It is unfortunate that competitive nursing colleagues often play similar games. In another study a nursing clinical director stopped progress on a nurse's study for months to demonstrate her own power and expertise. The clinical director, who served on the hospital nursing research committee, would not approve this study, citing "lack of scientific merit." She claimed that the investigators were not attempting anything new and that their methods were flawed. The investigators received a two-page, single-spaced list of questions generated by her to be answered and defended before the committee. Not one member of the committee had directed a funded research study, and most had never been involved in research. As a result, the principal investigator had to educate the committee about research, as well as respond to their questions, many of them tangential at best. Although the study was ultimately approved, the delay of 3 months, during the summer (a time of high productivity for investigators in academia), put the study significantly behind schedule. The nursing clinical director who created such serious roadblocks had been a project manager and research assistant on a federally funded study. However, overlooked and perhaps not important to her, the study under review by the hospital research review committee had already been approved and funded by four national organizations.

It is important to determine the actual function of the institutional research review group (Chenitz, 1985). Usually it assesses the protection of human subjects and the feasibility of conducting the research in the institution. Review of the scientific merit of the study is often done, but it generally is not the primary responsibility of the group. It is important to know the committee members and their research knowledge and experience.

You can go through the proper channels and maintain relationships and communication, but often you cannot counteract the behaviors of individuals who see themselves as research or practice experts who are sometimes in competition with you. Situations like the example just cited are not uncommon. Other commonly experienced problems involve physicians who cannot comprehend why a nurse is investigating a problem.

Home Site Political Issues

Researchers often contend with political issues in their home institution, which receives monies for the research. Some common problems are allocation of scarce resources (especially space and support services), release time to do the research, and un-colleague-like behaviors of co-workers. The need for space to do the research and the need for support services, such as secretarial services, are often the first issues to be resolved in any newly funded study.

Securing the space needed to conduct the research often requires education of the administration, money to underwrite the cost of the space, and political pull. If the conduct of funded research is a relatively new activity for the institution, the administration may not understand your need for space. One investigator was informed that because she did not have an animal colony, she did not need research space. She was expected to store her equipment, supplies, and data forms in her existing—and already overcrowded—office and carry data forms back and forth from home to her office in a suitcase. The situation was eventually resolved through several discussions with the chief executive officer of the organization.

Because institutional space costs money, you will be far better able to negotiate space needs if your research is funded. If the institution receives indirect cost recovery from the study, the indirect costs should cover your space needs. But sometimes the indirect cost recovery is inadequate to pay for the space needs, or there may not be any available space. Sometimes this problem can be addressed in the proposal and additional monies secured for space rental for the duration of the study. Sometimes the space issue is political. An analysis of organizations often reveals individuals who have no funding but have ample research space, whereas other, well-funded investigators have little or inadequate space. Sometimes this has to do with the timing of space allocation—who needed it first—and sometimes it is a statement of value and control by the head of the organization. Allocation of space sends a powerful message. In some instances, being an organization player or a confidante to the chief or to those in control of resource allocation will count far more than one's merit as a nurse researcher.

Another political issue often encountered at the home site involves negotiating release time to conduct the study. If the study has received major funding, a proportion of the principal investigator's salary has been included for this person to be released to conduct the study. In theory, the organization hires or finds someone to conduct that portion of the investigator's work paid for by the research grant. Sometimes it actually works this way. Some investigators ignore this completely and are funded for 100% or more of their salary. Obviously the funding sources do not know that the investigator is committed for more than 100% of salaried time. This approach is used when there is an incentive to do so because it brings more money, resource, or power to the investigator or the department. Alternatively, some organizations provide no incentive and instead set up disincentives. In these situations, the investigator may be funded for 30% of the time that is to be allocated to the study. Rather than assisting the investigator to find help in relieving the workload, the organization simply assumes that the individual will conduct the study in addition to the current workload—and the organization uses the 30% salary support of the investigator for other purposes. The investigator, concerned with maintaining the success of the investigation, is compelled to assume an extra-heavy workload—an intolerable situation, even in the short run.

POLITICS IN DISSEMINATION OF RESEARCH FINDINGS

Just as politics affects the choice of a research topic and the conduct of the work, so it colors the dissemination of the research findings. Here the issues generally center on three questions:

1. Where should the findings be disseminated?
2. Whose names should appear on the publications and in what order?

3. Who should participate in the research presentations?

The study findings should influence the decisions on where to publish and present the results. It seems clear that study results with broad public policy implications should be disseminated to the broadest possible audience, but even these situations may be fraught with political overtones. A nursing study demonstrated a reduction of 27% in hospital charges and a reduction of 22% in physician charges when low-birth-weight infants were discharged from the hospital early and received home follow-up by nurse specialists (Brooten et al., 1986). The nurse researchers submitted the study results to the *New England Journal of Medicine* because they knew that papers published in this respected journal tend to receive broad attention in the lay professional press. Although the research was published and received national and international media coverage, this did not stop nursing colleagues, including some in rather powerful positions, from criticizing the investigators for publishing their findings in a medical rather than a nursing journal. Other nurse researchers have reported similarly that the response to their requests for help from the national professional association in further disseminating their research findings has been negative. Here, too, the response has been that the findings were "reported in a medical rather than a nursing journal." Such a myopic view does not help to highlight nursing's contribution to improving health care with multiple audiences.

The politics involved in deciding whose names should appear on publications and in what order and who should make presentations is common to all investigators. The principal investigator of a study has the role and responsibility for oversight regarding the rigor, integrity, and successful conduct of the study. This includes dissemination of the study findings. Though the principal investigator is first author on the main findings, coinvestigators may be first authors on secondary findings from the study. Inclusion of additional coauthors generally depends on their contributions to the manuscript. A general rule is that a coauthor must have made a significant contribution to the manuscript's development and submission. Principal investigators should be listed as authors of all manuscripts resulting from studies they have conducted. Their authorship demonstrates oversight and agreement regarding the validity of the data presented and conclusions drawn from work they headed.

Each research team or each principal investigator ultimately has to decide how to handle these issues. With a team approach, the work usually receives broader dissemination, and more people can potentially gain from the effort. The cost of inclusion is generally minimal; the cost of exclusion is generally much greater. One guiding rule for principal investigators, however, is to control their own data. It is not uncommon for associates to publish or present study results as their own, without attribution to the team or the principal investigator. These situations can be minimized if the rules regarding publication and presentation are established at the start of the study, agreed to, recorded, and reviewed periodically during the course of the study. Problems can also be minimized if the principal investigator is the only one with access to the most current study results. This point became clear in one situation in which a physician coinvestigator planned to present the preliminary findings of a study headed by nurses at a medical research conference as his own work. He was stymied because the principal investigator was the only member of the team with the most current findings and would share them only during the routinely held meetings of the team.

Politics is an ever-present part of research, from choice of the question through conduct of the work and dissemination of the findings. For those who would still see research as apolitical, pure, and holy, we respond: NOT HARDLY!

REFERENCES

Brooten, D. (1984). Making it in paradise. *Nursing Research, 33*(6), 318.

Brooten, D. (1997, February). *Nursing research in a managed care environment.* National Institutes of Health presentation, Washington DC.

Brooten, D., Kumar, S., Brown, L., Butts, P., Finkler, S., Bakewell-Sachs, S., Gibbons, A., & Delivoria-Papadopoulos, M. (1986). A randomized clinical trial of early hospital discharge and home follow-up of very low birthweight infants. *New England Journal of Medicine, 315,* 934–939.

Brown, L., Hollingsworth, A., & Armstrong, C. (1990–1991). *Factors affecting milk volume in mothers of VLBW infants.* Funded by grants from the Nutrition Center, Children's Hospital of Philadelphia, and International Sigma Theta Tau.

Brown, L., Meier, P., Spitzer, A., Finkler, S., Jacobsen, B., & Spatz, D. (1995–2000). *Breastfeeding services for LBW infants: Outcomes and cost.* Funded by a grant from the National Institute of Nursing Research (grant No. R01NR03881), National Institutes of Health, Washington, DC.

Brown, L., Spatz, D., Hollingsworth, A., & Armstrong, C. (1992). Promoting successful breastfeeding of mothers of LBW infants. *Journal of Perinatal Education, 1,* 20–24.

Chenitz, W. C. (1985). The politics of nursing research. In D. Mason & S. Talbott (Eds.), *Political action handbook for nurses: Changing the workplace, government, organizations, and community* (pp. 307–314). Menlo Park, CA: Addison-Wesley.

Clemen-Stone, S., Atwood, J., Barkauskas, V., & Dumas, R. (1988). The cluster concept in nursing research. *Nursing Outlook, 36*(4), 193–197.

Mechanic, R., & Dobson, A. (1996). The impact of managed care on clinical research: A preliminary investigation. *Health Affairs, 15*(3), 72–89.

Naylor, M., Brooten, D., Brown, L., & Borucki, L. (1991). Institutional yield on research: A case study. *Nursing Outlook, 39*(4), 166–169.

Suplee, C. (1991, September 26). Sex study is scrapped due to political concerns. *Philadelphia Inquirer, 324*(88), 14A.

UNIT III CASE STUDY

The Healthy Work Environment as Core to an Organization's Success

Joanne M. Disch and Sue M. Towey

With the rapid restructuring of the U.S. health care system and the persistent uncertainty as to where health care is going, change is a constant—and not only purposeful change toward a particular end. Rather, health care is reeling in a world of mergers, acquisitions, start-ups, takeovers, divestitures, integrations, and disintegrations. The result is that organizations are often reversing their strategic positions within a short period or suddenly finding themselves unable to survive as independent institutions or as undesirable components of a delivery system.

Employees of health care organizations have been caught in the crossfires of these events. Downsizing, layoffs, work redesign, and restructuring are the norm. Books such as *Surviving Corporate Transition* (Bridges, 1993) and *Healing the Wounds* (Noer, 1993) address the pain of the work environment, and the authors offer suggestions as to how to overcome the trauma of layoffs and revitalize downsized organizations. Given the uncertainty and anxiety within the work environment, it is understandable that employees ask, "What *can* I count on?"

In the past several years, during which profound change has occurred within our medical center, the leadership team has come to believe that the only thing which can truly be counted on is ourselves and how we treat each other. Creating a healthy work environment is one thing for which we can hold ourselves accountable. *People can accept an outcome if the process is fair.* While we cannot prevent all of the outcomes from organizational redirection, we can help our colleagues and ourselves go through it.

Policy and procedure manuals line the shelves of nursing leaders' offices and patient care unit conference rooms. The pace of change and the work to be done no longer afford the time to read about how to conduct the business of patient care but, rather, challenge us to possess the *personal power* to work and relate in a manner that has personal and interpersonal integrity (Hagberg, 1994). As a result of our experience of change, chaos, and uncertainty, we have been challenged to rethink the meanings of the words *policy, politics, and power* and how we define and operationalize them. Our challenge was to create and articulate policies and procedures that would create meaning in a way that is inclusive of the "felt experience" of leaders and staff. The intent of the Healthy Work Environment Initiative was to identify policies and strategies that would operationalize the vision of healthy relationships that would create a healthy organization and health care system (Kreitzer et al., 1997).

GENERATION ONE: UNIVERSITY OF MINNESOTA HOSPITAL AND CLINIC

In 1992 the staff of the University of Minnesota Hospital and Clinic (UMHC) embarked on a journey to position the institution for survival within the Twin Cities. Known throughout the country as a community with one of the most advanced markets for managed care, the Twin Cities had been the site for decades of health-maintenance-organization activity and numerous hospital closings. Though the remaining hospitals in the area had been honing their skills to compete effectively within a managed care environment, UMHC had not been doing so. Consequently, in 1992, the strategic planning process and reorganization began.

UMHC was not alone in its struggle to survive. Academic health centers in general have been especially affected by managed care, given their tripartite missions of patient care, education, and research. Reuter and Gaskin (1997) describe how academic health centers are challenged with the increased costs associated with education and research, the decreasing revenues, the increased competition for managed care patients, and the lack of systems to deliver patient-focused care efficiently.

This journey—with its learnings—has been described elsewhere (Disch, 1996; Scott, 1997). However, certain key factors should be mentioned. They enable significant change to occur while preserving a focus on the human side of change.

1. Though a consulting firm was engaged, the control for the design, decision-making, and change process was retained by senior management.
2. A broad-based group of administrators, managers, and informal leaders formed the nucleus of the work teams, thus enabling a wide array of employees to participate.
3. The medical staff was engaged from the beginning in several ways: jointly funding the strategic planning process; cochairing the cost-reduction initiative; cochairing and actively participating in the work teams; communicating progress; and being responsible in certain areas for specific outcomes.
4. The chief executive officer of the institution remained actively involved and kept everyone accountable for the outcomes.
5. Considerable effort was directed toward assisting employees in the change process— for example, devising opportunities for them to participate; sharing information; listening

to their concerns; and working with them as they made the transition to new practices, new roles, or new organizations. In retrospect, and even at the time, we realized that more can always be done, but a firm resolve existed to maintain a focus on people throughout the process (Bridges, 1993).
6. Within nursing, work on the Healthy Work Environment Initiative was unfolding and would prove to be a cornerstone and focus for all efforts. With time, this philosophy and concept have expanded throughout the organization.

During a process of such considerable organizational upheaval, the politics of change brings out new leaders. If the organization is to survive, these individuals must be visionary and resolute. They must hold constant to the principles and values of the organization and yet help the employees to create new policies and practices (Jeska, 1996).

THE HEALTHY WORK ENVIRONMENT INITIATIVE

In the late 1980s a work group of staff nurses and nursing leaders came together to explore ways in which they could address the burgeoning issue of abuse in the workplace. Studies have shown that abuse and violence are escalating, and for health care workers there are particular issues (Kreitzer et al., 1997):

- Caring for patients and their families is inherently demanding in physical, mental, emotional, and spiritual dimensions.
- Health care workers experience a range of emotions that may not be acknowledged or dealt with openly and constructively.
- Bureaucratic structures and traditional patterns of behavior reinforce stereotypical attitudes and practices.
- The organization's culture and leadership may reflect a rigid and impersonal style.
- The myriad changes ascribed to managed care have probably generated some degree

of loss, grief, anxiety, and uncertainty among the staff.

A survey within UMHC at the time indicated that more than 60% of the nursing staff stated that they had experienced abuse within the workplace.

An ad hoc group of interested nursing staff came together to address the issue. Four principles formed the underlying foundation for this initiative:

1. Abuse, neglect, and violence are learned behaviors with rewards.
2. These behaviors can be unlearned.
3. The patterns are cyclical and reinforcing; they are passed from generation to generation.
4. We can control ourselves, not others. Thus we can change only ourselves, not others.

From discussions among the staff and leadership, an expansion of the original focus emerged. Though the initial goal was eliminating abuse and violence from the workplace, it became apparent that the goal was not sufficient. Eliminating abuse and violence would not, of itself, result in a work environment that fostered positive growth and performance. Thus the work group refocused the discussion and described the characteristics of a desirable work environment. The document "Characteristics of a Healthy Work Environment" was created, and it has served as the focal point for all work since that time (see Box, p. 335). Kreitzer (1996) described the work that was subsequently done to incorporate the values associated with the healthy work environment throughout the nursing organizational structure.

Several activities were instituted to operationalize the principles inherent within the document.

LEADERSHIP TRAINING. Members of the nursing leadership team participated with an outside consultant in a series of work sessions geared toward creating environments that would support open communication, mutual respect, and trust.

PRIMARY NURSING RENEWAL. Nursing staff and leadership within individual patient populations participated in ongoing focus-group work to learn how to create healthy work environments within their particular areas.

BEHAVIORS OF A RESPECTFUL WORK ENVIRONMENT. A companion document to "Characteristics of a Healthy Work Environment" was developed to describe concretely the desired behaviors within the environment. See Box, p 336.

STAFF SUPPORT SPECIALIST. A clinical nurse specialist with skills in psychiatric-liaison activities focused her efforts toward being an advocate for a healthy work environment: providing support, education, and feedback to staff and the leadership team to develop personal power and healthy interpersonal relationships that would improve the health of the environment.

CENTER FOR CAREER DEVELOPMENT AND RENEWAL. This resource, led by a person skilled in change theory and organizational health, was created to assist all staff in dealing with career change, transition, the stress of job changes, and layoffs.

COMPETENCY ASSESSMENT. Specific competencies were identified for "managing change" and "contributing to a healthy work environment," the belief being that these skills were needed in today's health care environment every bit as much as technical competency, e.g., electrocardiographic monitoring and infection control.

THE ASSIST PROGRAM (Assist Staff in Stress and Trauma). This program, headed by staff with expertise in counseling or mental health, helps staff in dealing with stress, abuse, or trauma in the workplace. This program educated and communicated to the staff the personal and professional expectation (policy) of the need to address the emotional debriefing and process necessary in the business of health care delivery. This program was initially used regularly by staff, but as they learned the value of this

University of Minnesota Hospital and Clinic

Characteristics of a Healthy Work Environment

In a healthy work environment:
- I am viewed as an asset
- people call me by name
- my contributions and talents are acknowledged and recognized
- communication is open, direct and honest

In a healthy work environment, I have:
- time for creative thinking and reflection
- opportunities for personal and professional development
- resources are available to promote maximum contributions of staff to patient care and professional development

In a healthy work environment, I feel:
- safe
- gender sensitivity
- a balance between autonomy and team
- valued
- respected
- trusted
- nurtured
- stimulated
- challenged
- permission to take care of myself
- balance between my work and personal life
- commitment to the philosophy and mission of the organization

In a healthy work environment:
- risk taking is facilitated
- new ideas are supported
- innovation is fostered
- mistakes are OK
- diversity is embraced
- humor is valued
- I look forward to coming to work

Nursing
EMPOWER Project Committee
8/92

Reprinted by permission

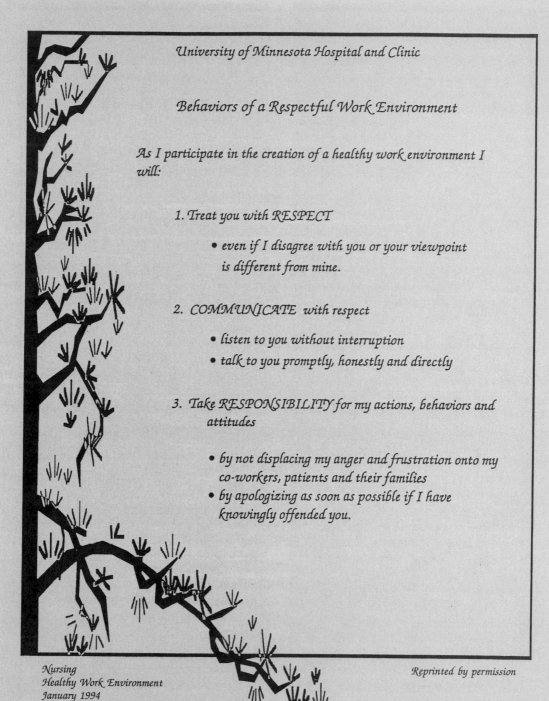

University of Minnesota Hospital and Clinic

Behaviors of a Respectful Work Environment

As I participate in the creation of a healthy work environment I will:

1. Treat you with RESPECT

 • even if I disagree with you or your viewpoint is different from mine.

2. COMMUNICATE with respect

 • listen to you without interruption
 • talk to you promptly, honestly and directly

3. Take RESPONSIBILITY for my actions, behaviors and attitudes

 • by not displacing my anger and frustration onto my co-workers, patients and their families
 • by apologizing as soon as possible if I have knowingly offended you.

Nursing
Healthy Work Environment
January 1994

Reprinted by permission

process, many were able to develop immediate support from their work area colleagues.

QUALITY MONITORING. Through the Quality Improvement Council, nursing staff developed a panel of indicators reflecting the health status of the environment. On a periodic basis, staff were asked to rank themselves and their work unit in such areas as respect ("I am treated with respect by my peers"; "I treat my peers with respect") and communication ("In my area, communication is open and honest").

CONCURRENT INITIATIVES

Concurrent with the work that nursing was doing in the institution, other areas also were instituting initiatives to address the work environment. For example, the Hospital Staff/Medical Council adopted a *disruptive behavior policy* that includes a formal mechanism for addressing inappropriate medical behavior. The *employee assistance program* was expanded to offer more services, and *workshops and other resources* were set up by the human resources department to help staff learn new skills and ways to deal with the changes occurring.

TRANSITION THEORY

Much of the work done within our organization in helping staff adapt to the changes stems from the work of William Bridges (1993), who describes the process of change as one moving from an ending, through a neutral zone, to a beginning. All changes create loss, even when the change is obviously for the better. Losses include the loss of attachments, of turf, of structure, of a future, of meaning, and of control. Usually there are tradeoffs, but one observation is that losses are felt emotionally, whereas the gains are more often experienced cognitively. This ending is important, however, because unless one gives up the old, one cannot embrace the new. Strategies for helping followers during this phase are based on theories associated with loss and grief: listening, acknowledging the pain, giving people time, recognizing

that people experience things differently, and being present.

The second phase—the neutral zone—encompasses tremendous uncertainty—situations in which individuals may be "disoriented and confused, hopeful one moment and despairing the next, a little crazy, very alone, and unable to communicate effectively with others" (Bridges, 1993, p. 59). In the current environment within health care, where the common wisdom is that "if you've seen one integration, you've seen one integration," the neutral zone can be daunting. The leader's role in this phase is particularly challenging and important, because it is during this period that the leader must step out ahead and provide direction and hope where little of either may be evident. This period is often likened to "taking followers through the wilderness." Conversely, it is during this phase that the greatest opportunities for creativity and excitement exist, because the old rules have been discarded and the new ones not yet codified.

Strategies for helping within this phase include the following:

1. Creating structure and predictability through *interim procedures and policies,* as well as temporary lines of authority, to provide direction between the known past and the unknown future
2. *Fostering group cohesion* wherever possible so that people can draw strength from each other
3. *Anticipating that old issues, myths, and rumors will surface* and allowing them to be aired, discussed, and acknowledged
4. *Reminding people* again and again why the particular change is necessary
5. Creating new *communication channels,* using them and being honest in the messages, which may only mean finding innumerable ways of saying, "I don't know"
6. *Minimizing unnecessary changes* whenever possible

7. *Reminding and showing people what they CAN count on*—often only each other in times of extreme organizational upheaval

In the third phase—the beginning—the framework and components of the new order of things emerges, such as the vision, direction, operational plans. The multidimensional plan needs to include some specifics, communication, leadership, training, incentives, and rituals. However, whereas the communication in earlier phases needed to be fact based, this phase requires it to be more evocative and compelling so that a sense of promise and hope is evident.

GENERATION TWO: FAIRVIEW-UNIVERSITY MEDICAL CENTER

In 1996 it became apparent that, in spite of major reductions in cost and improvements in service, UMHC would need to partner with another organization to obtain the needed primary care base and to survive. On January 1, 1997, the Fairview Health System of Minneapolis bought the UMHC facilities and integrated the UMHC and Fairview Riverside Medical Center, thus creating Fairview-University Medical Center (F-UMC). F-UMC is one entity, consisting of two campuses, the University campus and the Riverside campus, facing each other across the Mississippi River.

The creation of F-UMC has been notable for a number of reasons. First, it enabled the Fairview Health System to "round out" its services. With the merger, Fairview was suddenly able to offer the high-tech, highly specialized services of a quaternary medical center, internationally known for some of its programs (e.g., transplantation, cardiovascular services, oncology).

Second, coupled with numerous other changes in the environment, it meant that Fairview Health System had to rethink its overall strategy, mission, and vision. The new mission reflected the incorporation of a teaching hospital and the partnership with the Academic Health Center at the University of Minnesota:

Fairview's mission is to improve the health of the communities we serve. We commit our skills and resources to the benefit of the whole person by providing the finest in health care, while addressing the physical, emotional and spiritual needs of individuals and their families. We further pledge to support the research and education efforts of our partner, the University of Minnesota, and its tradition of excellence.

Similarly, the vision for the organization changed:

Fairview, with its partners, is the health system of choice, renowned for excellent clinical care and community health services integrated with education and research to help individuals, families and communities continually improve their health throughout all stages of life.

What has not changed are the four core values underpinning all activities throughout the system: *dignity, integrity, service,* and *compassion.* Work under way, however, suggests that two more values may be added as a result of the new relationship with the Academic Health Center. These are *innovation* and *collaboration,* strong components of the culture at UMHC and the University.

Third, it enabled the citizens of Minnesota to retain access to the state's teaching hospital, although in a different configuration.

Fourth, as with all integrations, it has required tremendous effort to bring together not only the two cultures, UMHC and Fairview-Riverside, but the myriad of subcultures that normally exist within complex organizations. Moreover, for the employees and the medical staff of Fairview-Riverside, this was not their first integration. For many, it was their third or fourth.

BRINGING TOGETHER TWO NURSING STAFFS

Margaret Wheatley (1992, p. 133) speaks of the importance of "simple governing principles: guiding visions, strong values, organizational beliefs—the few rules individuals can use to shape their own behavior." During a time when all elements of the environment are in flux and staff are asking, "What *can* we count on?" the answer may be only these few core rules—and each other. A prevailing focus for the leadership team was the principles inherent within the Healthy Work Environment Initiative.

Associated with any merger are a number of issues to resolve. For this particular merger, the special challenges consisted of blending a community health care system and an organization with national and international ties; of bringing together generalists and specialists; of reconciling practices from a public institution and a private institution; and of working with employees covered by different labor contracts (e.g., nurses were covered by union contract at Fairview but not at the University).

Against this backdrop, nursing leaders began the work of bringing the nursing staffs together. Two major directions were established: (1) bringing the nursing leadership staff together and (2) integrating the nursing staffs caring for particular patient populations.

Months before January 1, 1997, nursing leaders began meeting to develop strategies for integrating the two leadership teams. Workshops and retreats were held so that individuals from both campuses could share perceptions, misperceptions, myths, and fears about each other. Work was also directed toward identifying similarities, creating common objectives, and establishing a shared vision and framework. The principles of the Healthy Work Environment Initiative were the prevailing guidelines that were used, along with a strong commitment by the leadership to accomplish the work with consideration for the human side of change.

In December 1996, decisions were made regarding the nurse manager positions. Using the principles of the Healthy Work Environment Initiative, the incumbents helped shape the process that would be used, as well as the criteria that formed the basis for selection. Attention was paid to working with individuals not selected for positions, some of whom were assisted in finding other positions within the organization and some in making the transition to other employment.

Key groups began meeting. Clinical specialists, accountable to the director for nursing practice and research, came together, as did the nurse managers with the director for patient care delivery, the assistant nurse managers, and so forth. The Nursing Action Group, an advisory body to the vice president of patient-family services/chief nurse executive, was reorganized to include nursing leaders from both campuses to shape the course that nursing would pursue. The Staff Nurse Group on the University campus, a group of staff nurses who met monthly with the chief nursing executive, continued to meet but refocused their efforts toward identifying ways in which they could uniquely assist their peers in dealing with integration.

On the Riverside campus, the nurse executive met with staff nurse groups established through the Minnesota Nurses Association contract. On both campuses, decisions were made regarding such issues as nursing practice, staff development, and research. Where possible, the groups were integrated. When that was not a possibility, separate groups on each campus were established.

LEARNINGS AND REFLECTIONS

Several principles have emerged as the work has progressed.

1. Either/or thinking must be eliminated. Few options are right or wrong, good or bad, black or white. Collins and Porras (1994) discuss the "tyranny of the OR and the genius of the AND." Their point is that visionary companies operate with a mindset that challenges their employees to practice in a way that seems paradoxical and yet is highly effective: preserving a cherished ideology and stimulating change; promoting quality while being efficient; and practicing ethically while being sound financially. For nursing, an application would be to foster a strong nursing presence within an organization while advancing a pervasive interdisciplinary spirit. In the experience here, the best of both cultures had to be preserved. Whereas the literature on mergers suggests that there are "winners" and "losers," this group was committed to exerting their political strength toward *not* embracing that philosophy. Rather, the goal would be to create a new culture for nursing.

2. **Information is power, but relationships are the key.** Networks and linkages, connections and relationships, form the basis for support during turbulent times. Max dePree (1989, p. 23) comments that "we would like a work process and relationships that meet our personal needs for belonging, for contributing, for meaningful work, for the opportunity to make a commitment, for the opportunity to grow and be at least reasonably in control of our destinies." Again, there may be little in a situation that can be guaranteed. How individuals work together and provide support to each other *is* within the group's control.

3. **People can accept an outcome if the process is fair.** Spending time in identifying a process, adhering to it, changing it when necessary—and explaining why the change was necessary—are all components of a commitment to the process and to the individuals involved. Communication must be face to face, frequent, and interactive, with listening a key component. What people cannot accept is verbally wrapping change in a value (Larkin & Larkin, 1996), rather than embodying it consistently over time in action.

4. **Sufficient time, attention, and resources must be targeted toward supporting the work of the human side of change.** In addition to the time needed for communication, time is necessary for creating an infrastructure with policies, practices, new rituals, and traditions.

5. **The responsibility of leaders during these times is to make meaning out of what is happening, to help manage the transitions and chaos, and to sustain hope.** "We instinctively reach out to leaders who work with us on creating meaning. Those who give voice and form to our search for meaning, and who help us make our work purposeful, are leaders we cherish, and to whom we return gift for gift" (Wheatley, 1992).

A Case Study

By ourselves we suffer serious limitations. Together we can be something wonderful. — Max DePree

This is a story of the lived experience of "moving, merging, and leading" during the times of moving psychiatric inpatient units to a new campus within the first months of the creation of Fairview-University Medical Center. The issues encompass real-world change and the need for a nursing community to lead with integrity and respect during chaos and uncertainty.

This case study demonstrates the application of the policies, procedures, and vision created by the Healthy Work Environment Initiative begun several years earlier because operational policies, politics, and leadership powers were uncertain. The power now had shifted from external policies and procedures of the professional practice site to the internal personal power of all the leaders and staff involved. The formal and informal education provided to nursing leadership and staff nurses had been made explicit to guide this process of cocreation and problem solving *together,* as a team (Hagberg, 1994; Heider, 1985).

HISTORY AND CONTEXT

In the 1970s and early 1980s the UMHC psychiatry units were an innovative place to work. Dramatic new therapies were developed and groundbreaking advances in care were instituted. There was a sense that the future of psychiatric care was being created. In the fall of 1990 the nurse manager of the psychiatry units excitedly shared plans for the creation of a new, remodeled psychiatric center. With time, however, the practice and fiscal challenges of the 1990s brought about national changes in reimbursement and care delivery. Support for mental health services waned. Locally, changes were also occurring. The proposed remodeling was deferred. Managed care was evolving, and in November 1995 the announcement was made that the university teaching hospital would be merged with the Fairview Healthcare System.

Within the group, the years of uncertainty took their toll on the psychiatric health care team as many left. With the announcement of the merger, many felt unable to change their work status because of personal financial responsibilities, but the departure of experienced staff and leadership accelerated. The slow and insidious breakdown of the old and familiar practices within psychiatry contributed to a great sense of loss, and a grieving process for all those involved in these clinical areas emerged. For some, it was difficult to maintain hope, because their professional future was unknowable.

CREATING A TEAM

On December 2, 1996, only weeks before the official merger, a new leadership team was needed to maintain clinical integrity and programing. The new administrator who would lead the unit would not be named for a month. A staff support specialist—a psychiatric clinical nurse specialist (CNS) working with organizational change and staff crisis—was asked by nursing administrators to provide clinical supervision.

The interim leadership team was immediately developed to provide clinical supervision and communicate transition plans to the staff. An eclectic team consisting of the staff support CNS, the nurse manager of the child-adolescent unit, and a staff educator working with the unit formed the nucleus, along with an internal consultant. This team began to accept responsibility for collectively managing during this critical time, addressing the complex issues of clinical supervision, staff support, and communication about the multiple issues of integration. The date of moving the unit from the University campus to the Riverside campus, and of integrating the two psychiatric patient populations and staffs, was to be in the late spring of 1997.

With the appointment of the CNS, who had worked as a staff nurse on the unit 5 years before, the staff expressed some relief—but mostly great anger at their perception of abandonment by administrators whom they thought were concerned only about their own survival and not that of staff members. One highly skilled and experienced staff member stated that she was angry that administration had not shared the "plan" for the future, or if there was not a plan, that the administrators were incompetent. The staff members were tired, mistrustful, angry, and grieving, and they were fearful about their future as psychiatric nurses and as employed nurses.

Not only did the members of this developing leadership team not have answers, they were still learning the questions; the needs went well beyond clinical supervision. The staff members who had continued on the psychiatric units were mature, self-starting, and autonomous practitioners. Some were offended with the role of an interim leader and felt the need for more answers to questions about potential choices as to jobs with the merger and about the need for staff resources on a daily basis, in light of the wide fluctuations in the daily census. To add to the complexity, many of the hospital senior management team had still not been named; current administrators could not make policy decisions, and future leaders did not know who they were. Psychiatrists were creating or maintaining a stable leadership infrastructure. Conversations heard on the units between the physicians and the nurses frequently included aspects of their own job searches and attention to "getting off a sinking ship," as many perceived the merger. In spite of all the unknowns, critically ill patients were continuing to be admitted and were receiving thoughtful, expert care from the care team (Bridges, 1993).

EXPANDING THE TEAM

On January 2, 1997, the newly appointed director of behavioral services met with the interim leadership team. She immediately addressed the numerous personnel and practice issues, among them the potential and imminent shortage of staff. For example, because of severance opportunities for staff in association with the merger, there would be such a severe reduction in the number of paraprofessionals that there would not be sufficient staff to keep the units open beyond February. The move, originally intended for May, was moved up to February 28. This decision to put the date of the move on a "fast track" was met with appreciation and relief, but it increased anxieties and fears about choices for the future (i.e., layoff, early retirement, seniority with the union, transfer with the unit).

The director appointed a program director to manage the details of the move. Only a few weeks into these new, extensive responsibilities, the program director had a serious leg fracture—and was replaced with a head nurse from an adult psychiatric unit on the new campus. The staff knew and highly respected her as a person and as a clinician, and she joined the leadership team.

Two weeks before the move, the process of rebidding, according to the provisions in the nursing union contract, took place. The decision had been made earlier, when the creation of F-UMC was planned, that nurses on the Riverside campus, who were covered by a contract with the Minnesota Nurses Association, would remain so and that nurses moving to the Riverside campus would become members. Nurses on the University campus had voted against union representation 4 years previously and thus would retain that status. Nurses' optioning to move to the University campus would be covered by F-UMC policies, not a union contract.

This process used by the union at Fairview Riverside was new to the University hospital staff. Although they did not actually have information about their options until the day before the rebidding, surprisingly and happily the day of the rebidding went smoothly. This full-day activity actually seemed to be a day of very respectful healing because all staff members realized the complexity of the "fast track" plans. It was a day that modeled shared leadership and team learning among the nursing staff, the human resources staff from both campuses of the new hospital, and the interim leadership team.

BARRIERS

Some of the greatest challenges were to provide timely information, give human resources support, and maintain nursing and paraprofessional coverage of the units.

INFORMATION. Given the short time line of the move, the interim leadership team did not have answers about choices available to staff in a timely manner. Senior administration leaders were unable to give some of the answers because of the change in organizational policies and procedures resulting from the merger, some of which were still being developed. Though a lack of information may have been understandable, it was nonetheless extremely stressful to those involved.

HUMAN RESOURCES. Because the University Hospital nurses were nonunion and the Fairview nurses were unionized—a most unusual situation—policies to be used for integrating seniority as a result of the merger were difficult to develop. The human resources staff was unable to give answers to many critical questions asked by the nursing staff. Questions included the definition of seniority, the number of job openings within the psychiatry unit, benefits, and the number of part-time and full-time positions available. Salary ranges, although not the focus of concern, were available. The details regarding future human resources policies would take months to negotiate, and it was hoped that the result would be a blending of the best of both organizations. Unfortunately, staff mistrust and anger rose because each human resources representative had individual perceptions and beliefs regarding the prevailing policies.

NURSING AND PARAPROFESSIONAL UNIT COVERAGE. Continuing to maintain enough staff to continue to provide competent nursing care for the patients on the units had been a challenge for months. The staff nurses from the University hospital had been mature, creative, and autonomous in their management of staffing issues during the past months and worked readily with leadership staff to ensure that patient needs were met on a daily basis.

SUSTAINING HOPE DURING THE "DARK NIGHT"

The real world of health care is filled with uncertainty, and yet the resiliency of the human spirit of the staff and their ability to "dance with the chaos" was remarkable. The human reactions to the perceived injustice and "abuse" by the system were understandable, because staff members were unable to make decisions until they knew the options.

It was difficult for all to hear the information, or to acknowledge the lack of it, and not become frustrated or angry that no one could "take charge" or have more control over the outcome of the situation. The pain, loss, and grief over the "dominoes falling" in the merger were difficult to manage. It was challenging not to project anger onto "someone—anyone" who could have prevented this pain. The situation felt very much like a natural disaster in that we could watch the destruction, knowing that there would be more but not being able to stop it. Consistently, we found that hope was sustained moment by moment, in individual and group interactions in which people could be supported and heard, problems could be solved, and the next issue could be tackled. At times the shared experience of absurd but humorous "moments" made it possible to maintain some balance in ambiguous and paradoxical situations.

Once the dates were set for the moving and the rebidding, staff members were offered the opportunity to learn about other areas of nursing practice outside psychiatry. Many of the medical-surgical units were eager to have skilled psychiatric nurses on their staff, because the patient in the acute care setting is physically, emotionally, and spiritually complex. The staff began to experience the possibilities of personal and professional change because their specialty skills were valued in new and different settings in the health care system.

VIGNETTES OF SITUATIONAL LEADERSHIP

Every day new challenges emerged that needed to be addressed. Examples of situational leaders emerged; Max DePree (1989) would call them "roving leaders"—those indispensable people who are available in our lives when we need them. For example, on the second Monday after the merger, when paychecks were due, one of the interim leaders arrived on the adult psychiatric unit to discover that no one had taken the pay cards to human resources. When asked by a staff member whether she was there to do so, the leader calmly responded yes and proceeded quickly and quietly to ask another leadership team member what to do with time cards. Three of the interim leadership team then learned together how to do pay cards in a totally new system.

On another occasion, the interim clinical supervisor was called very early by unit staff with questions on how to provide staff coverage after electroconvulsive therapy (ECT). Providing this basic clinical practice herself for a few hours provided an ideal way for the supervisor to assess intuitively the clinical practice, morale, and needs of the staff.

BRINGING CLOSURE: A CELEBRATION

The leadership team continued to take the lead from the mature staff in helping to facilitate their needs in "closing the unit" (Achterberg, Dossey, & Kolkmeier, 1992). The days before the move were filled with both tears and laughter. The team and the patients all seemed to operate at an unusually peaceful level. There was an unspoken "knowing" that they were part of an "end of an era" in the history of nursing and psychiatry.

The final days of the unit, and the work to be done, brought a new sense of shared purpose and meaning to the staff community. Tears and laughter were elicited by reminiscing about the history of the unit, psychiatry, and the department. An old ECT box, ignorantly called the "hit man" by the manufacturers, was found in a corner of a treatment room and given to the current medical director of the ECT program with shared laughter. It was also a time of realization and pride that many of the major scientific breakthroughs in humane treatment and psychiatric knowledge were a part of our history.

On the evening of the last patient departure from our facility, the staff held a wonderful potluck supper in the old patient community room. The large pool table was transformed into a lovely buffet table. This event was attended by current and past unit staff, administrators, social workers, chaplains, nursing and medical school faculty, psychiatrists, residents, and many others who had a connection to this once-famous unit. It was truly a celebration of the end of an era in health care.

CURRENT STATUS OF STAFF

Months later, the staff members are settling in. Though the first analogy would be of a family moving in together, the members of which don't know each other very well, later observations would suggest a family with good times and bad, agreements and arguments, but pulling together over time.

Some specific updates are as follows:

- Staff members who did not support the move and thought there would be no place for them in the new organization are expressing enthusiasm for their new roles in the new organization.
- A master's prepared staff psychiatric nurse was seen several months after the move, looking bright, happy, and energetic. This nurse had chosen to relearn medical-surgical nursing and smilingly said, "There is life after psychiatry—in fact, change is good."
- One medical-surgical nurse manager shared that a former effective psychiatric nurse still needs mentoring because she had not worked in that environment for several years, but that she is eager to learn, is doing well, and likes her new job.
- One of the nursing staff who chose to work in medical-surgical nursing shared that she had learned to laugh at herself and her fears and felt hope and excitement for her future.
- One former psychiatric staff nurse shared a great relief in being able to move on and said that "it should have happened 5 years ago."
- A nurse who chose to take a severance package rather than apply for open positions had the summer off and was interested in returning to work in the fall.

- A few staff members who selected severance have taken part-time positions in the new unit.

CONCLUSION

Many of the lessons learned paralleled the writings of Bridges (1993) and the principles associated with the Healthy Work Environment Initiative, which many of the interim leadership team members had been active in helping to create. Though much work has been accomplished, much remains. Organizational change promotes personal transformation, which shapes organizational change. The experience can be difficult and draining, but is also survivable and growth producing. Much has been learned along our journey:

- The power of *presence—being there* for one another
- The need to be flexible to change expectations of self, others, and the organization
- The need to learn literally to live in the present moment
- The need to solve problems one moment at a time
- The ability to work with staff, organization, patients, and units in a crisis mode
- The importance of continually reviewing past processes cognitively with staff to remember that most of the conditions that created this situation were beyond any human control
- The need to use the knowledge of the grieving process to work with a grieving staff—physicians, registered nurses, all staff, and self
- The importance of remembering that grieving can be *very hard* and takes time and energy
- The need for priority commitment to personal self-care
- The importance of finding at least one personal confidant with whom one can express anger, cry, and laugh without judgment
- The need to celebrate small wins

- The importance of encouraging the staff members to take care of themselves in all ways
- The provision of career development resources for all staff members so that they feel able to make personal choices
- The importance of bringing food—eating together
- The need to keep a sense of humor about life's paradoxes
- The knowledge that information is power—but relationships are the key

References

Achterberg, J., Dossey, B., & Kolkmeier, L. (1992). *Rituals of healing.* New York: Bantam.

Bridges, W. (1993). *Surviving corporate transition.* Mill Valley, CA: William Bridges.

Collins, J. C., & Porras, J. I. (1994). *Built to last: Successful habits of visionary companies.* New York: Harper Business.

DePree, M. (1989). *Leadership is an art.* New York: Dell Publishing.

Disch, J. (1996). Strategies for nursing in managed care. *The managed care challenge for nurse executives.* Chicago: American Hospital Association/American Organization of Nurse Executives.

Eisler, R. (1987). *The chalice and the blade.* San Francisco: Harper.

Hagberg, J. (1994). *Personal power.* Salem, WI: Sheffield.

Heider, J. (1985) *The Tao of leadership; Leadership strategies for a new age.* New York: Bantam.

Jeska, S. B. (1996). *Applying leadership competencies for nurse executives: The managed care challenge for nurse executives.* Chicago: American Hospital Association/American Organization of Nurse Executives, pp. 51–64.

Kreitzer, M. J. (1996). *Creating a healthy work environment: The managed care challenge for nurse executives.* Chicago: American Hospital Association/American Organization of Nurse Executives, pp. 65–74.

Kreitzer, M. J., Wright, D., Hamlin, C., Towey, S., Marko, M., & Disch, J. (1997). Creating a healthy work environment in the midst of organizational change and transition. *Journal of Nursing Administration, 27*(6), 35–41.

Larkin, T. J., & Larkin, S. (1996). Reaching and changing frontline employees. *Harvard Business Review,* 95–104.

Noer, D. M. (1993). *Healing the wounds: Overcoming the trauma of layoff and revitalizing downsized organizations.* San Francisco: Jossey-Bass.

Reuter, J., & Gaskin, D. (1997). Academic health centers in competitive markets. *Health Affairs, 16*(4), 242–252.

Scott, L. (1997). Can marriage of academic, community hospitals work? *Modern Healthcare, 27*(11), 26–32.

Wheatley, M. (1992). *Leadership and the new science: Learning about organization from an orderly universe.* San Francisco: Berrett-Koehler.

Unit *IV*

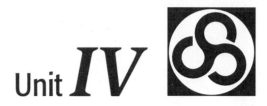

POLICY AND POLITICS IN GOVERNMENT

Unit IV

describes politics and policy in the sphere of government. Chapter 21 provides a comprehensive discussion of contemporary issues facing government—not only as they relate to health policy, but as they relate to the broader social issues that directly or indirectly affect the health of individuals, families, and communities. The vignette that follows this chapter discusses the impact that the Temporary Assistance for Needy Families Act is expected to have on child health and demonstrates the relevance of this change in U.S. welfare policy to the daily practice of nurses.

Nurses need to understand the legislative and regulatory processes explored in Chapter 22 in order to know how to influence the legislative and executive branches of government at the local, state, and federal levels. Particular emphasis is on the regulatory process, which is often overlooked. Yet many of the most significant influences on practice emanate from regulations that are developed after legislation is passed. Chapter 23 discusses the judicial branch of government and analyzes when and how nurses can use this route to change policy.

The next three chapters describe issues and processes in local (Chapter 24), state (Chapter 25), and federal (Chapter 26) governments. They contain examples of issues about which nurses need to be concerned and descriptions of how nurses have used their political skills to influence the development of public policy at each level of government. The vignette following Chapter 25 recounts the journey of a geriatric nurse practitioner who became a legislator and leader in the Wisconsin Assembly. The vignette that follows Chapter 26 is an interview with one of the most powerful nurses in Washington, D.C., during the past two decades—Sheila Burke, RN, former chief of staff to retired Senator Robert Dole. She shares her experiences and lessons learned in "rising to the top."

One way to take a leadership role in developing public policy is by being appointed to public office. Chapter 27 provides guidelines for how nurses can go about securing a political appointment. The vignette that follows describes two nurses in New Jersey who were appointed to high-level positions in the Department of Health and the factors that led to their leadership positions.

Influencing the development of policy occurs directly and indirectly. Participation in party politics is one avenue for indirect influence. Political parties and how to get involved are described in Chapter 28. Direct lobbying of policymakers is the topic of Chapter 29. It explores effective ways to convince elected officials to support your issues and outlines tips on telephoning and visiting legislators, letter writing, and testifying. Another indirect method of shaping policy is through electing candidates who support nursing's concerns and issues. Chapter 30 discusses selecting and becoming a candidate for public office and participating in election campaigns. The content of this chapter is illustrated by a vignette of a nurse who has successfully managed campaigns. The unit ends with a case study by a nurse legislator in Montana. Her humorous and instructive story illustrates the realities of being a policymaker and running for office.

Chapter *21*

CONTEMPORARY ISSUES IN GOVERNMENT

MARY WAKEFIELD, DEBORAH B. GARDNER, AND SHARRON GUILLETT

HISTORICAL PERSPECTIVE

Throughout the 1980s the relationships among local, state, and federal governments underwent significant change. With an expanding federal deficit and a struggling economy, more demands were placed on shrinking resources. While fiscal remedies were sought, the rhetoric of the 1980s, including "read my lips, no new taxes," fueled voter resistance to tax increases. Federal government and state officials were sensitive to voter sentiment; instead of raising taxes to meet growing needs, the federal government withheld federal dollars and pushed more of the fiscal burden onto state and local governments. In response, state governments initially helped to fill the funding void facing localities by extending increased financial support to them, but by the end of the decade, many states were experiencing budget shortfalls of their own and consequently reduced support to local governments.

In this environment, surging health care costs became particularly burdensome. During the 1980s, inflation in medical services rose significantly in comparison with the cost of other goods and services. The average annual rate of increase in health care costs from 1980 through 1989 was 10.3%. This growth rate in health care spending captured the attention of American businesses. In 1990, businesses spent an average of $3,000 per employee for health coverage—an increase of 24% from 1989. The

health care costs paid by business consumed 45% of corporate operating profits (Health Care Crisis, 1990).

Also affected by rapid increases in health care costs were state and federal governments. In 1989 the National Governors' Association, overwhelmed by Medicaid costs that increased from 9% of state budgets in 1980 to 14% in 1990, took the lead in advocating health care reform. One of the most contentious interactions between state governors and the Congress occurred in 1989, when the former demanded a freeze on new Medicaid expansions. Though the governors acknowledged that a real need for expanding services existed, they lacked the money to support those expansions.

At the end of the 1980s and on the threshold of the 1990s, the federal government was long on rhetoric and short on action in devising a plan to reform the health care system. Under tremendous fiscal pressure, states were left to their own devices and advanced various reform plans. The Oregon rationing plan (see Unit II Case Study) was one of the most hotly debated proposals; however, many states subsequently initiated their own plans for health care reform.

HEALTH CARE IN THE 1990s

In the early 1990s, bipartisan consensus developed around the need to produce a balanced federal budget and eliminate the expanding deficit. Since the federal government has not collected enough revenue to cover all federal spending, money is borrowed to pay for the deficit and accrues as the federal debt. In 1996 the debt hovered around $3.6 trillion. Federal debt is problematic for policymakers because money spent on interest payments means less money available for other federal programs, including health care. Additionally, when the government is obliged to borrow a lot of money, interest rates are driven up, affecting everything from home mortgages to interest rates on car loans.

Though the 1990s began with a Republican in the White House and a Democrat-controlled Congress, by 1992 the political landscape began to reverse with Democrat William Clinton's election to the Presidency. Two of Clinton's first objectives were to enact deficit reduction legislation and reform the nation's health care system. In 1993, after significant political battles, President Clinton succeeded in passing a deficit reduction package with spending cuts and increased taxes, the latter applied primarily to the wealthy. Since then, the federal deficit has been gradually decreasing. However, rising costs in federal programs such as Medicare and Medicaid continued to put pressure on spending and contributed to the deficit.

In the mid and late 1990s the Administration and Congress coalesced around the need to eliminate the deficit and balance the federal budget. Whereas deficit reduction occurs through spending cuts and generating revenue (i.e., raising taxes), with few exceptions the latter has generally remained politically unpalatable. Consequently, the creation of new federal programs and spending for old ones were considered within the context of impact on the federal budget. Interestingly, and quite unexpectedly, by the end of 1997 balancing the federal budget appeared to be an easier task because of consistent strong and unexpected economic growth as well as low inflation. However, by this time, major changes in federal spending were enacted.

HEALTH CARE REFORM

Various compulsory health insurance legislation has been proposed in the United States since the early twentieth century, beginning with legislation advocated by Theodore Roosevelt and the Progressive Party in 1912 (Wilson, 1993). Although many presidents since then have proposed significant health "reform," none of the proposals compares with that of President Clinton. From the beginning of his Presidency, he expressed strong support for legislation to expand health care coverage. The Democrat-controlled Congress viewed health care reform as a priority in light of rising costs and increasing numbers of uninsured persons. However, by the time the President's Health Security Plan was abandoned in September of 1994, tremendous opposition had developed. The bill was seen as too complicated, too costly, and highly regulatory, and public support had substantially eroded. Organizations from insurance companies to the American Medical Association opposed the bill.

Many opinions were expressed regarding the demise of the Health Security Plan, ranging from perceptions that the bill was too complicated, to concerns that the plan was hatched in secret by a team knowledgeable about policy but neophyte in terms of political reality. Others believed that the Clinton plan failed primarily because of misinformation (Fallows, 1995). Yet the story of health care reform efforts in the early 1990s was not that simple. Three daunting obstacles thought to help explain the failure of the Clinton plan are (1) the fact that health care policy problems are genuinely complex, (2) ideological conflict blocks consensus development, and (3) the best-organized interests in health care benefit from the present system (Starr, 1992).

Part of the complexity in reforming health care was the interaction of two opposing yet valid issues: inadequate access and rising health care costs. Pressure to provide universal "access" to health care began in the 1960s with the passage of Medicare and Medicaid. This was the first time legislation was enacted ensuring that selected population groups would have access to health care. In the early 1970s, the political impetus for further expanding access was complicated by fiscal pressures associated with rising costs of providing that health care (Hoefler & Thai, 1993). By 1990 the United States spent 13% of the Gross Domestic Product on health care while 15% of the population, 37 million people, were without insurance for regular health care. In the same year, opinion polls found that 90% of the American public believed that fundamental change or a complete rebuilding of the health care system was needed (Pew Health Professions Commission, 1995). These circumstances led President Clinton, in 1993, to propose major health care reform through the Health Security Act.

The strategies to meet the competitive goals of improving access and quality while containing costs were the focus of many political conflicts. The primary strategy was through "managed competition within a budget" (Weissert & Weissert, 1996). The Clinton plan had provisions similar to other health care proposals developed in 1993 and 1994, including consumer choice among competing health plans, the establishment of health insurance purchasing cooperatives, a standard benefit package, premium subsidies for low-income families, and a universal mandate. The Clinton plan also identified payment for health coverage through an "employer mandate." That is, to cover all Americans, employers were to pay 80% of the employee insurance premium, with employees making a 20% contribution (Starr, 1995). Coverage would be government subsidized for those who were unemployed or worked for small firms. Private insurance companies would continue to offer coverage, but the government would "manage" the way insurance companies competed for business.

Federal oversight would be operationalized through a national health board that would set standards and oversee compliance with new requirements, many of which were designed to encourage managed competition. Managed competition is a purchasing strategy designed to group public and private purchasers together in coalitions called health insurance purchasing cooperatives or alliances. Through participation in mandatory regional health or corporate alliances, each company or region would devise a list of standard benefits, to be offered at the same price to all customers. These health alliances would negotiate the best price and service from competing health plans. Each year people would have the opportunity to compare and choose a health insurance plan. Choices would include fee-for-service plans that let them continue to see the physician of their choice. To address the issue of cost, the government would set an overall limit on the amount of money that could be spent on medical care each year, while giving insurance companies and health plans latitude to spend the money as they thought best (The President's Health Security Plan, 1993). This limit was the "budget" in Clinton's strategy for "managed competition within a budget." Clearly the complexity of reforming multiple facets of the health care delivery system posed a massive challenge to policymakers.

The second obstacle to health care reform, identified earlier, is the extent to which ideological conflict blocks consensus development. According to many political historians, ambivalence about government intervention and its likely effects is rooted in our country's foundational belief that government must not become too powerful (Weissert & Weissert, 1996). The degree of government intervention and regulation in the health care sector of the economy was perceived as the crucial ideological issue regarding national health insurance (Wilson, 1993). In addition to ideology, the desire of members of Congress to win reelection and their relationship with the occupant of the White House are political factors that have an impact on most policy discussions.

The third obstacle to health policy reform, according to Starr (1992), concerns interest groups. There were a number of examples of power wielded by key organized interest groups during the health care debate. For example, business interests moved from the point of asking the Administration to spearhead sweeping health reform to preferring that the government make only incremental changes. Their initial interest in reform resulted from burgeoning costs in providing health care coverage. From 1948 to 1990, business spending on health coverage rose by an average of 15.6% a year. Initially, Clinton approached the need for health care reform from the need to control health care costs, winning the support of business leaders. In terms of small-business owners, the Clinton administration anticipated opposition and limited their obligations. In fact, most small businesses would have seen declines in health care costs under the Clinton plan. As health care inflation eased, businesses worried less about health care cost containment and more about the political implications of an expansion of government authority in the health care market. The growing opposition of special interest groups, particularly the millions of dollars spent by the Health Insurance Association of America on media, including the now famous *Harry and Louise* television commercials, coupled with lobbying and campaign contributions, helped to create public anxiety and political paralysis (Starr, 1995). Starr argues that, under these conditions, the ideological and interest-group opponents of reform were able to change the subject from health care to government. A referendum on government was not a debate that would be won.

Though most of the attention focused on the President's Health Security Plan, which proposed managed competition "within a budget," other policy approaches were offered by Members of Congress, including "single payer" and "play or pay" systems. A single-payer approach is a form of universal coverage where private doctors and hospitals would provide care but the government would take over all medical payments and finance them with taxes. In contrast, the play-or-pay strategy, supported by many Democrats, required companies either to buy health insurance for their workers or to pay into

a public fund to insure health care workers not insured through their employers. Using this approach, additional provisions would have to be made to insure the unemployed. The Clinton version of managed competition was an effort to integrate these two approaches. Yet managed competition, as it was operationalized in the Health Security Plan, was heresy to many Congressional Democrats (Fallows, 1995). Ultimately, the lack of consensus and the infighting among Democrats, and between Democrats and Republicans, confused the public and also slowed momentum for reform. In spite of the initial impetus for reform, ideological conflicts, organized special interests, and the perceived complexity of the bill effectively blocked comprehensive reform.

STATE HEALTH POLICYMAKING

In the vacuum left by the failure of comprehensive national reform, using an incremental approach, all states have moved in some way to address the goals of improving access and quality while containing costs. The critical policy issues debated and shaped at the state level are identified in four broad areas: oversight of managed care, expanding health insurance coverage for children, promotion of home- and community-based alternatives for the elderly, and redesigning of the health care work force.

In the area of managed care, just about every state has enacted small group insurance reforms (2 to 50 employees) to improve access. Thirty-nine states have enacted guaranteed issue laws. That is, states have mandated that health plans offer and issue coverage to any employer group that applies for coverage. At least 45 states have guaranteed renewal—a requirement that health plans offer to renew coverage of an employer group before expiration of a policy except for reasons such as fraud or nonpayment of premiums. With the 1996 passage of the Health Insurance Portability and Accountability Act at the federal level, many more states will focus on individual market reforms (The Forum for State

Health Policy Leadership, The National Conference of State Legislatures, 1997).

States continue the practice of mandating insurance coverage for certain types of situations and conditions to ensure access and quality. For example, in 1997, 29 states required insurers to cover inpatient stays after the birth of a child, 16 states passed laws regarding reimbursement for emergency care services, and 7 states mandated coverage for bone marrow transplants to treat cancer (Health Policy Tracking Service, 1997). Further, as the 105th Congress expanded coverage for children in the budget legislation of 1997, all but 8 of the 50 states were already implementing expanded care. Thirteen states had established state-financed insurance programs for children, 26 had expanded Medicaid beyond mandated levels, and 24 had initiated private Caring Programs for Children, sponsored by Blue Cross/Blue Shield. States used a variety of revenue sources to pay for the programs, including tobacco taxes, alcohol taxes, and federal Medicaid waivers. However, most of the state programs serve relatively few children (The Forum for State Health Policy Leadership, National Conference of State Legislatures, 1997).

In addition to addressing access and quality, states turned to managed care as a way to control costs in Medicaid programs. By 1997, 46 states had some type of waiver program in place which allowed states implementing managed care to restrict beneficiary choice of provider by requiring enrollment in certain health plans or accessing certain providers.

With market-driven rather than federally driven changes in health care under way, state interest in "conversions"—the sale of nonprofit hospitals to for-profit entities—became an intense issue. Even with new laws strengthening state oversight of such transactions, the trend toward high-profile acquisitions and joint ventures remains strong. Observers argue that the motivating force behind conversion mania is the need for the nonprofit facilities to raise capital that will keep them competitive in today's "health care as business" environment. Many state legislators became concerned that

the nonprofit facilities, long protected by tax breaks and rewarded with charitable contributions, fairly value the assets they transfer and that buyouts not lead to a deterioration of community services (National Conference of State Legislatures, 1997).

In 1996 Nebraska had the only law increasing the authority of the attorney general and the health department to review hospital sales and keep the public informed of the details. A year later, 20 states followed suit, although with little uniformity among the laws.

Home care and community-based alternative for care of the elderly is another critical issue on which states are focusing. To better serve the 80% of elderly populations who live in their own homes or community, some states are strengthening their network of home- and community-based services, with Medicaid an increasingly important funding source for these services.

Finally, because of budget pressures and persistent medical underservice, states have been forced to identify strategies to change the geographic and specialty imbalance in their health care work force. By 1997, 15 states passed legislation specifically to encourage or mandate the creation of family medicine departments in state-supported schools, and more than 40 states created special grants for family physician training. Financial incentives to medical students and residents are increasingly targeted to those who plan to practice primary care in medically underserved areas. As many as 12 states are looking to develop state health work force councils to assess/address state work force needs and to exercise authority in allocating state funds (The Forum for State Health Policy Leadership National Conference of State Legislatures, 1997).

Many of the health care reform issues have not changed, and they continue to challenge both state and federal governments. However, the number and types of strategies for developing an efficient and effective health care system have increased as states "experiment" with different models and expanded roles. Given the interdependency of states with the federal government, successful efforts to achieve increased efficiency and effectiveness in the health care system can best occur through collaborative efforts.

ACCESS TO HEALTH CARE

The failure of the Clinton Administration to build support for the Health Security Act did not indicate that cost, quality, and access problems were unimportant to legislators. On the contrary, members of both political parties in the House and Senate recognized the importance and urgency of holding down rising health care costs and increasing access to health care. The debate centered not on the validity of the issues themselves but on the policy approaches recommended to address them. Subsequent to the failure of Clinton's broad reform initiative, Congress pursued incremental approaches to resolving issues of cost and access. Legislative activity in the late 1990s primarily focused on expanding health care insurance coverage as a means to expand access. Two groups, in particular, were targeted: (1) people who lost health insurance as a result of either changing employment or preexisting conditions and (2) children who were Medicaid eligible but not participating and children who were ineligible for Medicaid but whose families were unable to afford health insurance.

Despite the attractiveness of supporting expanded access for both working people who lose health insurance and for children, there were competing concerns that warranted attention. For example, some members of Congress were concerned that government intervention would result in forcing insurance companies to raise premiums, further increasing the number of uninsured persons. Concern was also voiced regarding whether employers would take advantage of expanded insurance made available through the government and drop employer-based coverage, thereby increasing the burden on the government and ultimately the taxpayer. Despite these concerns, expanding employee access to health was generally supported.

Ultimately, incremental reform addressing access to care through the Health Insurance Portability and Accountability Act (HIPAA) was enacted in 1996. The prime objectives of this law were to make health insurance portable and continuous for employees changing employment and to prohibit insurance companies from rejecting coverage of individuals with preexisting conditions. These provisions were rooted in the least controversial elements of the Health Security Act proposed by President Clinton. Additionally, HIPAA mandated a demonstration project allowing 750,000 people to establish medical savings accounts, raised the tax deduction for health insurance, and clarified penalties for fraud and abuse by providers. It was estimated that between 21 and 25 million people would benefit from provisions of this law.

Building on the success of HIPAA and sensing strong public support, Democrats declared increasing access for the nation's 10 million uninsured children a "top priority" for 1997 and challenged Republicans to do the same. From a political standpoint, ensuring health care coverage for children was difficult to oppose. This was especially true in the latter part of the 1990s, when changes made in Medicaid standards resulted in the elimination by many states of all but the poorest children from their programs, without an offer of alternative solutions. Other factors also contributed to the heightened interest in expanding health care coverage for children. First, children continued to be the largest group of Americans without health insurance, accounting for one of every four uninsured persons in 1995 (Johnson, DeGraw, Sonosky, Markus, & Rosenbaum, 1997). Second, 9 of 10 uninsured children had working parents who earned too little to afford insurance but too much to qualify for Medicaid. Finally, the number of uninsured children remained high despite the expansion of Medicaid, in part because of the decline in employer-based coverage, a trend likely to accelerate because of structural changes in the work force (Employee Benefits Research Institute, 1997).

Expanding coverage to children presented unique concerns. For example, though the American Academy of Pediatrics reported that uninsured children were less likely to seek and receive necessary care, no causal link between having insurance and positive health outcomes has been established (Holahan, 1997). Nor was there evidence that parents would avail themselves of the insurance provided. A case in point was the high percentage of Medicaid-eligible children not enrolled in the program. Finally, there was concern in Congress that guaranteeing children the right to health care would create another middle-class entitlement, in direct opposition to President Clinton's statement in 1996 that the era of "big government" was over. Nonetheless, by mid-1997 there was strong Presidential and bipartisan Congressional support for expanding federal coverage to the nation's uninsured children. The debate moved from whether to increase access to insurance to how, and how much coverage should be provided. Eventually, $24 billion was provided through the Children's Health Insurance Program (CHIP) for expanded child health care coverage, with states having significant authority to determine the services that would be provided.

Expanding child health care coverage and enhancing health insurance portability for employees are typical incremental legislative responses to health policy problems. Reticent to embrace sweeping reforms after the political backlash against the Clinton Health Security Plan, Congress preferred smaller, politically palatable changes.

MEDICARE

With support building throughout the 1990s to balance the federal budget, large federal programs experiencing significant growth captured the attention of policymakers. Social Security, followed by defense spending, interest on the national debt, and Medicare were the largest components of the federal budget. Spending on other federal programs such as education, foreign aid, and welfare paled in comparison. The government having paid more than $1 trillion for health care in 1995 (Health Spending Projections, 1996) and with Medicare bankruptcy looming, the attention of policymakers

turned specifically to the nation's largest health care programs, Medicare and Medicaid. (See Chapter 5 for a description of Medicare and its impact on federal spending.)

Contributing to a projected increase in Medicare spending were demographic trends indicating that whereas 9% of the population was older than 65 years of age in 1960, the number was expected to increase to 20% by 2030 with the retirement of the baby boom generation beginning in 2010. In addition to demographic changes, utilization patterns of various health services changed markedly in the past 10 years. For example, the home health benefit became the fastest growing part of the Medicare program, rising from $3.7 billion in 1990 to $12.7 billion in 1995 (Leon, Neuman, & Paremte, 1997). This increase amounted to an average annual growth rate of 38%, reflecting a surge in volume of services. It came as no surprise, then, that costs associated with the home health benefit received considerable attention and that plans to move it to a prospective payment system were advocated in the mid-1990s. Additionally, investigations in the latter part of 1997 identified a significant factor contributing to the steep increase in home health costs—fraud (Office of the Inspector General, 1995).

With the dual pressure to decrease Medicare spending growth and reduce the federal deficit, a number of policy options have been considered. Discussions surround how much money needs to be saved in the Medicare program, what actions should be implemented to achieve those savings, and what changes in the program itself should be made to ensure its solvency.

These issues became the subject of much policy debate with a number of Medicare changes proposed in the fiscal year 1996 Balanced Budget Act, and with political rhetoric during the 1996 Congressional and Presidential election campaigns. Congressional Republicans proposed substantial restructuring of Medicare to slow the rate of growth. The changes included shifting Medicare from a solely government-regulated program to one that relied more heavily on market-based competition. Central to Medicare reform was a proposal to move it from an open-ended entitlement program to a defined contribution program whereby the government would set a payment amount per beneficiary for the purchase of health insurance. Basically, instead of being entitled to a predetermined set of benefits, beneficiaries would be entitled to a predetermined amount to pay for their health care. Whether the payment amount was adequate to cover needed health care would not be guaranteed. Moreover, Republican Members of Congress were strongly advocating the inclusion of Medical Savings Accounts (MSA) as a choice for Medicare beneficiaries. MSAs are personal savings accounts set aside to pay for health care expenses. Contributions would be made to these accounts by employers, individuals, or the government. The contributions would be excluded or deducted from taxes, and funds not used in the MSA could accumulate or even be used for nonhealth purchases. Republicans believed that MSAs provided consumers with an increased financial stake in buying health care and thus would encourage them to be smart shoppers. In fact, MSAs shift financial risk to beneficiaries if the MSA deductible exceeds the balance in the account. Meanwhile, Democrats predicted that MSAs would tend to attract mostly healthy people, and consequently a smaller pool of less healthy individuals would be left behind, resulting in increased insurance costs for beneficiaries remaining in traditional programs. In spite of antideficit rhetoric, many congressional Republicans supported MSAs, knowing that MSAs would likely add two billion dollars in costs to the Medicare program over 5 years (Congressional Budget Office, 1997).

These proposals provided political fodder for the election campaigns, with Democrats contending that Republicans were cutting and therefore substantially jeopardizing Medicare. Republicans responded by telling the public that they were not advocating cutting the Medicare program. Rather, they were proposing decreases in the rate of spending and Democrats were unjustifiably scaring the elderly. In the midst of this political clash, Medicare took center stage in the Presidential campaign. With public polls

indicating that the Democrats' message was more convincing, President Clinton vetoed the Balanced Budget Act to "save" Medicare.

After the 1996 elections, Medicare solvency and balancing the federal budget remained serious policy concerns. However, while Congress and the administration proposed Medicare changes, they proceeded cautiously. Most savings that were eventually obtained came from reducing provider payments, rather than substantially increasing beneficiary cost sharing or reducing benefits.

Receiving significant attention in 1997 was the fact that whereas Medicare had created the Medicare risk contract program in 1982 to capitalize on savings associated with health maintenance organizations (HMOs), such savings had yet to materialize. Specifically, HMOs were paid a flat fee for each beneficiary, in contrast to the traditional fee-for-service (FFS) Medicare program. HMO payments were set at 95% of the average cost of treating patients through the FFS system. Data collected since this payment strategy was implemented indicate that Medicare was paying, on average, about 6% more for beneficiaries who chose the HMO option than they would had those beneficiaries remained in the FFS system (Gage et al., 1997). Given the payment structure, Medicare managed care plans had a real incentive to enroll the healthiest beneficiaries, a point easily illustrated.

In 1996 the most expensive 10% of Medicare beneficiaries cost the Medicare program $37,000 per enrollee. In contrast, the healthiest 90% of Medicare enrollees cost an average of $1,400 annually. The Health Care Financing Administration (HFCA) paid Medicare managed care plans about $4,500 for each enrolled retiree. Clearly, the financial incentive would encourage HMOs (Komisar, Reuter, Feder, & Neuman, 1997) to enroll healthy senior citizens. Furthermore, the number of beneficiaries enrolling in managed care was increasing rapidly, exacerbating the overpayment problem. In 1997, five million seniors enrolled in HMOs; by 2002 more than one third of the population is expected to receive care through HMOs. As these numbers increase, absent a correction in the payment formula, managed care will continue to cost rather than save the Medicare program money.

For those HMOs that have costs below the payment levels they receive, HCFA mandates that the savings must be used to decrease beneficiary premiums and copayments or to increase benefits, or the excess payments must be returned to Medicare. The latter option is rarely, if ever, selected, and HMOs competing for Medicare beneficiaries have often used these savings to add very substantial benefits beyond the traditional FFS system. These benefits range from prescription coverage to elimination of co-payments.

Managed care organizations sought to block Congressional efforts to reduce reimbursement, but most policymakers were interested in stemming these losses. In 1997 the Administration and Congress expanded the variety of health plans from which beneficiaries could choose. Adding preferred provider organizations, point-of-service care, and provider-sponsored networks would increase choices available to seniors and potentially help hold down Medicare spending by increasing competition. With the addition of new plans, Medicare beneficiaries have an increased need for information so that informed choices can be made. As HCFA's orientation changed from one of serving as just a payer for services to an informed purchaser of services, HCFA's expectations for information regarding plan performance and beneficiary satisfaction increased.

MEDICAID

Medicaid captured the attention of the states and the federal government because of its rapid growth between 1988 and 1992. During this time, spending increased 22.4%, having a significant impact on state and federal budgets. Through program expansions, enrollment increased from 22 million recipients to 29.8 million recipients. Between 1992 and 1995, growth in Medicaid spending increased at an average annual rate of 9.5%. Through the National

Governor's Association, governors asked for regulatory relief from federal mandates, indicating that they could not manage costs without significant changes in the program. In response to budgetary pressure, the Congress proposed repealing the Medicaid program in 1995 and replacing it with block grants to states. This strategy would have given states a fixed amount of money as well as broad spending flexibility. Adamantly opposed to a block grant approach, President Clinton recommended keeping the Medicaid program as an entitlement but placing a cap on per-enrollee spending and enhancing state flexibility. Though setting caps would help to limit spending, this strategy did not address the programmatic changes needed to avoid exceeding these caps.

Ultimately the Congress sent the President a block grant proposal as part of the Balanced Budget Act of 1995, which Clinton then vetoed. With Medicaid mired in controversy, the Republican-controlled Congress decided to move Medicaid reform to a later time and proceeded, instead, with the less controversial welfare reform package. In 1996, pressure to enact Medicaid changes lessened considerably with a significant drop in the rate of spending growth to 3.2%. This unanticipated decrease in rate of growth was likely due to increased enrollment of beneficiaries in managed care plans, lower general and medical price inflation, and an improved economy. By 1996, 12.8 million individuals were enrolled in Medicaid managed care, constituting 38.6% of Medicaid recipients and up from 2.7 million in 1991 (Liska, Marlo, & Shah, 1996; PPRC Update, 1997). These numbers increased as states obtained waivers of federal statutory requirements allowing them to undertake managed care demonstration programs. Before the 1990s, states were allowed to operate managed care plans but only if certain requirements were met. As states extend managed care, expand coverage, and improve access, program outlays will not necessarily decrease. However, with less immediate impact on the federal deficit, incentives to alter the Medicaid program markedly diminished. Though it is too early to predict the impact of moving Medicaid populations into managed care on cost, quality, and access, research likely will inform future state and federal initiatives.

HEALTH POLICY ISSUES IN THE 1990s: BALANCING COMPETING CONCERNS

Environment

I want an America in the year 2000 where no child should have to live near a toxic waste dump, where no parent should have to worry about the safety of a child's glass of water, and no neighborhood should be put in harm's way by pollution from a nearby factory. [President Clinton, August 1996]

In 1996, world population reached 5.8 billion, an increase of 80 million people over the previous year. This burgeoning of the population, combined with expanding technology and industry and accompanied by hazardous chemical and biologic byproducts, has led to a deterioration in the quality of food, water, land, and air (World Health Organization, 1997). Transcending national borders to reverse environmental damage and protecting the environment from future pollutants has been a public policy issue for more than 20 years. The U.S. Government established the Environmental Protection Agency (EPA) in 1970 to address environmental concerns. In the 1990s a philosophical shift occurred in the focus of environmental policy, linking environmental protection with protecting and promoting public health. This linkage is evident in the EPA mission statement to "protect public health and to safeguard and improve the natural environment—air, water, and land—upon which human life depends" (EPA, 1996). Authority for implementing most environmental regulations falls within the jurisdiction of the EPA. This authority was the subject of significant political challenges, and in the mid to late 1990s, after taking control of Congress in 1994, Republicans attempted to roll back regulations they perceived as too onerous on business, especially environment-related laws. Though regulatory relief is

often welcomed, the American public became increasingly uncomfortable with the proposed weakening of the EPA. Environmental policy was afforded additional visibility during the 1996 Presidential campaign, when President Clinton effectively wove public concern regarding the Republican Party's willingness to abandon environmental protection into his reelection campaign. In 1996 President Clinton identified five environmental initiatives: (1) cleanup of toxic waste sites, (2) cleanup of abandoned urban industrial projects, (3) public protection from environmental "criminals" who continue to pollute the air, ground, and water, (4) expansion of individuals' rights to have information about what is present in the environment that is potentially harmful, and (5) making water safe and clean. Addressing health through environmental legislation was evident in bills such as the Food Quality Protection Act and the Safe Drinking Water Act of 1996 and in the implementing regulations associated with the Clean Air Act.

In the mid to late 1990s, air quality became a major health concern. Respiratory diseases linked to air pollution, such as chronic obstructive pulmonary disease and asthma, ranked among the three principal causes of workdays lost and were associated with the deaths of almost three million people a year worldwide (World Health Organization, 1997). Armed with numerous scientific studies on the impact of ozone and particles in the air, the EPA proposed two rules in late 1996 to regulate acceptable levels of these pollutants. On the particulate standard, the EPA estimated that tiny particles result in more than 64,000 premature deaths a year. New, more stringent regulations would prevent these deaths, as well as more than 250,000 cases of aggravated asthma and 60,000 cases of bronchitis. The Clean Air Act regulations of 1996 ignited a heated high-stakes debate in Congress, primarily between Republicans who support industry and are typically opposed to regulation and Democrats who tend to favor tighter controls and support environmental groups. Republicans contested the new rules, stating that more than 200 studies failed to demonstrate that the new standards would result in any appreciable benefit. Furthermore, the cost to industry of implementing these regulations would be exorbitant. However, because Republicans failed to garner support for their antiregulation position in the 104th Congress and were portrayed as enemies of the environment and health, they avoided taking a direct confrontational approach on the Clean Air Act regulations. Instead, the Republican strategy in the 105th Congress was to have the Senate Environment and Public Works Committee conduct hearings on the proposed regulations in an effort to build opposition. Though Republicans were the major dissenters related to the clean air regulations, some Democrats (generally those from coal- and oil-producing states) also opposed the new standards. Nevertheless, the EPA and the Clinton Administration stood firm in support of the new rules.

In addition to partisan politics, the political overlay of environmental policy also involves special interest groups. For example, environmental groups charged that the Clean Air Act rules do not go far enough in protecting the public. In contrast, industry supporters spent millions of dollars to influence public opinion, claiming that the new rules were too stringent and would outlaw such activities as backyard barbecues. A public opinion poll conducted by an independent firm shortly before the rules were to go into effect indicated that industry tactics did not convince the public. Respondents strongly supported stricter rules on air quality regardless of the cost (U.S. Newswire, 1997). This battle over regulation is an excellent example of how interest groups, government agencies, political parties, and individuals wrestle with and ultimately define public policy. Additionally, incidents such as large oil spills or massive fish kills focus public attention on environmental issues. The public, when faced with these incidents, applies pressure on Congress to ratchet air and water quality standards to tighter and tighter levels. At the same time, industrialists will continue to pressure their

representatives to set "reasonable" standards that will not adversely affect their respective markets. Balancing these competing concerns of the environment and the nation's local and global economies will continue to challenge policymakers in the new millennium.

Education

Health and education are joined in fundamental ways and with the destiny of the Nation's children. To help children meet the educational and health and developmental challenges that affect their lives, education and health must be linked in partnership. [Secretary Riley and Secretary Donna Shalala, 1993]

In the 1990s education emerged as a prominent policy issue. A poll conducted for the Coalition for America's Children in the latter part of 1996 reported that 8 of 10 voters were concerned about education and would consider a candidate's position on educational reform when casting their ballot. The reasons for this national concern can be explained by highlighting a few facts:

- A 1993 survey found that 42 million Americans (22%) could not read (National Right to Read Foundation, 1997).
- Industry estimates $300 billion is being spent on employee remediation (National Right to Read Foundation, 1997).
- The *Journal of the American Medical Association* reports that 33% of patients receiving prescription drugs cannot read the labels.
- In 1994 there were 3.7 million (11.5%) 16- to 24-year-old Americans who had not completed high school and were not in school (U.S. Census Bureau, 1994).

A wide range of educational programs are funded through federal initiatives, but responsibility for the control and direction of elementary and secondary education rests with state and local governments. However, because a well-educated populace is perceived as essential to a competent work force and U.S. businesses' ability to compete both nationally and internationally, both state and federal governments are concerned with shortcomings in the educational system. Though this is a bipartisan issue, no agreement exists on appropriate strategies for improving education outcomes. Without agreement, education reform will continue to be debated.

Fueled by strong lobbying efforts from child health advocacy groups, support has grown around the belief that to be ready to learn, children must be healthy. As a result, it is likely that state and federal education policy will incorporate strategies designed to ensure children's health, rather than viewing health and education as separate policy arenas. Individuals and organizations interested in one arena will increasingly forge relationships with individuals and organizations committed to the other. The growth and success of school-based health centers (SBHCs) is evidence of this. SBHCs grew exponentially in the 1990s, increasing from 40 in 1985 to more than 900 in 1996. These health centers provide children with physical examinations, immunizations, and treatment for illness and injury, as well as acute management of chronic conditions like asthma. Student health has been a concern for almost a century, beginning with Lillian Wald's experiment in 1900 in placing nurses in public schools. Traditionally, schools have focused on health education, physical education, health screenings, and healthy environments. SBHCs are a natural expansion of these concerns and forge the link between education and health. Just as children must be healthy to learn, they must be educated to achieve and maintain optimal health (National Health and Education Consortium, 1997). Policies and programs will increasingly reflect this orientation as policymakers look for cost-effective ways to improve the health and educational outcomes of the nation's children. An example is a program instituted in 1996 by the Secretary of Health and Human Services, Donna Shalala, called Girl Power. This program educates girls between the ages of 9 and 14 years to prevent the loss of self-esteem, decline in academic performance, and onset of risky be-

haviors leading to health problems, such as tobacco use, drug use, and teenage sexual activity (Shalala, 1997). Demonstrating a public-private partnership, Secretary Shalala's program in 1997 established a partnership with the Girl Scouts of America to get the message of Girl Power to the local level. This joining of resources demonstrates how the federal government often chooses to work with and through nongovernmental organizations to implement policies and programs.

Violence

The Centers for Disease Control and Prevention (CDCP) (1997) views violence as a public health issue because of its tremendous impact on health and well-being. Violence also has an impact on the health care system by increasing costs and straining emergency care systems. In the early part of the 1990s, the rate of violent crime rose to 732 of 100,000 individuals annually affected (Department of Justice, 1990). In an attempt to reverse this trend, a number of legislative initiatives, including the Crime Bill, the Brady Bill, and the Violence Against Women Act, were enacted, and in the first half of 1996 the Bureau of Justice Statistics reported a 3% decrease in overall crime for the nation (Department of Justice, 1997a). With highest rates for teens and young adults, the homicide rate declined by 7%. Though the overall decline in violence is encouraging, brief descriptions of juvenile violence, domestic violence, and street gang violence highlight why the best efforts of policymakers continue to be challenged.

Juvenile Violence. According to the CDCP (1997), suicide and murder take the lives of American children less than 15 years of age at rates higher than those of their counterparts in the remainder of the industrialized world. Among the top 10 leading causes of death in American children, homicide and death during the course of legal intervention (e.g., police chases and apprehensions) rank third among 5- to 14-year-olds and second among 15- to

24-year-olds (National Center for Health Statistics [NCHS], 1995).

In 1993 more than two million juvenile arrests were made for violent crimes such as aggravated assault, robbery, forcible rape, homicide, and manslaughter (Department of Justice, 1994). A national survey of victims of violent crimes reported that one fourth of the serious violent crimes were perpetrated by teenagers (Department of Justice, 1997c). The potential for continued violence is highlighted in survey results of inner city high school students revealing that 35% carried firearms regularly or occasionally (Department of Justice, 1994).

The majority of homicides committed by juveniles involve handguns (Blevins, 1995). In 1994, former Surgeon General Joycelyn Elders called gun violence the country's leading health issue. Underscoring the public health epidemic related to firearms are statistics indicating that more teenagers in the United States die from firearm injuries than all natural (non-injury-related) causes combined (NCHS, 1993). In injury-related deaths, the risk of dying from a firearm injury has increased by 77% for teenagers 15 to 19 years of age since 1985. If the present trend continues, firearm-related deaths are predicted to be the leading cause of injury-related deaths by 2003 (CDCP, 1996). For black males, age 15 to 24 years, firearm homicide is already the single leading cause of death, accounting for more than three times the deaths related to motor vehicle accidents.

In addition to the tremendous toll in lost lives, firearm injuries have a significant impact on the economy as well. Studies indicate that, on average, it costs $20,000 to treat one gunshot wound victim; the total national direct costs of gun violence in 1995 were estimated at $4 billion (Kizer, Vassar, Harry, & Layton, 1995).

A number of bills have been introduced in Congress that specifically target the growing problem of youth violence. The CDCP, as a lead agency in injury control, has taken an active role in researching youth violence and the policy solutions needed to address correlative risk factors: poverty, discrimination, lack of educational and employment opportunities, and family violence.

Domestic Violence. In addition to juvenile violence, concern regarding domestic violence has also captured the attention of federal policymakers. Statistics convey the extent of the problem in terms of financial costs, economic costs to businesses, and loss of life. In terms of personal injury, during 1996 almost four million women reported having been physically abused by their husbands or boyfriends, and 42% of women murdered were killed by their intimate male partners (Family Violence Prevention Fund, 1997). Additionally, a survey conducted by the Department of Justice found that domestic violence accounts for 15% ($67 billion dollars) of crime costs per year. Respondents to a survey of Fortune 1000 companies reported that domestic violence had a significant negative impact on their companies in the areas of work attendance (48%), medical and insurance costs (44%), and productivity (49%) (Roper & Starch, 1994).

Gang Violence. The third area of concern to policymakers involves violent crimes committed by gang members. A nationwide problem, street gangs are not confined to urban areas. In fact, 68% of municipal and county jurisdictions with a population less than 25,000 reported gang activity. In larger populations as many as 98% of reporting jurisdictions cited gang activity (Wiley, 1996). Gangs even exist in remote Indian Territory. More than 7,000 different gang sets have been identified across the country, many of which are engaged in drug trafficking. President Clinton equated gang activity in the mid-1990s with mob activity in the 1920s. Clinton recommended initiatives to address this growing problem, including legislation that would allow federal prosecutors the discretion to prosecute juveniles as adults. Other initiatives included evicting drug dealers and perpetrators of violent crime from public housing and holding gun peddlers accountable for selling guns to children and adolescents. Though violence has been characterized in part as a public health problem, most of the policy interventions treat this issue as a law enforcement problem. No doubt a broader discussion of the issues and possible solutions would greatly benefit from more health care providers' engaging in and informing the policy discussion.

Welfare Reform

As political pressures continued to build through the 1990s to balance the federal budget and delegate greater power to the states, the most sweeping welfare reform law since the 1960s was enacted. Welfare, which represents a major federal social entitlement and expenditure program, was profoundly altered in 1996 through passage of the Personal Responsibility and Work Opportunity Act (P.L. 104-193). Congressional leaders spoke of this legislation as an effective way to stop welfare dependency and strengthen families by discouraging single parenthood and building in work requirements.

Historically, welfare has primarily consisted of six major components: (1) Aid to Families with Dependent Children (AFDC), the basic income support for poor families; (2) Emergency Assistance (EA), the short-term emergency services and benefits to needy families; (3) Job Opportunities and Basic Skills (JOBS), an employment and training program; (4) the Supplemental Security Income (SSI) program; (5) child support, protection, and nutrition; and (6) the Food Stamp Program. The new welfare law moved much of the responsibility for these programs from the federal government to the states. With a fixed block grant from the federal government, states now have major discretion over eligibility, benefit levels, and program rules. Other parts of the Act tightened eligibility standards for SSI and the Food Stamp Program (Steuerle & Mermin, 1997).

The centerpiece of the welfare reform law was the replacement of AFDC, EA, and JOBS with a new federal single-block entitlement to states—Temporary Assistance for Needy Families (TANF). The welfare reform legislation restricted state use of TANF funds by limiting federal support for welfare benefits and encouraging work. Federal TANF requirements included a limit of 5 years of assistance to a family. Further, states were required to increase the percentage of TANF families who are also working, with virtually all TANF families working after having received benefits for 2 years. Finally, each state was mandated to maintain 80% of its own recent AFDC spending level. In 1995, state AFDC spending totaled $10 billion and varied from a low of $120 per month in Mississippi to about $550 per month in California and New York (Ku & Coughlin, 1997).

Under TANF, the federal government provided each state with an annual block grant, the amount of which is predetermined for 6 years on the basis of the individual state's AFDC spending before enactment of the new law. Thus the higher the historic spending level, the more generous the TANF funding from the federal government. With declining caseloads and associated costs, federal block grants for 1997 were expected to be sufficient to finance the federal share of cash assistance at pre-1996 levels in nearly all states. This resulted in a "bonus" to states in the first year of implementation. However, according to this formula, states with historically low welfare expenditures (yet often with significant need) continued to receive the least amount of funding.

The new block grant structure provided states with different incentives to spend state funds. Under AFDC, any additional money states chose to spend was matched by federal funds. Under TANF, additional money states chose to spend in order to expand coverage for groups ineligible for TANF would not be matched with federal dollars. Therefore, while TANF increased state autonomy in decisions concerning benefit levels or work requirements, it concurrently reduced federal funding resources. According to the Congressional Budget Office (1996), the bill was projected to save $55 billion in the next 6 years. The reality is that federal spending for AFDC has steadily declined since the early 1980s, from 0.50% to 0.25% of the Gross Domestic Product. Reductions in welfare spending are due to cuts in the food stamp program, the SSI program, and assistance to legal immigrants, rather than the creation of TANF. Because of these reductions, opponents of welfare reform predicted that low-income disabled children, working poor families, and the elderly poor would be most affected (Zedlewski & Giannarelli, 1997).

Another change resulting from this welfare legislation was the severing of the traditional linkage of Medicaid to welfare programs. Medicaid is a major component of the federal safety net. In 1995, 41 million people were insured by Medicaid at a cost of $151 billion. The Congressional Budget Office (1996) estimated that the new welfare law would lower federal spending on Medicaid by 1% in the year 2002 and save a total of $4 billion over 6 years (Ku & Coughlin, 1997).

Although the welfare reform law does not change Medicaid directly, changes in welfare will indirectly affect Medicaid eligibility and funding because Medicaid and TANF eligibility were not linked. Health insurance coverage could be maintained for former welfare recipients and for the working poor, who often occupy jobs that lack private health insurance, and the states now have the option to adopt more generous Medicaid criteria. Finally, decoupling of Medicaid from welfare may encourage participation in the work force because single women with children no longer have to choose between working and Medicaid eligibility (Fubini, 1997).

However, one potentially negative outcome related to the decoupling of Medicaid from welfare is increased complexity in determining eligibility for various welfare programs. Confusion may result in denial of assistance to people who need it. For example, to prevent loss of Medicaid health insurance coverage because of tighter welfare eligibility, the new law requires states to apply AFDC eligibility criteria (from before the 1996 welfare reform) to determine Medicaid eligibility for families with children, regardless of TANF changes. How to reach the growing number of low-income parents and children who continue to be eligible for Medicaid but not for TANF is a key concern. Now that Medicaid

eligibility cannot be determined solely by welfare eligibility, the problem of uninsured children may be exacerbated. For example, in 1994, 2.7 million children under age 11 years were eligible for Medicaid but were not enrolled; they represented 45% of the total population of uninsured children. Welfare reform may increase the percentage of uninsured children from 20% to 30% within the next 5 years (Fubini, 1997). Finally, many welfare supporters fear that if state spending on Medicaid grows rapidly, fewer resources may be available for other social support areas, including TANF. Thus the separation of Medicaid from welfare may be an artificial distinction for state budgets, and obtaining adequate support for the needy may become a very difficult task.

In terms of the SSI program, major changes took the form of a substantially narrower definition of disability. Rather than having an individual assessment, children must now demonstrate one of the "listed" medical impairments to qualify for federal SSI benefits. The Social Security Administration estimated in 1996 that 135,000 children would lose SSI grants because of these changes (Fubini, 1997). In 1996, HCFA estimated that by 2002, some 315,000 low-income children who would have qualified under the old welfare law will not qualify under the new law (Fubini, 1997). Welfare reform reduced total benefits provided to disabled children by more than $7 billion over 6 years (Super, Parrot, Steinmetz, & Mann, 1996). Traditionally, SSI participation was linked to Medicaid eligibility, and approximately 80% of these children will still be eligible for Medicaid through other criteria. However, with Medicaid eligibility assessed separately and with new administrative procedures, delays may occur in gaining access to SSI (Ku & Coughlin, 1997).

Major welfare spending reductions in P.L. 104-193 came from the food stamp program. Specifically, the welfare reform bill cut $27.7 billion from the food stamp program over 6 years, including $3.8 billion for immigrants. Though food stamps remain an entitlement, individual allotments were reduced. When the new law is fully implemented, food stamp benefits will decrease by almost 20%, the equivalent of reducing the average food stamp benefit from a level of 80 cents per person per meal to 66 cents per person per meal (in 1996 dollars). These reductions affect all recipients, including families with children, the elderly, and the disabled. About 2% of savings from the food stamp program comes from provisions to reduce fraud, abuse, and administrative costs. Hardest hit by these changes are those with the lowest incomes—below half of the poverty line. This group absorbs 50% of the food stamp cuts, phased in over 6 years.

Perhaps the harshest provision of this legislation is the limiting of food stamp use to 3 months over 3 years for most unemployed individuals between the ages of 18 and 50 years who are not raising minor children. There are no hardship exemptions to this limit, and food stamps continue only if an individual in this category worked at least half time or is in a training program. However, the legislation provided no new money for workfare or training programs. It is estimated that, in an average month, one million jobless individuals, willing to work if work were available, will be denied food stamps under this provision (Congressional Budget Office, 1996).

As part of welfare reform, state waiver authority was expanded to allow for changing the food stamp benefit structure. A new range of options were granted to states, including an option for states to terminate benefits for either custodial parent who does not cooperate in collecting child support, or for parents who do not make required child support payments (Fix, Passel, & Zimmerman, 1996).

Among the most important health-related measures in the welfare reform law are those affecting immigrants. To trim welfare spending by $54 billion over 6 years, the government was to deny $24 billion in benefits to legal immigrants (Super et al., 1996). Some of these provisions were immediately challenged after their enactment. As a result of political backlash, primarily from states with high immigrant popu-

lations, P.L. 104-193 was changed in the 105th Congress. For example, the 1996 deadline set to eliminate SSI benefits to disabled legal immigrants was delayed at a cost of $10 billion over 5 years.

Trends indicate that the number of elderly and disabled legal immigrants receiving cash aid doubled between 1990 and 1996, with nearly 75% of these immigrants residing in California, New York, Florida, and Texas. Approximately 895,225 legal immigrants receive SSI, and 1,414,000 receive food stamps (Wolf, 1997). The rise in immigrant participation in welfare programs is thought to be due to the growth in numbers of immigrants and not to the increase in the propensity of immigrants to use welfare. Nevertheless, these trends prompted some policymaker interests in trimming benefits to this population.

Before the enactment of welfare reform, noncitizen immigrants legally admitted to the United States were entitled to Medicaid coverage on the same terms as native and naturalized citizens. New changes limit the eligibility of noncitizen immigrants for Medicaid coverage and other public assistance programs. Specifically, under the new law, states can decide whether to provide Medicaid and preventive health services, among other programs, to legal immigrants. However, most legal immigrants entering the United States before August 1996 were to lose SSI. Many who lost SSI would still qualify for Medicaid through other criteria, such as medically needy provisions. Immigrants in states such as Texas, with stringent medically needy provisions, are more likely to lose Medicaid coverage. Immigrants entering after August 22, 1996, are banned from Medicaid for all but emergency services and from many other programs for the first 5 years in this country. The Congressional Budget Office (1996) estimated that more than 300,000 noncitizens could lose Medicaid eligibility by 1998 (Ku & Coughlin, 1997). Congressional supporters of these provisions argued that the benefits cutoff was necessary to prevent abuse by immigrants who bring their relatives to the United States, who are then eligible for SSI and other welfare programs.

Politically, welfare reform policy divided Republicans into two factions: those who wanted to cut benefits as planned and those facing reelection in states with heavy immigrant voter populations. Because of increased naturalizations and voter registration, immigrants make up the nation's fastest-growing voting block. Meanwhile, Democrats, who have traditionally benefited most from immigrant support, attempted to portray the Republicans in 1996 as heartless in their efforts to cut the budget at the expense of vulnerable populations (Carney, 1997). Meanwhile, President Clinton signed the welfare reform legislation with serious reservations. On the eve of the 1996 Presidential election, Clinton was under pressure to make good on his promise to "reform" welfare as we know it. Promising to "fix" the most objectionable parts of this legislation, President Clinton partially fulfilled that commitment in the balanced budget bill signed in July 1997. The 1997 budget legislation passed with three key changes: (1) SSI benefits were restored to about 500,000 elderly and disabled legal immigrants who were in the country when the welfare bill was signed in August 1996; (2) children who lost disability payments were allowed to retain Medicaid; and (3) $4 billion in additional funds was approved to help welfare recipients find work. As a result of these changes, many concerns regarding massive increases in poverty rates diminished.

As a result of welfare reform, more than 1 million people left the welfare rolls during 1997, most of whom had skills that allowed easier job placement. Since then, states face greater challenges in placing long-term welfare-dependent adults with little education or job skills, or an unwillingness to comply with the new requirements. While stringent welfare provisions are phased in, most states have kept spending levels constant, transferring savings from falling caseloads into such services as childcare and job training (Vobejda & Jeter, 1997).

Declining welfare rolls may not offer a true picture of whether the law has succeeded.

Moving people off public assistance and helping families lift themselves out of poverty would be the goal of responsible social policy. The success of this historic legislation to revamp the nation's welfare laws will take years to determine.

Homelessness

Homelessness, often the result of circumstances that push people into poverty and force vexing choices among food, shelter, and other basic needs, poses particularly complex challenges to policymakers. In the United States, 760,000 people are homeless on any given night, and 1.2 to 2 million people experience homelessness during the year (National Coalition for the Homeless, 1997). Currently the fastest growing group of the homeless are families with children, at 45% of the homeless population (National Coalition for the Homeless, 1997). A study of 20 U.S. cities found that, in 1996, 29% of all requests for emergency shelter went unmet because of a lack of resources (Waxman & Hinderliter, 1996). Although one fifth of the homeless population is employed, housing is frequently not affordable. A full-time minimum-wage job does not cover the costs of a one-bedroom unit at "fair market rent" in 45 states (Kaufman, 1996). Additionally, there are few or no shelters of any type available in many rural areas of the United States (National Coalition for the Homeless, 1997).

Similarly, poor health is closely associated with homelessness. In fact, the rates of both chronic and acute health problems are extremely high among the homeless population. Approximately 20% to 25% of the single adult homeless population has some form of severe, chronic mental illness. People who are homeless are usually uninsured and often lack access to the most basic health services for their complex health care needs (National Coalition for the Homeless, 1997).

In response to the needs of this population, in 1985 Congress enacted the McKinney Act, creating a wide range of services for the homeless, including emergency services, primary health services, housing, mental health and substance abuse programs, and training and education. Funding for McKinney Act programs increased to $1.475 billion in 1995, but subsequent funding has declined. For example, for fiscal year 1998, President Clinton requested $1.098 billion, a 26% decrease in funding. Advocates for the homeless believe that McKinney Act programs are underfunded and are thus unable to reach large numbers of homeless individuals and families. Similar to many other discretionary programs, funding for services for the homeless is affected by efforts to decrease federal spending. With the priority of balancing the federal budget by 2002, decreased funding for welfare and SSI benefits is predicted to increase poverty. Policy consequences may well increase the number of homeless individuals and families, placing additional stress on an already-strained safety net (National Coalition for the Homeless, 1997).

CAMPAIGN FINANCE IN THE 1990s

Special interest groups, including those representing health interests, actively participate in the political process through campaign contributions to political parties and candidates. The perceived impact on policymakers of large financial contributions from wealthy individuals, corporations, and labor unions has grown increasingly controversial. The broad campaign finance question concerns the amount of influence that large contributors have on the Congress and the President and whether the policy process is affected by these contributions. Political parties, by their nature, form broad coalitions to obtain financial resources. Interest groups invited to support political parties and individual candidates are concerned with a narrow range of policies—those which affect them directly. In general, the public is ambivalent about the potential impact of these interest groups on the making of public policy. On one hand, interest groups advocating for their own special interests are perceived to do so at a cost to the general public's interest. On the other hand, competing

interest groups may tend to balance each other and, in doing so, preserve the public's interest (Pfiffner, 1995).

As early as the 1830s, Congress recognized that the financing of political campaigns would be a contentious subject. Since then, legislating significant change in campaign finance has usually been the product of highly publicized scandals, Watergate being one example. More recently, in 1971, Congress consolidated earlier reform efforts in the Federal Election Campaign Act (FECA), which sought to (1) limit the disproportionate influence of wealthy individuals and special interest groups on the outcome of federal elections, (2) regulate spending in campaigns for federal office, and (3) deter abuses by mandating public disclosure of campaign finances. Through FECA, more stringent disclosure requirements were imposed on federal candidates, political parties, and political action committees (PACs).

After reports of financial abuses in the 1972 Presidential campaign, Congress amended FECA in 1974 to set limits on contributions by individuals, political parties, and PACs. The 1974 amendments also established a central administrative agency, the Federal Election Commission (FEC), to enforce the law, facilitate disclosure, and administer public funding of campaigns. Six FEC commissioners, appointed by the President, serve staggered 6-year terms.

Further amendments to FECA were made in 1976 after a Constitutional ruling in the U.S. Supreme Court case *Buckley v. Valeo*, which limited contributions to candidates but did not limit candidates' expenditures. Candidate expenditures were interpreted by the courts as constitutionally protected speech. Most recently, the Supreme Court ruled in *Colorado Republican Campaign Committee v. FEC* that political parties, PACs, and other groups can make unlimited "independent" expenditures on behalf of candidates (Rubin, 1997). An independent expenditure is money used for a communication that expressly advocates the election or defeat of a specific candidate and must be made independent—*without consent or request*—from the candidate's campaign. For example, separate from any candidate, the American Nurses Association or the National Rifle Association could purchase radio advertising time to communicate an opinion about a political issue or candidate. There is no limit on how much money can be spent through an independent expenditure, but the amount and the source of the funds must be reported. Though the FEC provides a central administrative authority, campaign finance laws are difficult to enforce, especially given the complex legal interpretations of campaign finance laws.

Complicating campaign finance is the use of "soft" money—funds raised by the national party committees that are exempt from federal limits and from some disclosure laws. As the amount of "soft" money continues to grow, there are questions concerning the effectiveness of the FEC in regulating election spending (Center for Responsive Politics, 1997). In 1979, Congress passed laws that weakened the FEC's ability to monitor compliance with the law. For example, the FEC was prohibited from conducting random audits of candidates, parties, and PACs. For individuals and organizations concerned about campaign finance, random audits were seen as a powerful deterrent against violations and a means of monitoring compliance with campaign finance laws. Currently the FEC audits political committees only in cases where discrepancies are identifiable in campaign finance disclosure reports. Generally speaking, the ability of the FEC to move quickly or powerfully on potential violations is seriously handicapped. For example, the FEC may suggest only a financial penalty and then must negotiate with the violator over the amount of the penalty through a conciliation agreement that is, at minimum, a 30-day process. Uncooperative respondents may try to delay the process, often exceeding the 90-day maximum conciliation period. If negotiations fail to produce an agreement, the FEC can seek court judgment against the respondent, but the case is subject to a *de novo* trial, which means that the FEC must introduce evidence and begin the case again. Additionally, court action

can be a huge drain on FEC resources. Compounding the problems of FEC effectiveness is the reality that the President appoints the members, and Congress and the President determine the budget for this regulatory agency (Federal Election Commission, 1996). The FEC may be a good example of the view that regulatory agencies eventually become the captives of those whom they regulate—in this case, elected officials.

In 1994, campaign finance reform advocates were guardedly optimistic when a majority of freshmen elected to the Congress promised to end "business as usual" in Washington. In fact, the campaign finance system, perceived to allow huge amounts of special interest money to affect elections and influence legislation, was one of the major issues that freshmen promised to change. Two years later, a public opinion poll found that 83% of Americans still wanted Congress to pass campaign finance reform (Common Cause, 1997). Yet the failure of a 1996 bipartisan campaign finance reform bill with numerous changes, including a ban on PAC contributions to federal candidates, continued more than a decade of deadlock over campaign finance reform.

In addition to political fundraising scandals, a major reason campaign finance reform remains on the political agenda is the increasing amount of money needed to run for political office. For example, total expenditures for federal campaigns in the 1995–1996 election cycle were approximately $2.3 billion, plus an additional $400 million in "soft" money. In contrast, 20 years ago, total campaign expenditures were approximately $309 million (Doherty, 1997). Soft money contributions of $100,000 and $200,000 are prevalent (Common Cause, 1997). The largest single soft money contribution on record is a $2.5 million donation from Amway Corporation to the Republican National Committee in 1994. Similarly, tobacco interests contributed $1.5 million in soft money to the Republicans during the first 6 months of 1995. The top three soft money contributors were Philip Morris, RJR Nabisco, and Brown and Williamson

Table 21-1 Contribution Limits

	CANDIDATE OR CANDIDATE COMMITTEE PER ELECTION	NATIONAL PARTY COMMITTEE PER CALENDAR YEAR	TOTAL PER CALENDAR YEAR
Amount individual may give*	$1,000	$20,000	$25,000
Amount multicandidate committee may give†	$5,000	$15,000	No limit
Amount other political committee may give	$1,000	$20,000	No limit

*Exception: If a contributor gives to a committee knowing that a substantial portion of the contribution will be used to support a particular candidate, then the contribution counts against the donor's limit for that candidate (first column on the chart).

†A multicandidate committee is a political committee with more than 50 contributors that has been registered for at least 6 months and, with the exception of state party committees, has made contributions to five or more candidates for federal office.

From Federal Election Commission (August 1996).

(Rosenberg, 1997). The tobacco industry's contributions, made at a time when health issues related to smoking were under discussion in the policymaking arena, are a clear example of how huge soft money contributions can be perceived to influence government decision making.

In addition to "soft" money fueling political machinery, PACs play a significant role. PACs are organizations created to raise and contribute money to candidates, and they are typically created by corporations, associations, industries, or other groups with shared policy interests. Many health-related organizations have PACs, including the American Nurses Association. Campaign contributions to candidates from individuals and PACs are referred to as "hard money" and are subject to federal limits and other regulations. Table 21-1 shows how the limits apply to various participants in federal elections. Table 21-2 reflects 1996 total PAC contributions by major health care organizations identified in the top 100 federal contributors.

Substantial PAC contributions from various health organizations indicate that the 1990s is a time of extraordinarily high stakes for the health care industry. In fact, specific interest groups such as the insurance industry and physicians have dramatically increased political contributions, targeting their support to congressional members in key positions. According to a 10-year study, the health insurance industry gave

Table 21-2 1996 Contributions from Health Care PACs

RANK (OF ALL PACs)	AMOUNT ($)
9 American Medical Association PAC	4,344,254
25 National Committee to Preserve Social Security and Medicare	2,314,060
47 Texas Chapter, American Medical Association	1,425,804
59 American Hospital Association PAC	1,256,055
78 Physical Therapy PAC	1,030,468
79 National Association of Social Workers PAC	1,026,189
80 American Nurses Association PAC	1,004,132

Based on data available on-line from the Federal Election Commission as of June 25, 1997.

From Federal Election Commission (1996).

more than $25.5 million in PAC and soft money contributions to congressional candidates between July 1985 and June 1995 (Common Cause, 1996). House Ways and Means Committee members—key players in decisions affecting the Medicare program—received 2.4 times more PAC money from the health insurance industry and physicians than did the average Member of the House of Representatives during the same period. Also during this time, physicians gave $23.1 million dollars in PAC and soft money contributions overall, and hospitals and nursing homes gave $9.7 million.

From 1993 through 1995, health organization contributions were higher to Congressional Republican than Democratic candidates. The Senate majority leader and House majority and minority leaders were also recipients of large health care PAC contributions. These targeted activities make it clear that contributions by health care PACs and individual contributors are perceived as critical to influencing health care policy development.

Through the 1996 elections, Congressional and Presidential campaigns were marred by unethical and illegal practices of members of both political parties. In response, congressional committees and a Justice Department task force probed a range of issues in 1997, including whether national security may have been compromised by foreign contributions. Advocates of campaign finance reform continue to express concern that the infusion of more money into campaigning inappropriately contributes to the American public's mounting distrust of government and *both* political parties (Doherty, 1997). Absent substantive changes in campaign finance reform, health care special interests will continue to seek influence through political contributions.

EMERGING HEALTH POLICY ISSUES

On the verge of the twenty-first century, emerging health care issues will demand more attention from policymakers. For example, policy surrounding genetics and telemedicine and, more broadly, ensuring quality in the health care system will have the attention of both state and federal governments.

Genetics Testing (Privacy/Confidentiality)

According to the Institute of Medicine (1994), 3% of all children are born with severe disorders that are presumed to be genetic in origin. Challenging policymakers on a number of fronts, several thousand single-gene diseases have been

described and the ability to diagnose genetic disease has increased dramatically in the past 20 years. These developments have accelerated markedly since the inception of the National Institutes of Health (NIH) Human Genome Project in 1991. From the outset, researchers recognized that increased genetic information would raise a host of complex ethical and policy issues for individuals and society as a whole. The government, as a major funding source for genetic research, was deeply concerned with the ethical issues surrounding genetic research, and in 1995 President Clinton established the National Bioethics Advisory Commission (NBAC). The NBAC provides advice and makes recommendations to the National Science and Technology Council and other appropriate government entities about (1) the appropriateness of governmental programs, policies, guidelines, and regulations related to bioethical issues arising from research on human biology and behavior and (2) applications of that research. It is in the latter capacity that the NBAC recommended a ban on human cloning. After the Commission's recommendation, the President endorsed a bill banning human cloning in the United States for 5 years. The NIH, also concerned about ethical, legal, and social implications, established programs to investigate these issues, collectively referred to as ELSI. In addition, NIH Office for Protection from Research Risks has developed guidelines for protecting the privacy, autonomy, and welfare of individuals involved in human genetic research. Though testing is currently confined primarily to research environments, testing and counseling increasingly will be part of health care.

In addition to ethical considerations, federal-level policymakers focused their attention on issues related to protections against discrimination and violations of privacy. Congress was particularly concerned that genetic information or even employee requests for genetic testing could be used by employers to deny jobs and by health insurers to deny coverage to individuals on the basis of their genetic maps. Policymakers responded to this concern by introducing a number of bills in the latter part of the 1990s to prohibit such actions. Other specific bills were also proposed to address the conditions under which DNA samples could be obtained, stored and analyzed. Typically, policy related to reproductive issues is a source of contention between political parties, with abortion a particularly good example of this dissension. Though genetic research and its applications certainly have reproductive implications, there seems to be bipartisan support for legislation protecting genetic privacy, banning cloning, and dealing with related issues.

Privacy/Confidentiality

Traditionally patient privacy has been protected by professional codes of ethics; however, increasing technology and marketplace demands are eroding these protections. In a 1993 report the Office of Technology Assessment concluded that the security system in place failed to address privacy in an increasingly "borderless" computerized society.

Medical record information is routinely shared by insurers, educational institutions, civil and criminal justice systems, social welfare and other government agencies, rehabilitation programs, public health agencies, researchers, credit bureaus, and the media. This is not necessarily undesirable. In fact, Vice President Gore established the Information Infrastructure Task Force (IITF) to articulate and implement the Administration's vision for the National Information Infrastructure (NII). As a consequence, the health care community is increasingly committed to using the NII to collect, aggregate, and disseminate medical information on a nationwide basis in an effort to provide better care at less cost. Examples of computerized system benefits include decreasing costs and delays associated with processing claims, receiving test results, ordering medications, and scheduling appointments. Nevertheless, benefits of advancing information technology must be balanced against the threat to individual privacy, which, although not an absolute right, is a highly valued

freedom accorded to Americans in the U.S. Constitution.

In 1994 the Institute of Medicine called on Congress to enact prescriptive legislation to ensure confidentiality and the protection of privacy in personally identifiable health data. Although the 104th Congress considered the issue of protection of confidentiality and privacy in discussions of the Medical Records Legislation Act, no comprehensive health data confidentiality legislation was enacted. However, Congress did begin to address the issue in other ways. For example, the Health Insurance Portability and Accountability Act (HIPAA), enacted in 1996, encouraged the development of a health information system with uniform guidelines for transmitting health-related data. Through this legislation, the Secretary of Health and Human Services was charged with the task of establishing standards, including security standards, to facilitate those transmissions. Additionally, HIPAA established the National Committee on Vital and Health Statistics to advise the Secretary on these matters. Absent Congressional action by 1999, HIPAA requires the Secretary to issue privacy standards before transmission standards can be implemented. More recently the National Research Council (Leary, 1997) stating that medical records were "vulnerable to misuse and abuse," called for the creation of incentives to ensure that health care employees protect patient information.

According to the National Information Infrastructure Task Force (Gage et al., 1997), the nation is still some years away from full computerization of the patient record used for clinical care but is moving "swiftly" in that direction. Many private sector organizations are helping to develop policy by adopting voluntary standards and codes based on the principles of fair information established by Vice President Gore's National Information Infrastructure Task Force (1995). These principles include (1) a person's reasonable expectation of privacy regarding access to and use of personal information should be ensured; (2) personal information should not be improperly altered or destroyed;

and (3) personal information should be accurate, timely, complete, and relevant for the purposes for which it is provided and used.

With advances in computer technology, protecting privacy transcends industries beyond health care. In early 1997, at a Senate-convened conference on privacy in the information age, Chairman of the Federal Reserve Board, Alan Greenspan, stated:

> The central dilemma in these discussions almost always involves fundamental choices about how to strike prudent balances between the needs of individuals for privacy; the needs of commerce to bring us new products and new ways to communicate; and the needs of the authorities to provide for the effective administration of government and to ensure the public safety. These are not easy choices. . . . We need to be aware that the balances we strike in one era may need to be reexamined as technology and circumstances change.

Without question, technology will continue to serve as a catalyst for ongoing vigilance and specific policy action designed to protect patient privacy and confidentiality.

Telemedicine

In one form or another, telemedicine has been practiced for more than 30 years. However, early on, most telemedicine programs had few policy implications. Generally, clinical applications did not cross state borders, and if they did, they involved federal government agencies that were not bound by state licensure or liability policies. Recent advances in communications technology development, coupled with changing incentives in the health care marketplace, have resulted in increasing interest in expanding potential use of telemedicine technology.

As with other emerging technologies, *telemedicine* has not been precisely defined, and the term is often used interchangeably with *telehealth*. The U.S. Department of Commerce (1997) defined telemedicine as the use of electronic communication and information technologies to provide or support clinical care at a distance. The term telehealth usually refers to diverse health-related activities that can be linked through technology to create a common infrastructure, such as health professionals' education, community health education, public health, research, and administration of health services. Almost all the telemedicine activities funded by federal agencies have broader telehealth applications (U.S. General Accounting Office, 1997).

Application of telemedicine technology has the potential to impact access to care, quality of health services, and health care costs. For example, in remote rural areas, where a patient and the closest health professional may be hundreds of miles apart, telemedicine may mean access to health care. Telemedicine has the potential to improve the delivery of health care by bringing a wider range of services such as radiology, mental health services, and dermatology to underserved communities in both urban and rural areas. In addition, telemedicine may help attract and retain health professionals in rural areas by diminishing professional isolation. Telemedicine affects not only how and where health care is delivered but also who delivers it and who pays for it.

Though many believe that telemedicine may be a cost-effective service, to date there are few "hard data" to support this opinion. Nevertheless, nine federal agencies ranging from the Bureau of Prisons to the Department of Defense, to the federal Office of Rural Health Policy, invested approximately $646 million in telemedicine initiatives for fiscal years 1994 to 1996. Also reflecting support for the application of telehealth technology, more than 40 states have some type of telemedicine initiative under way and funded by federal agencies, the private sector, and/or states themselves (U.S. General Accounting Office, 1997). With substantial state and federal investment, coupled with the potential to increase access to care, policymakers are interested in a range of issues including the value-added capability of telemedicine application, clinical and technical standards, and reimbursement for services rendered through application of this technology. Lack of evaluative information, however, has been a significant barrier to the broader deployment of telemedicine.

Given the range of activities, and the federal investment in telemedicine, Vice President Gore identified telemedicine as a key area in the development of the NII. Since 1992 the Information Infrastructure Task Force (IITF) has examined broad, innovative uses of NII on certain market segments. In 1994 the IITF created the Health Information Application Working Group, with a subgroup that focused on telemedicine. Health care was selected because of its impact on the economy and the well-being of each American. In 1995 Vice President Gore asked the U.S. Department of Health and Human Services to take a greater leadership role in developing cost-effective health applications for the NII. Subsequently the Commerce Department joined forces with Health and Human Services to form the Joint Working Group on Telemedicine (JWGT).

The JWGT is a government-wide entity focusing on telemedicine and includes more than eight member departments and agencies. The JWGT is charged with assessing the role of the federal government in telemedicine and coordinating telemedicine activities across federal cabinet agencies. Part of this mission involves (1) developing specific actions to overcome barriers to effective use of telemedicine technologies, (2) developing a working inventory of federal telemedicine projects available, and (3) evaluating federally funded telemedicine projects through the development of an evaluation framework and uniform data collection instruments (U.S. Department of Commerce [Telemedicine Report], 1997). Embedded within these tasks are multifaceted policy concerns.

The jurisdictional issue related to licensure is one of these policy concerns because telemedicine challenges the traditional structure of professional practice, which involves face-to-face encounters between clinicians and patients. By breaking the physical link, telemedicine raises complex questions about where a telemedicine practitioner should be licensed if the practitioner and the patient are located in different states. Currently, responsibility for licensing and regulating health professionals lies with state governments. For example, although most states allow physicians an exception to consult with licensed physicians from other states, state consultation exceptions are not uniform. Furthermore, state consultations do not appear to offer protection for an out-of-state clinician unless a consultation is requested by or otherwise involves an in-state clinician (Institute of Medicine, 1996). The complexity of different state licensure standards and the costs of obtaining and maintaining multiple licenses have led telemedicine advocates to propose federal legislation that would either create a national telemedicine license or replace state licensure with a national system. With renewed interest in protecting states' rights and the potential for states to lose revenues currently obtained through licensure fees, replacing state licensure with national licensure is a complicated policy solution. However, the Supremacy Clause of the Constitution mandates that even state regulation designed to protect vital state interests must give way to paramount federal legislation. Should Congress desire to license the practice of telemedicine, it could legally do so.

Complicating changes in state licensure are special interest groups affected by licensure changes. For example, a new level of competition is introduced when consumers, primary care providers, or health plans can access providers in other states. In addition to the JWGT, the National Council of State Boards of Nursing, the Federation of State Medical Boards, and other organizations are exploring telemedicine's impact on practice liability, licensure, and reimbursement (U.S. Department of Commerce [Telemedicine Report], 1997). In 1997 the state boards for nursing began exploring a driver's license approach to nurse licensure: the nurse is licensed in one state and can practice in any but is held to the laws of whatever state she is practicing in.

Another policy concern relates to the lack of security and privacy standards for telemedicine technologies. With the proliferation of computer-based patient information systems and databases, these concerns relate especially to acute treatment of individuals with acquired immunodeficiency syndrome, mental illness, or substance abuse. For example, unlike traditional medical records, with most interactive telemedicine consultations, the practitioner and patient interactions are often recorded in total. In this context, clinicians have less discretion to remove sensitive information that they might not otherwise record. Privacy from the patient's perspective can be of concern for a number of reasons, including something as basic as the patient being unable to "see" anyone else viewing the session with the clinician at the other end of a consultation (U.S. Department of Commerce [Telemedicine Report], 1997).

Public and private policies limiting reimbursement for telemedicine services are regarded by telemedicine advocates as a major obstacle to widespread use of telemedicine. How such policy concerns are resolved affects the benefits, costs, and sustainability of telemedicine programs (Institute of Medicine, 1996). In the public sector, HCFA has different policies that cover telemedicine in the Medicare and Medicaid programs. Under Medicare, standard medical practices are reimbursed that do not require face-to-face contact between patient and practitioner, including telepathology and teleradiology. In fact, teleradiology is currently the most widely applied and reimbursed form of telemedicine. Most private sector third-party payers take a "wait and see" reimbursement approach by following Medicare's lead. Consequently the interventions HCFA chooses to reimburse through Medicare have potential and broad ramifications for the application of this technology. The challenge of expanding and sustaining support for telemedicine at the federal level rests in the ability to demonstrate value-added cost-savings characteristics (Cunningham, 1997). Telemedicine reimbursement through the Medicaid program is based on state policy and thus varies from state to state, with accompanying variation in coverage of

health professionals and services. As of 1997, nine states reimburse for telemedicine services through their Medicaid programs.

In the private sector, interest in telemedicine primarily stems from (1) potential for expanding market share in rural, underpopulated areas, (2) decreasing costs associated with professional travel, (3) patient transfers between hospitals, and (4) duplication of records. Conversely, telemedicine presents concerns for payers regarding issues such as efficacy, quality, costs associated with purchasing, maintaining and using technology, volume of care, and potential overutilization. Thus, regardless of cost savings, the increased access to health care through telemedicine technology may generate greater expenditures for payers (U.S. Department of Commerce [Telemedicine Report], 1997).

On another policy front, concerns about safety and effectiveness challenge the widespread use of telemedicine. Although system components such as software may be regulated for safety, the entire system has not been evaluated for its ability to provide diagnostic information safely. The rate of change in technology is a complicating factor that makes the development of standards difficult. However, a lack of technical, educational, and practice standards can lead to situations that could adversely affect patient safety. Whereas agreement exists that standards are needed, there is less agreement on who and how these standards should be generated. Several groups have engaged in generating clinical practice guidelines. Both the American Medical Association and the American Telemedicine Association have urged medical specialty societies to develop appropriate practice parameters. The American Academy of Ambulatory Nurses has developed practice standards for telephone-based nursing practice, and the American Nurses Association has developed general guidelines for professional nursing in telehealth. Meanwhile, the federal government, through the JWGT, is exploring the federal role in standards development.

Paradoxically, as some governmental policies such as reimbursement pose problems for telemedicine, other policies encourage telemedicine. Twenty bills were introduced during the 103rd Congress, and 15 bills in the 104th Congress supported telemedicine. Enactment of the Telecommunications Act of 1996 resulted in federal provisions that ensure universal communications services for the provision of health care in rural areas, at affordable rates. In addition, this legislation required federal agencies to report to Congress regarding current telemedicine initiatives, including patient safety, effectiveness, and the legal, medical, and economic impact. Telemedicine was further moved into the mainstream of health care through the provision in the Balanced Budget Act of 1997. This legislation provides Medicare Part B payments beginning in 1999 for consultation via telemedicine technology when the beneficiary resides in a rural county designated as a health professions shortage area. Newly created reimbursement streams generally trigger new practice patterns. This and other telemedicine provisions enacted in 1997 create an increasingly favorable environment for telemedicine. With continued advances in telemedicine technology, the challenge for policymakers is to craft legislation flexible enough to encourage the application of technology to health-related activities while ensuring that it is safe and secure and offers value-added service in a cost-effective manner.

Quality of Health Care

In September 1996, shortly before the Presidential election, President Clinton signed an executive order to create the Presidential Advisory Commission on Consumer Protection and Quality in the Health Care Industry. At a White House press conference in March 1997, President Clinton explained that the commission would make recommendations on how to preserve and improve quality in the health care system.

This 32-member commission, named from a pool of approximately 1,000 nominations, made this commission the most sought-after task force of President Clinton's tenure to date. Keen interest in the Commission indicated growing concern about potential threats to quality of health care as a result of massive change under way in the health care system. The President's significant concern regarding quality was evident by his naming of two cabinet members as chairs—Secretary Donna Shalala, of the U.S. Department of Health and Human Services, and Secretary Alexis Herman, of the U.S. Department of Labor. Sensitive to possible charges that the commission was a partisan initiative, both Democrats and Republicans were included and representation was broad based, including individuals from labor and business and health care providers—three nurses, consumers, and managed care and insurance representatives. Many health issues could potentially benefit from the visibility and work of a presidential-level commission, but it is noteworthy that President Clinton chose to focus on quality. Quality has long been the least visible of the cost-access-quality triad, and media accounts of consumer backlash against managed care have fueled concerns regarding possible erosion of quality of care and patient safety. These perceived threats to quality were attributed in part to cost pressures on health care organizations and providers. Whether the commission's work ultimately encourages consensus and charts needed strategies for preserving and enhancing quality in health care remains to be seen. Nevertheless, the President was betting on success by naming leadership that was close to him rather than structuring the commission at arm's length.

Coupled with the commission initiative, in 1997 Secretary Shalala made quality one of the priority areas for the U.S. Department of Health and Human Services. Her plan included highlighting and coordinating policy related to quality health care throughout the departmental agencies. For example, HCFA created the Health Care Quality Improvement Program, which reoriented the focus of HCFA's work to ensure quality in federal health programs, including deemphasizing structure and process measures as a basis for certification and emphasizing outcome indicators. In addition, peer review organizations (PROs) were asked to incorporate continuous quality improvement concepts into their now-cooperative efforts with HMOs and hospitals. This orientation differs significantly from the traditional work of PROs, which focused on policing providers through individual case review.

Paralleling the administration's interest in quality, numerous legislative initiatives were offered during the 105th session of Congress. One example offered by Senator Jim Jeffords, Chair of the Senate Labor and Human Resources Committee, was the Health Care Quality and Consumer Protection Act of 1997. Many of the provisions in this bill mirrored other Congressional proposals. Jefford's bill would require that comparative information be available that describes each health plan's services, cost-sharing requirements, and quality indicators, including measures of enrollee satisfaction and health outcomes information. The bill went so far as to stipulate the quality assurance program components, including review by an external organization. Also included were provisions that addressed payment for emergency services, grievance and appeals procedures, access to specialists and services, patient physician communications regarding medical treatment options, and establishment of a health quality council charged with providing expertise in quality measurement, in purchase and delivery of health care, and in advising on the health needs and requirements of health plan participants. Though legislation such as Jefford's was designed to take a broad approach to ensuring quality in health care, many of the bill's sections were prescriptive and specific. Nevertheless, casting a wider net to deal with quality concerns was preferred over legislation designed to protect consumers on a treatment-by-treatment basis. That is, laws passed with overwhelming support to force health plans and insurance companies to cover set lengths of stay for various procedures, including giving birth, though

politically popular, were criticized as inappropriate policy strategy for addressing quality of care.

Heightened interest in health policy that protects consumers and promotes quality is likely to continue into the next century. As long as change characterizes the health care delivery system, ongoing assessment and related intervention will be part of the policy equation for future policymakers. Policy initiatives may take many forms, including changing accreditation and licensure requirements, prohibiting payment schemes shown to put quality of care at risk, and ensuring that consumer's are informed about performance and able to exercise choice among plans and providers. Nursing has tremendous expertise to bring to this critically important policy discussion around quality of care.

CONCLUSION

The state of the nation's health is a result of a confluence of factors, including actions taken years earlier. Achieving significant improvement of the public's health is a formidable task, in no small part because of the various levels of activity (local, state, federal), multiple players, and pervasive underlying social problems. As Henry Kissinger notes, "A frustrating paradox is faced by policy makers: when their scope for action is widest, their knowledge is often minimal and when their knowledge is greatest, their scope for action has frequently disappeared" (Kissinger, 1988, p. 15).

The scope of action for health care is expansive. What knowledge exists regarding how to solve problems in health care is often rejected because of political ideology, fiscal constraints, and power struggles. The lesson for nurses intent on forging solutions to our health care problems is not that the task is insurmountable; it is only that the health care tapestry is woven with a myriad of patterns, threads, and colors. In addition to understanding nursing's position within the health care system, a macro view of health care must also be acquired.

REFERENCES

Andrews, L., Fullerton, J., Holtzman, N., & Motulsky, A. (1994). *Assessing genetic risks.* Washington, DC: Institute of Medicine, National Academy Press.

Blevins, J. (1995). Firearm violence: Youth and minorities. Available: www.LAPSR.org

Carney, D. (1997, May 17). Republicans feeling the heat as policy becomes reality. *Congressional Quarterly, 5,* 1131–1136.

Center for Responsive Politics. (1997). *Justice delayed, justice denied: Designed to fail* (on-line). Available: www.crp.org/pubs/justice/justice3.html

Centers for Disease Control and Prevention. (1997). *National summary of injury, mortality data, 1987–1996* (on-line). Available: www.cdc.gov

A citizens guide to the federal budget. (1996). Washington DC: U.S. Government Printing Office.

Clinton, W. (1996). *State of the Union* (on-line). Available: www.whitehouse.gov

Common Cause. (1996). *Politically insured, doctor recommended* (on-line). Available: www.ccsi.com/~comcause/news/medical.html

Common Cause. (1997). *Common Cause news update: Bipartisan campaign finance reform bill* (on-line). Available: www.ccsi.com/~comcause/news/update.html

Congressional Budget Office. (1996). *Federal budgetary implications of H.R. 3734, the Personal Responsibility and Work Opportunity Act of 1996.* Washington, DC: U.S. Government Printing Office.

Congressional Budget Office. (1997). *CBO estimate of president's budget plan for Medicare.* Washington DC: U.S. Government Printing Office.

Congressional Research Service. (1997). *Medicaid reform.* Washington, DC: The Library of Congress.

Cunningham, R. (Ed.). (1996, September). Budget pressures ease, but welfare bill jolts Medicaid. *Medicine & Health Perspectives.*

Cunningham, R. (Ed.). (1997, April 14). Regs awaited as telemedicine braces for life after subsidies. *Medicine & Health Perspectives.*

Department of Justice. (1990). *Crime in the United States: Uniform Crime Report* (on-line). Washington, DC: Author. Available: www.ojp.usdoj.gov/bjs

Department of Justice. (1994). *Crime in the United States: Uniform Crime Report* (on-line). Washington, DC: Author. Available: www.ojp.usdoj.gov/bjs

Department of Justice. (1997a). *Crime in the United States: Uniform Crime Report* (on-line). Washington, DC: Author. Available: www.ojp.usdoj.gov/bjs

Department of Justice (1997b). *Gang activity: Statement of Steven R. Wiley, chief of Violent Crimes and Major Offenders Section, FBI, before the Senate Committee on the Judiciary* (on-line). Washington, DC: Author. Available: www.ojp.usdoj.gov

Department of Justice. (1997c). *National Crime Victimization Survey* (on-line). Washington, DC: Author. Available: www.ojp.usdoj.gov/bjs

Doherty, C. J. (1997, April 12). Inquiry on campaign finance: Burning with a short fuse. *Congressional Quarterly,* 767–770.

Employee Benefits Research Institute. (1997). *Structural work force changes add to decline in employment-based health insurance coverage, EBRI finds* [press release]. Washington, DC: Author.

Environmental Protection Agency. (1996). *The new generation of environmental protection* (EPA 200-B-94-002). Washington, DC: Author.

Fallows, J. (1995). *A triumph of misinformation* (on-line). Available: www.theatlantic.com

Family Violence Prevention Fund. (1997). *What you can do: The facts.* (on-line). Available: www.fvpf.org/fund

Federal Election Commission. (1996). *The FEC and the federal campaign finance law* (on-line). Available: www.fec.gov/pages/fecfeca.ht.

Fix, M., Passel, J., & Zimmerman, W. (1996). *Summary of facts about immigrants' use of welfare* (on-line). Available: www.urban.org/immig/borjas.htm

Fix, M., Passel, J., & Zimmerman, W. (1997). *The use of SSI and other welfare programs by immigrants* (on-line). Available: www.urban.org/testmon/fix.htm

The Forum for State Health Policy Leadership, The National Conference of State Legislatures. (May, 1997). *Current state health policy issues* (Issue Brief No. 076720). Washington, DC: Authors.

Freedman, A. (1997). Chaffee claims the middle on clean air standards. *Congressional Quarterly, 55*(7), 422–423.

Fubini, S. (Ed.). (1997, February). Medicaid under welfare reform. *Healthcare Trends Report, 11*(2), 1–2, 16.

Gage, B., Kenney, G., Liu, C., Moon, M., Nichols, L., Sulvetta, M., Zuckerman, S. (1997). *Medicare savings: Options and opportunities.* Washington, DC: The Urban Institute.

Greenspan, A. (1997). Federal Reserve Board speech, March 7, 1997 (on-line). Available: http://www.

bog.frb.fed.US/BOARDDOCS/SPEECHES/1997030 7.htm

Health Policy Tracking Service. (1997, January). *Major state health care policies: Fifty state profiles, 1996* (5th ed.). 444 N. Capital St., N.W., Suite 515, Washington, DC 20001.

Health Spending Projections. (1996). Congressional Budget Office. Washington DC: U.S. Government Printing Office.

Hoefler, J. M., & Thai, K. V. (1993). The politics and economics of health care finance: Tough questions and no easy answers. *Journal of Health and Human Resources Administration, 16*(2), 121–143.

Holahan, J. (1997). *Expanding insurance coverage for children* (on-line). Available: www.urban.org

Institute of Medicine. (1994). *Telemedicine: A guide to assessing telecommunications in health care.* Washington DC: National Academy Press.

Johnson, K., DeGraw, C., Sonosky, C., Markus, A., & Rosenbaum, S. (1997). *Children's health insurance: A comparison of major federal legislation.* Washington, DC: George Washington University.

Kaufman, T. (1996). *Out of reach: Can America pay the rent?* National Low Income Housing Coalition, 1012 14th St. NW, No. 1200, Washington, DC 20005.

Kissinger, H. (1988) *Knowledge and power.* Occasional Paper of the Council of Scholars (Report No. 6). Washington, DC.

Kizer, K. W., Vassar, M. J., Harry, R. L., & Layton, K. D. (1995). Hospitalization charges, costs, and income for firearm-related injuries at a university trauma center. *JAMA, 273*(1), 1768–1773.

Komisar, H., Reuter, J., Feder, J., & Neuman, P. (1997). *Medicare chart book.* Menlo Park, CA: Henry J. Kaiser Family Foundation.

Koszezuk, J. (1997, April 12). Nonstop pursuit of campaign funds increasingly drives the system. *Congressional Quarterly,* 770–774.

Ku, L., & Coughlin, T. (1997). *How the new welfare reform law affects Medicaid* (on-line). Available: www.urban.org/newfed/anf_a5.htm

Leary, A. E. (1997, March 6). Panel cites lack of security on medical records. *New York Times,* p. A1.

Leon, J., Neuman, P., & Paremte, S. (1997). *Understanding the growth in Medicare's home health expenditures.* Kaiser Medicare Policy Report, Washington, DC.

Liska, D., Marlo, K., & Shah, A. (1996). *Medicaid expenditures and beneficiaries: A Report of the Kaiser Commission on the Future of Medicaid.* Washington, DC: Kaiser Commission.

Medicaid Facts. (1997). *Medicaid enrollment and spending growth.* Washington, DC: The Kaiser Commission on the Future of Medicaid.

National Center for Health Statistics. (1993). Available: www.CDC.gov\nchs

National Center for Health Statistics. (1995). Available: www.CDC.gov\nchs

National Center for Health Statistics. (1997). Available: www.CDC.gov\nchs

National Coalition for the Homeless. (1997, March). *Who is homeless?* (on-line). Available: http://nch.ari.net/who.html

National Conference of State Legislatures. (1997, August 4). Nonprofit hospital conversions remain topic on state agendas. *State Health Notes, 18*(258), 1 and 6.

National Health and Education Consortium. (1997). Membership brochure.

National Information Infrastructure Task Force. (1997). *Options for promoting privacy on the National Information Infrastructure* (on-line). Available: www.iitf.nist.gov/ipc/privacy.htm

National Right to Read Foundation. (1997). *Literary statistics in America* (on-line). Available: www.jwor.com/nrrf/researc3.htm

Nonprofit hospital conversions remain topic A on state agendas. (1997, August 4). *State Health Notes, 18*(258) 1, 6.

Office of the Inspector General. (1995). *Variation among home health agencies in Medicare payments for home health services.* Document No. OEI-04-93-00260. Washington DC: U.S. Department of Health and Human Services.

Pew Health Professions Commission. (1995, December). *Critical challenges: Revitalizing the health professions for the twenty-first century.* San Francisco: UCSF Center for the Health Professions.

Pfiffner, J. P. (1995). *Governance and American Politics: Classic and current perspectives.* New York: Harcourt Brace College Publishers.

PPRC Update. (1997, March). *Medicaid moves to managed care* (No. 15.) Washington DC: Physician Payment Review Commission.

The President's Health Security Plan. (1993). New York: Times Books.

Riley, R. W., & Shalala, D. E. (1993). *Joint Issue Statement on Health and Education.* Washington, DC: U.S. Government Printing Office.

Roper, A., & Starch, R. (1997). *Women's work program.* New York: Liz Claiborne.

Rosenberg, L. (1997). *The campaign finance game: They win, we lose* (on-line). Available: www.lwv.org/~marchapril/winlose.html

Rubin, A. (1997, April 5). The language of campaign finance, from bundling to tax checkoffs. *Congressional Quarterly*, pp. 785–790.

Sanchez, R. (1997, June 11). U.S. soars in 4th-grade assessment. *Washington Post*, p. AO1.

Shalala, D. E. (1997). *Secretary Shalala unveils new girl power! Girl Scouts partnership* (on-line). Available: www.dhhs.gov

Starr, P. (1992). *The logic of health-care reform.* Knoxville, TN: The Grand Rounds Press.

Starr, P. (1995). *What happened to health care reform?* (on-line). Available: http://epn.org/prospect/20/20star.html

Steuerle, E., & Mermin, G. (1997). *Devolution as seen from the budget* (on-line). Available: www.urban.org/newfed/anf_a2.htm

Super, D., Parrot, S., Steinmetz, S., & Mann, C. (1996). *The new welfare law* (on-line). Available: www.cbpp.org/WECNF813.htm

U.S. Bureau of the Census. (1994). *Vital and health statistics.* Washington, DC: U.S. Government Printing Office.

U.S. Department of Commerce. (1997, January 31). *Telemedicine report to the Congress.* Washington, DC: National Telecommunications and Information Administration.

U.S. Department of Health and Human Services. (1991). *Healthy People 2000.* Washington, DC: U.S. Government Printing Office.

U.S. General Accounting Office. (1997, February). *Telemedicine: Federal strategy is needed to guide investments* (Report No. NSIAD/HEHS-97-67). Washington, DC: Author.

U.S. Newswire. (1997, May 29). *Poll shows public supports stricter clean air standards.* Washington, DC: Author.

Vobejda, B., & Jeter, J. (1997, August 22). Though welfare rolls are down, true test of reform is just starting, experts say. *The Washington Post*, p. A13.

Waxman, L., & Hinderliter, S. (1996). *A status report on hunger and homelessness in America's cities: 1996.* U.S. Conference of Mayors, 1620 Eye St., NW, Suite 400, Washington, DC 20006.

Weissert, C. S., Weissert, W. G. (1996). *Governing health: The politics of health policy.* Baltimore: The Johns Hopkins University Press.

Wiley, S. (1997). Statement of Steven R. Wiley, Chief Violent Crimes and Major Offenders Section, FBI, before the Senate Committee on the Judiciary.

Wilson, T. M. (1993). Congress and the politics of compulsory health insurance. *Journal of Health and Human Resources Administration, 14*, 64–84.

Wolf, R. (1997, March 24). States take up welfare slack. *USA Today*, p. 1.

World Health Organization. (1997). *World Health Report 1997: Conquering suffering—enriching humanity.* Geneva, Switzerland: Author.

Zedlewski, S., & Giannarelli, L. (1997). *Diversity among state welfare programs* (on-line). Available: www.urban.org/newfed/anf_a1.htm

VIGNETTE

Impact of the New Welfare Law on Child Health

Mary R. Haack and Christine M. Wallin

Jane Brown, a public health nurse, works with young children at risk for and with disabilities. She has been working with the Jones family for the past several months, since the birth of their youngest children, twin girls who were born 10 weeks prematurely. Often when Jane visits, Ms. Jones's younger sister, Barbara, is in the home. Barbara lives with the Jones family but spends a lot of time at her boyfriend's house, several blocks away in the same neighborhood. During her last visit, Barbara tells Jane she thinks she is approximately 3 months' pregnant and asks why some babies are born early.

Jane tells Barbara it is important to get prenatalcare and asks whether she has seen a physician or midwife. Barbara states she has no money to see a physician and does not have a Medicaid card. Jane tells Barbara she should make an appointment at the clinic at a nearby hospital where her twin nieces were born, and offers to call the clinic today. The social worker at the clinic can assist Barbara in applying for Medicaid. Barbara seems hesitant and states she needs to speak with her boyfriend before making an appointment. When Jane asks why, Barbara tells her that he is infected with human immunodeficiency virus (HIV) and is adamant that she not tell anyone. She fears someone at the clinic might know her and word will get out. Jane explains that her visit is confidential and tells her it is very important that she be tested so that she and her unborn baby can be treated if necessary.

Jane knows through previous conversations with Ms. Jones that Barbara has been using "crack" cocaine for the past several years. She decides to broach the subject with Barbara at this time, asking her if she has been smoking, drinking, or using drugs since she realized she was pregnant. Ms. Jones urges Barbara to trust Jane and tell the truth. Barbara admits to using cocaine occasionally but knows she should stop while she is pregnant. She states that she needs help but is fearful that she will be reported to Child Protective Services if she seeks treatment. Again, Jane offers to call the clinic and speak with the social worker on Barbara's behalf. Barbara finally agrees and Jane makes the call.

Unfortunately, Jane finds that there are no clinic appointments available for the next 3 weeks and additionally that the social worker is on vacation until the following week. Jane makes a prenatal appointment for Barbara in the first available slot but does not share her history with the clinic at this point in time because of Barbara's grave concerns regarding confidentiality. She tells Barbara when her appointment is and promises to call the social worker about the Medicaid, HIV status, and drug issues next week.

When Jane finally reaches the social worker the following week, she is helpful but not hopeful. She tells Jane that she can help with the Medicaid process, but the physician is responsible for ordering HIV testing and detoxification services. These will have to wait until Barbara's appointment, in 3 weeks. If her HIV test result is positive and she needs drugs for treatment, she will need to have her Medicaid card in hand before any pharmacy will dispense the drugs, and that could take up to 2 months. Additionally, there is at least a 3-month waiting list for detoxification services. The social worker promises to help Barbara as much as she can, but she is one of many pregnant women needing specialized health care services.

As a pediatric specialist, Jane Brown is understandably frustrated with the numerous barriers she has encountered. She knows that many of the possible poor birth outcomes for Barbara and her baby can be prevented with prenatal care, drug treatment, and zidovudine (AZT) therapy (should Ms Jones be infected with HIV). With critical periods in pregnancy and fetal development passing by, the prospect of getting services in time dim. Jane Brown asks her supervisor why it is so difficult to get care for a woman who obviously needs many health care services. She is told that the community is still struggling with the implementation of the federal welfare reform bill and the transition to Medicaid managed care.

Welfare Reform

The Personal Responsibility and Work Opportunity Reconciliation Act of 1996, the welfare reform law, is predicated on the notion that too many families rely on public support who should be working and depending on themselves. As a result, the following changes were enacted July 1, 1997: Aid to Dependent Children (AFDC) was abolished and was replaced with Temporary Assistance for Needy Families

(TANF). Job Opportunities and Basic Skills (JOBS), the work and training program for welfare recipients, was abolished, but welfare recipients will be required to participate in work activities within 2 years. Under the old law, states received federal funds on an open-ended, entitlement basis. With the new law, states will receive a capped block grant, TANF, which has been set at $16.4 billion nationally. Small supplements will be available to states with high rates of population growth, and bonuses will be available to states that demonstrate a net decrease in out-of-wedlock births. States may transfer up to 30% of the welfare block grant fund into either the Child Care and Development Block Grant or the Title XX Social Service Block Grant (Rosenbaum & Darnell, 1996b). As a consequence of welfare reform, many parents will successfully enter the work force and care for their families. However, others will be unable to cope on their own, and their children will suffer. Families headed by drug-dependent mothers will be likely candidates to fail.

Families with Substance Abuse Problems

States may use *the* Personal Responsibility and Work Opportunity Reconciliation Act of 1996 to encourage drug-dependent women to seek substance abuse treatment, to improve their parenting skills, and to improve their lives in general. Or the law may be used to drive families with substance abuse problems farther away from intervention and place children at greater risk (Feig & McCullough, 1997).

Welfare reform addresses substance abuse primarily as a criminal problem rather than a health problem and, as such, offers several options that states may adopt to deny welfare or Medicaid. States may choose to deny benefits if, during application for public assistance (Section 115), the applicant states in writing that he or she, or *any member of the applicant's family,* has been convicted of a felony involving drugs or (Section 902) if the applicant tests positive for drugs. Welfare recipients may lose their benefits if at any point it comes to the attention of the case worker that the woman has been convicted

of a drug-related felony offense. A woman may also lose SSI and food stamps if the case worker discovers that the recipient has not met the terms of probation, parole, or sentence of any felony conviction (U.S. Department of Health and Human Services [Center for Substance Abuse Treatment], 1996).

Breaking the Link Between Cash Assistance and Medicaid Eligibility

The shift away from welfare as an entitlement to a block grant has important implications for health care for women and children because the new law effectively breaks the link between Medicaid and welfare benefits. As a consequence, eligibility for Medicaid benefits is no longer automatic for welfare recipients, as it was under AFDC. States must establish a separate Medicaid application process designed to preserve Medicaid eligibility for persons losing welfare benefits, but there is evidence that the welfare reform law will result in the failure of many otherwise eligible children and families to apply for Medicaid (Rosenbaum & Darnell, 1996a). These changes will greatly impact access to health care services because families will be unable to pay for services.

In most states a pregnant woman with a substance abuse problem who meets the income eligibility requirements for Medicaid will qualify for prenatal care even if she is denied income assistance (Rosenbaum & Darnell, 1996a). However, families might not realize or be informed that health insurance is still available and thus may never apply for benefits. In mandatory-reporting states, a substance-using mother may also fear that she will be reported to Child Protective Services. Though the failure of a substance-using mother to enroll in Medicaid may save Medicaid some managed care dollars in the short term, the long-term costs to the health care system will outweigh any savings.

Outcomes Related to Untreated Maternal Substance Abuse

The national price tag for treating infants exposed to drugs in utero is estimated at up to

$3 billion annually (U.S. General Accounting Office, 1990). Short-term human costs are evidenced by premature and low-birth-weight infants, whereas long-term costs include chronic illness and developmental disabilities. The U.S. rankings of twentieth in infant mortality and thirty-first in low birth weight are directly related to lack of prenatal care and prenatal use of alcohol, drugs, and cigarettes (Racine, Joyce, & Anderson, 1993). In addition, 8 of 10 babies abandoned at birth are left because of maternal drug use (Shalala, 1996). HIV infection in most children results from prenatal transmission from an HIV-infected woman. Most such women are intravenous drug users or have an intravenous drug–using partner (Centers for Disease Control and Prevention, 1993). Median hospital costs for babies exposed to drugs in utero range from $1,100 to $8,450 higher than for babies who are not exposed to drugs in utero (U.S. General Accounting Office, 1990). Inpatient care for one child with acquired immunodeficiency syndrome is estimated to cost $34,713 per year. When multiplied by the number of women in need of drug treatment who are receiving public assistance, estimated to be between 600,000 and 1,000,000, the costs are staggering (U.S. Department of Health and Human Services [Center for Substance Abuse Treatment], 1996).

Welfare Reform and Medicaid Managed Care

The implementation of welfare reform comes at a time when states are grappling with the delivery of Medicaid services within a managed care environment. Responses to managed care and welfare legislation vary by state. In the past, many agencies segregated services and populations along federal or state categorical funding lines. But the emergence of managed care, funding cuts, and welfare reform has heightened the need for collaboration and coordination among community agencies. Though a number of states have begun to develop strategies for cooperation that address the barriers encountered by women with substance abuse problems, many states continue to struggle with collaboration issues. In some states, social services agencies purchase treatment services from alcohol- and drug-treatment providers. Other states have begun to take steps to link Medicaid and welfare reform efforts to current state alcohol and other drug prevention and treatment programs. In a number of states, however, strategies (or the lack of strategies) for cooperation do not begin to address the problems encountered by substance-dependent women.

The greatest barriers to health care are the most hidden. Failure of a state to coordinate laws and policies relating to the welfare act, Medicaid, managed care, and other public benefit provisions will mean that there is no process for families excluded from health care in one program to learn about or obtain coverage through another program. Failure to train the front-line personnel, such as nurses, to inform applicants that they have a right to prenatal care and drug treatment, and to guide applicants to those benefits, will mean that needy families will never claim care.

Implications for Nurses

The reform of the welfare system and the shift to Medicaid managed care arrangements have everything to do with economics and very little to do with high-quality care for vulnerable women and their children. Though the welfare law is intended to limit cash assistance and require recipients to participate in work and work-related activities, it also has the potential to separate needy mothers and children from essential health care services paid for through Medicaid benefits. This is especially true for high-risk mothers with substance abuse problems, and their children. The obstetrical and developmental risk imposed by maternal use of alcohol and other drugs, perhaps more than any other risks, are preventable. Yet the welfare reform legislation and the transition into Medicaid managed care create barriers that impose lengthy delays and limit referrals to specialty providers, expensive pharmacy and laboratory services, or inpatient services that are essential to these women and children.

Nurses have established models of care designed to overcome barriers identified in the vignette. Dr. Shoni Davis, a psychiatric mental health specialist, has established Perinatal Treatment Services, a comprehensive program for substance-using women and their children in Seattle, Washington. In Tampa, Florida, Shirley Coletti has created PAR Village, an exemplary therapeutic community for mothers with substance abuse problems and their children. And in the District of Columbia, which has the highest infant mortality and morbidity rates, Dr. Ruth Lubic, a certified nurse-midwife, and Dolores Farr, Executive Director of Healthy Babies, are providing leadership in the development of a comprehensive one-stop service center for childbearing and childrearing families that will provide a full scope of maternity services with linkages to the hospital system, well child care, drop-in services for abused and abusing women and families, legal assistance, and Head Start services.

On a practical level, nurses have much to learn from these nursing leaders. Each has had to design her program within the limits of the existing political and financial environment and to balance those realities with the best possible clinical care. It is no longer enough that nurses master their clinical specialty; they must be aware of potential conflicts that exist between policies such as welfare reform and good clinical care. Primary care providers and case managers need norms and standards of practice that can be legally enforced when their clinical judgment conflicts with actuarial standards imposed by the changing health care environment. The adoption of legally enforceable standards for clinical practice will require data that document the impact of the law on vulnerable women and children. Nurses are ideally situated to direct or participate in such research endeavors.

Not everyone can create innovative models of care, but every nurse can have an impact on improving services for women and children. For example, Jane Brown, in our vignette, could begin by discussing the matter with her colleagues who have similar frustrations in gaining access to necessary services for their clients. Next, Jane could contact the U.S. House and Senate via the Internet at www.house.gov and www.senate.gov to find the names and addresses of her state congressional representatives and the committees on which they currently serve. Jane and her colleagues could draft a letter to the appropriate Congressional representatives of their state, with detailed descriptions of the challenges they face on a day-to-day basis. In addition, Jane could write to the public health agencies in the neighboring counties and suggest that they, too, share their "stories." She could provide them with a sample letter and the names and addresses of their state representatives. Because Jane lives and works in the District of Columbia metropolitan area, she could also invite her Congressional representatives to spend a day with her "on the road" so that they could experience at first hand what she and many other public health nurses face each day as they make their rounds.

References

Centers for Disease Control and Prevention. (1993). *HIV/AIDS Surveillance Report, 5*(3), 2–3.

Children's Defense Fund. (1996, September 23). *Summary of the new welfare legislation.* Washington, DC: Author.

Feig, L., & McCullough, C. (1997). The role of child welfare. In M. R. Haack (Ed.), *Drug-dependent mothers and their children: Issues in public policy and public health.* New York: Springer.

Haack, M. R., Budetti, P. P., & Darnell, J. (1993). *Analysis of resources to aid drug-exposed infants and their families.* Washington, DC: Center for Health Policy Research, George Washington University.

Racine, R., Joyce, T., & Anderson, R. (1993). The association between prenatal care and birth weight among women exposed to cocaine in New York City. *Journal of the American Medical Association, 270,* 1581–1586.

Rosenbaum, S., & Darnell, J. (1996a). *An analysis of the Medicaid and health related provisions of the Personal Responsibility and Work Opportunity Reconciliation Act of 1996.* Washington, DC: Center for Health Policy Research, George Washington University Medical Center.

Rosenbaum, S., & Darnell, J. (1996b). *Medicaid Section 1115 Demonstration Waivers: Approved and proposed activities.* Washington, DC: Kaiser Commission on the Future of Medicaid.

Shalala, D. [Secretary of the Department of Health and Human Services]. (1996). C-Span. Washington, DC.

U.S. Department of Health and Human Services, Office of the Assistant Secretary for Planning and Evaluation and the Public Health Services, National Institute on Drug Abuse. (1994, July). *Substance abuse among women and parents.* Washington, DC: Author.

U.S. Department of Health and Human Services, Substance Abuse and Mental Health Administration, Center for Substance Abuse Treatment. (1996). *Alcohol and drug treatment: Policy choices in welfare reform.* Washington, DC: Author.

U.S. General Accounting Office. (1990a). *Drug-exposed infants: A generation at risk.* Report to the Chairmen, Committee on Finance, U.S. Senate (GAO/HRD-90-138). Washington, DC: Author.

U.S. General Accounting Office. (1990b). *Prenatal care: Medicaid recipients and uninsured women obtain insufficient care* (GAO Publication No. HRD 87-137). Washington, DC: Author.

Washington State Department of Social and Health Services Research and Data Analysis. (1996, July). *First Steps program outcomes.* Olympia, WA: Author.

Washington State Department of Health. (1997). *The ABC's of First Steps 1997 manual* (940–001). Olympia, WA: Author.

Chapter *22*

LEGISLATIVE AND REGULATORY PROCESSES

SHEILA ABOOD AND PAMELA MITTELSTADT

The making of laws is a lot like the making of sausage—not necessarily a process you want to watch too closely.

THE PATH OF LEGISLATION AND INFLUENCING THE PROCESS

Nurses who understand the path of legislation can influence the system and the development of sound health and public policy for their patients, their families, and the profession of nursing. This chapter will describe the federal path by which a bill becomes a law. For state law we have used Michigan to illustrate the legislative path. Though the pathway may differ slightly from state to federal level and from state to state, the basic process is the same.

Introduction of a Bill

The legislative process is complicated by many rules and procedures. The member of Congress or the state legislator who understands this process will most likely be more successful in the passage or defeat of a bill than one who is an expert on the substance of the bill. (We will refer here to members of Congress and state legislators as members of the legislature.) Moreover, the numerous players in the executive branch, the members of the legislature, constituents, and special interest groups, and the many complex steps in the passage of legislation, make it far easier to defeat a bill than to pass one.

Bills can be introduced only by a member of the legislature, although the idea can come from anyone, including constituents. Sometimes, legislation is introduced in both the Senate and the House of Representatives simultaneously as companion bills. Every bill introduced into Congress faces the 2-year deadline of the Congressional term. Of the thousands of bills introduced annually, Congress takes up relatively few. During the 1993–1995 term, 8,544 public bills and joint resolutions were introduced; of these, only 465 became public laws (Davidson & Oleszek, 1996). Of the approximately 4,400 bills filed during a 2-year session in the Michigan Legislature, between 600 and 700 will be enacted (Browne & VerBurg, 1995). Proper consideration of bills requires organization, time, and hard work. Legislators and legislative committees spend many hours of work on each bill before the bill is sent to the floor of either house for consideration. The floor debate on a bill, seen by a visitor, is only one of the stages of the legislative process.

Legislators introduce bills for a variety of reasons: to declare a position on an issue; as a favor to a constituent or a special interest group; to obtain publicity; or to prevent a political attack. Once a bill is introduced, the legislator can claim he or she has done something about an issue without continuing to work on the bill, blaming the committee or other members of the legislature if no action is taken. Passage of a bill requires continuous work and nurturing.

Influencing the Introduction of a Bill

Nurses can influence the introduction of bills as constituents and, more often, as members of professional associations that lobby the legislature. They can call attention to the problems in the funding of health care, such as the need for more services for uninsured children or the need for reimbursement of nursing services. Legislators like to work with organized groups, such as the American Nurses Association (ANA) or state nurses associations, that represent a constituency or a position on a bill.

Frequently associations are asked to assist in the drafting of legislation and in lobbying members of the legislature. In recent years, coalitions of interested organizations have been established to present a united front, a clear message, and a strong constituency to persuade legislators of the need for legislation on a particular issue. Sometimes this is a process that may stretch over a number of legislative sessions. It took a period of 6 years to pass the Health Professional Recovery Program legislation, which brought about significant reform in Michigan's licensure and discipline laws. During that time the Michigan Nurses Association actively worked with other health professional associations and staff from the Bureau of Occupational and Professional Regulation to develop legislation that provided a new nondisciplinary approach to working with health care professionals who are chemically dependent or mentally ill. Providing input at the very beginning of the legislative process and working with other interested groups ensured that nurses' concerns were addressed in the reform laws. After enactment of the law, members of the Michigan Nurses Association continued to work closely with the Michigan Department of Commerce and with the Health Professions Recovery Program to keep registered nurses aware of the changes in the disciplinary process. Efforts included extensive consultation to groups and individuals, publication of materials explaining the program, and sponsorship of a presentation by officials of the Department of Commerce. ("1995: A Successful Year . . .," 1996).

Identifying the appropriate sponsor to introduce a bill is also critical to its success. Generally, it is best to ask a member of a committee that has jurisdiction over a program or issue addressed in the bill. For example, in the U.S. Congress, the Senate Finance Committee has jurisdiction over the Medicare program and decides which legislation gets sent to the full Senate for a vote. Legislation that provides for direct reimbursement of nurse practitioners under Medicare would have a healthier prognosis if it were introduced by a member of the Senate Finance Committee.

Committee Action

Committees are the centers of policymaking and public education both at the federal and state levels. Committee procedure provides the means for members of the legislature to sift through an otherwise overwhelming number of bills, proposals, and complex issues. Committee consideration usually consists of three standard steps: public hearings, markups, and reports. It is at the committee stage that proposed legislation is given the most intensive consideration. It is in committee where conflicting points of view are discussed and where legislation is actually hammered out.

After a bill is introduced and given an identifying number, an appointed leader of the house will refer it to the committee that has jurisdiction over the bill. A broad subject like health care can cut across the jurisdiction of more than one committee. In this situation, the speaker of the house will identify the appropriate primary committee and may also send the bill to other committees. The primary committee retains the predominant responsibility for guiding the referred legislation to final passage. Referrals to more than one committee can have a positive effect by providing opportunities for greater public discussion of the issue and multiple points of access for outside interest groups, but this can also greatly slow down the legislative process (Davidson & Oleszek, 1996).

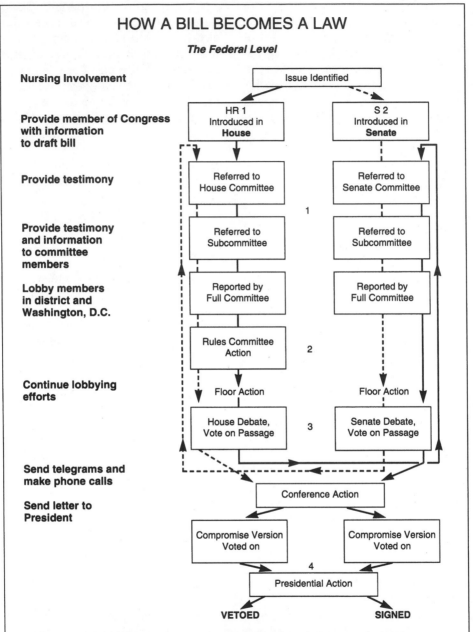

HOW A BILL BECOMES A LAW

The Federal Level

Nursing Involvement

Issue Identified

Provide member of Congress with information to draft bill

HR 1
Introduced in
House

S 2
Introduced in
Senate

Provide testimony

Referred to
House Committee

Referred to
Senate Committee

1

Provide testimony and information to committee members

Referred to
Subcommittee

Referred to
Subcommittee

Lobby members in district and Washington, D.C.

Reported by
Full Committee

Reported by
Full Committee

Rules Committee
Action

2

Continue lobbying efforts

Floor Action

Floor Action

House Debate,
Vote on Passage

3

Senate Debate,
Vote on Passage

Send telegrams and make phone calls

Conference Action

Send letter to President

Compromise Version
Voted on

Compromise Version
Voted on

4

Presidential Action

VETOED   **SIGNED**

[1] A bill goes to full committee first, then to special subcommittees for hearings, debate, revisions, and approval. The same process occurs when it goes to full committee. It either dies in committee or proceeds to the next step.

[2] Only the House has a Rules Committee to set the "rule" for floor action and conditions for debate and amendments. In the Senate, the leadership schedules action.

[3] The bill is debated, amended, and passed or defeated. If passed, it goes to other chamber and follows the same path. If each chamber passes a similar bill, both versions go to conference.

[4] The President may sign the bill into law, allow it to become law without his signature, or veto it and return it to Congress. To override the veto, both houses must approve the bill by a $2/3$ majority vote.

In Congress, a bill is usually referred by the committee chairman to a subcommittee. For example, the Ways and Means Committee of the House of Representatives refers most Medicare bills to the House Ways and Means Subcommittee on Health. If the subcommittee wishes to take action on the bill, it will schedule a hearing to discuss the substance of proposed legislation. In the end, committees and subcommittees select the bills they want to consider and ignore the rest. In this way committees perform a gatekeeping function by selecting from the thousands of measures introduced in each session those which merit floor debate.

A committee can handle a bill in several different ways:

- Approve a bill with or without amendments
- Rewrite or revise the bill and report it out to the full House or Senate
- Report it unfavorably, which allows it to be considered by the full House or Senate, but with a recommendation that the bill be rejected
- Take no action, which kills the bill (Congressional Quarterly's Congress . . .," 1993)

In the Michigan Legislature, a comprehensive committee system has evolved in each house as a means of dealing with the large number of bills introduced during each 2-year session. The chairs of the committees control the work of the committee and, by negotiating with their members, establish the agenda for considering the bills. The primary workhorse committees in the Michigan legislature are the 29 standing house committees and the 18 standing senate committees. Unlike Congress, where the responsibilities of each standing committee are defined by the rules of each house, the names, functions, and number of members of the standing committees of the Michigan legislature may vary somewhat with each legislative session. Changing leadership and shifting state and regional agendas drive those changes. Committee work in the Michigan legislature includes the review and screening of proposals as legislators and staff check with both affected interest groups and constituents, and conduct multiple analyses of the potential impact of proposals. Committee members also network widely with legislators whose districts are affected by any bill. The negotiations and compromises necessary to get a bill passed are most often made at this point in the process.

The committee at the state level has several options for action, including taking no action. A committee's refusal to consider or report a bill can be overridden by a discharge motion; if this is approved by a majority of members of the chamber, the bill is sent to the floor for consideration by the full body (Browne & VerBerg, 1995).

Hearings

Hearings are conducted for the purpose of educating committee members and the public on a bill and to offer the opportunity for opposing views to be discussed. Sometimes a hearing is conducted to generate publicity for an issue or to provide oversight of an existing program or agency, such as the U.S. Food and Drug Administration. "Committee oversight" refers to the process in which the committee watches over and monitors a federal or state program to protect the interests of the citizens and to ensure that the laws are being correctly implemented by the agency.

Nurses can influence the process at this point by requesting the opportunity to testify at bill hearings. Frequently committees prefer to relate to large organized groups that have a position on the issue rather than to individuals. The ANA frequently testifies on behalf of its members on various health care issues. If there is no opportunity to testify at the hearing, written testimony can usually be submitted by organizations and individuals.

The committee process can also be influenced at this time by meeting with and writing to the members of the committee about the bill. Concerns expressed by constituents are given serious consideration. Lobbyists will meet with all members of the committee to express the views of their clients. Professional associations often activate a grassroots network of members, asking them to contact the committee members with their concerns.

The hearing process at the state level is almost identical, and so is the importance of an organized approach to presenting testimony. When several representatives of nursing plan to testify on a bill, it is more efficient and effective for them to coordinate their response, raising different aspects of an issue rather than repeating the same points. It is also important for the various representatives to emphasize the issues where there is agreement, so that a unified message can be presented to the committee members. A hearing room packed with a supportive audience makes a powerful statement to legislators about support for a particular issue.

Markup

When the hearings are concluded, the subcommittee meets to mark up the bill—that is, to consider all the provisions in it, amending some and deleting others. At a committee's markup session, the committee makes its final decision about the content and form of the bill. The result can be a weakened or a strengthened bill. Pressure from outside interest groups is often intense at this stage. Under Congressional "sunshine rules," markups are conducted in public, except on national security or related issues. After conducting hearings and markups, a subcommittee sends its recommendation to the full committee, which may conduct its own hearings and markups, or it may ratify the subcommittee's decision, or take no action, or return the bill to the subcommittee for further study.

Committee Report

The rules of the U.S. Senate and House dictate that a committee report accompany the bill to the floor of either house. The report, written by committee staff, describes the intent of legislation—its purpose and scope. It explains any amendments and any changes in current law, estimates the cost of the bill to the government, contains a minority report if some members were opposed to the bill, and sets out documentation for the legislative intent.

The legislative intent of the bill is extremely important, especially for the government agency that will implement and enforce the law. Sometimes the report contains explicit instructions on how the agency should interpret the law through regulations, or the report may be written without great detail. Sometimes an agency will interpret the law narrowly, particularly, if a law is written vaguely. For example, when certified nurse midwives received reimbursement authority under the Medicare program, the agency chose to reimburse them only for maternity services, not for all the services that are covered by Medicare and that they are legally able to deliver. This was a narrow interpretation of the law and was not the intent of the members of Congress.

The committee report is also important because it offers those interested in the bill an opportunity to promote or protect their interests. Committee staff frequently include report language suggested by special interest groups if it is congruent with the bill.

Floor Action in the House and Senate

A bill reported out of committee is referred to the floor of the house for consideration. If the bill is not controversial, it may be dealt with expeditiously. Otherwise it is placed on a calendar for future consideration. The rules governing the type of calendar on which a bill is placed and subsequent floor procedures differ greatly between the two federal houses and state houses.

Debate begins once the bill is brought to the floor for consideration. Rules govern the time allotted for debate and for each member, with time parceled out for proponents and opponents of the measure. When the debate has ended, amendments to the bill are brought to the floor, and debate on these amendments follows. These amendments usually provide a way to shape the bill into a form acceptable to the majority.

When the bill moves to the floor, interest groups continue to lobby the opponents, the proponents, and particularly the undecided legislators, attempting to influence the outcome of the vote. This process is usually begun after the introduction of the bill, when lobbyists meet with the members of the referring committee to gather support for the measure, and continues until the bill is signed into law. The grassroots network is also reactivated when the bill moves to the floor to contact the members of the legislature from their own districts. Members listen attentively to their constituents, and lobbying should continue until the moment of the vote, especially with undecided members. Lobbyists are known to wait outside the cloakroom in the "lobby" to catch the attention of members as they move in and out of the chambers.

A vote on the bill is taken after the debate and amendment process is completed. There are three methods of voting:

1 A voice vote calls for the volume of members answering yea or nay.
2. The division vote requires a head count of those favoring and those opposing an amendment.
3. The recorded teller vote records each legislator's name and position taken on the vote. Recorded votes are the most valuable to lobbyists and constituents because they document how the member voted—helpful information in determining continuing support for a legislator and as a predictor of a legislator's future stand on issues.

Conference Action

Before a bill can be sent to the executive branch for consideration, an identical bill must be passed in both houses. Frequently the bills considered by the houses are not identical, so members of each house must meet to resolve the differences. This is often where much of the hard bargaining and compromising takes place in the passage of legislation. Conferees, usually senior members of the committee with jurisdiction over the bill, are appointed by the leaders of the two houses.

The conference offers another opportunity for groups and individuals to persuade members to support a position on the controversial measures in the bill. Frequently there is controversy over the amount of funding being given to a federal program. For example, authorization for levels of funding for nursing education programs can differ by tens of millions of dollars. Clearly supporters of the program would lobby for the bill with the largest amount of funding.

When an agreement has been reached on the controversial provisions of the bill, a conference report is written explaining the differences considered in resolving the issue. The conference version of the bill must then be approved by both chambers.

Executive Action

After identical bills have been passed by the chambers, the bill is ready to go to the executive branch. The executive (state governor or the U.S. President) has the power to sign the bill into law or to veto it. The executive may return the bill to the chamber with no signature and with a message stating his or her objections. If no further action is taken, the bill dies. The houses may decide to call for another floor vote to overturn the executive's veto. A two-thirds vote is required to override the veto in the U.S. Congress and in many states. Under the Constitution, a bill may become law without the President's signature in one other way: it becomes law if the president does not sign it within 10 days from the time he receives it, provided Congress is in session. Presidents occasionally permit enactment of legislation in this manner when they want to make a political statement of disapproval of the legislation but do not believe that their objections warrant a veto. If Congress adjourns before the 10-day period expires, the unsigned bill does not become law. In this case the bill has become a pocket veto ("Congressional Quarterly's Congress . . .," 1993).

Authorization-Appropriation Process

As one begins to understand the legislative process and to analyze individual pieces of legislation, it is important to know the distinction between authorizing legislation and appropriating legislation. Because a considerable amount of Congressional activity is concerned with decisions related to spending money and because many of those decisions have a direct impact on health care and nursing programs, it is especially important for nurses to be familiar with the authorization-appropriation process. Programs and agencies such as the Nurse Education Act, Scholarships for Disadvantaged Students, the National Health Service Corps, the National Institute of Nursing Research, the National Institutes of Health, and the Agency for Health Care Policy and Research are all subject to the authorizing and appropriating process.

Before any of these programs can receive or spend money from the U.S. Treasury, a two-step process usually occurs. First, an authorization bill allowing an agency or program to exist or continue must be passed. The authorization bill is the substantive bill that establishes the purpose and guidelines for the program and usually sets limits on the amount that can be spent. It gives a federal agency or a program the legal authority to operate. Authorizing legislation does not provide the actual dollars for a program or enable an agency to spend funds in the future. Renewal or modification of authorizing legislation is called reauthorization. Second, an appropriation bill must be passed. The appropriation bill enables an agency or program to make spending commitments and to spend money. In almost all cases an appropriation bill for an activity is not supposed to be made until the authorization for that activity is enacted. No money can be spent on a program unless it first has been authorized to exist. Conversely, if a program has been authorized but no money

is provided (appropriated) for its implementation, that program cannot be carried out (Collender, 1991).

Today, much of the federal government is funded through annual enactment of 13 general appropriations bills. Whether agencies receive all the money they request depends, in part, on the recommendations of the authorizing and appropriating committees. Each house has authorizing and appropriating committees with differing responsibilities. For federal nursing education and research activities, the authorizing committees are the Senate Labor and Human Resources Committee and the House Commerce Committee. The appropriators for federal nursing education and research programs are the Senate and House appropriations committees and their subcommittees on labor, health and human services, and education.

The two-step authorization-appropriation process is designed to concentrate the policy-making decisions within the authorizing committees and the precise spending amounts within the appropriations committees. The authorization-appropriation process is determined by Congressional rules that, like almost all Congressional rules, can be waived, circumvented, or ignored. For example, the failure to enact an authorization does not necessarily prevent the appropriations committee from acting. If an expired program is likely to be reauthorized—for example, the Nursing Education Act—it may receive funds that must then be spent in accordance with the expired authorizing language.

The Nursing Education Act, Title VIII of the Public Health Service Act, was last authorized in 1992 for a 2-year period, and there has been growing concern within the nursing community regarding its future. Fortunately, members of the House and Senate committees have continued to fund the eight programs that make up Title VIII, despite the lack of reauthorization. Through the yearly appropriations process, it is evident that Congress has continued to support nursing education (Tri-Council for Nursing, 1996).

CASE EXAMPLE   The Health Insurance Portability and Accountability Act

Political Environment and Background

The passage of the Health Insurance Portability and Accountability Act of 1996 (Public Law 104-191) was preceded by a lengthy national debate over the need for comprehensive health care reform and access to basic health care services for all U.S. citizens and residents. This debate was driven by the need to contain health care costs and the growing number of people who had no health insurance coverage. In 1991 the American Nurses Association released *Nursing's Agenda for Health Care Reform,* a plan that addressed access to health care, cost containment, and quality. Endorsed by more than 75 nursing organizations and associations, it sent a unified message to policymakers about the essential components that nurses envisioned in a reformed health care system. (See Appendix C.)

Health care reform continued to dominate the political debate throughout the early 1990s, and shortly after election in 1992, President Clinton announced that health care reform was at the top of his national agenda. The Health Security Act of 1993, which sought to guarantee health care coverage for all Americans, was introduced in Congress, but the President and the Democratic leadership were unable to generate bipartisan support for the plan. It was criticized as being too complex, too expensive, and too bureaucratic, and by the autumn of 1994 Clinton's comprehensive health care effort had collapsed (Davidson & Oleszek, 1996).

The midterm Congressional elections in November 1994 changed the majority in Congress and gave control of the 104th Congress (1994–1996) to the Republicans. The change in leadership and the emphasis on the "Contract with America" resulted in a less ambitious and less focused health care agenda for the 104th Congress. There was a return to the incremental approach to health care reform. Many members of the legislature pledged to address pieces of the last session's comprehensive health care reform bills; however, during the session few of the proposals moved beyond a subcommittee hearing.

Health insurance reform was one health-related issue that stayed on the legislative agenda in both the House and the Senate. Private health insurance was seen as a place to start a modest reform of the existing health care system. By the spring of 1996 the House of Representatives and the Senate had passed differing versions of legislation addressing health care insurance. Both versions supported the concept of "portability," the ability of workers to move from one job to the next without losing their health insurance. The legislation aimed to provide working Americans with more security about their health care coverage, even if they had a preexisting medical condition that might not otherwise be covered. It had taken more than a year for these two bills to move through the legislative process, enduring along the way presidential campaign politics, partisan fighting in Congress, and opposition from powerful interest groups.

Strategizing in the Senate

The Senate bill (S 1028), sponsored by Senators Nancy Kassebaum (Republican) and Edward Kennedy (Democrat), was the first significant health insurance measure with bipartisan support to make it out of committee in the 104th Congress. The bill had been introduced early in the session and referred to the Senate Labor and Human Resources Committee. However, it did not reach the Senate floor for a vote in 1995, largely because it was considered to be a magnet for controversial amendments that would add complexity, making it much more difficult to pass.

Early in the process, determined not to repeat the history of the failed Clinton health initiative, the sponsors, Kassebaum and Kennedy, put together a plan based on their years of legislative experience and knowledge. To secure the backing of the business and health care groups, they vowed to fight any attachments to their bill that might hinder final passage, even amendments that they strongly supported. For a while, that strategy worked. The legislation gained momentum and 50 Senators across the political spectrum signed on as cosponsors. After a hearing before the Senate Labor and Human Resources Committee, the bill was approved unanimously by the committee on August 2, 1995. At this point in the process, it became stalled by several obstacles. First, there was vigorous opposition from segments of the health insurance industry which maintained that the group-to-individual coverage guarantee would cause premiums to increase for everyone. Conservative senators, who shared the insurance industry's concerns, placed "holds" on the bill. (A hold allows a senator to prevent a bill from coming to the Senate floor for a vote, but only as long as the majority leader allows it.) President Clinton's endorsement of the bill and media coverage of the "holds" applied pressure on the opponents to give in, but only after they had won time to organize their opposition. Another challenge came from supporters and health care interest groups who feared that adding controversial floor amendments would add costly federal mandates and jeopardize the final passage of the bill. The sponsors held firm, and when the bill finally came to the full Senate for a vote, it was successfully ushered through with an overwhelming vote of 100 to 0 (Langdon, 1996b).

House Action

The House version of health insurance reform was passed by the House of Representatives on March 28, 1996. Three existing health care bills introduced earlier in the session were melded into one bill (HR 3103). Though it was similar to the Kassebaum-Kennedy bill, the House bill was much broader in scope. It included limits on damages for medical malpractice, tax deductions for the self-employed, and a provision calling for the creation of medical savings accounts (MSAs). (MSAs are tax-preferred savings accounts that employers would set up to help defray medical expenses. They are coupled with a high-deductible health insurance policy that would pay costs after the deductible was reached.)

Compromise and Reconciliation in the Conference Committee

The major differences between the House and Senate bills proved to be difficult to resolve. Preconference jockeying delayed the start of formal negotiations to reconcile the two bills. It took weeks of negotiations between Senator Kassebaum and the principal House sponsor, Ways and Means Committee Chairman Representative Bill Archer, for the two legislators to reach an agreement to drop the provisions on medical malpractice, while keeping a scaled-down MSA program. This compromise position turned out to be unacceptable to Senator Kennedy, who was opposed to MSAs in any form. Using Senate rules to block the naming of the conferees and to delay the convening of the conference committee, Senator Kennedy negotiated with Chairman Archer. They eventually worked out an agreement on a tightly constrained pilot program for MSAs to be available to a limited population for a limited period of 4 years. The Kennedy-Archer settlement was significant, but several other issues remained to be resolved by the conference committee (Langdon, 1996a).

House and Senate conferees worked out details of the insurance portability provisions. They also dealt with a Senate provision, not included in the House bill, that proposed to require health insurers to treat mental illness like any other illness. It would have prevented insurers from imposing limitations on mental health coverage that are not imposed for physical illnesses. Business groups adamantly opposed the mental health parity provision, arguing that it would raise health insurance costs and result in a scaling back of benefits. In the end, the conferees dropped that controversial provision. Senator Pete Domenici, who had sponsored the amendment, said he would push the mental health parity issue in a stronger, stand-alone bill later in the year. The conference report on HR 3103 was adopted by the House and Senate in the first week of August, and the legislation was signed into law by President Clinton on August 21, 1996, officially ending the struggle to pass the most basic reforms on the health care agenda (Langdon, 1996b; Nather & Darling, 1996).

ANA Endorsement of the Health Insurance Portability and Accountability Act

ANA endorsed this legislation as a first step toward the ultimate goal of making appropriate health care accessible for all Americans. Though the bill is not a substitute for comprehensive health care reform, still a strong priority of ANA, it was the first significant health insurance measure to be reported out of a Congressional committee with bipartisan support. Through letters to every member of Congress, ANA urged the members to heed the message of a strong, bipartisan coalition among health care providers, business leaders, organized labor, and consumers that the bill be kept free of controversial amendments in the interest of passing reforms all could agree on. ANA actively opposed the inclusion of MSAs because of concerns that MSAs without safeguards in a comprehensive reform plan could be seen by some employers as an inexpensive alternative to offering comprehensive health insurance coverage. ANA participated in a press conference with Senator Kennedy to express concerns about the inclusion of MSAs in the bill. Through fact sheets and articles in ANA publications, nurses around the country were kept informed about the progress of the bill as it moved through both the House and the Senate. In addition, ANA activated

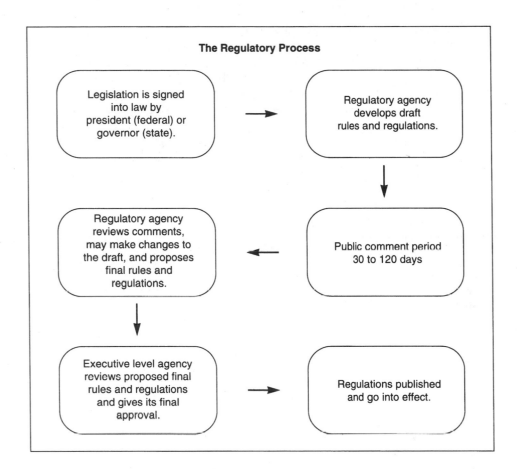

The Regulatory Process

Legislation is signed into law by president (federal) or governor (state).

→

Regulatory agency develops draft rules and regulations.

↓

Regulatory agency reviews comments, may make changes to the draft, and proposes final rules and regulations.

←

Public comment period 30 to 120 days

↓

Executive level agency reviews proposed final rules and regulations and gives its final approval.

→

Regulations published and go into effect.

its grassroots network, the Nurses Strategic Action Team (NSTAT), and thousands of individual nurses responded by contacting their members of Congress about this legislation ("Health Insurance Reform Enacted," 1996).

NURSES AND THE REGULATORY PROCESS

As important as it is to become skilled at influencing the legislative process, it is equally essential to be astute about the regulatory process. Regulations have a direct impact on a nurse's work and professional life. As changes in health care financing and delivery structures are driving changes in the current health care provider licensing system, many states are consider-

ing changes in the regulation of nursing, from amending the nurse practice act to accomplishing a major overhaul of the entire licensing system. Many of these changes will take place in the regulatory arena.

Though some regulations may be developed or amended without new legislation, other regulations fill out the details of new or amended laws. The development of such regulations takes months and sometimes years. It is this important step—the development of regulations—that may be overlooked by organized groups and individuals working to influence policy and the political process.

In 1995 legislation was introduced that reflected new efforts by Congress to limit federal regulations. This legislation proposed to change radically the procedures that federal agencies use to produce new regulations and to modify or revoke existing regulations that are determined to be unnecessary or overly burdensome. Proposals included detailed risk assessments and cost-benefit analyses before new rules could be imposed, retroactive reviews, and a period for Congress to block new regulations. These proposals raised concerns that regulatory overhaul would undermine health, safety, and environmental regulations already in place and delay the development of new regulations. The regulatory reform issue became a very real concern for nurses around the country as they realized that a major regulatory overhaul would severely limit the Occupational Safety and Health Administration and could repeal essential workplace standards—for example, the "bloodborne pathogens" regulations. To voice the concern of the nursing community, NSTAT, the ANA's grassroots network, was activated, and nurses responded by contacting their Senators and Representatives to urge a less radical approach to reform the regulatory process. The regulatory reform proposals of the 104th Congress were suspended after Senate Democrats and Republicans failed to reach a compromise on the details of these bills ("Senate Filibuster Derails Efforts . . .," 1995). Future Congressional debate and action is anticipated on regulatory reform because it is an issue that has generated bipartisan support and interest, especially in the business community.

Defining Government Regulations

A major role of government regulation is an interpretive one. As laws are passed by Congress and state legislatures, they rarely contain enough explicit language to guide their implementation completely. It is the responsibility of the administrative agencies to promulgate the rules and regulations that fill in the details of those laws. The health policy positions of the executive or legislative branch of government will determine the laws that are passed, but once enacted, laws and their accompanying regulations will shape the way health policy is translated into programs and services. Regulations may clarify definitions, authority, eligibility, benefits, and standards. Their development is shaped not only by the law but by the ongoing involvement and input of professional associations, providers, third-party payers, consumers, and other special interest groups.

The administrative agencies, usually part of the executive branch of government, may enact, enforce, and adjudicate their own rules and regulations, assuming functions of all three branches of government: legislative, executive, and judicial. Agencies are created through legislation that broadly defines their structure and function. They must develop their own regulations that set policy to govern the behavior of agency officials and regulated parties; spell out their procedural requirements, such as rules governing notices of intent, comment periods, and hearings; and develop enforcement procedures. For example, the Food and Drug Administration sets and monitors standards for food and tests drugs for purity, safety, and effectiveness, and the Environmental Protection Agency controls health risks from water-borne microbes in drinking water through the development and implementation of regulations.

The promulgation of regulations is guided by certain rules. Key among these at the federal level, with parallels in most of the states, is the requirement that the agency responsible for implementing a law publish a draft of a rule or set of rules in the *Federal Register.* The publication of proposed rules offers an opportunity to those with an interest in the rules and regulations applicable to implementing a particular policy to react to the draft rules before they become final. Commenting on draft rules is one of the most active points of involvement in the entire legislative process (Longest, 1997).

Regulation at the State Level

In Michigan an administrative department such as the Department of Community Health Services or the Department of Commerce is assigned the responsibility of developing the rules for a particular section of a law (*Administrative Rules,* 1997). For instance, a rule may specify what criteria must be met for someone to be considered a "qualified health professional," or, as recently happened, the Michigan Board of Nursing may propose rules changing licensure requirements for registered nurses in Michigan.

The Board of Nursing, after drafting new administrative rules requiring 25 hours of continuing education contact hours earned (during the two preceding years) for nursing relicensure, held a series of public hearings around the state, giving institutions, individual nurses, and nursing organizations, like the Michigan Nurses Association and the Michigan League for Nursing, an opportunity to present their views and comment on the proposed rules. During the hearings, much controversy was raised regarding the proposed rules and the requirements they would impose on all nurses in the state. Individual nurses, representatives from schools of nursing, and a number of nursing organizations and other interested groups presented testimony at the hearings. Many individual nurses wrote letters to the Michigan Board of Nursing and to their state legislators about the proposed rules. The Board of Nursing considered all the testimony received and subsequently revised the rules to accommodate many of the recommendations. The revised rules provided a variety of ways for nurses to meet the mandatory continuing education requirements ("Revised Rules for Licensure," 1995). The revised rules were then finalized by the Board of Nursing and sent to the Legislative Service Bureau for certification to ensure proper form, language, and classification and then on to the Office of Regulatory Affairs for certification to ensure that they satisfy all constitutional and legal standards. After certification by the Office of Regulatory Affairs, the revised rules were referred to the Joint Committee on Administrative Rules (JCAR), a legislative committee of five senators and five representatives, for final approval.

The JCAR held committee hearings on the rules, where interested parties and individual

HOW TO INFLUENCE LEGISLATIVE AND REGULATORY PROCESSES

- Become informed about the public policy and health policy issues that are currently under consideration at the local, state, and federal levels of government.
- Become acquainted with the public officials and elected officials that represent you in the legislative arena at the local, state, and federal levels of government. Communicate with them regularly to share your expertise and perspective on health care and nursing issues.
- Call, write, or send a fax or E-mail message to your legislator, stating briefly the position you wish him or her to take on a particular issue. Always remember to mention that you are a registered nurse and that you live and vote in the legislator's district.
- Request that legislation be introduced or a regulatory change made. Offer your expertise to assist in developing new legislation or in modifying existing legislation/rules.
- Become active in your professional association and work to activate a strong grassroots network of members who are prepared to contact their elected representatives on key health care issues.
- Attend a public hearing on a bill or regulation to show support for an issue, or actually testify yourself.
- Build your own political resumé—become active in local politics in your area.
- Volunteer to work on the campaigns of candidates who are knowledgeable and supportive of nursing's perspective on health care issues.
- Seek appointment to a government task force or commission and have the opportunity to make legislative, regulatory, and public policy changes.
- Seek election to public office or employment in an administrative or executive agency.
- Explore opportunities to be involved with the policy and legislative process through internships, fellowships, and volunteer experiences at the local, state, and federal levels.

nurses had additional opportunity to offer testimony. Members of the JCAR were lobbied by both supporters and opponents of the rules in their final format. When considering proposed rule changes, the JCAR may vote to approve or to disapprove proposed rules, or the committee members may ask the department to withdraw the rules and make specific changes. The JCAR itself cannot amend the rules. In the case of the continuing education rules, the JCAR voted to approve the rules as proposed by the Board of Nursing.

Once the JCAR passes rules, they are filed with the Secretary of State, Office of the Great Seal, and become official. The Board of Nursing rules took effect on March 31, 1997, for those seeking relicensure in 1999 ("Revised Rules . . .," 1995). In Michigan there is another way to pass administrative rules. In an emergency situation, Michigan has a constitutional provision allowing the Office of Regulatory Affairs, part of the executive branch of government, to pass rules without the approval of the JCAR (*Administrative Rules,* 1997).

CONCLUSION

By participating in the legislative and regulatory processes of government, nurses can improve access to and the delivery of health care services. They can also affect the practice of their profession in both state and federal programs. Understanding these processes is an important first step in being able to use them to the fullest extent.

REFERENCES

Administrative rules: Help. (1997). [On-line]. Available at: http://www.migov.statemi.us/rules/help#ruledef.

Browne, W. P., & Verburg, K. (1995). *Michigan politics and government: Facing change in a complex state.* Lincoln, NE: University of Nebraska Press.

Collender, S. E. (1991). *The guide to the federal budget.* Washington, DC: Urban Institute Press.

Congressional Quarterly's congress and the legislative process. (1993). Washington, DC: Congressional Quarterly.

Davidson, R. H., & Oleszek, W. J. (1996). *Congress and its members* (5th ed.). Washington, DC: Congressional Quarterly.

Health insurance reform enacted. (1996, August 30). *Capitol Update, 14*(16), 1–2.

Langdon, S. (1996a). Kennedy and Archer call truce: Insurance conference begins. *Congressional Quarterly Weekly Report, 54*(30), 2122–2123.

Langdon, S. (1996b). Kennedy, Kassebaum steer insurance bill to safety. *Congressional Quarterly Weekly Report, 54*(31), 2197–2200.

Legislative summary: Health insurance and accountability act. (1996, August 28). *Health Legislation and Regulation, 22*(35), 2–7.

Longest, B. B., Jr. (1997). *Seeking strategic advantage through health policy analysis.* Chicago: Health Administration Press.

Nather, D., & Darling, L. (1996, August 12). Clinton to sign health bill after Aug. 19: Final version drops drug patent measure. *BNA's Health Care Policy Report, 4*(33), 1289–1290.

Nursing's agenda for health care reform. (1991). Washington, DC: American Nurses Publishing.

Revised rules for licensure. (1995, September). *The Michigan Nurse, 68*(8), 11.

Senate filibuster derails efforts to limit federal regulations. (1995). *Congressional Quarterly Almanac,* 3–3. Washington, DC: Congressional Quarterly Press.

1995: A successful year for nurses. (1996, January). *The Michigan Nurse, 69*(1), 16.

Tri-Council for Nursing. (1996). *Funding recommendations for nursing education, nursing practice and nursing research* [Brochure]. Washington, DC: Author.

Chapter *23*

NURSING AND THE COURTS

VIRGINIA TROTTER BETTS AND DAVID KEEPNEWS

SHAPING POLICY BY A PROFESSION

One critical arena in which public policy is shaped is through the courts. The legal and judicial system is one through which the American people have traditionally sought vindication of their rights. Legislative initiatives and administrative regulations are often affirmed or invalidated through the courts. The details and circumstances under which employees can bargain collectively have often been matters of court rulings. Existing rights spelled out through statute, such as antitrust laws (which are designed to protect consumers from anticompetitive business practices) are enforced through the courts, as are professional scope-of-practice and licensing laws.

Court processes and judicial law are often thought of by nonlawyers as arcane, inaccessible, or highly technical areas better left to legal experts to address and understand. But just as nurses have learned that they can and must shape legislation and regulations that affect nursing, nurses can and must understand how judicial decisions also affect nursing practice and roles and how, especially through their professional associations, they can positively impact such legal decisions.

As activists interested in achieving particular policy outcomes, nurses need to consider their broadest set of alternatives in developing a plan for success in policy development and imple-

The views expressed in this chapter do not necessarily express the views of the Department of Health and Human Services of the United States.

mentation. Policy analysts, social activists, and legal scholars differ as to the effectiveness of using the judicial branch of government and its action instrument, the courts, to bring about social change. Nevertheless, the courts can be an appropriate arena for policy action by organized nursing and should be more widely considered and utilized.

ROLE OF THE COURTS IN SHAPING POLICY

The Judicial System: A Brief Overview

The United States has two major, parallel court systems—federal and state. The federal courts have jurisdiction over matters that involve the U.S. Constitution, federal legislation and regulation, and rights conferred under federal law. Federal courts can also hear complaints that arise between parties in different states if a significant monetary amount is in dispute. The trial courts for the federal system—which is the entry point for most federal cases—are district courts; there are 94 federal judicial courts located throughout the United States and its territories. Federal courts of appeals are organized into 11 circuits plus the District of Columbia Circuit Court and the Federal Circuit Court (Want, 1997). The U.S. Supreme Court is the court of last resort for federal cases.

Each state has its own court system, which generally interprets the laws of its state and the state constitution. State courts can also hear some claims that arise under federal law or the U.S. Constitution. Generally, the state court system includes trial-level and appellate courts, with a high court (usually the state supreme court) as the court of last resort. Often, trial courts are further subdivided on the basis of subject matter, amount in dispute, or another specific legal issue. On certain matters, decisions of a state supreme court may be appealed to the U.S. Supreme Court.

Evolution of the Courts

As the U.S. court system has evolved, there have been varied periods of judicial activism in shaping social policy for the nation. The first era of judicial activity (from 1776 through the 1930s) established the very principles that gave form to judicial influence. Judicial review—the power of the courts to determine acts of thelegislative and executive branches as valid or invalid—was established by the U.S. Supreme Court through its historic decision in *Marbury v. Madison* (1803). Judicial review has evolved into one of the most important powers belonging to the courts because it grants courts the power to make law by striking down other laws, thus exerting tremendous influence over governmental activities. Another doctrine that has increased the prominence of the courts as a force in social policy is the legal maxim of *stare decisis.* *Stare decisis*—"let the decision stand"—sets the course for judicial precedents by adhering to previous findings in cases with substantially comparable facts and situations (Filippatos, 1991). Prior decisions bind not only because they make good sense but also because they embody rules of law that make expectations of life and law predictable. Armed with these two weapons of influence, courts have increasingly become lawmakers rather than mere law interpreters.

As the legislative and executive branches of government slowly responded to public demands for social reform, the U.S. Supreme Courts of 1953 to 1968 and 1969 to 1986 extended the concept of individual liberties and civil rights. Their decisions found expanded rights in the Constitution and the Bill of Rights, including the right to enforce contractual rela-

tionships free from discrimination and the right to privacy in making health decisions.

The current Supreme Court (1987 to the present), seen as more conservative in its ideology than the prior two Courts, has disregarded some precedents and, in some ways, has narrowed the scope of the Bill of Rights (Chermerinsky, 1991). This translates into a narrowing of individual rights, giving rise to an increased necessity for activists to turn to legislators for protection of those rights or to develop new strategies for action. For example, when the Supreme Court declined to include disabled persons under the umbrella of existing civil rights statutes, Congress was lobbied heavily to enact the Americans With Disabilities Act in 1991.

Impact Litigation: Establishing Rights

A strong tradition, particularly in the past several decades, has been to utilize the courts to establish new rights or to provide clarification of existing rights under the Constitution or a particular statute. Litigation that seeks to have a broad social impact in this manner is often referred to as "impact" litigation. A particularly prominent example is *Brown v. Board of Education,* a 1954 case in which the U.S. Supreme Court struck down school segregation and mandated that states begin a process of desegregating their public schools. The Court found that segregated public school education constituted a state policy of inferior education for African American children and that it thus violated the Equal Protection Clause of the 14th Amendment to the U.S. Constitution.

Another example of utilizing the courts to establish social policy is *Roe v. Wade,* in which the U.S. Supreme Court in 1973 found that women had a right to the medical procedure of abortion during the first two trimesters of pregnancy. The Court made this ruling on the basis of its interpretation of various amendments to the Constitution that, it found, conferred a right of self-determination in seeking a medical procedure to terminate pregnancy. Though *Roe v. Wade* has been modified and narrowed in some respects by subsequent Supreme Court decisions, the basic right to choose abortion established by the Court in 1973 has remained intact.

In more recent years, another series of cases has focused on establishing rights in another area—the right to die. The courts have established the right of patients to refuse life-sustaining treatment. More recently, advocates of the right to die by suicide have sought to establish physician-assisted suicide as a legal option for terminally ill patients. These advocates have challenged existing state enforcement actions against physician-assisted suicide or pushed state-level initiatives to establish such a right, as in Oregon. In 1997 the U.S. Supreme Court ruled for the first time on the issue of physician-assisted suicide. It rendered a unanimous decision, finding that there is no constitutional right to assisted suicide. However, the justices offered three different opinions, which signaled a recognition that both the specific issue of assisted suicide, and the broader issue of care of the terminally ill, will continue to be the subject of debate and reflection throughout American society (*Washington v. Glucksberg,* 1997; *Vacco v. Quill,* 1997). The Court basically returned the issue to the states to determine policy on assisted suicide and reaffirmed the distinction between withdrawing life-sustaining treatment and providing active assistance in committing suicide. Justice Stephen Breyer, in his concurring opinion, suggested an approach to the question of assisted suicide that "would use words roughly like 'a right to die with dignity.'. . . [A]t its core would lie personal control over the manner of death, professional medical assistance, and the avoidance of severe physical suffering—combined" (Breyer, 1997).

Courts as Enforcers of Existing Legislation

The courts are commonly used as a means to enforce existing legislative and regulatory requirements and processes. For nurses, this means that the courts can be a source through which nurse practice acts or other relevant laws are enforced.

For example, in 1992, the Alabama State Nurses Association and the Alabama Board of Nursing—with the support of the American Nurses Association (ANA) and the Emergency Nurses Association—sued local hospitals that sought to place emergency medical technicians in the emergency department to provide nursing care. The nurses alleged that such assignment violated the Alabama Nurse Practice Act by allowing individuals to practice nursing without being appropriately educated and licensed. The nurse plaintiffs prevailed in the suit, and the hospitals were forced to end this practice.

In Oklahoma the state board of nursing, supported by the Oklahoma Nurses Association, sued a hospital over its practice of using unlicensed assistive personnel (UAP) to provide some technical aspects of nursing care. This private hospital had sought to utilize an exception to the state's nurse practice act that permitted UAP, under some circumstances, to provide care within public health programs; the hospital argued that, because it served indigent patients, including Medicaid recipients, it should fall within this exception. The Board of Nursing challenged the hospital. The board lost at trial, and the case went to appeal. ANA submitted an *amicus curiae* brief in support of the Board of Nursing. The appellate judge remanded the case back to the lower court, and the matter was subsequently settled before going to trial again. Thus, though this case produced a less definitive legal result than, for instance, the Alabama case discussed above, it does represent an example of the use of the courts to seek enforcement of the state nurse practice act.

Antitrust Laws

Federal and state antitrust laws are designed to protect consumers by prohibiting anticompetitive business practices. These laws have their roots in the turn of the century, when large and powerful businesses combined into alliances and agreed on prices, distribution, and other market-sensitive areas, effectively eliminating competition between them and eliminating newer companies from entering the market to the detriment of the consumer. Antitrust protections have been an area to which nurses and others have looked for relief from practices that block their full participation in the health care marketplace. Federal antitrust laws are enforced through two federal agencies, the Federal Trade Commission (FTC) and the Antitrust Division of the Department of Justice (DOJ). Individuals can also bring antitrust suit in federal court, although the cost of a private antitrust action can be extremely high. Several states have parallel antitrust laws, which are generally enforced through the offices of the state attorney general and through private lawsuits in state court.

Although for many years health professionals were essentially free from antitrust scrutiny under an exemption for "learned professions," the past two decades have seen increasing enforcement of and interest in antitrust laws as they apply to the health care industry. Courts have invalidated such practices as agreement by a county medical society to set fees for medical procedures *(Arizona v. Maricopa County Medical Society)*. Increased merger activity among hospitals, insurance companies, and health systems has brought scrutiny from antitrust enforcement agencies. In recent years, the DOJ and FTC have issued joint guidelines for antitrust enforcement in the health care industry, intended to offer general guidance on which practices are and are not likely to trigger action by these enforcement agencies (U.S. Department of Justice and Federal Trade Commission Statement of Antitrust Enforcement Policy in Healthcare, 1996).

One case in which nurses brought an antitrust action to confront anticompetitive business practices involved a group of certified nurse midwives in Tennessee. In 1980 these nurse midwives were forced to close their newly opened family-centered nursing practice and midwifery services after meeting the concerted resistance of several Tennessee physicians, hospitals, and a prominent physician insurance company. The nurse midwives were barred from receiving hospital privileges, physician supervision, and an opportunity for collaborative practice. After 9 years from closure of their practice and extensive litigation, the nurse midwives won settlements against some but not all of the defendants *(Nurse Midwifery Associates v. Hibbett et al., 1990)*.

Liability (Torts, Product Liability) as a Means to Effect Social Change

Another area of the law that presents nurses with a means to effect change is the tort system. Tort law (laws through which individuals and corporations are held financially accountable for acts or omissions that cause injury to others) is often what nurses think of first when the subject of "legal issues in nursing" is raised. Indeed, one aspect of tort law includes professional malpractice issues. But this area is broad, and nurses can often use it to address problems and issues that affect them and their practice.

For instance, health care workers have at times successfully sued their employers for failure to take reasonable measures to protect employee health and safety—such as failure to provide reasonable security measures, which resulted in injury to health care workers, or failure to switch to needleless systems, resulting in nurses' becoming infected with human immunodeficiency virus or hepatitis B virus from needle sticks. The impact of such legal actions has implications beyond any individual plaintiff because other employers may be influenced to take measures to provide protection for employees to avoid potential future liability.

Antitobacco advocates have also made much use of tort and product liability law. Through both individual lawsuits and class actions *(see below)*, opponents of tobacco as a consumer product have sought to hold that industry accountable for illnesses and deaths caused by tobacco use. These legal efforts have also helped publicize important and previously undisclosed information about the industry and its practices and about the health outcomes of tobacco use, adding ammunition to both legal and political efforts to limit access to tobacco.

Class Action Suits

Class action suits have been another means through which advocates have sought to make an impact on health, safety, and social justice issues. Such suits seek to vindicate the rights of an entire class of individuals who share a common interest that gives rise to the suit and who seek a common outcome. Generally, such suits are brought on behalf of a large group by a smaller number of class representatives. Class action suits have been brought on behalf of recipients of silicone breast implants, of citizens of a geographical area who have suffered ill effects from the dumping of toxic wastes, of female employees of a public university system who have suffered wage discrimination, and of airline flight attendants who have been injured by secondhand smoke.

Challenging Inappropriate Government Action

The U.S. Constitution and state constitutions offer citizens and residents a number of protections, including protection from unreasonable government action in a number of areas. For instance, the government cannot take an individual's property or liberty without due process. Individuals are free from unreasonable searches and seizures. All individuals are guaranteed equal protection under the law. These guarantees have been made more specific as they apply to the actions of government agencies through a federal Administrative Procedures Act and similar acts at the state level that define the processes for and restrictions on administrative action. In addition, administrative agencies are generally limited to acting within the parameters set for them by legislation.

Together, these constitutional and legislative protections provide a basis for challenging inappropriate or unreasonable government action—or, perhaps more accurately, action by a government agency that an individual or group believes or alleges to be inappropriate or unreasonable. For instance, in 1987, when the National Labor Relations Board (NLRB) set out seven specific bargaining units within the health care industry (including one unit composed only of registered nurses), the American Hospital Association challenged the rules in federal court by charging that it was beyond the NLRB's authority to issue them (*American Hospital Association v. NLRB,* 1991). That challenge eventually went to the U.S. Supreme Court, which upheld the NLRB's authority and the health industry's bargaining rules themselves.

In 1988 a coalition of providers challenged rules by the U.S. Department of Health and Human Services that would have prohibited providers in federally funded family planning clinics from discussing abortion as an option for pregnant clients or from offering such clients referral to an agency that performs abortions (Regulations on Title X–Funded Family Planning Projects Issued to Regional Health Administrators of the U.S. Department of Health and Human Services, February 1988). Although the challenge to these rules continued, the issue was resolved on the second day of President Clinton's first term in 1993 when the president signed an Executive Order removing these gag rules.

ACTING "DEFENSIVELY"

Though court decisions can have a positive impact on issues that concern nurses and other health care advocates, they can also have an adverse impact. Nursing is sometimes faced with trying to react to, address, and mitigate the impact of a negative court decision. Probably the most prominent recent example of such a decision is the U.S. Supreme Court's decision in *NLRB v. Health Care and Retirement Corp.* (1994) (see Chapter 19). In that case the Supreme Court invalidated the NLRB's rationale for finding that nurses were not "supervisors" under the National Labor Relations Act simply because they directed the work of others. A finding that a nurse is a "supervisor" under the Act would mean that she is exempt from the collective bargaining rights conferred by that Act. *Health Care and Retirement Corp.* specifically concerned licensed practical nurses who directed the work of nurse's aides; however, the implications of the decision applied to registered nurses (RNs) as well. In this case the NLRB had ruled, as it had ruled in similar cases, that the nurses involved directed the work of others, not "in the interests of the employer" (as the National Labor Relations Act requires as part of its definition of a supervisor), but "in the interests of the patient." The Supreme Court rejected this distinction and held that it could not be used by the NLRB as a basis to find that nurses who direct the work of others are not supervisors.

The decision understandably caused a great deal of concern among nurses because it eliminated the reasoning by which the NLRB had found most nurses to be eligible for collective bargaining. Because supervisors (as defined by the National Labor Relations Act) do not have the right to bargain collectively, the potential implications of the decision jeopardized the collective bargaining rights of many, if not most, RNs.

Since the time of the decision, however, the ANA has worked to mitigate its impact. It has challenged employers' efforts to claim that large numbers of nurses are ineligible for collective bargaining and has supported the NLRB in its decision to find alternative approaches to ruling that directing the work of others in providing patient care does not make RNs ineligible for collective bargaining. Nurses in Montana, at Bozeman Deaconess Hospital, won a big victory when the NLRB issued a decision finding that the hospital had committed unfair labor practices and ordered it to bargain with the Montana Nurses Association (MNA) (*Bozeman Deaconess Hospital* [322 NLRB No. 196], 1997). Bozeman Deaconess Hospital withdrew its recognition and refused to bargain with MNA, claiming that all the RNs were supervisors and not covered under the National Labor Relations Act. The hospital argued that it was the day-to-day responsibilities of *all* RNs that warranted their designation as supervisors.

The NLRB found that the hospital had committed unfair labor practices and ordered Bozeman to recognize and bargain with MNA. The NLRB concluded that the responsibility of the RNs to assign and direct other employees does not require independent judgment but is routine. The NLRB recognized that the "RNs' status as professional employees carries with it responsibility for making expert judgement in assessing the conditions and needs of the patient." However, "having made those determinations, the RNs' additional responsibility for directing employees to perform the appropriate tasks to care for the patient in a routine manner," which successfully resisted an employer's claim that all RNs were "supervisors" and thus ineligible for collective bargaining. At Providence Hospital in Anchorage, Alaska, nurses opposed the hospital's refusal to bargain with the Alaska Nurses Association (*Providence Hospital v. NLRB,* 1997). The hospital claimed that the bargaining unit was not appropriate because it contained charge nurses and others whom they claimed were "supervisors." The NLRB found in the nurses' favor, in agreement with the ANA. The U.S. Court of Appeals for the Ninth Circuit ruled two to one (upholding the February 1996 decision by the NLRB) that charge nurses at Providence Alaska Medical Center in Anchorage are not supervisors and therefore are eligible for collective bargaining.

THE ROLE OF *AMICUS CURIAE*

Amicus curiae (friend of the court) briefs provide an important tool for advocacy groups to make their views known on a case with broad implications even when they are not parties to that case. An *amicus curiae* brief is filed (with the court's permission) by a group with an interest in the case in order to advise the court on how it should rule; generally it offers the court a group's unique knowledge of and perspective on the issue before it.

Nursing has used this avenue to make its policy preferences and professional viewpoints known in appellate-level federal and state cases throughout the country. In *NLRB v. Health and Retirement Corp.*, discussed above, ANA filed an amicus brief with the U.S. Supreme Court in order to offer its unique perspective as the nation's largest professional and labor organization for registered nurses in explaining why direction and oversight of ancillary personnel is an integral aspect of nursing practice and not a "supervisory" function. More recently, ANA joined with the American Medical Association and other nursing and physician groups to offer the perspective of health care providers regarding physician-assisted suicide by filing a joint *amicus curiae* brief in *Washington v. Glucksberg* and *Vacco v. Quill.* The ANA has also made its voice heard in cases regarding appropriate bargaining units for hospital employees; the right of publicly employed nurses to speak out on the job regarding safe patient care; and the right of Medicare recipients enrolled in HMOs to receive adequate services and procedural protections (*Grijalva et al. v. Shalala* [966 F. Supp. 747; D. Ariz. 1996]). The ANA has also addressed criminal prosecution of pregnant women for drug or alcohol abuse (*Whitner v. South Carolina* [22 Fam. L. Rep 1427; S.C. 1996]) and the issue of what constitutes a "serious health condition" under the Family and Medical Leave Act (*Victorelli v. Shadyside Hospital* [decision pending]). The *amicus curiae* brief is a particularly useful and attractive option for nurses to use in speaking out on important legal issues that affect the profession or on those for which the profession has important concerns, even where they are not party to the action itself.

PROPOSING LEGISLATION TO ESTABLISH LEGAL RIGHTS

Because Congress and the state legislatures are sources of (respectively) federal and state law, legislative authority provides the foundation for future legal action. In other words, laws passed at the federal or state levels create legally enforceable rights that, when necessary for implementation, can be actionable through the courts. For instance, the Americans With Disabilities Act (ADA) provides for equal treatment for disabled Americans and bars discrimination in a number of areas, including employment and public accommodations. For example, a person with a disability who is able to perform the essential aspects of a job with reasonable accommodation cannot be fired or denied a promotion on the basis of her or his disability. Though many would argue that the ADA merely applies principles of equality and fair play that are basic to principles of American law and public life, it also creates specific actionable rights through a specific statutory scheme. Similarly, the Family and Medical Leave Act (FMLA) grants specific rights for employees to take unpaid leave under certain circumstances in order to receive or provide care to a family member (see Chapter 10). The FMLA, signed into law by President Clinton after being vetoed previously by President Bush, was strongly supported by ANA. The Act defines a number of new and important parameters for families' rights.

Another example of proposing and passing legislation granting a right is the Boren Amendment. Through the Boren Amendment, Congress gave providers of Medicaid services a right to receive payment at a level comparable to that paid by private insurers. As a result of the Boren Amendment, many health care institutions have sued their state Medicaid programs in order to force them to pay higher rates. (Many state governments objected to the obligation imposed on them by this law, and repeal of the Boren Amendment—an objective of the National Governors Association and others who seek to turn greater control of the Medicaid program over to the states—was achieved with the enactment of P.L. 105-33, the 1997 budget bill. What effect this repeal will have on Medicaid reimbursement rates remains to be seen.)

Using a similar strategy in 1996, New York nurses developed and supported state legislation to grant professional licensing boards the power to seek judicial interventions to prevent the unauthorized practice of a profession. For instance, under rights granted by this proposed legislation, the board of nursing would have been able to seek to stop the use of UAP, who would then be practicing nursing without a license. This legislation would have given nurses a significant tool to use in preventing the dangerous, inappropriate use of UAP by health care institutions. Unfortunately, the bill, passed by the state legislature, was vetoed by New York's governor.

PROMOTING NURSING'S POLICY AGENDA

Health care is experiencing rapid and chaotic change in which the rules of the game are being developed more in closed corporate boardrooms than in the halls and auditoriums of public policy assemblies. Thus nursing needs a greater range of effective strategies to achieve its preferred outcomes. Organized nursing must become comfortable, proficient, and well prepared to be successful in all policy arenas and at all levels of government.

Understanding litigation as a winning strategy, enhanced risk-taking skills, and sufficient resource building for expensive litigation must be developed by organized nursing on a proactive basis. Nowhere may this become more important than at the state and local levels, where here-and-now issues of material interest ripe for litigation and judicial decision will occur that may affect the whole of nursing or all health care consumers. In addition to many of the current nursing/litigation issues heretofore mentioned, nurses must prepare to address effectively a variety of evolving professional concerns such as managed care panel development, private insurer reimbursement, enforcement of the Nurse Practice Act in ways that expand and protect nursing practice, and achieving the right of nurses to form professional corporations. Using the courts and the judicial process may be the action of choice for resolving each of these concerns with a "nurse friendly" solution.

Organized nursing, at the national, state, and local levels, must prepare nurses to evaluate issues and opportunities to promote health and social policy though the judicial system. When achieving nursing's policy objectives is likely to be best accomplished through the courts, nursing must be ready, willing, and able to play and win in that arena of government.

ACKNOWLEDGMENTS: We wish to thank Linda L. Minich for her invaluable research and support in the preparation of this chapter.

REFERENCES

Alabama Nurses Association, Alabama State Board of Nursing, et al., v. Samuelson and the Alabama State Department of Public Health. (1992). Case Nos. CV-92-2275 and CV-92-2477.

American Hospital v. NLRB. (1991). U.S., 111 S. Ct. 1539.

Arizona v. Maricopa County Medical Society. (1982). 457 U.S. 332.

Breyer, S., concurring opinion in *Washington v. Glucksberg,* U.S. Supreme Court, No. 96-110.

Brown v. Board of Education. (1954). 347 US 483.

Chermerinsky, E. (1991, June 16). Rehnquist's court: Activism from the right, *Courier Journal,* D1-4.

Filippatos, P. (1991). Doctrine of *stare decisis* and the protection of civil rights and liberties in the Rehnquist court. *Boston College Third World Journal,* 335–377.

Marbury v. Madison. (1803). I Cranch 137.

NLRB v. Health and Retirement Corp. (1994). 114 S. Ct. 1778.

Nurse Midwifery Associates v. Hibbett et al. (1990). 918 F. 2d 605 (6th Cir.).

Roe v. Wade. (1973). 410 US 113.

Vacco v. Quill. (1997). U.S. Supreme Court, No. 95-1958 (117 S. Ct. 2293, 65 U.S.L.W. 4695 [June 26, 1997]).

Want, R. (Ed.). (1997). *Federal-state court directory.* New York: Want Publishing.

Washington v. Glucksberg. (1997). U.S. Supreme Court, No. 96-110 (177 S. Ct. 2258, 65 U.S.L.W. 4669 [June 26, 1997]).

Chapter *24*

LOCAL GOVERNMENT

JUANITA V. MAJEWSKI AND MARJORY C. O'BRIEN

El Paso, Texas: *Hospitals Serving the Poor Struggle to Retain Patients*
— *The New York Times,* September 3, 1997

New York City: *New York's Law on Lead Paint Removal Compromises Safety*
— *The New York Times,* December 20, 1995

New York City: *One Creature's Free Meal Is Another's Death Knell: A Devious Plan to Eliminate Lyme Disease*
— *The New York Times,* July 29, 1997

New York State: *Chautauqua County Offering Variety of Programs for Pregnant Teens*
— *Dunkirk Observer,* April 20, 1994

New York State: *Broome County Radon Risk Among State's Highest: Higher Exposure to Gas Can Cause Lung Cancer* — *Binghamton Press & Sun Bulletin,* July 28, 1997

Commonly filed under Health Issues, these headlines represent a growing concern for local governments. How are local governments structured and what are their responsibilities for health care?

Increasing media attention on national and state governments and their relationships with big business and special interests has heightened citizens' interest in and understanding of these levels of government. Taking local governments largely for granted, we tend to know more about these higher levels than we do about our own local governments—the counties, cities, towns, villages, and school districts in which we reside. Localities, however, have great authority over many aspects of our daily lives. Nurses who understand the structure and function of local governments can participate in and influence decisions that affect not only their immediate community but also the larger society.

IMPORTANCE OF LOCAL GOVERNMENT

Local government is the vital link between citizens and the state or nation. Providing services and carrying out policies prescribed by state and national government, local governments distribute billions of local, state, and federal dollars to community agencies. In their role as administrative agents, cities and counties often have the authority to modify application of centrally determined policies because of different social, economic, and cultural patterns of localities.

The obligations of local government grow continually in scope and importance. Public education, public health, potable water supply, sewage disposal, police protection, solid waste management, and recreation are among the services provided principally by local governments. The quality of life in a community is directly affected by decisions about these services.

Localities, those government units closest to popular control, are profoundly influenced by their constituency. Citizen pressure often results in changes in local policy and may ultimately affect state or national policy. Issues that are common to many municipalities become increasingly significant and pass from local to higher-level governments for action. They become state or national concerns not because they are statewide or national in nature but because growing local concerns demand response on state and national levels.

The impact of the devolution of responsibility from the federal government to state governments and, ultimately, to local governments can be seen in the growing concern over the loss of federal and state funds for uncompensated care provided by community-supported public hospitals. Through the years a system of "safety nets" had been developed to transfer revenues from the federal and state governments, and from private-pay and third-party reimbursement, to public hospitals to compensate for what in 1995 amounted to $17.5 billion—6% of hospital expenses—in uncompensated-care costs (Mann, Melnick, Bamezai, & Zwanziger, 1997).

According to one study uncompensated care is primarily concentrated in southern states with many tax-supported small public hospitals and relatively restrictive Medicaid programs (Fishman, 1997). However, uncompensated care is an issue for many large urban areas, as well. In El Paso, Texas, and elsewhere, the competition for Medicaid patients by private providers who increasingly see Medicaid reimbursement rates as comparable to managed-care or capitation rates, has led to a severe decline in revenues available for public hospitals. Yet it is these hospitals that continue to provide for the bulk of uninsured people seeking both routine and emergency health care.

> But public hospitals do more than just care for the uninsured. They also protect community health overall, offering important but money-losing services like trauma centers and burn units, treating public health threats like AIDS or drug-resistant tuberculosis, and creating outreach programs for high-risk pregnancies, violence prevention or immigrant health. [Lewin, 1997, p. A1]

FORMS OF LOCAL GOVERNMENT

There is wide variation in the number, size, and type of local governments throughout the nation, but a fairly common format does exist.

The structures and responsibilities of local governments have undergone continual growth and change, but present-day forms of government essentially reflect colonial models established by the original settlers. Counties and townships, created by the states to administer basic state functions within geographic subdivisions, are often described as involuntary units. As counties grew, additional duties and powers were delegated. In contrast, cities and villages are described as voluntary units created by the state at the request of the residents to meet particular needs.

Our system of local governments is complex, not only because of the varied models that evolved, but also because of enormous differences in population, wealth, geography, climate, and cultural influences. The pattern and functions of localities is further complicated by overlapping authority of units, particularly in large urban centers. There is no commonly accepted definition of a local government; in practical use the term simply refers to a particular local community. The U.S. Census Bureau, however, has developed detailed criteria that a unit must meet to qualify as a local government body. These criteria are categorized into four major types: counties, municipalities, towns and townships, and special districts.

County Government

Generally, counties are the largest local governments in most states, although these units are called parishes in Louisiana and boroughs in Alaska. The number of counties varies widely among states; however, there is no relationship between the number of counties and the population or size of the state—Connecticut and Rhode Island have no counties.

Early duties of the counties were few and practical: to provide citizen protection and to maintain law and order. To ensure reliable travel to county jails and courthouses, counties additionally became responsible for the construction and maintenance of roads. Today, counties administer a vast array of additional services: health, social services, election law, sanitation, and parks and recreation. Services that are outside the jurisdiction of the county governing body are administered by "row officers," who are separately elected. These may include sheriffs, prosecuting attorneys, county clerks, treasurers, coroners, and judges. County governments vary in form: the elected board or commission, the board of supervisors, the county executive or county manager, and the mixed county board.

ELECTED BOARD OR COMMISSION

The most prevalent form of county government, this body performs both executive and legislative duties. Members might oversee services jointly or separately as heads of departments. Some boards focus strictly on policy development and appoint managers to run departments. In some states, members are elected from geographic districts apportioned according to population, whereas in other states all members are elected at large.

BOARD OF SUPERVISORS

This is the oldest form of county government and, despite functional disadvantages, continues to be fairly prevalent. The board is composed of supervisors who are elected as town officers in town elections and who serve collectively to manage the county's executive and legislative functions.

COUNTY EXECUTIVE OR COUNTY MANAGER

Most often found in urban areas, this form of government has an elected board that is responsible for policy and legislation. In addition, there is either an elected executive with broad executive power or a board-appointed manager, with no independent authority, who is responsible for administrative functions and is accountable to the board.

MIXED COUNTY BOARD

These boards are most common in southern states. Elected judges and county representatives perform executive and legislative duties. The judges officiate in judicial capacities in addition to their normal governing roles.

Municipalities

Municipalities exist in all 50 states and are called by many names including cities, boroughs, and villages. Functionally, municipalities carry out some functions as instruments of the state and perform some operations to benefit primarily their own residents. Although they are less inclusive of territory than counties, many municipalities exercise more power and provide more services than do county governments. The powers are defined by state charters and statutes to spell out the differences between villages and cities. Four basic forms of municipal government have evolved: mayor-council, commission, council-manager, and mayor-manager.

MAYOR-COUNCIL

This form of municipal government is the most common and can exist in two different ways: weak mayor-council or strong mayor-council. The weak-mayor system is the oldest form of local government, and nearly every municipality functioned under this plan into the nineteenth century. The council, elected either by district or at large, has both executive and legislative powers. The mayor, also a member of the council, may be elected directly by the voters or selected by fellow council members. Under this form, power is fragmented. Authority over administrative and appointive decisions is held by the council, and the mayor has limited or no veto power. This form remains in many municipalities today, especially in villages and smaller cities.

Rapid urban expansion in the nineteenth century frequently paralyzed the decision-making process of the weak mayor-council system as disputes arose over priorities. Failure of councils to act and the power void in the office of mayor gave rise to the political machine and its boss, able to provide a variety of needed services in return for votes. Reforms led to the development of the strong-mayor plan, in which the mayor, elected by the voters, is the chief executive and administrative head and the council is the policymaking body. Most contemporary large cities and some medium-sized cities employ this form.

COMMISSION

This model gained wide popularity after its adoption by Galveston, Texas, in 1901. The corrupt incumbent government, unable to handle the crisis that followed a destructive tidal wave, was suspended by the state legislature and replaced by a five-member commission. All executive and legislative authority was vested in the commission, with each member responsible for administering a different department; one member was designated as mayor but had little additional power. Several variations of the commission plan evolved, but, like the weak mayor-council model, the absence of checks and balances hampers decision making and action when serious disputes arise among commission members. Many cities subsequently reverted to strong mayor-council government or the newer council-manager plan. Despite the drawbacks, some small to medium-sized cities still use some form of commission government, with Miami, Florida, among them.

COUNCIL-MANAGER

Another solution to inefficient government, the council-manager form models private business and relies on an appointed professional manager for administrative control. The elected council sets broad policy, and the position of mayor, if it exists, may be filled by one of the council members or be elected by the people. In most cases the mayor is relegated to a minor role and functions in a ceremonial capacity.

This form gained great momentum after it was adopted in Dayton, Ohio, in 1912 after a destructive flood. It is prevalent in municipalities with populations of 10,000 to 200,000 people but also occurs in larger cities, including Dallas, Phoenix, and San Diego. The arrangement is attractive to those who seek to eliminate the politics of city administration by vesting authority in qualified professionals. However, managers may be subject to pressures from current or potential council members, on whom continued employment depends.

MAYOR-MANAGER

The newest improvement in city government, this form provides a strong system of checks and balances. The elected mayor appoints a chief administrator and concentrates on executive duties of budget preparation, appointments, and certain veto powers over council actions. The council retains policymaking power.

Towns and Townships

The term *town* is used informally to refer to communities large or small in rural or suburban areas. In a formal application of the term, however, town government is that which originated and still exists in some New England states. When this country was developing, New England settlements refused to be governed by royal charters, as were other, urbanized areas of the colonies. Fiercely independent, the settlements established town meetings at which all in attendance voted to enact laws, levy taxes, appoint officials, and make other administrative decisions. The number and kinds of issues voted on directly at modern town meetings have been greatly reduced, but towns tend to have a larger number of elective offices. Rural areas, known as plantations in Maine and locations in New Hampshire, are included in the use of this term.

Townships may be rural in nature and function, being simply organized and supplying few services. Urban townships are adjacent to highly urbanized areas and may have populations greater than those of some small cities. They are granted more self-governance and are increasingly becoming units of urban government.

Towns and townships, like villages and counties, have a variety of elected officials with specific administrative responsibilities: clerk, receiver of taxes, assessors, judges, and superintendent of highways. Except for the level of participation, townships operate like municipalities, providing similar types of services and retaining revenue-raising authority. In general, there is no separate executive branch. The town board or council is composed of a supervisor and members elected at large and is similar to the weak mayor-council structure. As administrator and chief financial officer, the supervisor is responsible for day-to-day operations but has no veto power or independent authority for policy.

Special Districts

Special districts, which provide a variety of single or limited services, are the most numerous of local governments and exist in all states but Alaska. School districts whose budgets are not part of a municipal budget are the most predominant of the special districts and those with which most people are familiar. They are properly regarded as governmental units with the power to tax, borrow, and spend public funds for a specific service. Budgets, policy, programs, and appointments are the responsibility of an elected board of local citizens who serve without salary. The superintendent of schools attends meetings and works with the board. In some communities, positions on the school board are viewed as prestigious or powerful, and races for a seat on the board generate a good deal of competition, controversy, or both. In addition, greater interest is shown in these positions in recent years because of the desire of parents or other interest groups to control policy, curriculum development, and budget expenditures.

Other major types of special service districts are fire protection, water supply, and soil conservation. They, too, have power to tax, borrow, and spend public funds and are governed by boards whose elected or appointed members are called commissioners. These districts are not always recognized by citizens as units of government, and people may take note of them only when the assessment appears on their tax notices.

Demand for greater numbers and varieties of services continues as new suburban areas develop and special districts proliferate to meet the needs and wants of a community. Only those who reside within the boundaries of a specific district can be taxed for that service. Districts can be very parochial, serving very few, or so broad that portions of, or entire, local governments may be involved. For example, citizens in heavily populated subdivisions within a rural area may request sidewalks or street lighting. If the majority of property owners agree, these amenities are installed and only those who derive the benefit are taxed. Sewer districts are an example of more expansive special districts, which may require the cooperation and participation of towns, villages, and counties. A public hospital district often serves at least one city and the surrounding rural area.

LOCAL GOVERNMENT RESPONSIBILITY FOR HEALTH CARE

The provision of health care services is often overlooked in an examination of the responsibilities of local government. The federal government is recognized as the entity responsible for setting broad health policies and for funding research into disease prevention and protection from environmental hazards. State government provides many of the same health functions as the federal government and also acts to implement state and federal policies.

Public health services, which began in response to epidemics and the need to control the spread of disease through isolation and quarantine and later through sanitation, were well established as state responsibilities by the end of the nineteenth century. The first public health agency in the country, however, was the New York City Department of Health, which was established in 1866 in recognition of the need to ensure public health and the protection of its large and growing population as a societal responsibility (National Institute of Medicine, 1988).

The growth and influence of state health departments, and later their local county public health offices, have kept pace with the expansion of knowledge about disease transmission and the impact of the environment on the health of individuals and society. Sanitation and immunization responsibilities expanded into clinical care and health education. Contemporary public health issues such as acquired immunodeficiency syndrome (AIDS), access to health care for the indigent, injuries, teen pregnancy, control of high blood pressure, smoking, drug and alcohol abuse, toxic substances, and Alzheimer's disease are debated at the national and state levels, but it is most often at the local government level that policies are implemented and action occurs.

Local government, particularly at the state and county level, is also responsible for other health-related services such as those provided by the county coroner or medical examiner, state and county laboratories, offices for the aging and long-term health care facilities. Perhaps most important is the local government's provision of health and mental health services through public hospitals and clinics.

Much of the discussion about access to health care focuses on financial barriers. As state and federal government policies move toward greater reliance on block grants and capitation as ways of reducing government funding and excessive regulatory control, this discussion will intensify. Though the 1996 federal welfare reform bill, the Personal Responsibility and Work Opportunity Reconciliation Act, did not convert Medicaid into block grants, it did eliminate the link between cash assistance under the Aid for Dependent Children program and Medicaid eligibility, making it more difficult for this population to gain access to needed services. Nonfinancial barriers, including geographic isolation and lack of transportation, shortage or lack of health care providers, legal restrictions on access to service, and a growing lack of individual awareness of the importance of preventive health care, are becoming an even more important focus of local government. Children, adolescents, and women needing family planning or obstetrical services are seen as particularly vulnerable to these barriers (Klerman, 1992). The solution proposed by many is expansion of school-based health care. What other institution, they ask, is so universally accessible (Goldsmith, 1991)?

School districts are a form of local government with the power, as noted earlier, to tax, borrow, and spend public funds to provide a community service. They are also policymaking institutions and are subject to requirements of both state and federal governments. Most states require schools to provide periodic health examinations, specific screening services, health assessments, health referrals, and immunization compliance. Federal government requirements for school health services is included in the Individuals With Disabilities Act, originally the Education for All Handicapped Children Act of 1975 (P.L. 94-142), which requires schools to guarantee a free, appropriate, public education in the least restrictive environment to all students regardless of their disability. This has often been judged to include provision of health and social services limited only by the needs of the student.

School-based health clinics operate under a variety of models, from limited in-house services provided by the school nurse to affiliation with a university hospital or a health maintenance organization. These school-based clinics rely on knowledge of the local community, which may indicate a need to provide other services, from health education to mental health screening and prenatal services to pregnant teenagers.

Nurses remain the primary caregivers in all school-based programs. In many cases, they are also the initiators of expanded services through their interaction with students and their awareness of community problems. Nurses serve as community health educators, as coordinators of health and social services, and as advocates for the needs of the community. They serve as the early warning system for environmental hazards like lead poisoning and as statisticians alert to the ever-changing patterns of youth behavior and its impact on a healthy society.

TRENDS IN LOCAL GOVERNMENT

The many forms of local government are, or should be, engaging in self-scrutiny and strategic planning. Duplication and overlapping of services by different levels of government, which are contiguous or geographically inclusive, create fiscal burdens for localities and become increasingly difficult to sustain. Sharp declines in federal assistance, and the elimination in 1986 of revenue sharing, contributed to budget shortfalls for many jurisdictions. The ability of states to allocate additional resources to localities is limited. In addition, some contemporary governors propose sharp reductions in state aid to force local solutions paid for with local resources.

During the 1980s and 1990s, many regions of the country experienced unprecedented economic growth, while, at the same time, some large cities were faced with loss of viable economic bases. Some of those localities have been on the cutting edge of developing strategies to address the impact of business/industry relocation and major population shifts.

Changes already taking place in our society require reevaluation of the scale and mix of services as well as how they will be financed. Various solutions and concepts are being promoted by elected and appointed officials, planners, government analysts, economists, and other experts. Based in large part on economies of scale, these proposals are introduced under a variety of names and designs—consolidation of services, regionalism, metropolitan government, city-states, and government mergers being among the most common. All plans share a common goal: to make governments more efficient and cost-effective and to promote economic revitalization. Resistance to such proposals is not uncommon: neither citizens nor those who hold power want to lose local autonomy.

Some plans are fairly simple, such as a regional planning agency to forge consensus among communities to provide maintenance of roads and highways that pass through many different localities. Other plans are emotionally volatile, as in mergers of city police precincts or of sheriff and local departments where one jurisdiction lies within another. Residents fear losing protection, and departmental personnel fear loss of jobs. Mergers of public hospitals generate

similar fears, especially when the loss of small local hospitals limits access by underserved populations.

At the other extreme is the vision of collaborative networks of local governments such as those configured in Indianapolis, Indiana; Baltimore, Maryland; Minneapolis–St. Paul, Minnesota; Charlotte-Mecklenburg, North Carolina; and Dallas–Fort Worth, Texas. Common themes in these metropolitan regions include strategies to address education reform, poor and underserviced populations, environmentally sensitive land use, and the health and housing needs of our aging population. For example, in Charlotte-Mecklenburg during the 1980s, many firms began to relocate to the area, creating an expanding regional economy. Growth provided many opportunities but began to threaten those very qualities that attracted growth: livability of the area and economic vitality. Eight critical issues—growth assumptions, environment, public services and facilities, development, neighborhoods, citizen involvement, urban design, and local government—were identified in strategic planning that involved business, neighborhood leaders, developers, and civic leaders. The resulting "2005 Plan" is a long-range land use plan that incorporates the vision of providing opportunity for economic mobility for all segments of the population (Kemp, 1993).

In the 1980s, civic and political leaders in Indianapolis, Indiana, determined to make Indianapolis a "city of distinction," and today that city is a strong, united community that operates under its "uni-government" system. Most of Indianapolis and Marion County government functions have been consolidated and are managed by a local legislative body responsible for policy and budgeting for all city-county units. The mayor administers through a strong "cabinet" relationship and literally speaks for the community in all competitive relationships. Under this system, cost savings have not been significant, but this was not a primary goal. It is agreed, however, that the intent to operate efficiently and effectively has been realized (Pierce, 1993).

Today, as in the past, restructuring local government might be the answer to ensuring basic needs. New organizational forces and greater interdependence among the various levels of government are promoted by public officials, economists, and planners. Some experts who believe there are too many local government units have long advocated such action. The various models of consolidated governments or shared services that exist in such metropolitan areas as Dallas–Fort Worth, Texas, which incorporates two cities, and Charlotte-Mecklenburg, a city-county planning approach, appear at the present time to be thriving and successful.

INFLUENCING LOCAL GOVERNMENT

As nurses comprise the largest group of health care providers, we recognize our responsibility to speak out and act on behalf of those to whom we deliver care. We have developed skills and organized our numbers to achieve lobbying successes at state and national levels of government. Like the public in general, however, we have not always recognized the power of local governments and the important role those levels have in shaping public policy.

The growing number of services provided by local governments and the changes taking place in federal-state-local relationships require that we turn our attention to working with and within local governments. The opportunity to have an impact on local government decisions is, in fact, much greater than in the state and federal governments (which tend to be more complex and distant). Access to officials is easier simply by virtue of geography, and, more important, these officials may well be neighbors, members of our religious communities or clubs, professional colleagues, or co-workers in a volunteer school or community project.

Gathering Information

To be effective in influencing local government, one must first have a good understanding of how local systems operate. The form of government determines in large measure who wields power and in what context that power is exercised.

Attending meetings of the city council, town or village board, or county legislature is one way to learn not only how that governmental body works but also what the current issues are. Meetings of local planning boards, zoning boards, and school boards are open meetings. Minutes of these meetings are public record and are available at the municipal hall; public libraries often have a copy of the community boards' proceedings.

Knowledge of the political climate and the power brokers is important. Some localities, because of perceived stability or benign neglect, see little competition for elected office and have long-term incumbents. This occurs most in small, long-established communities with little change in population. In newer areas, there is a greater cross section of people, significant grassroots activity, and more individuals who vie for elected and appointed positions. In either case, basic information is essential:

- Which members of the elected body have the most power, both formal and informal?
- Who, outside the government unit, has influence and should be considered when devising strategy—a former public official, members of a powerful family, an influential business leader?
- Is there a political dynasty controlled by a politically entrenched family or powerful interest group?
- What strategies have resulted in successful grassroots initiatives?
- Is there evidence of a spoils system in which appointments to powerful boards or committees are granted on the basis of political connections rather than on merit?

This kind of information is more difficult to gather. The extent to which any of these conditions exist in different communities varies, but an understanding of these dynamics increases the possibilities for achieving policy goals.

Formulating a Plan

The form of government and nature of the specific issue will determine which tactics are best to achieve change in local policy. For example, if you want to protest a budget that freezes the hiring of nurses, you must know where to lodge the protest. In a hospital operated by a small city, in which the government is a weak mayor-council form and the mayor holds no real power, you must organize to lobby the council members. In a health department run by a county with an elected executive and council, there is shared power and strong checks and balances. Both the county executive and the council must be targeted.

Enlist support of those who share the same or similar positions on the issue. If the issue is one of widespread concern or has a negative impact on a large segment of the community, numbers alone can be most effective. So often, officials do not respond to persistent or impassioned pleas until large numbers support a cause. Elected officials who have not identified and addressed a concern are put on notice by large-scale citizen efforts. Their reelection is threatened when they fail to serve their constituencies.

Movements typical of this kind of activity often fall into the "NIMBY" (not in my back yard) category. Projects such as landfills, construction of 200- to 300-foot cellular transmission towers, and group homes for drug or alcohol recovery or for mentally impaired persons are examples. In the case of group homes, nurses can play a valuable role in mustering support for the project by educating the public and helping to allay their fears, which are generally grounded in lack of understanding.

Numbers are not and should not be the sole approach. In many instances, expert support is extremely valuable in persuading local decision makers. For example, rural landfill operations can be a source of revenue for a community, and officials may decide, despite many objectors, that a company with a record of well-maintained sites may be a compatible enterprise. Possible contamination of ground-water supplies by effluent and runoff can be documented by hydrologists, environmental conservation officers, or soil and water conservation experts. Nurses can seek out such experts and act as facilitators to educate their local board about the possible health hazards (see Chapter 34, vignette on environmental justice).

Deciding on using numbers, experts, or a combination of both depends to some extent on the form of government and who in that unit will be targeted. For example, a protest against a budget that replaces nurses with unlicensed personnel must know where to focus activity. In a hospital operated by a small city with a weak mayor–strong council unit, grassroots lobbyists should organize to influence the council members. A county with an elected executive and council has shared power and strong checks and balances. Both the county executive and the council must be targeted.

Remember that legislation and policy development are incremental, building and changing during the course of many information-sharing and negotiating sessions. Rarely is a proposal adopted in its totality, but small successes do make a difference. Laying the foundation for further change and developing a support base for future initiatives are necessary and valid short-term goals.

Getting Involved

Nurses can influence government in a variety of ways, individually or collectively, with professional colleagues or citizens, in small groups or large. There are a number of paths from which to choose:

- Serving on volunteer committees of community, school, or church events results in developing new skills and fine-tuning others. This also creates a network of local people who can provide informal information or who might become part of an issue advocacy group.
- County and city hospitals, community health services, elder services, and emergency treatment centers are often major employers in a community. Nurses in these facilities can participate in the resolution of problems

confronting them or the populations they serve.

- Testifying at public hearings or speaking out on issues at meetings of local government bodies are opportunities for nurses to become recognized as experts.
- Coalitions and citizen movements are increasing. There is strength in numbers, but choose carefully which efforts to support because some groups employ tactics of emotion and misinformation. Well-intentioned, informed groups are a good place for a nurse to develop competency in influencing policy decisions.
- Nurses can take the initiative to form committees to study a problem and make recommendations to local officials.
- Advocacy and expertise can be demonstrated by responding to health concerns with letters to the editor or to the officials who have jurisdiction over the matter. Video editorial comments are part of the growing information system available on some networks and provide an opportunity to reach even wider audiences.
- The local electoral process provides several ways to influence who will make policy. Nurses can join local party committees to have a voice in the candidate selection process. They can work on the campaigns of candidates who share their values and goals.
- A local nurses' political action committee (PAC) is an effective way to create a stronger presence by endorsing candidates and organizing nurses to work for them. Monitoring voting records is also an important function of a PAC.

As nurses become more involved and visible in a wide range of community activities, they become more proficient and will, in fact, be sought for their expert opinion and often approached to serve on boards or commissions.

Nurses should actively seek appointment to local boards and committees and become part of the decision-making teams. Health facilities and hospitals are logical units for nurses to become members of the board of directors. Planning, zoning, and conservation boards are powerful authorities, as are school boards. Remember, too, that the many special districts discussed earlier are units of government and are managed by elected or appointed members. There will be much specific information to learn in such positions, but nurses should be confident that they have many skills and talents that will benefit their local governments and communities.

Becoming a decision maker as a member of a community board can be the first step to running for office. A network of supporters becomes established, new skills in management and communication are developed, and knowledge of broad issues can be used as preparation for higher office.

We are accustomed to hearing about exorbitant levels of spending needed to win elections at the federal and state levels. Candidates for office in large cities or counties may even have to spend large sums to be viable. The smaller cities, towns, and villages do not require such vast financial resources. Candidates rely on extensive networks of family, co-workers, and neighbors to spread their message. The candidate's achievements may already be well known. Leaflet distribution, ads in local papers or trade publications, and door-to-door campaigning by the candidate and spokespersons are the tools used effectively in races at these levels. These activities often become opportunities to invigorate neighborhoods and generate cooperation and camaraderie.

It is not uncommon for local government officers to run for higher office. In fact, local government is regarded by many as the training ground for state and national office. Many public officials attain their first positions in local office by accident rather than by design. That is, they move from community activism to elected office because of their involvement in issues. Others, particularly those from families with extensive involvement in political activity or public office, make decisions early on to follow that course.

Many nurses have been and will continue to be elected to office by the accidental route; this is good and it is important. Congresswoman Carolyn McCarthy of New York is a prime example. After the tragic death of her husband and the wounding of her son by a gunman who opened fire on a Long Island commuter train, Carolyn McCarthy successfully challenged her local congressman, who had voted against a major gun control initiative. Her one-issue campaign took this nurse to Congress, where she has been able to use her health care background to benefit her constituents.

Service on a local school board allowed another nurse to use her background and influence to convince other board members of the importance of seat belts on school buses and the need for monitoring environmental hazards in school buildings. It is hoped that more and more nurses will be convinced that holding public office is the manner in which they can influence public policy and will make early decisions to do so.

CASE EXAMPLE   Making a Difference in Local Government

Elementary and secondary schools are faced with growing populations of "at risk" students who fail to fulfill their physical and mental promise. Emotional and behavioral deficits are barriers to learning that have consequences for society as well as for the individual students, but too often communities have no comprehensive approach to addressing these issues.

When a small rural school district established its federally funded Safe and Drug-Free Schools Committee, the elementary school nurse volunteered to serve. The nurse advocated early intervention and prevention programs for the primary grades. For the first 3 years, however, all the initiatives supported by the committee targeted the high school population. This was due to the proportionately higher representation of high school staff, highly visible pressing problems at that level, and lack of understanding of the effectiveness and value of early intervention versus crisis intervention in later years. Goals in serving the high school were to provide support to students at risk of academic failure or dropping out of school. The approach was fragmented, with a variety of programs but no long-term evaluation or follow-up.

The nurse continued to educate committee members as a body and individually about the need for a long-range plan for all students, kindergarten through twelfth grade, with a focus on early intervention. Information about a particular primary-level program with documented success for 25 years was strongly recommended by the nurse. Support was built formally and informally, and the committee eventually funded the recommended program as a 2-year pilot project. The program has been positively evaluated by elementary level teachers whose students had fewer school adjustment problems and who were helped.

A broad-based holiday celebration, also initiated by the school nurse, was planned and carried out by a subcommittee of the Safe and Drug-Free School Committee. Business, government, churches, and the school district cooperated in providing both in-kind service and financial support for a family-oriented, intergenerational drug- and alcohol-free New Year's Eve event. Attendance was double the number for which the steering committee had planned and hoped. Postevent evaluations completed by attendees, vendors, and performers revealed strong support for the event to be held annually.

Though it is sometimes possible to accomplish sweeping change, this is not usually the case. Nurses acting as change agents must understand that achieving change requires patience, persistence, and an understanding of the incremental nature of policy development.

Establishing a support network will strengthen the chances of accomplishing a goal. This network should include both formal and informal power brokers. The school nurse targeted two committee members likely to be supportive of the need for comprehensive early intervention: a highly respected elementary teacher who was also a school board member in a neighboring district and an active parent of elementary students who had served several terms on the local parent-teacher association's board of directors. They, in turn, generated additional support. The principal of one of the elementary schools lent early support after reading program material provided by the nurse.

A knowledge of government structure and of some of the history, as well as an understanding of the informal power system and decision-making process, helped this nurse and members of the celebration subcommittee to get their effort off the ground. The most common form of town government, similar to the weak mayor-council form, was in place. Commitment to the event was accomplished informally by lobbying individual councilmen and then sending a project proposal to be acted on at an official meeting of the town board. The strong appeal of the program content provided momentum and generated community support.

CONCLUSION

Providing assistance and services to local residents, once the responsibility of local governments, was gradually assumed by the federal government through such programs as Social Security, Medicare, higher education grants, Housing and Urban Development funds, and the "war on poverty." During the 1990s, however, the funding for health and human services, as well as support for state and local government operations, came under attack.

Cutting services and raising property taxes are the choices with which many localities grapple because local taxing and borrowing limits are capped by the states. Economic factors dictate that governments become more efficient in their operations. Despite shrinking revenues, some citizens expect the same level of services or demand additional amenities.

Nurses and local governments both have long histories of intervening in social problems. Nurses should continue to expand their efforts to participate in policy development both as grassroots lobbyists and as elected or appointed officials. The nursing profession recognizes the importance of these endeavors, and nursing associations at the national, state, and district levels support nurses in such activities through political action and candidate training workshops. As always, nursing looks to the future, and we should determine now what our role will be in the governments of the future and position our profession to shape that role. Understanding and participating in local government is a critical foundation for those activities.

As the largest group of providers in the health care system, our responsibility as nurses in caring for and about people includes our skills, resources, and power to improve the socioeconomic and political climate for all. The more we understand local governments, the better equipped we will be to make sound decisions about how and toward whom we should direct our activities.

REFERENCES

Berry, J. M., & Portney, K. E. (1993). *The rebirth of urban democracy.* Washington, DC: Brookings Institution.

Eggers, W. D., & O'Leary, J. (1995). *Revolution at the roots: Making our government smaller, better, and closer to home.* New York: The Free Press.

Fishman, L. E. (1997, July/August). What types of hospitals form the safety net? *Health Affairs, 16,* 215–222.

Goldsmith, M. F. (1991, May 15). School-based health clinics provide essential care. *Journal of the American Medical Association, 265*(19), 2458–2460.

Gore, A. (1993). *The Gore report on reinventing government.* (Report of the National Performance Review.) New York: Random House.

Kemp, R. L. (Ed.). (1993). *Strategic planning for local government.* Jefferson, NC: McFarland & Co.

Klerman, L. V. (1992, Winter). Nonfinancial barriers to the receipt of medical care. *The Future of Children, 2*(2), 171–183.

Lavin, A. T., Shapiro, G. R., Weill, K. S. (1992, August). Creating an agenda for school-based health promotion: A review of 25 selected reports. *Journal of School Health, 62,* 212–228.

Lewin, T. (1997, September 3). Hospital's serving the poor struggle to retain patients. *The New York Times,* pp. A1, A20.

Liner, E. B. (Ed.). (1989). *A decade of devolution: Perspectives on state-local relations.* Washington, DC: Urban Institute Press.

Maier, P. (1997). *American scripture.* New York: Alfred A. Knopf.

Mann, J. M., Melnick, G. A., Bamezai, A., & Zwanziger, J. (1997, July/August). A profile of uncompensated hospital care, 1983–1995. *Health Affairs, 16*(4), 223–232.

National Institute of Medicine, Division of Health Care Services, Committee for the Study of the Future of Public Health. (1988). *The future of public health.* Washington, DC: U.S. Government Printing Office.

Oakley, A. (1994). *Issues confronting city and state governments.* Skokie, IL: PO Publishing.

Peterson, G. E. (Ed.). (1994). *Big-city politics, governance and fiscal constraints.* Washington, DC: Urban Institute Press.

Pierce, N. R. (1993). *Citi-states: How urban America can prosper in a competitive world.* Washington, DC: Seven Locks Press.

Chapter *25*

STATE GOVERNMENT

T̲ERRI G̲AFFNEY

Although activities of Congress may garner much of the nation's attention, the bulk of public policies governing nurses and nursing practice are created at the state level. It is at this level that nurses are licensed and nursing practice acts are established. In 1996 more than 100,000 bills were introduced in state legislatures across the nation. Of this number, approximately 25% affected nurses and nursing practice. The purpose of this chapter is to acquaint the reader with the structure and expanding role of state government so that more effective advocacy for appropriate public health policies can be achieved.

A law is defined as the body of rules and regulations governing people's behavior, as well as their relationship with others in society and with the state. Both federal and state governments have constitutional authority to create and enforce laws. State and local governments have the greatest authority to regulate health care through the state's police power, which allows states to protect the health, safety, and welfare of their citizens.

EXPANDING ROLE OF STATE GOVERNMENT

From the first attempts of the colonies to act collectively, the issue of limiting government by balancing power between the states and the central government has dominated intergovernmental politics in the American Federal system. [Philip Burgess, President, Center for the New West, Report of the Proceedings of the 1995 States' Federalism Summit]

The U.S. Constitution attempted to strike a balance between the federal and state governments. However, the balance of power began to shift from the federal system in favor of states when the 104th Congress came to power in 1994.

Since 1994, several proposals have been put forward advocating the transfer of selected limited functions from the federal government to state and local governments—a process now commonly known as devolution. The underlying assumption is that by giving the states greater responsibilities and freedom in these areas, a number of innovative approaches to public policy problems will be created.

In addition to understanding the history of state governments, it is important to understand the political climate in the states. Approximately 20 states have enacted term limits for state legislators—prohibiting their members from running for reelection beyond a prescribed number of terms. In addition, some elected officials will be affected by reapportionment, campaign finance reform, or both. These actions are creating state legislatures filled with novice statesmen. Members are quickly rising to leadership positions after 2 to 4 years in the legislature, in comparison with the 15 to 20 years' experience of their recent predecessors. Soon there will be a time when entire chambers have members with fewer than 6 years' experience.

These changes have huge implications for nurses and nursing practice. The current environment is creating a system in which less experienced and less educated legislators will be faced with making critical decisions. Inexperienced officials will be faced with implementing complex public programs such as welfare—even more so with the impact of devolution. To perform the best job as advocates for the needs of clients and the community, nurses must become knowledgeable participants in the policymaking process.

STRUCTURE OF STATE GOVERNMENT

The framers of the U.S. Constitution shaped the national government largely on their experience in state and local governments. Today, states remain centers of power and innovation. Though each state government is unique, there are many similarities. For example, each state government consists of three branches: legislative, executive, and judicial.

Legislative Branch

> Today, state legislatures are among the most revitalized and changed institutions in America with a vastly increased capacity to govern. [William T. Pound, Executive Director, National Conference of State Legislatures, Report of the Proceedings of the 1995 States' Federalism Summit]

State legislatures are the oldest part of our government—having existed before the U.S. Constitution was created. These legislatures levy state taxes, appropriate money, create agencies to carry out the tasks of government, and investigate these agencies to make sure they are following the law.

Almost every national policy innovation can be traced back to the states. For example, old-age-pension programs created by states were the models for the federal Social Security Act. More recently, state legislatures have reformed health care delivery systems, in spite of the struggles of Congress and the President. Finally, states have streamlined Medicaid, increasing coverage and stabilizing costs.

The organizational structures and procedures of state legislatures are diverse and complex. Each state legislature has two houses (except Nebraska, which has only one). As in Congress, the lower body is generally referred to as the house of representatives and the upper body as the senate. There are 7,424 state legislators. Nearly half of the lower houses have between 51 and 100 members. In contrast, 45 state senates have fewer than 50 senators each.

Most state legislatures meet on an annual basis beginning in January. They generally remain in session for 30 to 60 days. Currently 13 states do not have limits on the length of sessions. Seven states meet year-round—Illinois, Massachusetts, Michigan, New Jersey, Ohio, Pennsylvania, and Wisconsin.

Although most states hold short sessions—in comparison with their federal counterparts—more states have been calling special sessions to address specific issues of concern. For example, though the Kentucky legislature was not scheduled to meet in 1997, it convened in two separate special legislative sessions to address postsecondary education and insurance.

Because the majority of state legislatures meet part time, many legislators pursue other occupations. In addition to being citizen lawmakers, legislators may also be employed as lawyers, farmers, real estate agents, and registered nurses—to name a few. In 1996, there were approximately 75 registered nurses elected to state legislatures—a record high.

Each state legislature has a hierarchy of leadership positions. The lower house in each state has a speaker who presides over the body. This individual is a member of the majority party. All but one of the state senates selects a president. Lieutenant governors preside over the senates in 27 states.

State legislative sessions are generally short in duration but intensive in nature. Between January and February 1997, approximately 15,463 bills were introduced in state legislatures. Every state considered legislation with an impact on nurses in 1997, except for Kentucky, which did not meet in 1997. In the first 6 months of 1997, 49 states *considered* measures related to nurses, and 25 states *enacted* more than 60 bills related to nurses, including three new laws expanding nurses' prescriptive authority.

On the state level, bills move through a process similar to that of the U.S. Congress. A bill is introduced in one body, is assigned to the committee of jurisdiction, and begins its journey through the committee process. Standing committees play a major role in the legislative process. The goal of standing committees is to establish a system to deal effectively with the more than quarter million bills and resolutions introduced each year. Committee names vary from state to state. However, committees addressing health, insurance, regulation, and reimbursement issues can be found in each state legislature.

To further describe the legislative process, let's take the example of a state legislator who introduces a bill to expand health care services for children in the Medicaid program. This bill would likely be assigned to the committee that deals with Medicaid or insurance. The committee process may entail public hearings during which various interest groups may be invited to testify—thus presenting their view on an issue. The committee may (1) recommend the bill for approval and pass it to the full body, (2) defeat the bill, or (3) send the bill for further study. Once the bill is passed by the committee, it is sent to the full body for approval; if passed, it then moves to the second house and begins the process again.

Because states legislative sessions are short, there is generally a date by which each house must pass a bill to the other body or the bill is considered to have been automatically defeated. This date may be referred to as the "crossover deadline." After both bodies have passed the same bill, it then goes to the governor for signature. If either body amends the bill, the conference committee process begins. During the conference, both bodies select several members to negotiate a final version of the bill. The final version then goes back to both bodies for approval and to the governor for signature or veto. States may hold a veto session at the close of a regularly scheduled legislative session to reconsider bills vetoed by the Governor.

Though the legislative process is similar across the 50 states, each state develops its own rules and procedures. Most states publish a handbook that describes the legislative process. The most frequently cited source for this document is the state legislative bill room; however, you may also be able to obtain this reference by calling the state capitol. Another source of information is bill status and tracking services. Generally states have established a phone number that may be called to determine the status of legislation. Today, legislatures are also on-line. Thus, many bills and issues can be tracked via the Internet.

State legislatures have broad powers to provide for the public's health. Nurse practice acts, in particular, are specific state statutes passed by legislatures to define and regulate the practice of nursing within each state. Much of the recent legislation affecting nurses and nursing practice involves scope of practice and licensure issues. In the case of advanced practice nurses, many critical legislative issues revolve around prescriptive authority and reimbursement for services. So that the reader can sample the flavor of the legislation affecting nurses and nursing practice, the following activities are highlighted.

In 1997 Georgia and New Jersey both enacted bills that require health care professionals, specifically nurses, to wear identification badges when interacting with patients. The badges should reflect the status and training the health care professional has obtained. Massachusetts enacted similar legislation in 1996.

Several states addressed bills relating to advanced practice nurses. In 1997, Arkansas enacted Senate Bill 142, which provided that certified registered nurse anesthetists need to be only in *collaboration* with a licensed physician or dentist, and not under their *supervision*. Virginia enacted House Bill 2425, which provided Medicaid reimbursement to clinical nurse specialists providing services to recipients of medical assistance. Also in Virginia, Senate Bill 835 authorized registered nurses to pronounce death.

This same year, New Mexico enacted House Bill 939, amending the nurse practice act. The new law established prescriptive authority for clinical nurse specialists. The scope of practice for clinical nurse specialists included independent decision making in the area of specialty practice with the use of expert knowledge and the carrying out of therapeutic regimens related to the prescription and distribution of controlled substances included in Schedules II through V of the Controlled Substance Act.

Much activity takes place in state legislatures in a short time, which translates into limited time for analysis and debate. Consider the Maryland General Assembly, which meets each year for 90 days to act on more than 2,300 bills including the state's annual budget. A great deal of work must take place in a short time. Legislators welcome expert analysis that helps them sort through and understand the issues associated with this mass of legislation. Such an environment underscores the importance of nursing's involvement in the legislative process. Nurses are health care experts and can easily articulate the needs of the community.

In a collective effort, nurses have been extremely successful in shaping state health policy. Through the years, state nurses associations have been relatively effective in influencing state legislation.

- In 1996, five bills dealing with the level of nursing staff in hospitals were introduced at the request of the *Massachusetts Nurses Association* and heard by the Massachusetts Legislature's Joint Committee on Health Care. One bill would set staffing standards for hospitals by specifying how many nurses are required in hospitals, based on number of patients and severity of illness. Another bill would expand the Patient's Bill of Rights by giving patients the right to know hospital staffing levels. A third bill would require that a health care provider be identified by profession or status (e.g., registered nurse, licensed practical nurse) on a lapel pin. A fourth bill calls for mandatory data collection so that staffing levels can be tied to quality of care. Other state nurses associations have also focused on worker identification legislation, with both Washington and Iowa having bills introduced in their state legislatures requiring

health care facility workers to wear proper identification.

- At the request of the *Kentucky Nurses Association,* legislation was introduced in 1996 calling for the interim Joint Committee on Health and Welfare to conduct a study on health care safety and quality issues at health care facilities and their impact on patients and personnel.
- The *Florida Nurses Association* was successful in pressing for legislation that requires a task force to study the effects of the number of licensed nurses and the skill mix of licensed, technical, and nonlicensed nursing staff on services, including, but not limited to, length of stay, patient accidents, medication errors, and delays in surgical procedures.
- The *Pennsylvania Nurses Association* worked successfully with the House Health and Human Services Committee to recommend legislative language that would require the collection of "nursing quality indicators" by the state's data collection agency.

As you will note from the above examples, much of the work of the state legislature is actually accomplished in committees and study groups. Because legislatures meet for short periods, many bills are studied though the course of a year and hearings are held outside the legislative session. Thus nurses must be aware that the end of the legislative session does not mark the end of the process. Politically astute nurses will continue to study the activities of interim committees, attend hearings, and meet with state legislators—even when the session is completed.

Executive Branch

Although there are many strong and influential state legislators, they are often overshadowed by strong governors. Lamar Alexander, former governor of Tennessee, defines a governor's job as follows: "See to the state's few most urgent needs; develop strategies to address them; and persuade at least half the people that he or she is right." However, devolution—the reshuffling of government functions from the federal to the state level—has made the job of governor more complex. Today, governors are faced with increased responsibilities and the need to become more effective managers.

Governors hold critical positions in the state government environment. Most governors are elected for 4-year terms and are eligible for reelection. Currently, Virginia and Mississippi are the only states that do not allow governors to succeed themselves. Governors are responsible for presenting the state budget to the legislature and controlling spending. In many cases the governor's policy initiatives will be presented as part of the budget package. Governor William Weld (Massachusetts) proposed budget recommendations for fiscal year 1998 that provided drug prescription benefits to more than 50,000 elders and health insurance to an additional 13,000 currently uninsured children and adolescents. Governor Zell Miller (Georgia), in his proposed 1998 budget, announced plans to implement the recommendations of the Georgia Coalition for Health, related to Georgia's request for a Medicaid waiver.

Governors also have the power to veto bills, as demonstrated by Governor Lawton Chiles (Florida) when he vetoed House Bill 1543 in May 1997. The bill attempted to create a study of the health care delivery system in Volusia County. Though the governor believed the study to be worthwhile, he questioned several provisions of the bill, which caused him to question the "spirit of the study" as a whole.

In addition to the governor, the executive branch also consists of the lieutenant governor and attorney general. In some states the governor and lieutenant governor are elected as a team, whereas in approximately half the states the ticket may be split. The role and duties of the lieutenant governor generally consist of assuming the responsibilities of governor as needed and presiding over the senate. While holding limited constitutional power, this individual may have the ear of the governor and be able to effect compromises in the legislative arena.

The Honorable Jo Ann Zimmerman was particularly successful in influencing health and social policies during her tenure as Iowa's lieutenant governor (1987 to 1991). At the time of her election, the lieutenant governor also served as president of the senate. In this role Zimmerman cast tie-breaking votes on critical issues such as interstate banking, assigned senators to committees, assigned legislation to committees for deliberation, and developed the daily calendar for debate. Zimmerman was well equipped to serve in this capacity—being a registered nurse and having served two terms in the state house of representatives.

Not only should the office of lieutenant governor be respected for its independent powers and duties, in many cases the office is used as a steppingstone to other political office. As such, politically effective nurses should understand the role of the lieutenant governor in their state and cultivate a relationship with this individual in order to influence the executive branch.

The office of attorney general has gained much attention as of late. The attorney general represents the public's interest in all legal cases coming before the courts; however, it is important to note that the office of attorney general does not encompass the state supreme court. The attorney general is responsible for arguing the state's cases before the court. In addition, the office of attorney general provides legal support and consultation to state agencies, including the board of nursing. The board counsel may be an assistant attorney general.

The attorney general's office may also offer interpretations or opinions related to the nurse practice act. These opinions are meant to clarify the intent of legislation or regulations. Such requests may result from a blurring of the scope of practice as noted in North Dakota. In 1995 the North Dakota board of medical examiners and the board of nursing requested an attorney general's opinion on the question of whether a physician may assign tasks embraced within the definition of "nursing" to emergency medical services (EMS) personnel in a hospital setting on a routine, nonemergency basis. EMS personnel are not regulated by the board of nursing. The attorney general concluded that a physician cannot assign medical tasks within the scope of nursing practice to EMS personnel unless the EMS personnel are licensed by the board of nursing.

Attorneys general in several states have garnered much publicity as a result of the trend of not-for-profit hospitals to convert to for-profit entities. Typically, nonprofit conversions are dealt with in courts of law. These conversions generally occur when a nonprofit hospital seeks court approval to change its fundamental purpose. Opposition to such a conversion may lead to a court order. In 1996, Nebraska and California enacted legislation giving the attorney general's office more authority in monitoring these proposed transactions in an effort to protect the public's interest. The majority of states addressed this issue during their 1997 session; however, Rhode Island has the distinction of having enacted one of the toughest conversion laws.

STATE AGENCIES

Once the legislature creates a statute or law, it delegates the authority to implement and establish new regulations to meet the intent of the statute. This authority is usually delegated to the executive branch or may be delegated directly to an independent agency. State executive branch agencies may be divided into five categories and have many layers. The five categories are as follows:

- Agencies led by elected, constitutional officers, such as secretaries of state, treasurers, and attorneys general
- Agencies run by officials appointed by governors or independent boards with or without legislative confirmation, such as secretaries of human services and commissioners of health
- Professional licensing and regulatory boards, such as boards of nursing
- Public authorities and corporations, such as higher education assistance authorities
- Independent boards and commissions, such as councils of higher education, and public utilities commissions (Council of State Governments, 1995)

State agencies or departments oversee health, insurance, labor, and transportation, to name a few. As nurses, we are probably most familiar with the state agency that regulates nurses—the board of nursing.

The basis of the states' ability to regulate health providers is established in the U.S. Constitution, which dictates that the authority to regulate health care providers is a state function. Thus states regulate the professional practice of nurses, physicians, and other health care providers. Although state legislatures created the nurse practice acts, the acts in turn establish state boards of nursing as administrative agencies with the authority to develop and enforce regulations concerning nursing practice. Regulations on nursing practice are considered administrative laws that are legally binding. In these rules and regulations, specifics related to delegation, supervision, educational requirements, and scope of nursing practice can be found. However, it is important to note that statutes and regulations vary from state to state.

The mission of these regulatory boards is to protect the health, safety, and welfare of the public from incompetent health care providers. This mission is accomplished through the administration of responsibilities such as establishing criteria for practice, issuing licenses, regulating standards of conduct, investigating complaints against licensees, and promulgating rules that regulate nurses and nursing practice. Implicit in these major responsibilities for upholding public protection are (1) rule-making authority, (2) quasijudicial authority, and (3) administrative authority (Betts & Waddle, 1992). (See Box, p. 423.)

Another agency that has an impact on nurses and nursing practice is the department of health. Generally the mission of the department of health is to maintain the health of the community. The director of the department is appointed by and serves at the pleasure of the governor. Within the department of health are many divisions. These divisions may encompass health care data collection, administration of the Med-

> ## AUTHORITY OF REGULATORY BOARDS
>
> **Rule-making authority** provides for setting standards, as well as for due process requirements.
>
> **Quasijudicial authority** provides for enforcement of standards and outlines procedures for adjudication of contested matters.
>
> **Administrative authority** provides for elements needed to enforce standards, such as agency budget, personnel, and office management.

icaid program, public health programs, and hospital regulation.

The Massachusetts Executive Office of Health and Human Services (EOHHS), established in 1971, is the largest executive office in the governor's cabinet. The EOHHS oversees a total operating budget of nearly $8 billion. This figure represents 43% of the total state budget. Within EOHHS is the Massachusetts Department of Public Health (DPH). DPH assists communities in defining needs and identifying appropriate public health interventions. Separate from DPH is the division of medical assistance, the state agency that administers the Medicaid program in Massachusetts. It is interesting to note that the board of nursing is not housed within EOHHS but, instead, is located in the Office of Consumer Affairs and Business Regulation.

Virginia demonstrates a similar organizational structure. The position of secretary of the Virginia Department of Health and Human Services is a cabinet-level appointment. The secretary is responsible for the department of health, the department of medical assistance (which administers the Medicaid program), and the department of health professions (where the board of nursing is located).

Some believe that the governor's appointive power is his or her most important function. Through recruiting effective people and delegating appropriately, a governor can provide direction for the state government. This power is clearly noted in a governor's appointments to the board of nursing. In most states the members of the board of nursing are appointed by the governor. North Carolina is the only state whose board members are elected by their peers.

Nurses influence public policy through both political action and political appointments. In 1993 Governor Pete Wilson (California) named Sandy Smoley as the secretary of health and welfare (see Chapter 27). She was the first registered nurse to be appointed to the post. Smoley's responsibilities include managing the state's $12 billion health and welfare agency, which employs more than 40,000 individuals within 11 departments. Before her appointment, Smoley served as California's secretary of the California State and Consumer Services Agency.

Tricia Hunter, another California nurse, was also appointed by Governor Wilson to an administrative post. Hunter served as the special assistant to the director of the Office of Statewide Planning and Development. In this role she served as the administration's representative on the issue of malpractice.

Another precedent-setting nurse is Alexandra Liddy Bourne, who was appointed in 1996 as the deputy director of the Virginia Department of Conservation and Recreation. Her responsibilities included communicating with local soil and water boards about implementing strategies to protect the Chesapeake Bay. Bourne was well positioned for this role, having been previously elected to her community soil and water board.

Each of these nurses served in a unique capacity. Critical to their success in such challenging roles was their ability to communicate, solve problems, implement policy, and evaluate their actions. Again, the nursing process easily translates from the clinical environment into the political environment.

CHANGING ROLE OF THE BOARD OF NURSING

In the past several years, as the debate around licensure of health professionals and overlapping scopes of practice has evolved, much attention has been focused on the boards of nursing. In recent years, Arizona, Colorado, Maine,

Oregon, Utah, Virginia, and Washington have undertaken studies examining ways to improve their state licensure systems. Recommendations have arisen that include but are not limited to consolidation and restructuring of boards, increased public representation on boards, creating overlapping scopes of practice, establishing criteria for regulation of providers, and exploring continued competency. Colorado introduced legislation in 1996, although it did not pass, that would have privatized professional licensure.

In 1997 legislation was introduced in Nebraska, Connecticut, Arizona, and Oregon that calls for more studies of health care professional regulation in areas such as provider competency, scope of practice, and access to health care without diminishing public protection. Legislation enacted in Nebraska in 1997 provided for the sunset of the departments of social services, public institutions, health, and aging and of the office of juvenile services. In addition, three new agencies were created. The new agencies were health and human services, regulation and licensure, and finance and support—all to be managed by cabinet members appointed by the governor.

Judicial Branch

In recent years, state courts have become more prominent in state political life. Judges have begun applying their own state constitution more rigorously. In addition, there has been a revolution in state tort law—the law relating to noncontractual injuries to person, reputation, or property. Thus more malpractice suits are being brought by people who believe they have been injured as the result of faulty actions by doctors, hospitals, lawyers, and other professionals.

A recent example of such legal action involves a case that demonstrates how patients are placed at risk when hospitals cut costs by replacing registered nurses with unlicensed workers. In 1994 a 46-year-old Cincinnati, Ohio, woman died of surgical complications after hysterectomy. She had complained for several days of "incisional pain"; however, the hospital person-

nel to which she complained were not registered nurses but unlicensed personnel. The family filed a wrongful death suit and in 1996 agreed to a $3 million settlement from the hospital. This case highlights the critical nature of nursing's pursuit of the passage of worker identification legislation and adequate staffing levels.

Another example of the judicial system's interfacing with nursing practice involves the criminalization of health care providers. In one case, three Colorado nurses were arraigned to stand trial for criminally negligent homicide stemming from a medication error that resulted in the death of a newborn infant. The Colorado State Board of Nursing determined that the nurses were negligent and imposed strict sanctions, including the suspension of their professional licenses for a period of not less than 1 year, counseling, and formal reeducation in pharmacology. However, the district attorney argued that the nurses' actions constituted criminal negligence. Criminal actions against nurses are becoming more prevalent. This apparent trend is also being seen in other professions including medicine, firefighting, and law enforcement.

EMERGING STATE ISSUES

In the coming years, state policymakers will be grappling with emerging issues that affect nurses and nursing practice. Assessing the continuing competence of health practitioners is an issue that is gaining the attention of many state agencies. Although licensure boards strive to guarantee that individuals are competent when initially licensed, they have been less effective in ensuring competence throughout the licensing period. Approximately 20 states require continuing education credits for nurses as a condition of license renewal. However, there is little research that demonstrates a link between continuing education and competence. Generally states do not impose requirements on licensed professionals to demonstrate their continuing competence to practice. In 1995 the Pew Health Professions Commission called for states to require each health regulatory board to develop, implement, and evaluate continuing competency requirements to ensure the continuing competence of regulated health care professionals (Pew Health Professions Commission, 1995). In 1997, Ohio, Oklahoma, Vermont, Virginia, and Texas introduced competency legislation. The Texas legislation authorized the Texas Board of Nursing to develop pilot programs to evaluate the effectiveness of mechanisms designed to ensure maintenance of clinical competency by registered nurses. This was the beginning of a new wave of public policy focused on protecting the public from incompetent health care professionals. Expect to see more state activity—both legislative and regulatory—on the issue of ensuring competence in the future.

A second issue that will be gaining the attention of state lawmakers involves the blending of health care and telecommunications technology. The expanding use of telehealth now allows health care providers licensed in one state to provide consultations for patients located in a different state. This practice across state lines raises several complex regulatory and reimbursement issues. The Western Governors' Association, at its spring 1997 meeting, called for a "uniform state code for telemedicine licensure and credentialing," which would simplify the licensure process for health professionals. In response, the National Council of State Boards of Nursing, at its 1997 annual meeting, adopted a "mutual recognition" model of nursing regulation. Under this model, boards of nursing would work toward an agreement under which nurses would hold a license in one state and be able to practice in any state, provided they follow the laws and regulations of the state in which they practice. For nurses, this means they need be licensed in only one state. However, they still maintain the responsibility of understanding and adhering to the nurse practice act and accompanying regulations of the state in which they are practicing. North Carolina was the first state to enact legislation creating the framework for such a licensure model. Implementing a new model of licensure requires new laws and regulations.

Look for more boards of nursing and state legislatures to debate this issue in the future.

CONCLUSION

State governments continue to play a strong role in shaping nursing practice—through the development of laws, regulations, and other vehicles of public policy. During the past few years, the trend has been one of increasing state influence in implementing federal programs in the states. The difficulty arises as state legislatures are becoming more influential while, at the same time, growing numbers of freshmen legislators are being elected to office.

Meanwhile, change continues to reverberate through the health care delivery system. Today professional roles are becoming more blurred, regulatory boards are being held more accountable, and the environment in which health care services are delivered is changing. State governments, health care facilities, and employers remain committed to decreasing the cost of health care services while nursing remains committed to providing high-quality, safe care. In the past, state legislatures addressed issues related to scopes of practice and reimbursement for nursing services. In the future they will be expected to act on more complex issues related to the work force regulation.

To fulfill their role as patient advocates, nurses must continue to expand their role in the development of public policy, particularly to create a system that promotes the nursing profession and protects our clients. Nurses must understand the system they are attempting to change, be able to negotiate the legislative and regulatory process, and act collectively. Ultimately, nurses should strengthen their efforts to educate legislators and influence state legislation and regulations in order to increase the public's access to high-quality, cost-effective health care services.

REFERENCES

Aiken, L. (1994). *Legal, ethical, and political issues in nursing.* Philadelphia: F. A. Davis.

Betts, V., & Waddle, F. (1997). Legal aspects of nursing. In Chitty, K. K. *Professional nursing.* (2nd ed., pp. 421–442). Philadelphia: W. B. Saunders.

Council of State Governments. (1995). *State government organizational charts.* Lexington: Author.

Council of State Governments. (1996a). *The book of states, 1995–6 edition.* Vol 32. Lexington: Author.

Council of State Governments. (1996b). *Restoring balance to the American federal system.* Lexington: Author.

DeLoughery, G. (1991). *Issues and trends in nursing.* St. Louis: Mosby.

Hansen, K. (1997). Living within the limits. *State Legislatures, 23*(6), 12–19.

Kuhen, J. (1996, September 30). The new hands-off nursing. *Time,* p. 56.

Pew Health Professions Commission. (1995). *The report of the taskforce on health care workforce regulation.* San Francisco: Author.

Zimmerman, J. A. (1993). Working the executive branch: An inside view. In D. Mason, S. Talbott, & J. Leavitt (Eds.), *Policy and politics for nurses: Action and change in the workplace, government organizations and community* (2nd ed., pp. 444–447). Philadelphia: W. B. Saunders.

VIGNETTE
One Nurse's Journey to Becoming a Policymaker
Judy Biros Robson

One of my goals is to be an example to nurses, to show them that if a woman, if a nurse, has the ability, interest, and knowledge of the issues, she can win public office and influence health care decisions. The stakes are so high that nurses need to influence governmental decisions. — State Representative Judy Robson (1997)

It is a myth that women elected to public office must have substantial prior political experience. *If you want to do it, go for it!* My prior experience in a political campaign was addressing envelopes and dropping flyers in local campaigns. I had, however, always been drawn to politics: president of the district nurses' association, Congressional district coordinator for the American Nurses Association, board member in the League of Women Voters, and a nurse intern in a state legislator's office (as a requirement for a graduate nursing course). It was a big leap, however, to leave the security of college teaching to embrace the uncertainty of a high-profile political campaign. The context for this unusual step was a mixture of both personal and professional experiences.

Personally the roots of this political attraction took hold in the 1960s. As a young Kennedy idealist, I heeded his call to government service, which paralleled my attraction to nursing. I viewed both as a special way to meet the needs of the voiceless, the powerless, and the most vulnerable, and to make a difference.

Professionally I was ready to run. Though I had worked contentedly for 9 years as a nursing instructor, I frequently challenged students in a nursing trends course to become politically involved. "The political stakes are too high for a nurse to be a passive observer," I repeated for several years. The tables were turned when a legislative seat was unexpectedly vacated. A renegade thought then emerged: maybe I should practice what I preach and run for the seat.

At the same time the health care system, where I had practiced for more than 25 years, was "morphing" into an industry. Emerging terms such as *market shares* and *bottom lines,* reflected values that were challenging professional standards and nursing practice. It was becoming obvious that nurses needed to sit at the policy table during this time of change in health care.

Equally important to this decision were my previous experiences in a system that frequently undermined my role as a geriatric nurse practitioner in collaborative practice with a physician. For example:

- As part of my practice I would make home calls, after hospital discharge, on elderly patients. For instance, I would assess a bedridden client, Hattie, in her home, create and coordinate a plan of care, and be her advocate. This strategy avoided an expensive, uncomfortable ambulance ride by her to the clinic for the same assessment. These less costly nursing services were not reimbursable. Insurance would cover only the more expensive alternative: the ambulance ride and physician office visit.
- Vera was a lonely, chronically ill person who often conjured up attacks to get the attention of a city paramedic ambulance unit for treatment. At one point she was transported eight times in 1 month to the emergency department. Insurance would pay for the expensive, unnecessary trips to the emergency department but not my home interventions, which virtually eliminated these costly trips.
- As part of a comprehensive assessment, I would examine and counsel elderly patients during lengthy office visits. The physician would have to pop in, basically a "meet and greet," sign my prescription pad if necessary, and leave—ceremonial steps required by some federal regulation.

My collaborating physician and I lobbied state, federal, and private insurance companies about the cost-effectiveness and unique contribution of nurse practitioners and the value of preventive care. We even submitted an article to a state medical journal on our unique practice and the value of geriatric nurse practitioners. Our voices fell on deaf ears.

Equally frustrating was the powerlessness I felt as a nurse. It seemed we had few advocates: bureaucrats followed baffling policies or restrictive rules written by nameless people, oblivious of or indifferent to nursing.

I wanted change, but how could it be accomplished? While I waited, a possibility arose: an open seat for the Wisconsin Assembly. Men outnumbered women in the legislature four to one, and no woman had ever served my Assembly district. An open seat is a golden opportunity for women in politics to level the playing field.

Running for Office

Running for the Assembly, however, felt like working in the emergency department on Friday night after a tornado has devastated a trailer park. Initially I was in a reactive mode to the constantly ringing phone, incessant press inquiries, friendly advice on winning strategies— most of it conflicting—while I continued to teach full time in a difficult team-leading clinical rotation. I was naive and not prepared to handle the press or understand partisan politics, having landed in the center of this election bull's-eye. The stakes were high and pressure was intense.

The governor quickly called a special election within 6 weeks of the incumbent's resignation, one of the shortest election spans in Wisconsin history. This short time frame put me at a distinct disadvantage, which was the intended strategy. My opponent already had great momentum from high name recognition, and my time for campaigning was limited by a full-time teaching load. I was clearly the *underdog,* so much so that my own party fielded a candidate against me in the primary, a well-liked county supervisor and farmer.

To overcome the odds, I had to work harder and smarter. My campaign strategy was logical, a bit unorthodox, and hard work! The strategy was to identify those most likely to vote in a special election in the middle of June and visit as many of them as possible. After work and on weekends, I donned my white nursing shoes and knocked on the doors of regular, faithful voters. I complemented each home visit with friendly postcards, both before and after my personal visits.

I believe nurses are natural campaigners. We are people oriented and problem solvers by training, and we know how to listen. As a result, people trust us. Strangers invited me into their kitchen and easily shared conversations. I often found myself listening to detailed health problems instead of political issues. I listened, I cared, and people responded positively. To this day, they still remember my visit.

This campaign strategy was not without skeptics. Many friends urged me to abandon this unconventional door-to-door canvas and to follow a more traditional campaign like my opponent's: visit merchants or bankers downtown, and attend ice cream socials and church picnics. Their goal was to have me attend as many group activities as possible and be highly visible. Because I was inexperienced and in uncharted waters, it was hard to resist this well-meaning advice. Others argued that I stay focused on this fact: special elections with only one item on the ballot turn out few voters. The voters that do vote are dedicated. I stuck to my original plan to maintain the door-to-door effort and visit committed, faithful voters.

My opponent from the other political party was a formidable candidate. He was the executive director of the chamber of commerce, a former police captain, a school board member, and a legendary auctioneer. From these various public perches, he was able to garner visibility and press attention. As a nursing instructor, I had no such public platform. I was practically invisible to the media. He, on the other hand, as director of the chamber of commerce, was newsworthy while cutting ribbons or giving speeches at large community events. One afternoon, he even showed up on the stage at my son's high school graduation. I sat in the audience, steaming and demoralized. Then his front-runner status and glad-handing style began to work in my favor. Convinced he was a sure winner, his political party diverted resources earmarked against me to another, seemingly needier special election. This decision leveled the playing field for me. A cardinal rule in politics was violated: never underestimate your opponent.

My own county political party was equally unimpressed with my potential to win but finally became enthusiastic after I trounced the farmer, their anointed candidate, in the primary. Nonetheless the most enthusiastic volunteers were the nurses. I relied heavily on them: faculty members, Wisconsin Nurses Association members, and student nurses willing to do literature drops, mail, and call. To bolster *esprit de corps,* we called ourselves the white-shoe army and looked more formidable than we felt. It's tough to beat a nurse, we reasoned. A nurse running for political offices is more than a curiosity (not many run) because we have an intrinsically positive image. Nurses project a natural image of trustworthiness, honesty, and caring, qualities not often associated with politicians. This message sparked interest and ignited the campaign.

As election day approached, I began to feel grassroots momentum building. The tide was turning, despite apathetic coverage from the only newspaper in town. The paper regularly featured photos of my opponent at community events. The editor, a friend of my opponent, also regularly printed his supportive letters to the editor and withheld mine. We knew the letters were sent, because many friends sent us copies and because a whistle blower at the paper "snitched" about the backlog of letters. An attorney friend made a friendly personal visit to the editor, challenging the newspaper on its bias. Soon afterward, an avalanche of supportive letters to the editor were published.

To sustain this momentum and capitalize on the door-to-door effort, we organized a phone bank for a "Get Out the Vote" (GOTV) strategy. It's one thing to identify likely supporters, and another to be sure they vote on a hot June day. Phoners called likely prospects on the night before the election. On the afternoon of election day, volunteers cross-checked the precinct poll list with our supporters list and reminded voters again. Voter turnout was heavier than expected because of our GOTV efforts. Enthusiasm for my outsider status helped, as did nurses who spontaneously called nursing stations to remind nurses to vote after work.

Election night found nervous supporters, friends, and family huddled around the radio, waiting for news. The polls closed at 8 PM, and by 8:30 we knew that I had won. What satisfaction to see television and radio crews who were sitting at my opponent's campaign headquarters suddenly pack up their equipment and race over to my election-night headquarters! Three special elections were held in the state; I was the only Democrat to win and the only Democrat to win a special election in decades. I was an instant celebrity in political circles. The headlines in the paper the next day read: ROBSON WINS AN UPSET, with a large picture of me and my husband grinning like Cheshire cats.

Early Transition

On my first day in the capital, eager to start and yet overwhelmed with the reality of being elected to represent 50,000 people in five communities, I was stopped by the highway patrol for speeding, a symbolic foreshadowing of coming events. This bumpy transition from nurse to legislator was perhaps not as rapid as my driving but was hastened by immediate immersion into the hectic budgetary process. Many seasoned capital observers told me that this was the worst time to be elected. With 25 years of solid nursing skills behind me, I thought I was prepared for anything. Well, not exactly.

The transition from nurse to legislator was made more difficult by partisan egos. Though I nominally had an office in the state capitol, the opposing party, still upset over my victory, refused to vacate it. I felt parachuted into the middle of alien territory with little support: no office, no desk, no staff, and worst of all—no phone. Because of the work on the budget, orientation for new legislators was nonexistent. For several weeks I shared an office with a colleague, awkwardly working at his conference table. I naively thought that partisan politics ended with the campaign. In fact, partisanship colors every decision: office assignments, furniture, chairmanships, bill priorities, and fund raising. I had a lot more to learn.

The Budget Wars

The situation in the capital during budget deliberations is like war games. Budget building is the most time-consuming, intensive component of the 2-year legislative calendar. Everyone presses for advantage, scores points, collects personal favors, or outmaneuvers each other or the opposing party. Lobbyists swarm like locusts; legislators scurry for amendments; and leadership maneuvers for key votes to pass the budget bill.

I thought the worst was behind me when I left the operating rooms of temperamental surgeons who threw instruments and belittled nurses publicly. But the worst moments in surgery did not prepare me for the budget caucus: a partisan meeting set up so that members could discuss the budget bill, pending legislation or strategies for partisan advantage.

Any resemblance to group process is purely coincidental. The budget caucus is chaotic. Members represent a variety of constituencies and interests ranging from fishermen and dairy farmers to inner city youth. They all vie for attention and advantage. Their comments are sometimes pure theater, sometimes eloquent, and sometimes just plain nutty. Sometimes an angry legislator stalks off, shouting, "I'm off the budget." (Translation: I'm taking my bat and ball home until you play the game my way.) Another legislator whines, "I never get my amendments in the budget; leadership always sticks it to me." Or another legislator tearfully shouts, "When are we going to take care of our dairy farmers?" Or another regular cry rises: "What do Democrats stand for, anyway?" So it goes for days and weeks.

Our caucus met in a hot, windowless, sticky hearing room. The capitol building in Madison is beautiful marble that heats summer hearing rooms to oven temperatures. As the hours dragged from day to night and into morning, tempers flared. We were tired and sweaty and needed fresh clothes and healthier food. My nursing diagnosis: inadequate decision making related to stress, sleep deprivation, and junk food.

After another late, hot evening, I finally bellowed: "Why don't we move across the street to the air-conditioned hotel? It's healthier." Cold stares from leadership locked me into frozen silence. A buddy came up later and whispered that leadership preferred this hot room to speed up the budget process. I was afterward labeled the "nurse legislator."

This early baptism-by-fire, the biannual budgetary process, was great training for subsequent floor periods. I had to learn fast and hit the ground running during the next session, working on an ambitious agenda of health care in the district's interest. Bills signed into law included a loan forgiveness program for nursing students, insurance mandate for screening mammograms, immunization-law changes to improve compliance, a primary-health grant program for public health departments, academic credit transfer for associate-degree registered nurses, a task force on cocaine-addicted babies, grants for health care workers for assessment and treatment of cocaine-addicted babies, statute revisions to strengthen public health, emergency medical services legislation to improve the health-care delivery system, and independent prescriptive authority for advanced practice nurses.

This bill-passing process is challenging but fun. Winning is everything, and when you win, it feels terrific. The pomp and ceremony surrounding the governor's bill signing underlines this achievement. A variety of skills are required: tenacity, negotiation, people pleasing, and balancing on political tightropes. Such skills we depend on in nursing, whether negotiating with doctors about discharge plans, motivating difficult patients regarding a major life-style change, or soothing a hassled nursing team to maintain quality of care with fewer staff.

Prescriptive Authority Bill

Passage of an independent prescriptive authority bill for nurses was a textbook example of *how a bill becomes a law.* The legislative road to passage of bills is strewn with obstacles both formal and informal; this bill had a hefty share of both. Legislative rules may dictate the process, but politics can dictate success or failure because of political detours or personal intrigue. For example, a committee chair may hold up a bill not on merit but for leverage or revenge. Legislators, in turn, may vote for or against a bill because of a partisan label attached to the author. Striking a balance and keeping bills out of partisan potholes require agility.

Forging alliances was the first skill perfected on the road to passage of prescriptive authority. Before introducing a bill, I built coalitions and developed consensus outside the legislature. I wanted to avoid a repeat of the divisive "entry into nursing practice" bill. At that time, legislators heard nurses fight and criticize each other harshly during public hearings. Legislators hate being caught in crossfires, especially with nurses. Nurses took a credibility hit by not having their act together and by attacking each other in public. Legislators accused nurses of "turf guarding" and "elitism." Nurses defeated themselves and defeated the bill, which died in committee.

This time would be different: nurses would be unified and focused. I met with representatives from nursing organizations before introduction of the bill to flush out problems and to reach consensus. Months dragged on as we perfected the draft. One of the major sticking points was certification and master's degree educational requirements for an advanced practice nurse. We often discussed side issues: the changing role of nurses in primary care, definitions of scope of practice, and other legal issues. Although frustrated by the pace and tedium of this process, I remained committed to developing a consensus before I took the bill to the legislature.

In retrospect, this decision was wise. During the public hearings on the bill, nurses were focused and unified. We knew the process, stuck together, and supported each other. This unified front was essential to withstand the criticism and strong lobbying that would surely come later from physicians and pharmacists.

The bill, now law in Wisconsin, certifies advanced practice nurses—nurse practitioners and clinical nurse specialists—to prescribe medications according to their educational specialty, independent of physicians or protocols.

How a Bill Becomes Law

How a bill becomes law sometimes defies logic to outside observers. Bills advance along the road to law through a bumpy combination of key factors: timing, need, coalitions, a bit of luck, and effective political pressure. The introduction of prescriptive authority landed in the middle of the enthusiastic debate on health care reform initiated by President Clinton. Changing the health care system at the state level was at the top of the legislative agenda.

With this as background, prescriptive authority for advanced practice nurses fell naturally into the debate on health care reform, with the practical message that nurses improve access to primary care and provide cost-effective services. The message was backed up with years of nursing research describing patient satisfaction, professional outcomes, and cost-effectiveness. Prescriptive authority was viewed as a necessary and noncontroversial component of health care reform by legislators. In addition, the bill landed on politically friendly territory: the speaker of the state assembly was a baccalaureate-prepared nurse. He liked the bill and referred the bill to a friendly committee, which I chaired.

A Call for Nursing Action

A call to action! The bill needed cosponsors. The more legislators who sign up as cosponsors, the stronger the bill becomes. Nurses rallied and contacted legislators to explain the need for the bill and to ask for their support. Legislators' responses were positive because they had been cultivated through the years. Nurses, through their professional organizations or unions, had built an effective political network. The nurses worked on campaigns, invited legislators to special events, and endorsed them in the last election. The bill listed an impressive array of cosponsors from both parties, including a senator whose husband was a doctor. The Wisconsin Nurses Association had endorsed her in a tough reelection bid, and she remembered.

The next step is the public hearing. I was concerned about stiff opposition by the state medical society, a powerful legislative force. The medical society employs several lobbyists, and if an issue is a priority to them, additional contract lobbyists are hired. In contrast, the Wisconsin Nurses Association had one part-time lobbyist.

We waited anxiously for testimony from physicians asserting that this step by advance practice nurses would doom Western medicine, or that patients would be in harm's way if nurses were allowed to prescribe medications. Such testimony did not materialize. At the public hearing, the state medical society registered "neutral"—neither for nor against the bill. We were surprised and pleased with this position and met with the physicians later to work out some of their objections raised during the public hearing. The physicians' main concern focused on the need for additional pharmacology credits and the jurisdiction and composition of the committee designated to write the administrative rules for implementing the new law.

The bill passed the assembly unanimously and was promptly sent to the state senate for its own public hearings, debate, and vote. When the state assembly passed the bill unanimously, we expected smooth sailing in the senate. Not quite. The hospital association lobbyist suddenly emerged with a "harmless" amendment that would make the hospitals "more comfortable." This harmless amendment translated into institutional licensure, which would destroy the intent of the bill. Individual hospitals would have authority to certify nurses, rather than the Wisconsin Department of Regulation and Licensure and nursing professional organizations. We again rallied the nurses, via the Wisconsin Organization of Nurse Executives and the Wisconsin Nurses Association, and through our statewide newsletter, *NursingMatters*, sent to all registered nurses in the state. Protests from nurses bombarded the senate, which "deep sixed" the "harmless" amendment. The bill passed the senate.

The last hurdle was the governor. How could we get him to sign this bill? The Wisconsin Nurses Association executive director and I decided to invite the governor, up for reelection, to sign the bill at a Wisconsin Nurses Association workshop, Day at the Capitol. He agreed and we cheered. Several weeks later, with 1,000 enthusiastic nurses as background, the governor signed our bill into law.

Nurse as Legislator

When giving speeches to nursing organizations, I am often asked, "Do you miss nursing?" At first I was startled by the question, but now I reply, "I *am* practicing nursing!" I'm at the policy table instead of the bedside. I write and rewrite laws affecting nursing. I find ways to improve access to health care for children and the uninsurable. No, I don't monitor heart rates, but I do monitor policy that affects nurses, their patients, and public health.

Traits that help make a good nurse also help make a good public official. We are problem solvers. We have great people skills. We are team players. We are organized. We have lots of stamina.

Of course, the capital is not the hospital. Being a "political nurse" requires a few other skills and attitudes. Though nurses aren't born with the thick skin necessary to withstand the rough and tumble of political life, it is easy to grow. Politics is a tough game for anyone to play. And it is a game where winning is everything. A winner is toasted; a loser is ignored.

What are notable differences between clinical nursing in a health care institution and nursing in the legislature? A clinical nurse follows clear-cut medical procedures and strict standards of behavior. A legislator must learn the subtle art of deal making and gentle arm twisting. Nurses use nurturing, soothing words. Policymakers use tough, locker-room language.

Anyone moving into the public arena must be prepared to live in a fishbowl. Eyes will peer at you from all sides; you are no longer anonymous. Your personal life will be scrutinized, and your public life will be criticized. The hometown newspaper will print nasty attacks in letters to the editor and snooty, condescending editorials. You can't take the criticism personally. It is not about you, but about the issue. More often than not, it is a partisan potshot. People need to vent frustration, and elected officials are easy targets.

Nurses may be on call part of the time, but legislators are on call all the time. Whether you are rushing to the supermarket to buy groceries, going to church, or biking with your family, someone wants to give you their two cents' worth about this issue or that problem. There are no days off. Protecting personal time, ensuring family privacy, and coping with the life-style change require major adjustments.

An important aspect of the transition from nurse to legislator is the change in power you wield. All of a sudden, you can make things happen. You confront the rich and mingle with the famous. You talk to the governor and have calls returned personally by your congressmen. When the President of the United States comes to town, you are given VIP status: a seat behind him, a conversation, and a photo opportunity. You are called *Representative* and your mail is addressed to *The Honorable* . . . .

Some people let the privilege of office go to their heads. But good legislators balance the advantage of privileges without abusing them. Part of the balance is to remember that it is the office to which the titles belong, not you. Committee chairmanships, prized seats on the legislative floor, office assignments, nice office furniture, and special parking stalls are marks of seniority. Seniority at its best reflects tenacity and stability and at its worst, simply longevity in office.

Among other things, tenacity means that you reflect an identifiable set of values that you represent to your electorate and to legislative colleagues. Any legislator who starts to feel like a big shot, giving orders instead of taking them, soon remembers the thousands of "bosses" out there who have the power to fire you every 2 years at the ballot box.

In striving to represent your electorate, you have to remember you can't please all the voters all the time. As a legislator, you have to make tough choices on polarizing issues, such as abortion and gun control. On hot-button issues, you are bound to disappoint many voters. This hotseat may be tough for women legislators—and for nurses who are oriented to the business of people pleasing. We come to nursing because it is a helping profession. As an elected official, it can be painful to realize that some people have a mind-set *not to like* you or your job performance purely because of party affiliation or a single vote.

The Struggle of Political Women

As an elected official, I am supposed to be an equal to my male colleagues. I represent the same number of voters and enjoy equal pay. Yet there is the undeniable fact that women legislators do not have easy access to or carry equal clout in the power cliques that many male legislators move in.

Political women want to be treated as equals, but they don't necessarily want to play by the men's rules. Women want to establish inclusive power circles instead of the exclusive circuit of bars, private golf outings, and clubs. Women leaders tend to focus on team building and consensus rather than on the power trips sometimes characteristic of male politicians. Women's lack of appetite for raw personal power is probably one reason that politics remains male dominated.

Another reason for women's slow rise in politics is historical. Political man is a familiar figure in history—the chief, the premier, the dictator, who builds, battles, conquers, judges, and governs. Political women did not emerge in the United States until the 1920s, when the right to vote was extended to women. Newspaper editorials at that time reflected public opinion that women were too pure to vote and be contaminated by the dirty business of politics. The state capitol building in Wisconsin reflects this history. It was not until recently that the area adjacent to the state assembly chamber built a women's bathroom equivalent to the men's.

Women's slow political rise can also be attributed to the seniority system endemic in politics. Women didn't start making great inroads into politics until the 1970s. When we start out new to the field, we have to cue up patiently for senior statesman status.

Women nurses can help boost women's status in the political arena by running for office. Campaigning is a challenge, but it is exhilarating to meet new people, learn new skills, become more self-confident, and realize the potential power of nurses. Being a nurse legislator is rewarding. I made a difference, and you will too! Women like me often do not have substantial political experiences before we made the decision to run for office. If you want to do it, go for it! An army of thousands of white-shoes will support you and cheer you on.

Grassroots Lobbying

Obviously, not every nurse cares to seek public office, but we can also play two other important roles: campaign volunteer and lobbyist. "Lobbying" may sound like a mysterious activity that is foreign to regular folks. The truth is that regular folks are some of the most effective lobbyists. Regular folks can be even more effective if they follow three keys to effective lobbying: preparation, politeness, and perseverance.

Remember that our legislators need our votes. This fact makes you influential—sometimes more influential than dozens of well-paid, Armani-suited lobbyists prowling the halls of the capital with cell phones attached to their ears. (I often wondered if the cell phones actually work or simply serve as power symbols.)

Try to set up an appointment with a legislator on home turf so that we have his or her undivided attention, away from the trappings of power. Being awestruck by the velvet, gold, and marble surrounding the legislator's office is intimidating. Intimidation can reduce us to babbling adolescents happy to get a smile and a handshake. This person walks away with nothing to show for our efforts.

A legislative breakfast meeting with a group of nurses is a great opportunity to talk. Prepare for the meeting by prioritizing the message into three or four major themes. Get to the point, stay focused, and avoid side issues. Though you may be an authority, you don't have to give the legislator every detail of complex health issues. You will lose him or her in the details. Clarity of persuasion comes more often from billboards than from footnotes.

For example, when we lobbied on prescriptive authority, our message was that "a qualified nurse saves money and improves health care."

Avoid health care jargon: others don't know, want, or need our jargon. Anticipate possible arguments against your position and develop responses. Never deceive or mislead the legislator. Your word is golden. Threatening never works, and it could end your access or that of other nurses.

Try to personalize the issues by giving examples of how you, your co-workers, or your patients are affected. Tragic stories bring the point home. Stories of families coping with difficult situations are remembered and often repeated during floor debates. For example, testimony given by certified nurse midwives described a harried pregnant mother with a restless toddler in the office who had to wait in the reception area needlessly while the nurse tracked down a physician for a prescription for prenatal vitamins.

Lawmakers need to be told your stories: what is happening to your patients because of a shortage of nurses, what happens when hospitals use unlicensed personnel, what happens when patients have no health insurance, and what happens to the elderly patient when she is discharged early after a mastectomy.

Just as you shouldn't get sidetracked in your presentation with extraneous detail, do not let the legislator steer you to another topic. For example, if legislators suddenly ask what nurses think about the state lottery, steer them back to your message on health care.

When the meeting is wrapping up, ask the legislator for a commitment of action; a vote for or against a bill; or a promise to introduce legislation, cosponsor a bill, or help persuade another legislator. Failure to get a commitment will leave you with a dose of political junk food: "Sounds like a good idea," or "I've always been a friend of nursing." A cardinal rule of politics is never to break a promise. If you make a commitment, stick to it.

If the legislator is not supportive, determine the specific reason. Then you can follow up with more reasons why the legislator might change his or her mind. Follow-up is crucial in lobbying.

Whether the legislator was supportive or nonsupportive, send a thank-you note or make a follow-up call with additional information and more true-life stories to underline your point. A few calls or letters on an issue generate interest by a legislator; several calls, letters, and personal meetings generate a response.

In spite of women's initial disadvantage in negotiating the unfamiliar and often harsh world of politics, move in we must. Nurses have too much at stake not to become politically active. Nurses have shown they can be successful in the political arena. We have won elections against the odds, shepherded bills through legislatures, and shaped policy at the local, state, and federal levels. But our full impact has not been realized.

Think what influence we could wield with a united front: the sheer numbers of nurses working together to advocate prenatal care, responsible child-care, or money for child-abuse prevention programs. Nurses together and organized can control a large number of votes. You have yards to offer for campaign signs and contributions to offer to campaign funds. Elections are not won single-handedly. For every candidate running for office, there are a dozen or more hardworking, smart, selfless campaign volunteers.

Nurses carry a high degree of respectability and credibility within their communities. An endorsement by nurses can be at least as powerful as an endorsement by a labor union or business alliance. You have the potential to help or hurt a candidate's campaign. As soon as you realize this, your legislator will, too.

At nearly 2.2 million, nurses are the largest group of health care providers in the nation. Imagine a half-million nurses in white shoes rallying in front of the Washington Monument. Or 3,000 nurses parading up to their state capitol. The white-shoe brigade would be a force to reckon with.

Chapter 26

FEDERAL GOVERNMENT

Geraldine Polly Bednash, G. Brockwel Heylin, and Anne M. Rhome

The federal government's three branches function in ways that have enormous impact on both the delivery of health care in general and the practice of nursing in particular. Ranging from legislative actions such as approving funding for nursing education and research, to expanding authority for reimbursement to nurses who deliver advanced practice nursing care, to judicial decisions regarding health care regulations, the federal government affects nurses in major ways.

Through its programs for funding support or through its efforts to design structures for the delivery of health care or education, the federal government has created incentives or policies that affect both the characteristics of the nursing work force and the nature of nursing care. Federal reports, policies, and initiatives have served as stimuli in the development of new roles for health professionals and have funded the development of new technologies and care innovations that have changed the scope of practice (Fox, 1996). In the current market of health care delivery and of nursing education, policymakers have questioned the appropriate role that the federal government should play. For instance, the federal government in 1998 still provides substantial funding through Medicare for support of entry-level, nondegree nursing programs,

most often diploma programs. A diverse group of policymakers, however, have questioned the appropriateness of this practice and have recommended a redirection of these funds for other types of nursing education programs, most notably advanced practice nursing education. Reinhardt (1996) notes that, in the emerging market environment, questions should be raised about what he terms "interventionist policies" of the federal government to drive both the development of the health work force and the structure of the market environment.

Nurses, as part of their professional responsibility, need to be aware of the policymaking activities of the federal government. They also should be willing to contribute to the development of sound policy that will guide the delivery of effective and high-quality health care. Currently the legislative and administrative branches of the federal government have oversight or implementation accountability for a variety of programs that affect nursing education, practice, and research. Despite growing questions about the appropriate federal roles in the oversight of care delivery or the supply of nurses and other health professionals, the three branches of the federal government will continue to have a key role in the policies that guide nursing practice, education, and research.

This chapter will describe federal legislative, executive (administrative), and judicial branch authorities and activities that affect how health care is delivered, and nursing's role in the health care system.

The views expressed in this chapter are those of its authors and do not necessarily represent the views of the Board of Directors or the membership of the American Association of Colleges of Nursing.

EXECUTIVE BRANCH (Fig. 26–1)

Office of the President

As the highest-ranking popularly elected federal official, the President of the United States theoretically embodies the conceptual will of the people in terms of major policy goals and the scope, size, and direction of the federal government. Because of low voter turnout (less than 50% of the adult population in 1996) and the way the electoral system works, however, the president's mandate and power actually are much more limited. Though the president has some executive powers, for major policy initiatives he needs legislation to put programs into place and appropriations to operate them. For both, the president needs Congress more than it needs him. Congress can enact a law without the president's assent (by overriding a veto), but not the reverse.

Of course, this does not mean that the president is powerless. During the campaign for the office, the president may have caught the public's attention with messages of sufficient resonance to influence the priorities and objectives of the Congress. For example, President Ronald Reagan, a Republican, won a landslide victory and began his first term with momentum that encouraged a Democrat Senate and House to support his plans for tax cuts, defense increases, and a smaller government. And, although President Bill Clinton's massive attempt at total health care system reform in 1993 ultimately failed, he sharpened the public's sensitivity to inadequacies in health care coverage. In 1997 he signed into law a child health plan that established the first new entitlement program in more than 30 years.

Another strength of the president springs from the executive function as manager of legislated programs. As enacted, statutory language may be less than clear. The president and his executive staff make the policy decisions and write the regulations that interpret the statutes, which can be important for what the laws accomplish. In fact, detailed regulations may deny proponents of legislation what they thought they had won.

SUGGESTION: Once a bill has become law, interested people should make recommendations about its interpretation to the appropriate agency to help shape initial perceptions of the legislative language. Though rules ultimately will be published in the *Federal Register* as a proposal, waiting to comment on that proposal may not be as effective as ensuring that one's views are in the proposal when it is published. An agency may be reluctant to change the proposal to address comments.

With the members of the Cabinet, the President focuses policymakers in agencies on issues that fulfill the Administration's objectives. The President then determines which policies to embrace and develops strategies to move them through Congress. Because initiatives can begin in the White House or at the department level, those seeking to influence the development of federal policies should let both the president and the appropriate cabinet officer know of their concerns. For example, 1997 Medicare amendments greatly expanded the eligibility of nurse practitioners and clinical nurse specialists to be reimbursed for services outside rural areas. The ink was barely dry on the President's signature before nursing groups began to draft recommendations for federal officials who will implement the change.

SUGGESTION: To improve your chance of getting White House attention, show that your issue is a major policy concern for such reasons as its national scope, costs, and serious implications for public health. Do your homework and offer poignant, real examples. Avoid exaggeration, dire predictions, and technical jargon. Mention other groups or people who share your concerns. Avoid appearing turf oriented by framing the issue as a nursing issue; rather, show that it is one of health care. Cabinet-level issues relate to topics within an agency's statutory responsibility and often focus on how a particular program is performing or if there is an unmet need.

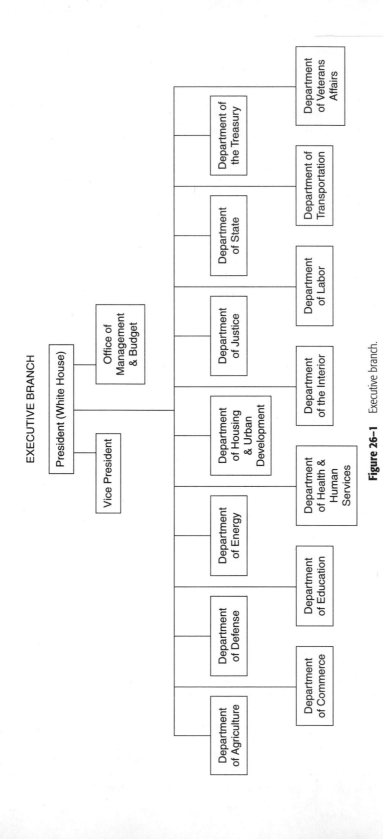

Figure 26-1 Executive branch.

Within the Office of the President, several offices are important to nursing. The Office of Policy Development analyzes and drafts major White House policy initiatives such as health care reform. The Office of Public Liaison provides links to the Administration for major interest groups such as nursing, labor organizations, women's groups, and minorities. The Office of National AIDS Policy serves as a monitor and advocate for people affected with acquired immunodeficiency syndrome (AIDS). The AIDS office also has an Interdepartmental Task Force on HIV/AIDS to foster communication on AIDS between federal agencies. (The Office of Legislative Affairs contains House and Senate liaison offices. These liaisons are the President's advocates before the Congress, and they develop strategies to move the President's issues. They usually do not deal directly with the public.)

OFFICE OF MANAGEMENT AND BUDGET

The President also oversees the Office of Management and Budget (OMB). For advocates of nursing and the health professions, OMB is very important. OMB reviews cabinet and independent agency budgets and negotiates spending levels for the coming fiscal year (FY) (Fig. 26–2). The federal fiscal year is from October 1 to September 30. The review process begins at the agency level more than 1 year before the beginning of the FY. For example, in late spring or early summer of 1997, managers of programs submitted to their agency or department budget office their recommendations for funding for FY 1999.

SUGGESTION: Those who want funding increased or shifted in various programs should inform the federal agency program managers by the end of May or beginning of June. To do so effectively, one must have detailed program knowledge and use concrete examples of achievements (or shortfalls). Recommending specific funding levels to the head of the department or agency can help. Getting funding for a program is difficult if

the executive agency responsible has not adequately provided for it in the President's budget presented to Congress.

Once the department or agency has finalized its budget proposal, OMB reviews it and either agrees or revises it and sends it back to the department or agency. The Cabinet office or agency head can contest an OMB decision by going to the President. At this point, public contact with the President may move the funding levels in a positive direction. The administration budget proposal is transmitted to Congress with the President's State of the Union message in late January for the fiscal year that will begin October 1. That budget often is not the final budget or appropriations figure for programs that are included, particularly if the President and the majority party in Congress are of different parties. For example, the Clinton Administration advocated sharp reductions in funding for the Nurse Education Act (NEA) for FY 1998 to a figure of about $10 million (from $65.3 million in FY 1997). Congress thought otherwise, with the House voting $67.1 million and the Senate voting $55 million for the FY 1998 NEA. House and Senate conferees agreed on $65.6 million for NEA for FY 1998.

OMB also reviews policy options and estimates their anticipated costs to the federal government if enacted as legislation. Within OMB's Health and Personnel Office there is a health division that deals with all U.S. Department of Health and Human Services programs, a human resources division for the U.S. Department of Education and Department of Labor, and a veterans affairs division. A relatively small OMB staff is responsible for a large number of agencies and hundreds of programs but may have no real sense of what those programs do or how important they are. Program advocates sometimes claim that OMB is primarily concerned with reducing federal expenditures. In the past, it has been difficult for interested people to get through to OMB staff and to educate them about programs.

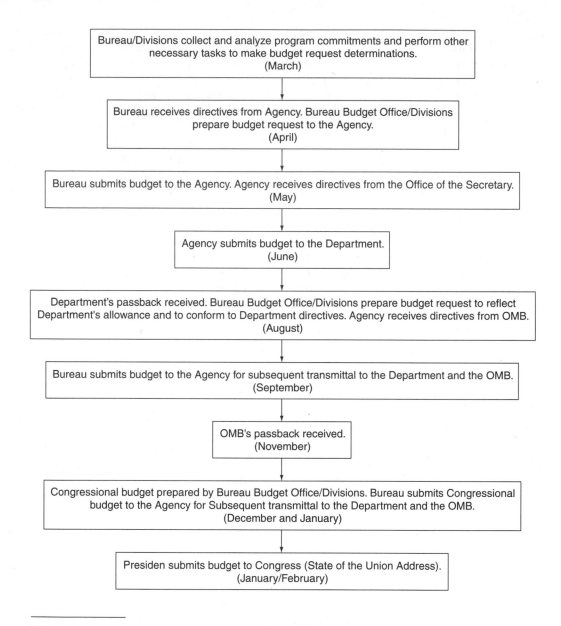

Bureau/Divisions collect and analyze program commitments and perform other necessary tasks to make budget request determinations. (March)

Bureau receives directives from Agency. Bureau Budget Office/Divisions prepare budget request to the Agency. (April)

Bureau submits budget to the Agency. Agency receives directives from the Office of the Secretary. (May)

Agency submits budget to the Department. (June)

Department's passback received. Bureau Budget Office/Divisions prepare budget request to reflect Department's allowance and to conform to Department directives. Agency receives directives from OMB. (August)

Bureau submits budget to the Agency for subsequent transmittal to the Department and the OMB. (September)

OMB's passback received. (November)

Congressional budget prepared by Bureau Budget Office/Divisions. Bureau submits Congressional budget to the Agency for Subsequent transmittal to the Department and the OMB. (December and January)

Presiden submits budget to Congress (State of the Union Address). (January/February)

*Dates given are estimated and are subject to change within any given year.

Figure 26–2 Budget formulation process.

VETO POWER

A discussion of the President's policy role would not be complete without looking at the power of the veto. When presented with a piece of legislation that has been sent to him by Congress, the President can sign it into law or allow it to become law without a signature under certain limited circumstances. The President can veto (reject) it by a message to Congress or can veto it by using a "pocket veto" for a bill passed at the end of a session of Congress. Under power recently granted, the President can veto specific provisions of legislation, using a line item veto.

The line item veto gives the President power to eliminate "pork barrel" projects (typically unbudgeted public works and road construction) from spending bills. This line item veto was an objective of the Republican-dominated Congress in 1994 and, ironically, was first used by a Democratic President in 1997. The power is certain to be the subject of court challenge.

The threat of a Presidential veto is a grave one for proponents of legislation, because to override a veto and make a bill become law without a Presidential signature requires a two-thirds majority vote in the Senate and the House. In the 105th Congress, with narrow majority margins of the political parties in each house and weakened control by parties over their members, overriding a veto can be extremely difficult.

SUGGESTION: Getting concerns included in a veto message is a step toward winning the issue. Was something missing from the bill? Was something in the bill that shouldn't have been? Give the President sound reasons why your issue should be part of the veto message.

POWER TO APPOINT

The President's power to appoint cabinet officers, senior government officials, and judges/justices also has a major impact on policy. For example, putting an advocate for children in a senior-level job will more or less ensure that children receive strong attention from the agency in which the official serves. For some positions, congressional approval of an appointment may be required. The confirmation process can be prolonged by personal bias and politics to the point that nominations may have to be withdrawn. The practice of allowing a Senator to put an anonymous hold on a nomination moving forward may also slow or kill a nomination.

SUGGESTION: Public support of a nominee may help to move a nomination forward both through the White House and before the Con-

gressional committees that have jurisdiction over the agency. Strong public opposition may stop the President from nominating, or the Congress from confirming, a nominee.

Cabinet Departments

Cabinet departments of special interest to nurses in terms of their policy role include the following:

- Department of Health and Human Services
- Department of Education
- Department of Labor
- Department of Veterans Affairs

DEPARTMENT OF HEALTH AND HUMAN SERVICES

The Department of Health and Human Services (DHHS) is a huge agency (Fig. 26–3); FY 1998 funding was $201 billion. It supports a wide variety of health sector programs focused on health promotion, Medicare, Medicaid, nursing and health professions education, rural health, AIDS, a malpractice data bank, maternal and child health, aging, substance abuse, mental health, clinical laboratory quality, health and biomedical research, and disease prevention and control. Many of the DHHS missions are important to nursing education, research, and practice. For example, DHHS funds the Nurse Education Act and the National Institute of Nursing Research.

U.S. Public Health Service. The Public Health Service Act is the statutory authority for many important DHHS functions, including nursing education, nursing and health services research, and rural health initiatives. There is a chief nurse of the U.S. Public Health Service, a rear admiral, who serves as a liaison on nursing practice with chief nurses of other federal agencies such as the army, air force, navy, Veterans Administration, and Department of Defense (DOD). Each of these entities employs large numbers of nurses. DOD supports the Uniformed Services University of the Health Sciences, which offers nurse practitioner and nurse anesthetist master's degree programs.

U.S. DEPARTMENT OF HEALTH AND HUMAN SERVICES

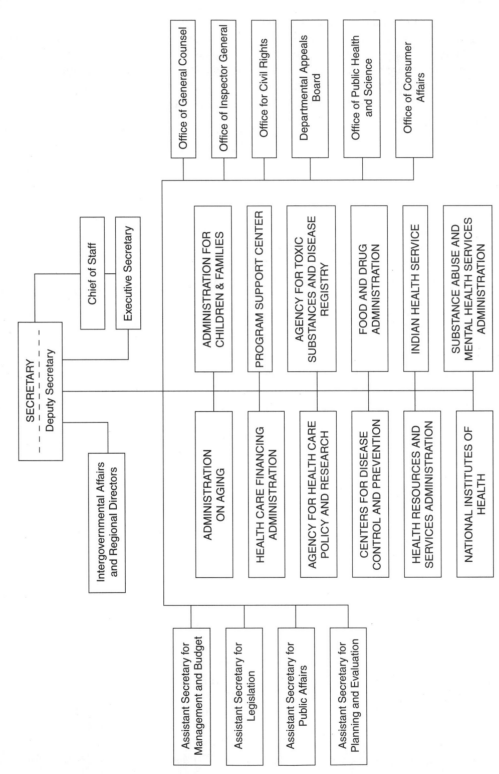

Figure 26-3 U.S. Department of Health and Human Services.

Office of Disease Prevention and Health Promotion. Within the DHHS Public Health and Science Office of the Assistant Secretary for Health is the Office of Disease Prevention and Health Promotion, which manages the National Coordinating Committee on Clinical Preventive Services (NCCCPS). The NCCCPS directs a clinical preventive services campaign and advises the Secretary of Health and Human Services on implementation of the objectives of Healthy People 2000. Healthy People 2000, released in 1990, is a comprehensive strategy for improving the nation's health through health promotion, protection, and prevention. It also sets age-related and special population objectives for health. The American Association of Colleges of Nursing and other major nursing organizations helped NCCCPS in its work by sharing information about the successes of the nursing profession in promoting health.

Health Resources and Services Administration. The DHHS Health Resources and Services Administration (HRSA) houses the Office of Rural Health, the Bureau of Primary Care, the Bureau of Maternal and Child Health, and the Bureau of Health Professions (BHPr) (Fig. 26–4). HRSA's Web address is *http://www.hrsa.dhhs.gov.* It includes a description of programs, grant opportunities, and applications for all HRSA entities.

Bureau of Health Professions (Fig. 26–5). The BHPr manages the Nurse Education Act (NEA) through the Division of Nursing. The NEA provides funds ($65.6 million in FY 1998) for programs and students in baccalaureate and graduate nursing education and includes a low-interest loan program for undergraduate and graduate nursing students. The NEA is the major federal program focusing on professional nursing education. NEA supports nurse-managed centers that serve as clinical training sites for undergraduate and graduate nursing students and deliver primary care to underserved populations. It funds nurse practitioner, midwife, and nurse anesthetist education programs and provides stipends for master's and doctoral students. It has a program for students from disadvantaged backgrounds, many of whom are

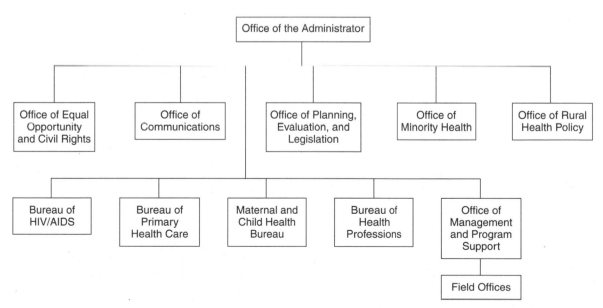

Figure 26–4 U.S. Department of Health and Human Services Health Resources and Services Administration (future).

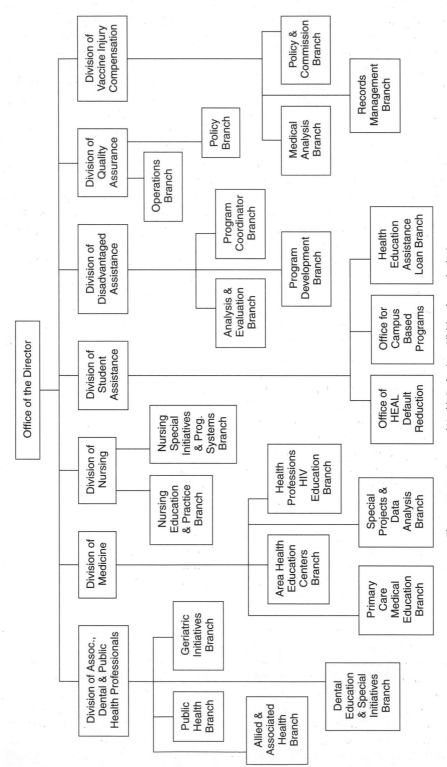

Figure 26–5 Bureau of Health Professions (divisional organization).

from minority groups. It also has money for programs to educate clinical nurse specialists and faculty for nursing schools.

DIVISION OF NURSING. The Division of Nursing also has a statutorily created 21-member National Advisory Council on Nursing Education and Practice (NACNEP) that is broadly representative of nursing education and practice. NACNEP advises the DHHS secretary on matters of policy regarding the NEA. Recent NACNEP papers have addressed the basic registered-nurse work force and the nurse-practitioner work force. Future work will address informatics and other topics of interest to nursing. NACNEP meetings are held several times a year and are open to the public. Time for public comment is provided at NACNEP meetings.

DIVISION OF STUDENT ASSISTANCE. The BHPr also manages the Division of Student Assistance, which runs the Scholarships for Disadvantaged Students (SDS) program. Thirty percent of SDS appropriations are required by law to go to nursing students. In FY 1998, this meant that more than $5 million went to nursing students, most at the baccalaureate level. SDS funds go to financially or educationally disadvantaged students. Schools with more students from underrepresented minority groups than the national average receive additional funds.

Bureau of Primary Health Care. The Bureau of Primary Health Care (BPHC) operates the National Health Service Corps—a scholarship and loan repayment program that places health professionals in "health professional shortage areas" (HPSAs). In FY 1998, this program received $78 million. Nurse practitioners and certified nurse midwives are eligible for this program, and in 1997 62 nurse practitioners and 11 certified nurse midwives received scholarships. The scholarship recipient must agree to serve a minimum of 2 years in the assigned community. The hope is that these professionals will want to stay in the area after their service commitment ends. BPHC also runs the NEA Section 846 program, which provides an education-loan payback for nurses who are willing to serve in an area of nursing shortage, such as rural health clinics,

Indian Health Service centers, and public hospitals. BPHC funds support community health centers, migrant health centers, and homeless and public housing health programs. The agency runs the individual assistance part of the Ryan White Comprehensive AIDS Resources Emergency (CARE) Act program. BPHC sponsors "Models That Work," a competition for privately initiated health service approaches to delivering primary care to underserved populations. In 1996 a nurse-run entity affiliated with the University of Pennsylvania was a winner of this competition. It focused on primary care delivery for a large public housing community. In addition, BPHC determines what areas of the country will be designated as HPSAs.

Bureau of Maternal and Child Health. HRSA's Bureau of Maternal and Child Health manages the Maternal and Child Health Block Grant programs, Healthy Start, emergency medical services for children, and AIDS service to women, infants, children, and youth (Ryan White CARE Act, Title IV).

Office of Rural Health Policy. HRSA's Office of Rural Health Policy (ORHP) is the focal point for answers to questions about rural health access, quality, financing, and data. ORHP manages the Rural Health Outreach Grant program ($32.5 million in FY 1998), which encourages innovative approaches to rural health care delivery in areas without traditional health services. ORHP manages the Rural Telemedicine Grant Program created under Section 330A of the Public Health Service Act. This $4 million program seeks to fund telemedicine networks that will increase rural population health access and will attempt to reduce the feeling of isolation of rural health practitioners. It also provides some funding ($11.7 million in FY 1998) for research on rural health issues. The National Advisory Committee on Rural Health meets three times per year to offer strategies and recommendations for improving health care access for rural residents.

National Institutes of Health and National Institute of Nursing Research. The National Institutes of Health (NIH) is another U.S. Public Health Service agency of major importance. NIH encompasses 19 research entities, including the National Institute of Nursing Research (NINR). NINR began its existence as an NIH Center in 1986. Because of the legislative efforts of the American Association of Colleges of Nursing and other nursing organizations, NINR moved up from center status to an institute in 1993. With appropriations of about $60 million per year, NINR provides grants for external (outside NIH) and intramural (with other NIH entities) nursing research and training of investigators. It leverages its funds by working collaboratively with other NIH entities. NINR's research focus is threefold: health promotion and disease prevention, acute and chronic illness, and nursing systems. These foci touch on reducing the incidence of low birth weight in babies, chronic disease symptom management, pain management, neurological conditions, patient care issues affecting older Americans, and structural care delivery and bioethical issues related to nursing care. Program priorities are women's health, minority health, home health for older adults, and collaboration with other sciences. The 17-member National Advisory Council for Nursing Research advises the NINR director on research matters. The Council meets several times per year, and its meetings are open to the public. NINR's on-line address is *http://www. nih.gov/ninr.* Other NIH entities are important for nursing as well: the National Institute on Aging, the National Cancer Institute, the National Institute of Child Health and Human Development, and the National Genome Research Institute. NIH's hospital, the Warren Magnuson Clinical Center, is a model of quality tertiary care. NIH also houses the National Library of Medicine, home of the MEDLINE research vehicles GratefulMed and PubMed (*http://nlm.nih.gov*).

Agency for Health Care Policy and Research. The Agency for Health Care Policy and Research (AHCPR) is another federal research entity of interest to nursing. AHCPR received $146.4 million in FY 1998. AHCPR's mission is to generate and disseminate information that improves health care delivery. Through its Patient Outcomes Research Teams, AHCPR evaluates effec-

tiveness of treatment strategies. "Evidence-based practice centers" are an initiative to assess the value of new health care technologies. AHCPR has funded the development of a series of clinical practice guidelines, two teams of which (pain and pressure ulcers) were chaired by nurses. In 1997 it created the National Guideline Clearinghouse to share practice guidelines electronically. AHCPR projects seek to discover which health care and medical procedures are cost-effective and have good outcomes. AHCPR is the designated lead agency (together with NINR and the Division of Nursing) to conduct an Institute of Medicine–recommended study of nurse staffing needs in hospitals. In conjunction with the American Academy of Nursing, AHCPR sponsors a senior nurse scholar in the agency to study the integration of clinical nursing care with critical issues of quality, cost, and access to health care. The AHCPR's 16-member National Advisory Council for Health Care Policy, Research, and Evaluation meets several times per year, and the meetings are open to the public. AHCPR's address is *http://www.ahcpr.gov.* A full description of AHCPR's program and grant opportunities can be found there.

Substance Abuse and Mental Health Services Administration. The Substance Abuse and Mental Health Services Administration (SAMHSA; $2.1 billion in FY 1998) is another key U.S. Public Health Service agency. SAMHSA provides services to prevent and to treat mental health problems and substance abuse through its Center for Mental Health Services, Center for Substance Abuse Treatment, and Center for Substance Abuse Prevention. It provides some money for training and research. Each center has an advisory council that meets several times per year. Meetings are open to the public. SAMHSA's web address is *http://www.samhsa.gov.*

Centers for Disease Control and Prevention. The Centers for Disease Control and Prevention (CDC), a DHHS agency, seeks to promote health and quality of life by preventing and controlling disease, injury, and disability ($2.3 billion in FY 1998). CDC has pledged to the public that it will base its public health decisions on scientific data and place the benefits to society above the benefits to the institution, thus giving it the reputation of being public health at its best. Because of CDC's focus on the community (rather than individuals) as its client, nursing's contributions have been many, especially in the establishment of guidelines on infection prevention (e.g., universal precautions and hospital precautions), and the areas of violence, adolescent and school health, infants' and children's health, women's health, and immunizations. CDC's web address is *http://www.cdc.gov.*

Food and Drug Administration. The mission of the Food and Drug Administration (FDA) is safe food and cosmetics, safe and effective medicines and medical devices, and safe products such as microwave ovens. Animal food and drugs also are within FDA control. FDA regulates products worth more than $1 trillion, has 1,100 inspectors and 2,100 scientists, and has jurisdiction over 95,000 businesses. FDA also monitors the effect of drugs that have been approved. Its MedWatch program follows up by advising health professionals with prescription authority about recently discovered effects of the use of approved drugs. MedWatch is important to nurses because they often are the first to learn of adverse drug reactions. FDA is funded by the U.S. Department of Agriculture and received $819.9 million in FY 1997.

Critics of the FDA contend that lives are lost and medical conditions remain unaddressed because the process for approval of new drugs and devices is costly and takes too long. For example, a U.S. House of Representatives report found that approval for a new drug took an average of 12 years and cost $350 million. Often cited are the practices of other countries that act much more quickly. In 1997, legislation to revise FDA procedure and speed up its processes was enacted. The FDA web site is *http://www. fda.gov.*

Indian Health Service. The Indian Health Service (IHS) is a DHHS agency, but the Department of the Interior provides funds for the IHS. The IHS is a $2 billion per year operation that provides hospital, dental, health, substance abuse, public health nursing, and other services to Indian Americans and Alaska Natives. Public health nursing represented $28.1 million of this expenditure in FY 1998. The IHS offers scholarships and loan repayment programs to attract nurses, especially Indian Americans, to practice at IHS hospitals and clinics. The IHS web address is *http://www.tucson.ihs.gov.*

Health Care Financing Administration. The Health Care Financing Administration (HCFA), a DHHS entity, administers the Medicare and Medicaid programs ($164.8 billion in FY 1997). Both programs reimburse providers for providing health care service to more than 72 million eligible beneficiaries. HCFA's mission is to ensure health care for beneficiaries by providing access to affordable and quality health care services; by protecting the rights and dignity of beneficiaries; and by providing clear and useful information to beneficiaries and providers to assist them in making health care decisions.

Medicare, the nation's largest health insurance program, provides insurance to people who are 65 years of age or older, people who are disabled, and people with permanent kidney failure. It provides hospital coverage and helps pay for the cost of physician and nursing services, outpatient hospital services, medical equipment and supplies, and other health services and supplies. Legislation authorizing Medicare and Medicaid is under the jurisdiction of the Senate Finance Committee, the House Ways and Means Committee, and the House Commerce Committee. HCFA's web address is *http://www.hcfa.gov.*

The Medicaid program, a joint venture between the federal and state governments, provides health care assistance for certain individuals and families with low incomes and resources. As a result, coverage and compensation for health-related services vary from state to state. The Omnibus Budget Reconciliation Act of 1989 allowed state Medicaid programs to cover services of certified pediatric nurse practitioners and certified family nurse practitioners. Most state programs have chosen to reimburse those providers.

HCFA also administers Medicare payments for educating medical residents, nurses, and allied health personnel. Since 1965, Medicare payments have been made to hospitals to reimburse a portion of the costs of nurse education to promote quality inpatient care for Medicare beneficiaries. Most are diploma programs, only about 109 of which still exist. Nursing education has shifted almost entirely to community colleges, senior colleges, and universities; yet Medicare reimbursement has not shifted. Nursing organizations are working to urge redirection of Medicare monies to the clinical training of advanced practice nurses, where the demand is more critical. Legislation must be enacted to make this policy change. (For a detailed explanation of the issue, see the vignette on the American Association of Colleges of Nursing's policy effort regarding Medicare funding of graduate nurse education in the Unit V Case Study.)

DEPARTMENT OF EDUCATION

The U.S. Department of Education provides billions of dollars each year for postsecondary education of students, including those in nursing. For many students, professional nursing education would be impossible without Federal Family Education Loans (Stafford Loans), Ford Direct Loans, Pell Grants, Perkins Loans, Federal Work-Study funds, and other programs managed by the Department of Education. Through programs for special populations and vocational education, the Department provides millions of dollars for community college nursing programs. The Department's web address is: *http://www. ed.gov.*

DEPARTMENT OF LABOR

The U.S. Department of Labor enforces the Occupational Safety and Health Act (job safety and health), the Fair Labor Standards Act (minimum wage and overtime laws), and the Employee Retirement Income Security Act (ERISA; requirements for employee benefit and retirement plans). Nursing has had interest for a long while in the Occupational Safety and Health Administration (OSHA), a Department of Labor agency that focuses on workplace issues. Its mission is to save lives and prevent injuries, protecting the health of the American worker. With nurses providing the majority of occupational health care, organized nursing has lobbied to establish the Office of Occupation Health Nursing and to maintain adequate funding for it. Nurses have been dedicated to establishing standards for the workplace (e.g., surveillance of blood-borne pathogens) and to urging OSHA to look at establishing standards for ergonomics and latex toxicology. The American Nurses Association (ANA) has been actively working to protect the health and safety of registered nurses at work for the past 15 years. The nursing community works primarily with the Department of Labor, DHHS, and Department of Education appropriations subcommittees to ensure adequate funding for OSHA's mission. The Department of Labor's web address is *http://www.dol.gov.*

DEPARTMENT OF VETERANS AFFAIRS

The Department of Veterans Affairs (DVA) is the major employer of nursing personnel in the United States. Through the Veterans Health Administration (VHA), the DVA employs more than 59,000 nurses in its 171 VHA-affiliated hospitals and its various clinics or other health care facilities. The VHA is the largest single U.S. employer of entry-level professional nurses and advanced practice nurses. A physician with the title of Undersecretary for Health directs the VHA. The highest-ranking nurse in the VHA has the title of Chief Consultant in the Nursing Strategic Healthcare Group (NSHG). This person advises the undersecretary and other key VHA and DVA officials on issues that relate to nursing in the DVA. The mission of the NSHG is to "function as a Center for Nursing Leadership by providing the linkages and opportunities for the enhancement of innovation and preservation of the caring dimension across the spectrum of Nursing Service Delivery" ("Department of Veterans Affairs Mission Statement," 1997).

The VHA has engaged in a variety of efforts to educate nurses and to promote innovation in the delivery of health care services. Professional nurses in the VHA serve in nursing faculty roles in many academic institutions. Moreover, the clinical settings in the VHA serve as training sites for a wide array of nursing clinicians.

The DVA has faced public pressure to save money and improve care by expanding ambulatory care services and reducing reliance on the traditional hospital. In 1997 the DVA undertook a comprehensive review of its roles in the education of health professionals and the types of resources and services provided to academic institutions that prepare nurses and other health professionals. The NSHG has studied the roles, responsibilities, and scope of utilization of professional nurses in the VHA nursing system. In 1997 the NSHG established the Innovations in Nursing Committee to make recommendations to help facilitate innovative nursing practice and to enhance the nursing presence in the VHA. Individuals from both within and outside the VHA were appointed to this committee by the Undersecretary to provide advice on nontraditional roles for nurses in the VHA.

A second NSHG initiative, the Nurse Qualifications Standards Task Group, studied the education and skill qualifications of the DVA nursing staff. Its charge was to make recommendations regarding the nursing qualifications and skill mix that would best facilitate meeting the DVA health care mission. This task group conducted a detailed review of the health care market in general and the types of nursing care requirements that have emerged for the DVA population served by the VHA. The VHA increasingly has sought to deliver community-based care to veterans and also has seen a growth in the proportion of patients that require geriatric-focused care. The recommendations made by the Nurse Qualifications Standards Task Group have the potential to create a model with a range and scope of innovation for the general health care market.

The VHA is searching for ways to meet the needs of an aging veteran population and to provide a cadre of qualified and experienced primary care providers to meet the general health care needs of the veterans of the VHA

(National Center for Cost Containment, 1997). In 1997 the NSHG looked at the VHA's use of advanced practice nurses (APNs) to provide recommendations on how to meet the VHA goal of increasing the employment of APNs by 200% by the end of 1999. This effort began with a review of the current employment settings, trends, and standards for APNs in the VHA. Marketplace competition for APNs is strong, and the findings of this task group are likely to indicate that aggressive recruitment is needed to increase the number of APNs in the VHA.

The VHA also wants to reform the agreements between the VHA and academic institutions as these organizations partner in the education of professional nurses. These agreements, termed "academic affiliation agreements," serve as the guide for the concurrent responsibilities and rights in these partnerships. Academic nursing programs, however, will experience growing pressure to articulate the clear benefits of these partnerships to the DVA. The forces driving the larger health care market are also now affecting the VHA, including concerns related to costs, efficiency, and effectiveness. They have produced pressures in the DVA sponsored health care facilities to assess all partnerships. Academic partnerships in the future likely will be required to develop clear links to the goals of improving efficiency and effectiveness of nursing care and to the goal of lowering the cost of health care delivery. The VHA has the Special Medical Advisory Group to advise the Secretary of the VA and the Undersecretary for Health relating to the care and treatment of veteran health; this body typically includes one or more nursing professionals.

The DVA has affiliation agreements for clinical training of nursing students with many schools of nursing. In the past, the DVA offered a variety of programs such as upward mobility and scholarships to provide financial support for nursing students who would later come to work for the agency. There was even a program for the DVA to pay nursing school faculty salaries in areas where the DVA was a major clinical training site and employer of nurses. The DVA has reduced this academic connection to the point where student assistance and support is available mainly to present DVA employees who are upgrading their skills. DVA continues to offer paid and unpaid traineeships for advanced practice nursing students without a service obligation. In addition, the Veterans Affairs Learning Opportunity Residency (VALOR) program for honor students in nursing programs continues. (The DVA nursing web site is *http://www.va.gov/Nursing.*)

Though all the agencies discussed above have a variety of responsibilities, they all are facing increasing pressure to do more with fewer staff and less money. They are interested in solving problems before they reach crisis proportions. And they all are becoming more consumer and client oriented.

SUGGESTION: Select those agencies that have missions relevant to your individual or organizational objectives. Get to know the appropriate staff and program cycles. Lobby for programs and funding (the agencies are prohibited by law from doing that). Work with those in Congress who have jurisdiction over those functions.

THE CONGRESS

The U.S. Senate and the U.S. House of Representatives possess the sole federal legislative power. Whereas the President may promote major policy initiatives, Congress can and often does make its own proposals. And if the will of the Congress is strong enough to override a veto, it can create laws that the President totally opposes. Members of the President's party in Congress often feel free to go their own way on issues because the U.S. Presidency is a weak office. Within the Congress itself, party is less important today because individual members may place their own objectives ahead of those of their party. The days of the well-oiled party machine that keeps everyone in line and cranks out party platform–mandated legislation are over.

Congress does not look like America: there is only one African American senator; she is one of nine female senators (of 100). The House has 51 female members of 435 members, and the number of members of minority groups in the House declined after the 1996 election. In the 105th Congress, there were two nurses, a registered nurse from Texas and a licensed practical nurse from New York, both in the House.

Among its many powers, Congress:

- Reviews the success or failure of legislated program operations (General Accounting Office)
- Conducts hearings on issues that may generate federal legislation
- Drafts legislation
- Estimates cost of proposed legislation (Congressional Budget Office)
- Enacts legislation to create programs (authorization)
- Determines budget levels
- Appropriates funds for federal operations
- Determines tax policy
- Decides entitlement policy (Medicare, Social Security, postsecondary Federal Family Education Loans and Direct Loans)
- Confirms or rejects Presidential nominees for high-level federal posts (Cabinet members, judges, members and some staff of commissions and boards)
- Influences executive agency operations with hearings and personal contact
- Votes to override Presidential vetoes
- Votes to ratify treaties that may affect nursing practice (i.e., the North American Free Trade Agreement)

Congress' legislative work depends on a collection of committees with jurisdiction over federal issues and agencies. Several committees may share jurisdiction of a particular issue, complicating and often slowing down the process. For example, Medicaid legislation in the House must go through the Ways and Means Committee and the Commerce Committee. The committees with jurisdiction over federal policy issues of interest to nurses are as follows:

Senate (Fig. 26–6)

1. *Appropriations Subcommittee on Labor, Health and Human Services, Education, and Related Agencies (of Appropriations Committee)*
   - Nursing Education and Research
   - National Institutes of Health
   - Health Services Research
   - Student Financial Aid
   - Nurse Education Act
   - Scholarships for Disadvantaged Students
   - Occupational Safety and Health Act
   - Affirmative Action and Equal Opportunity
   - Overtime (Fair Labor Standards Act)
   - Retirement (Employee Retirement Income Security Act)
   - Rural Health
   - National Health Service Corps
   - Public Health
   - Centers for Disease Control and Prevention
   - Food and Drug Administration
2. *Appropriations Subcommittee on Interior and Related Agencies (of Appropriations Committee)*
   - Indian Health Service
3. *Appropriations Subcommittee on Defense (of Appropriations Committee)*
   - Military Health Research
   - Uniformed Services University of the Health Sciences nursing program
4. *Budget Committee*
   - Budget issues
5. *Labor and Human Resources Committee*
   - Nursing Research
   - Nurse Education Act
   - Occupational Safety and Health Act
   - Rural Health
   - Public Health
   - Centers for Disease Control and Prevention
   - Substance Abuse and Mental Health Administration
6. *Public Health and Safety Subcommittee (of Labor and Human Resources Committee)*
   - Nursing Education
   - Nursing Student Aid

   - Nurse Education Act
   - Occupational Safety and Health Act
   - National Health Safety Corps
   - Public Health
   - Centers for Disease Control and Prevention
7. *Finance Committee and its Subcommittee on Health Care*
   - Medicare
   - Medicaid
   - Medicare support of:
     - Diploma Nursing Education
     - Graduate Nursing Education
   - Reimbursement for nurse practitioners and clinical nurse specialists (Medicare)
   - Telehealth/telemedicine
8. *Committee on Indian Affairs*
   - Indian Health Service
9. *Acquisition and Technology Subcommittee (of Armed Services Committee)*
   - Military Health Research
10. *Readiness Subcommittee (of Armed Services Committee)*
    - Uniformed Services University of the Health Sciences nursing program
11. *Committee on Veterans Affairs*
    - Veterans Affairs
12. *Veterans Affairs, HUD [Housing and Urban Development], and Related Agencies Subcommittee (of Appropriations Committee)*
    - Veterans Affairs
13. *Subcommittee on Agriculture, Rural Development, and Related Agencies (of Appropriations Committee)*
    - Food and Drug Administration

Other Senate committees and subcommittees of interest include the Aging Subcommittee (of Labor and Human Resources); the Subcommittee on Social Security and Family Policy (of Finance); and the Special Committee on Aging.

House of Representatives (Fig. 26–7)

1. *Subcommittee on Labor, Health and Human Services, Education, and Related Agencies (of Appropriations Committee)*
   - Nursing Education and Research

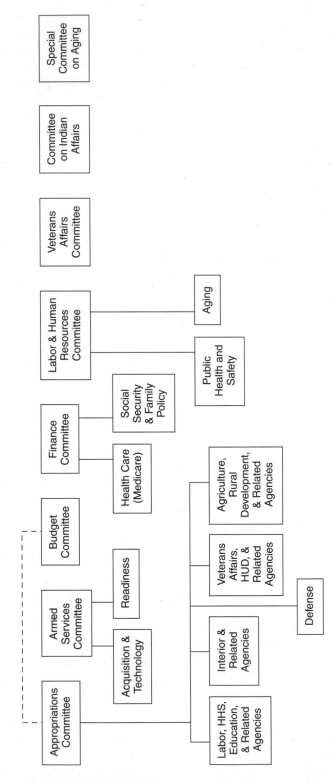

Figure 26-6 Senate committees and subcommittees of interest to nurses.

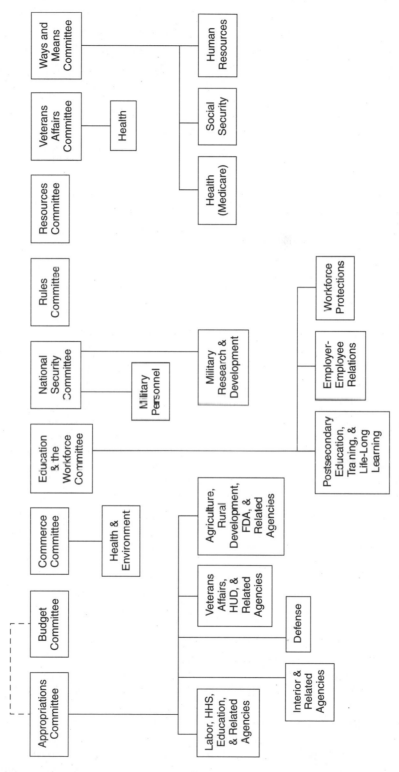

Figure 26-7 House of Representatives committees and subcommittees of interest to nurses.

- National Institutes of Health
- Health Services Research
- Student Financial Aid
- Nurse Education Act
- Scholarships for Disadvantaged Students
- Occupational Safety and Health Act
- Affirmative Action and Equal Opportunity
- Overtime (Fair Labor Standards Act)
- Retirement (Employee Retirement Income Security Act)
- Rural Health
- National Health Service Corps
- Public Health
- Centers for Disease Control and Prevention
- Food and Drug Administration

2. *Subcommittee on Interior and Related Agencies (of Appropriations Committee)*
   - Indian Health Service
3. *Subcommittee on Defense (of Appropriations Committee)*
   - Military Health Research
   - Uniformed Services University of the Health Sciences nursing program
4. *Committee on the Budget*
   - Budget issues
5. *Health and Environment Subcommittee (of Commerce Committee)*
   - Nursing Education
   - Nursing Research
   - National Institutes of Health
   - Health Services Research
   - Nursing Student Aid
   - Nurse Education Act
   - Scholarships for Disadvantaged Students
   - Rural Health
   - National Health Service Corps
   - Public Health
   - Centers for Disease Control and Prevention
   - Food and Drug Administration
   - Substance Abuse and Mental Health Administration
6. *Postsecondary Education, Training, and Life-Long Learning Subcommittee (of Education and the Workforce Committee)*
   - Student Financial Aid

7. *Employer-Employee Relations Subcommittee (of Education and the Workforce Committee)*
   - Occupational Safety and Health
   - Affirmative Action and Equal Opportunity
   - Retirement (Employee Retirement Income Security Act)
8. *Workforce Protections Subcommittee (of Education and the Workforce Committee)*
   - Overtime (Fair Labor Standards Act)
9. *Committee on Resources*
   - Indian Health Service
10. *Committee on Rules*
    - Rules
11. *Health Subcommittee (of Veterans Affairs Committee)*
    - Veterans Affairs
12. *Health Subcommittee (of Ways and Means Committee)*
    - Medicare support of:
      - Diploma Nursing Education
      - Graduate Nursing Education
    - Reimbursement for nurse practitioners and clinical nurse specialists (Medicare)
    - Telehealth/telemedicine
13. *Social Security Subcommittee (of Ways and Means Committee)*
14. *Human Resources Subcommittee (of Ways and Means Committee)*
15. *Military Personnel Subcommittee (of National Security Committee)*
    - Uniformed Services University of the Health Sciences nursing program
16. *Military Research and Development Subcommittee (of National Security Committee)*
    - Military Health Research
17. *Veterans Affairs, HUD [Housing and Urban Development], and Related Agencies Subcommittee (of Appropriations Committee)*
    - Veterans Affairs
18. *Subcommittee on Agriculture, Rural Development, Food and Drug Administration, and Related Agencies (of Appropriations Committee)*
    - Food and Drug Administration

House and Senate committee rosters can be obtained from their respective web sites (*http://*

www.house.gov/ and *http://www.senate/gov/).* Member office information, biographies, and E-mail addresses are also available on the Web sites. (Because committee and subcommittee jurisdictions change, it is wise to double-check before taking the time to arrange a visit, call, or send an E-mail message or letter.)

Legislative Policy Development

No matter what the subject, the professional staff of the Congressional committee or subcommittee that handles the issue probably knows more about that issue than the senator, representative, or anyone on that member's personal staff. Thus the discussion of technical matters about how a program works or does not work should first be directed to committee staff. On the other hand, the senator or representative and his or her personal staff certainly know more about what the thinking on that issue is or might be back in the home state or Congressional district. Similarly, information about a problem in the Congressional district or state that might need a federal solution should be brought first to the member or the personal staff.

Another general principle that applies to policy initiatives is that unless an issue is very important back in the home state or district, or the senator or representative is on a committee or subcommittee with jurisdiction over that issue, he or she won't care very much about it. The lawmaker might appear to care if the person discussing the issue is a constituent but will do little to move the issue. A constituent focusing on a member of the committee with jurisdiction is the most powerful connection; a nonconstituent focusing on an issue outside the member's frame of reference (committee or subcommittee assignment or home state or district) has the least impact.

SUGGESTION: Even sound information and logical presentations will have no effect unless the presenter offers material in a way relevant to the listener. This may involve looking at the health needs of the state or Congressional district, discovering that a serious health problem in the senator's family has turned him or her into an advocate or enemy of an aspect of care delivery, or framing the information to give a national view of its importance and cost. Everyone's view of health issues is not identical, so avoid telling everyone, whatever his or her interests, the same story. Instead, consider the person's frame of reference and cast the message accordingly.

Congressional Agencies

Performing a function similar to the Office of Management and Budget, the Congressional Budget Office analyzes legislative proposals to determine what, if any, costs they would generate if enacted into law. Congress' General Accounting Office, headed by the Comptroller General of the United States, reviews the operation of legislated programs to determine whether they are meeting their statutory objectives. The Library of Congress serves as a public repository of books and other materials and is open to the public. Its on-line reference service, THOMAS *(http://thomas.loc.gov),* provides legislative and other information relating to the legislative process. The Library's Congressional Research Service is available only to members of Congress to conduct in-depth studies of issues relating to legislative concerns. The Government Printing Office prints official documents, the *Congressional Record,* compiled laws, the *Federal Register* (available on-line at *http://www.gpo.ucop.edu),* and other federal materials.

Legislative Process

AUTHORIZATION

Authorization, the Congressional procedure to create or to extend programs, starts the program and then, for renewal, occurs every 3 to 5 years for most federal programs. Congress does not want a program to run without a periodic review of whether it is attaining its statutory objective. So it provides a 3-year life, after which time the program expires and must be renewed (reauthorized). This process can include hearings, reports from the General Accounting Office on the effectiveness or weakness of the program, outreach by committee staff for input from affected publics, and the like. At some point, a draft bill will be prepared, usually at the subcommittee level, followed by a markup (member's changes) and movement to the full committee, a report, a floor vote, and then referral to the other body. The other body may act on that bill or produce its own bill. If the two bills are not similar, differences must be resolved before the bill can be sent to the President. Authorization bills can start in either the House or Senate. For example, in the 104th Congress, a bill (S. 555) to reauthorize the Nurse Education Act went through hearings and passage in the Senate but failed to pass the House.

The theory is that a program that has expired cannot receive appropriations, but if an unauthorized program is on the path to reauthorization, it can be funded and can operate under the terms of its expired authority. Supporters of an unauthorized program, however, always fear that the absence of authorization could terminate program funding. Thus the program proponents strive to get authorization. (For example, the Nurse Education Act's authority expired with the beginning of FY 1995 on October 1994, but Congress continued its appropriations for FY 1995, FY 1996, FY 1997, and FY 1998. This enabled the Act to continue to function as support for nursing education programs and students. At the same time, there was progress in the 105th Congress, first session, but not success, toward a reauthorization of the Act and HPSA Title VII programs.)

BUDGET CYCLES

The House and Senate budget committees have the responsibility to prepare an overall federal budget by April 15 each year. The budget committees have an odd role: they decide spending ceilings for various federal government functions (health is Function 550; education is Function 500) and make allocations to the appropriations committees for those functions. However, the budget committees cannot prevent the appropriations committees from funding a particular program as long as the appropriations committees do not exceed the budget commit-

tees' ceiling set for that function. Sometimes a budget committee offers a list of programs for which it is not providing money and is promptly ignored by appropriators.

APPROPRIATIONS

Appropriations activity begins in the spring each year with hearings in the House and Senate appropriations committees. Each has 13 subcommittees with jurisdiction over all aspects of federal spending and revenue raising. The goal is to complete action on spending bills by September 30, when the new fiscal year begins. The Constitution requires that all spending bills begin in the House, so House procedures start first. After hearings, a bill is developed in an appropriations subcommittee and drafted in formal legislative language by the Office of Legislative Counsel. A key factor is the chairman's mark, those programs that the subcommittee chair has selected to be priorities in the funding language. Then a markup is held to give subcommittee members an opportunity to make changes in the draft bill. If the changes are accepted and the bill is passed, it moves to the full appropriations committee. Next, a report is prepared describing the funding levels and why particular choices were made. Appropriations reports often provide specific instructions as to how the funds are to be spent and what the committee's priorities are. If approved by the full appropriations committee, the bill moves to the floor for a vote. (In the House, a bill must also go before the Rules Committee.) If the other body is able to complete its similar procedure, after floor passage, a conference between the House and Senate will be held to resolve differences in the two bills. If the bills are identical, the bill will be sent to the President for signature or veto. Once the differences have been resolved, and each body has voted to accept the report on the conference agreement, the bill can be sent to the President.

SUGGESTION: Know the schedule and participate in the authorization and appropriations process for programs important to you. Work with the agency and increase your leverage by being a part of a larger coalition in favor of similar goals.

Input from the public to Congress and the President gives them valuable and detailed information about how federal programs affect particular populations and sectors of the health care delivery system in cities, towns, and rural communities across the country. Knowledge about policy and agencies alone is not enough.

THE JUDICIAL BRANCH

Judges are not supposed to make policy, but sometimes judicial interpretations of the Constitution or various laws have a policy effect. The U.S. court system consists of 94 federal district courts (each state has at least one; some have more), 13 U.S. circuit courts of appeals, the U.S. Supreme Court, and a number of other, specialized courts to deal with customs, patents, military cases, and the like. District courts are trial courts that may only indirectly affect health care policy. Courts of appeals resolve questions regarding agency regulations and may reach policy issues. The Supreme Court provides the ultimate interpretation of federal statutes and the Constitution. Beyond the federal system are state regulatory and court systems that may have a direct effect on nursing practice and reimbursement issues. (See Chapter 23.)

SUGGESTION: Those who are not parties to a particular judicial action, but who would be affected by the decision, may be able to provide valuable assistance to a court. Such concerned individuals or groups may be allowed to file a brief *amicus curiae* (friend of the court), offering additional contextual information about the issue facing the court.

CONCLUSION

The federal government plays an important role in nursing education, practice, and research. Although the amount of federal funds spent on nursing is small compared with the total federal budget and with the amount of money coming from the private sector and state governments, the federal funds provide seed money for initiatives that address current health care problems and research issues, and for changes in educational focus to meet the health care system's need for differently trained nursing professionals.

REFERENCES

Department of Veterans Affairs Mission Statement. (1997). Available: http://www.va.gov/nursing.

Fox, D. M. (1996). The political history of health workforce policy. In M. Osterweis, C. J. McLaughlin, H. Manasse, Jr., & C. J. Hopper (Eds.), *The U.S. health workforce: Power, politics and policy* (p. 31). Association of Academic Health Centers.

National Center for Cost Containment, Department of Veterans Affairs. (April 1997). *Utilization of advanced practice nurses (APN): Education levels, demographics, practice patterns, barriers to practice, job satisfaction.* Milwaukee: Author.

Reinhardt, U. E. (1996). The economic and moral case for letting the market determine the health workforce. In M. Osterweis, C. J. McLaughlin, H. Manasse, Jr., & C. J. Hopper (Eds.), *The U.S. health workforce: Power, politics and policy* (pp. 3–14). Washington, DC: Association of Academic Health Centers.

VIGNETTE
Rising to the Top: An Interview with Sheila Burke
Judith K. Leavitt

Sheila Burke is a nurse whose career at the highest levels of national policy and politics spanned 20 years. She probably has been closer to the seat of national power than any nurse in the last decades of the twentieth century. At the time of this interview, Sheila was serving as executive dean of the John F. Kennedy School of Government at Harvard University. She shares her perspective and lessons learned during her years in the Senate, to enlighten readers to the nuances and realities that such a position provides. Her hope is that more nurses will follow her journey.

Sheila began her career in public policy after graduation from the University of San Francisco School of Nursing. After graduation she worked as a staff nurse at Alta Bates Hospital, in Berkeley, California. Because of her experience as president of the California Student Nurses Association, she was recruited to New York to become director of program and field services for the National Student Nurses Association (NSNA). In that capacity she learned much about the policy process and grassroots organizing and mobilized students around nursing and health policy issues. She was mentored by organizational leaders within the NSNA and the National League for Nursing, as well as through the American Nurses Association. Subsequently Sheila decided to pursue graduate education. As she was preparing to leave NSNA, she was contacted by Congressional staff in Washington, D.C., whom she had come to know, and told that Senator Robert Dole was seeking to hire someone with expertise in health policy. She was encouraged to apply. Although Sheila knew little about the Senator except that he was a Republican and she a Democrat, and although she knew even less about Washington, she decided to interview for the position. Thus began a relationship that brought Sheila to what many in the media and policymaking termed the "most powerful staff position on Capitol Hill."

Lesson 1: Take Advantage of Unique Opportunities—However Unexpected. They May Never Come Again

Lesson 2: Timing is Everything—It Is Being in the Right Place at the Right Time

How did this rise to such a powerful position happen? Sheila's career and job responsibilities paralleled those of Senator Dole. When Dole was the junior Senator from Kansas, Sheila was his staff person. When the Senator became Ranking Member on the Senate Finance Committee, Sheila became deputy staff director, and finally, when he became Majority Leader in the Senate, she became first his deputy chief of staff and then his chief of staff. At the time she was one of only two nurses who served as chief of staff in the Senate. (The other was Mary Wakefield, who served Senators Quentin Burdick and Kent Conrad, of North Dakota.) During Senator Dole's campaign for the 1996 Presidency, Sheila served as a senior policy adviser and coordinated the debate preparations.

She describes life as a staffer as first and foremost being responsible to the Senator. "As a staffer, one is only as powerful as the person whom you serve." Her authority and influence came from the positions that Senator Dole occupied—the most powerful in Congress. Her success derived from staying with the Senator for a long time, from the networks she developed, and from the authority and independence that he gave. Clearly she had his full support and confidence, which enabled her to develop her own negotiating, administrative, and policy skills and influence.

Lesson 3: Referent Power Is a Vital Means to Move Policy Issues

As chief of staff, Sheila was in charge of the Senator's office personnel. That enabled her to influence workplace policy. For instance, she instituted a "family and medical leave" policy before it became federal law. However, her primary responsibility to the Senator entailed gathering and sorting through all pertinent information he needed to be able to make decisions about policy issues. To do so meant presenting competing points of view that facilitated his ability not only to make the best decisions but also to be prepared for the opposition. As part of the process, she would share her opinion on issues; sometimes the Senator agreed and sometimes he did not, but he always listened and respected her perspective. Ultimately the decisions were his to make, and it was his accountability to his constituents that mattered most. One such example was the Senator's position on reproductive choice. Sheila supported the prochoice position; the Senator was antiabortion. Sheila was able to voice her opinion, but it was the Senator's decision that counted—and it was her responsibility ultimately to support his decision. Her entire job was to help the Senator achieve *his* policy agenda.

Lesson 4: The Public Focus and Responsibility Is on the Elected Policymaker; It Must Never Be on the Staff

"To be in the Oval Office of the White House with the President and Vice President of the United States and a few selected leaders in Congress, when history is made, is an extraordinary opportunity," says Sheila. She related many such experiences as part of the "highs" of her position. To be 1 of 10 people with the President when final budget decisions were made, or when domestic and foreign policy crises arose, enabled her to be part of the process. She participated with Presidents Reagan, Bush, and Clinton during such historic occasions. She derived both personal and professional satisfaction from involvement in health policy issues such as legislation expanding home- and community-based health care; hospice care; and Medicare coverage for advanced practice nurses, including nurse midwives and nurses practicing in rural areas.

As special as such experiences were, Sheila painfully remembers other times, when her role as staffer was filled with disappointment. The demise of catastrophic health insurance, which she had worked so diligently to create, and the battles over health care reform and welfare legislation, left her frustrated. Personally, her role as chief of staff meant that she had moved from a position of anonymity to one of public scrutiny. Often her designation as "most powerful staffer on the Hill" had negative connotations. Reading about herself in the newspaper, with no ability to respond to inaccuracies and innuendos, was difficult to bear. She had to confront personal loss and death, especially traumatic when one is in the public arena. How did she do so in the public arena? The same way any of us does: she turned to friends and family for support. Sheila had the advantage of a boss who was consistently supportive.

Any demanding job requires sacrifice. This is especially true for staffers in Congress. Family and personal needs must often become secondary to the competing demands of work. With three small children (all born while she worked for the Senator), she claims she was never without guilt about her choices of time spent. Too many nights, especially during budget negotiations, she would run home to put the children to bed and then return to the Senate to work until midnight. The job meant limiting her social life, limiting her nursing involvement, and sacrificing time with her spouse. Sheila acknowledges how fortunate she was to be able to have help with her children and a family that accepted her job commitments. In addition, she had the option to stay home when it was necessary to care for her children. The Senator never questioned her decisions to do so.

Lesson 5: A Support Network Is Essential to Share the Celebrations and Ease the Disappointments of a Job in Public View

How does one balance one's identity as a nurse with responsibility as a staffer? For Sheila, the answer was always clear. Although she believes that she always approaches issues from a nursing perspective, her primary responsibility in the Senate was to her boss, to whom she owed her full support. What was often difficult, was that organized nursing did not present a united front on many issues. For instance, Sheila often met with nurses from Kansas whose position on health policy issues differed from that of the American Nurses Association. For the Senator, his constituents in Kansas mattered most. Politically, the Senator's positions often differed from those of the national nursing organizations. Again, Sheila's responsibility was to support the Senator. However, Sheila was often able to work closely with her nursing colleagues. One of her most positive memories was the support for Medicare coverage of advanced practice nurses in rural areas. The Senator, with Sheila's strong endorsement, took a leadership role in championing the legislation. Clearly it is easier and more effective for members of Congress to respond to nursing issues when there is consensus from different nursing organizations. Without consensus, nurses make it easier for policymakers to respond to separate interests.

Lesson 6: Limited Collective Action Enhances the Likelihood of Legislative Success

How does nursing prepare one for practice in public policy? Sheila identified five essential skills that are easily transferable and ensure competence in public policy:

1. **Communication:** the ability to impart complex information both verbally and through writing, in a clear and simple way. Sheila compares the process to patient teaching. In the public arena it is imparting complex information and ideas to folks who have limited knowledge and experience with the issues.
2. **Active listening:** the ability to concentrate on complex information and negotiations, identify covert needs and concerns, and process the interactions.
3. **Consensus building:** the ability to work with disparate viewpoints until consensus is achieved.
4. **Team building:** the ability to create a group effort that incorporates diversity of perspectives, abilities, and strengths.
5. **Strategic planning:** using the "nursing" process in formulation of policy and political goals.

Sheila compares the competing forces in health care institutions to the U.S. Senate. Many of her skills as a nurse were brought to bear in finding ways to maneuver around competing demands and to find ways to resolve issues.

For Sheila, there is so much that needs to be done to improve health care for Americans. When asked what her vision for health care is, she continually refers to the issue of access. "How can the richest nation in the world still have 41 million people without access to health care?" She plans to continue to work to find solutions for how to provide that access and how to finance it. Through her work on the Kaiser Commission to Improve Medicaid and her participation on the Commonwealth Commission on Health Care, she is committed to finding answers.

She believes strongly that nursing, as a profession, must never abandon involvement in the larger health issues: "We must fight to be relevant—relevant to the broader social issues, such as assuring health care for the most vulnerable, the most disenfranchised." The responsibility of professional organizations to educate their members about policy is paramount. Too many nurses are not adequately informed, and yet their voices are needed as policymakers try to sort out such complex issues.

Sheila's strongest advice is for individual nurses to become involved:

1. Become knowledgeable about the relevant health policy issues.
2. Become involved in the debate about the issues.
3. Know your legislators, and enable them to get to know you. Educate them; they usually do not have health care expertise.
4. Actively support those policymakers whose perspectives are similar to yours—in their campaigns, and when elected, as health advisers.
5. *Vote*—the most important action one can take.

In addition, Sheila has advice for nursing organizations:

1. Never burn bridges with policymakers who disagree with your position. You will need to cross the bridge at a future time.
2. Be bipartisan in focus, philosophy, and support.
3. Focus on education—of the public and of nurses. Most of the public still has a limited knowledge of nursing expertise.

As Sheila pursues a new phase in her career, she is guided by her professional education, her incredible experiences in the public arena, and her devotion to the health needs of Americans. She will continue to be a role model for nurses' involvement in public policy.

Chapter 27

POLITICAL APPOINTMENTS

BETTY R. DICKSON

When Lil Peters, ARNP, a psychiatric/mental health nurse, got the call from the Kansas Nurses Association to consider an appointment to the Hospital Closure Commission in her state, she accepted the challenge because she thought her patients should have a voice through her. Lil Peters was convinced that registered nurses should be involved in development of health policy and accepted the appointment. She said: "I wanted to influence the decisions that were made and to protect patients and their families. Nurses are often hesitant to get involved but, having served, I realize we need to participate in the decision-making process."

A political appointment powerfully affects almost every aspect of daily life. Shaping policy through a political appointment constitutes a journey that runs through America's smallest towns, increases in scope at the state level, and reaches its pinnacle through federal appointments, some of which are made at America's most famous address, The White House, 1600 Pennsylvania Avenue. It takes its form in the school board member who makes decisions regarding removal of asbestos from school property or the member of the state board of health who influences decisions regarding immunizations.

Senator Barbara A. Mikulski said: "Nurses must take their values and turn them into national priorities. They must take their beliefs and make them national policy. Your ideals, your values and your beliefs are only dreams unless you translate them into vehicles of real power" (Goldwater & Zuzy, 1990).

When nurses do not step forward to claim important political appointments, to participate on important task forces, or to serve in any influential capacity, someone else does it for them, thus denying the American public access to some of the best decision makers inside and outside of health care.

Lil Peters answered that call, as did Eunice Cole, RN, who is a member of the Board of Nursing Home Administrators in Washington; Linda Gholston, first registered nurse (RN) to chair the Mississippi State Board of Health; Dr. Davina Gosnell, the second RN to serve on the Public Health Council in Ohio; and many other nurses who understand the importance of serving the public.

What motivated them to serve? The four nurses have much in common. All are members of their state nurses associations and were nominated for their respective appointments by their association. Certainly professional involvement is a key motivator, and each potential candidate has personal or professional reasons for considering a political appointment.

Is there something you wish to change or a service you wish to add in your community? Is the local school board spending a disproportionate amount of dollars on administrative salaries instead of teachers' salaries? Is there a need for a school nurse in your child's school? Could your presence on the board change that? Is your ultimate goal eventually to seek political office, and can serving in a political appointment set the stage for future plans? Will serving in a political/public role enhance future advancement in your career? Or do you want to serve out of a sense of responsibility to your family or your profession?

Lil Peters did not seek the appointment to serve on a committee to close hospitals. Terri Roberts, executive director of the Kansas Nurses Association, said: "They were looking for someone who could not be easily swayed, had impeccable credentials, and was a strong person who also knew the hospital business. When we were asked to make a recommendation, my first thought was Lil. She matched all those qualifications and more. She did not disappoint the association. After it was over and two hospitals were closed, we felt that her influence was essential in making the process fair, deliberate and sensitive to the needs of patients and families."

Peters chose to accept the appointment for professional reasons: a concern for her patients and their families. Though she did not consider personal gain as a result of this appointment, certainly her contributions did not go unnoticed. Participation by a respected, qualified nurse in such a capacity turns a favorable spotlight on the nursing profession.

Consider the personal and professional gains of a political appointment. For example, a dean of a school of nursing, appointed to a hospital board, could provide the hospital with extensive nursing expertise, an understanding of the relationship between education and practice, and management and communication skills. In return, the dean would develop a better understanding of the need for more collaboration between faculty and service institutions.

FINDING THE OPPORTUNITIES

How does a nurse determine where the opportunities are? The types of political appointments run the gamut. For instance, a position on the state board of health affords an opportunity to develop policy, whereas an appointment to an election commission is a mechanism for carrying out state law.

Nurses can contribute at many levels, and the appointment doesn't necessarily have to be in health care. Beginning at the community level, nurses could serve on county health boards, task forces on redevelopment, even a local recreation committee to address policies to prevent children from getting hurt on the playing field. Community/county appointments could include the zoning commission, planning commission, hospital boards, boards of education, councils on aging, and economic development—the list is endless, and all these positions affect the quality of life where you live.

At the state level the list is broader. The following are categories of state departments in which citizens are appointed to the various boards that make policy decisions carried out by staff:

- *Licensure and regulatory boards.* It is under this category that you find boards of nursing, which make decisions affecting nursing practice and nursing education.
- *Commerce and economic development.* Tourism, industrial development, or banking could use the expertise of nurses. A nurse's knowledge of the health care system could provide industrial prospects considering relocation with valuable information about what they can expect for their employees' health care.
- *Conservation.* Environmental issues affect the health care of every community. A nurse could provide expertise regarding hazardous waste.
- *Corrections.* Nurses' expert health care knowledge could play a valuable role in policy decisions regarding the health care and education of incarcerated persons.
- *Education.* These boards provide the leadership for every public school district in the state. At this level, nurses could have an impact on policy decisions regarding school nurses, administration of drugs in the school, and health curriculum. A nurse's knowledge of budgeting and cost-effective management could benefit financial planning for school budgets.
- *Higher education.* Policy decisions at this level have an impact on all schools of nursing within the state. One example is the Mississippi

State College Board's approval of a request that changed the University of Southern Mississippi (USM) School of Nursing—previously a part of the university's College of Health and Human Sciences—into the USM College of Nursing, reflecting the growth in quantity and quality of nursing students on that campus.

- *Health and human services.* Policy boards in this category include public health, Medicaid, and mental health. These categories provide the most logical and frequent arena in which nurses serve.
- *Public safety.* Seat belt laws and seat belt requirements for children are determined in this division in most states, and nurses who have seen the destruction caused by nonuse can bring a significant perspective.
- *Transportation.* Policy regarding the size of trucks or dual trailer loads traveling the highways affects the safety of other travelers. Again, nurses have seen at first hand the impact of accidents involving these large vehicles.

These are only a few examples of the impact nurses can have through political appointments. Careful investigation within your state will provide the necessary information regarding each state department and the issues to be considered.

Identify the position or appointment that you wish to pursue. Finding information about such positions differs from state to state. In many states the governor's office publishes a manual on governmental appointments. In others, listings can be found in the secretary of state's office. Many states have on-line services via the Internet. Ask those friends you helped elect to public office for help. Call the agency in which you wish to serve. If it is a community appointment, contact the mayor or the county or district administrator.

Most state nurses associations, specialty organizations, and other professional organizations outside of nursing have appointment information. Your own legislator will assist a constituent in seeking this information. Other sources might be nonpartisan organizations like the League of Women Voters. There may be coalitions, such as Women in Government, to appoint specific persons to positions. Political parties may be responsible for some appointments.

DECIDING TO SERVE

The National Women's Political Caucus's *A Guide to Running a Winning Campaign* (1997) was designed for candidates seeking election to office but is a good resource for decision making for a political appointment. First, know there is always some level of hesitancy in deciding to serve. Personal questions must be resolved as part of the decision-making process:

- Can you take time away from your job or your family to meet the demands of the position?
- Will your employer support you?
- Will there be family support?

These questions must be answered with positive responses before one seriously considers pursuing a political appointment.

Then consider the following:

1. Why do you want to serve in this position? A good candidate is able to articulate why she is qualified for the job and why she should receive the appointment.
2. What are the strengths and weaknesses you would bring to the position? A candidate for a political appointment should have the ability to project her strengths and to minimize the weaknesses in presenting a good case for her candidacy.
3. What is your relationship to the community? Do you know your neighbors? Have you served in volunteer organizations? Having a solid base of support from your neighbors, your friends, and your fellow volunteers in local organizations will enhance your chances of success.
4. Where do you fit in the political spectrum? Are you a Democrat, Republican, or Independent? Party affiliation provides important linkages to valuable support from individuals and groups.
5. What is your education, background, and experience? Candidates should be able to

identify aspects of each that will qualify them for the position.

6. How is your health, family, and financial situation? Careful analysis should be given to each. Call a meeting of family members and have a frank discussion about their involvement in and commitment to your aspirations. Their support is as essential as being in good health and being able financially to serve.

Positive answers to all questions should not necessarily be the deciding factor. One nurse told me that she agonized over similar questions before deciding to be a candidate for a school board position. She listed the pros and cons on a sheet of paper. After making her list, the "cons" were longer than the "pros." She tore up the paper, tossed it aside, and simply said, "I've just got to do this!" And she did.

MATCHING THE CANDIDATE TO THE POSITION

In deciding on a position, consider the following:

1. Who makes the appointment? Is it the governor, the lieutenant governor, Speaker of the House of Representatives?
2. Are there educational or geographic requirements? In Mississippi the nurse practice act requires a baccalaureate degree as the basic degree for one board position and an associate degree as the basic degree for another. One position is designated for an advanced practice nurse, and another for a nurse educator. It also requires that each congressional district be represented. Many appointments require certain credentials (e.g., a physician or a nurse).
3. How often will meetings be held? If the meetings are on Saturday, will this impede your ability to serve? Will your employer provide the time for you to serve, or will you be required to take vacation time? What is the amount of time required?
4. Who are the stake holders who care about who gets this position, and what influence do you have with them?

5. Identify the qualifications needed for the appointment. Determine whether there is a match between your qualifications and the stipulations of the position. Carefully review the state or federal laws applicable to the appointment.
6. Do you have a chance of getting the position? What connections do you have with individuals and organizations that will make the decision?

THE IMPORTANCE OF POLITICAL AFFILIATION

Many states require party registration, and others do not. How active are you in your political party? Are you registered? Did you work on behalf of your party's candidates? A positive answer to these questions will identify you as an active party affiliate and will greatly influence the chances of a political appointment in an administration with the same party affiliation. When asked the secret to getting appointed, Barbara Lumpkin, political director of the Florida Nurses Association, was succinct: "Pick the right governor." Lumpkin is currently serving on the Florida Medicaid Reform Task Force. She attributes the Florida Nurses Association's political appointment success to a strong political action committee (PAC), which was established with a dues checkoff as part of membership in the association. The functions of PACs are addressed in Chapter 33; here it is important to note the usefulness of PACs in securing political appointments. They generally don't make the nomination (the parent organization does so), but having a strong PAC supporting your efforts strengthens your position.

THE ROLE OF ORGANIZATIONS

Each state nurses association, advocacy group, or specialty group differs in its methods of nominating candidates for political appointments. Working through an organized process facilitates the selection. For example, the Ohio Nurses Association (ONA) has a committee on qualifications to determine whether candidates are a match for certain positions in that state.

Dr. Davina Gosnell, RN, PhD, FAAN, dean of Kent State University School of Nursing, is serving her state in a 7-year-term on the Ohio Public Health Council. She was nominated by the ONA and is the second nurse to serve in that position. The membership of that board had consisted of six physicians and a pharmacist before the ONA pushed to change the law to mandate a nurse member on the board. Dr. Gosnell was the second nurse to serve in that position; the first was a nurse attorney. Earlier in her career, Dr. Gosnell was an employee of the state health department and had a keen understanding of the role of public health. She also was a consultant in home care and had worked in that capacity in all 88 counties of Ohio, thus ensuring her a large network of professional colleagues.

Working through the ONA, Dr. Gosnell was interviewed by the association's committee on qualifications as the committee looked for a match in the following categories: party affiliation, connections, and past political activity. Because she was a good match, her name was recommended to the ONA board and the appointment process began.

With Lil Peters, party affiliation was not important, but in the case of Davina Gosnell, it was necessary. Her governor is a Republican, as is she.

Carol Jenkins, ONA executive director, said that her association is actively involved in getting members appointed to various positions. Every RN member of the board of nursing was nominated by ONA. Jenkins added, "Because we have a system in place, we know immediately of ongoing appointments and have been successful in ensuring that our members are appointed."

Most candidates must undergo a careful review by the office making the appointment. In Mississippi, candidates for the board of nursing and other political appointments made by the Republican administration are often checked at the county level for their party affiliation, and approval is requested from the county chairman and legislators in that community. It is essential to know who these people are and to ask up front for their support. It is also important to keep key persons informed and to maintain effective communication with them. Once the appointment is made, occasional contact with these persons will ensure a favorable endorsement for other appointments.

GETTING NOMINATED

After the qualifications have been met, the next step is getting nominated. State statutes identify who can nominate persons to certain positions. North Carolina is the only state where nurses are elected to the board of nursing. Most other states do so by appointment. Consider which organizations can nominate by statute in your state. Are you a member of that organization? Find out about the organization's nomination process and express your desire to be a candidate through a personal letter including your resumé. Your letter should articulate how you meet the qualifications for the position. If nominations are not necessary from identified organizations, mail your letter to the agency head or to the governor. Always copy or fax the letter to your legislator.

Having the support of more than one organization strengthens your chance for nomination. Linda Gholston, RN, was nominated for her position on the Mississippi State Board of Health by the Mississippi Hospital Association with cooperation from the Mississippi Nurses Association (MNA). In 1990 she became the first nurse appointed to the Mississippi State Board of Health. During her first term, she served 2 years as the first nurse and first woman to chair what in years past had been an all-physician board. Gholston made further history when, after her initial appointment by a Democratic governor, she was reappointed by a Republican governor, thereby serving under two administrations with different political parties.

"MNA nominated me for a second term," said Gholston. "Many considered that second term unprecedented because of the Republican governor's option not to reappoint those of us who were originally appointed by a Democrat." But Gholston's reputation as a leader secured her another term on the board. One of her accomplishments was initiating the first board retreat. She invited another nurse, from the Texas Department of Health, to facilitate the 2-day event. "The strongest outcome of that retreat was to learn to function as a board. Board members began to see that our responsibility was to set policy, as opposed to micromanagement of the department. And they were led through that process by nurses. It also led to a better board-staff relationship."

Today the Mississippi State Board of Health is composed of three nurses, several physicians, and several lay persons. Many in the nursing community credit the increase of nursing appointments to Gholston's leadership. Because she was so eminently qualified, she opened the door for other nurses to serve. When the Mississippi legislature passed the statute regulating health maintenance organizations, the fiscal responsibility regulation was assigned to the insurance department and the quality segment to the department of health. Gholston was later appointed to a committee of the board that will recommend standards for quality assurance for health maintenance organizations. This committee assignment continues to ensure nursing's influence in this critical aspect of health care.

Moving the Nomination

Once your name has been placed in nomination, it's time to rally every political connection available. Identify your personal, political, and professional networks. Ask contacts in those networks to write letters on your behalf. Furnish these people with a sample letter of your qualifications and include the correct title, address, and telephone and fax numbers of the person responsible for making the appointment. Make this process as easy as possible for your supporters.

With the backing of the Washington State Nurses Association (WSNA), Eunice Cole, past president of the American Nurses Association

and of WSNA, was appointed to numerous positions throughout her long career, including the Washington State Public Health Improvement Board.

"Nurses can provide leadership skills; they are good listeners, and their care and concern for patients and the public at large are legend," said Cole, who retired in the spring of 1997. She continues to serve the public in retirement through her recent appointment by the governor to the Washington State Board of Nursing Home Administrators. She was nominated by WSNA and supported throughout the process.

Preparing for Confirmation

Before confirmation, it is essential to know the job description and expectations of the position.

If there is notification of a confirmation hearing by a legislative body after your provisional nomination, it is important to know what will be expected. Ask these questions:

- What do I need to bring?
- What questions will I be asked?
- Should I have representation or sponsorship at the confirmation hearing?

Usually the candidate will be notified by the agency of meeting dates, agendas, and task forces on which you will be expected to serve.

Once Appointed—Relationship With Supporters

Once you are appointed, what is your allegiance to those who put you there? It is critical to thank your supporters, including your legislators. If yours is a public appointment, your allegiance must be to the constituents served. If it's to a hospital board, your responsibility is to the patients and your community. It is important that you retain your autonomy if the appointment is of a regulatory nature, in which issues of confidentiality must be considered.

However, if your state nurses association or another group was instrumental in your nomination and subsequent appointment, it is a good idea to meet with the board or staff members periodically to keep them informed and listen to their concerns. If your assignment is to represent a specific group on a task force where input from the organization was requested as a part of the appointment, close communication is necessary to convey the ideas of your supporters to the task force.

Organizational Support–Using Coalitions

One of the most influential coalitions at the federal level is the *Coalition for Women's Appointments,* through the National Women's Political Caucus Leadership Development, Education and Research Fund, in Washington, D.C. The purpose of this coalition is to promote women for top-level policymaking positions in the federal government. Members of the coalition share the believe that, regardless of the outcome of the November elections, unprecedented opportunities are present for women, and it is in the nation's interest for women to participate in greater numbers at the highest levels of our government. The coalition is committed to seeking out women of every racial and ethnic group, of all ages and income levels, and from every part of the country.

The member organizations of the Coalition for Women's Appointments reflect the diversity of women in their professional lives, areas of expertise, and ethnic and racial backgrounds. Eleven bipartisan task forces are organized by substantive areas of government service. They consist of representatives of member organizations as well as individuals who bring knowledge and expertise to this effort.

The primary focus of the coalition and its task forces is on those full-time jobs for which the President nominates and the Senate must confirm—Cabinet secretaries, undersecretaries, assistant secretaries, agency directors, commission heads, and federal judges, among others. The typical nominee will have exceptional professional qualifications as well as strong political ties.

The task forces are charged with recommending to the coalition the prospective nominees that they deem most qualified and appropriate for Presidential appointments. The recommendations of the task forces will be considered and acted on by the full coalition. Those women selected for support by the coalition will then be actively promoted and assisted in achieving the top positions for which they qualify. Additionally, applicants will indicate whether they would like to be referred for corporate and state positions. The coalition will maintain a database of qualified women interested in these positions.

This group has worked since 1976 to gain access to the Presidential appointments process for qualified women. The efforts of the Appointments Project, the first of its kind, increased the number of women appointed to the senior-level positions in the Carter Administration to 13.5%, an increase over the Ford Administration. The effort to increase the percentage of qualified women appointees continued through the Reagan and Bush Administrations, with a high of 20% during the Bush Administration. In 1992, President Clinton set a record when over one third of his selections for top 400 Senate-confirmed positions were women. [Coalition for Women's Appointments, 1997, p. 1]

The American Nurses Association (1997) prepared a document entitled *Seeking Federal Appointment: A Guide for Nurses.* It outlines valuable criteria for seeking a federal appointment, including reasons that nurses should consider serving. "It is no surprise that officials often look for more than professional ability and topical expertise in filling posts. A demonstrated commitment to the elected official's goals—such as participation in his/her campaign—can be a very important factor in obtaining an appointment" (American Nurses Association, 1997).

EXAMPLES OF NURSES APPOINTED

Pat Ford-Roegner, RN, MSW, regional director of the U.S. Department of Health and Human Services, manages the Office of the Secretary in eight states.

Ford-Roegner's appointment came during the first term of the Clinton Administration. She attributes her success in obtaining a federal appointment to having years of national political experience: she knew key staff in the Department of Health and Human Services through the Clinton Campaign and through her role as political director of the American Nurses Association. She had strong affiliations with women's organizations, nursing, labor, and others in the health care field, and they were key to her appointment. She said: "Those groups comprise quite a large constituency. Federal appointments in the Clinton Administration required support from both the cabinet secretary and the White House through the White House Personnel Office. Many of those with whom I had worked during the Presidential campaign were working in the office of First Lady Hillary Clinton. They were instrumental in ensuring that my application went through the process."

Letters of support on behalf of Ford-Roegner's nomination came from members of Congress, labor, women, nurses, and physicians and were considered extremely important in securing this key appointment.

Ford-Roegner stated: "I think most people are surprised at how few appointments are available, which makes it important for the candidate to be very specific about the position in which one is interested. In my case, I indicated that I would take a regional appointment and identified specific positions in which I was interested. Homework is essential. Nurse candidates should not be hesitant about the follow-up process. I called weekly to check on the progress of my appointment."

Although Ford-Roegner's appointment was to a full-time position with the federal government, nurses do not have to be in full-time positions to influence policy. American Nurses Association President Beverly Malone, PhD, RN, FAAN, Mary Wakefield, PhD, RN, FAAN, member of the Virginia Nurses Association and former chief of staff for North Dakota Senator Kent Conrad, and Marta Prado, RN, member of the Florida Nurses Association, were appointed in March 1997 to the President's Commission on Consumer Protection and Quality in the Health Care Industry.

A MODEL THAT WORKED

Gaining the support of coalitions at the state and federal levels is critical. One example of how coalition members worked together is the Mississippi Nurses Association (MNA) Nursing Organizations Liaison Committee. Beginning in 1993, representatives from as many as 22 nursing organizations began meeting at the invitation of MNA to participate in the development of legislation and to work together toward obtaining nursing political appointments. Since that time, this group has been successful in influencing the Mississippi legislature to pass every legislative bill the group developed. Additionally, every RN member of the Mississippi Board of Nursing came from MNA, acting either alone or in conjunction with one of the participating organizations. The coalition also succeeded in placing an RN on the Mississippi Board of Health and in other influential positions.

PERSONAL REFLECTIONS

During the volatile 1970s, I owned a small weekly newspaper in southern Mississippi and covered local politics like a blanket—meetings of the board of aldermen, board of supervisors, school board, zoning board, circuit court, and chancery court. It was there that I learned the influence yielded by elected and political appointments. I saw at first hand how those persons influenced my life, my children's lives, and my community. I also saw the caliber of persons serving on those boards: many were uneducated, some were more qualified than others, and very few were women. None were nurses. Having worked with nurses for 8 years, I know now how refreshing it would have been to look across the board table and see one sitting there. It would have made a tremendous difference.

I interviewed a powerful judge once who explained to me his tough stand in not excusing persons from jury duty. It appeared to me that those persons trying to be excused from serving were the more educated, the more influential, and the more economically advantaged. I asked why. His explanation: "They think they're too busy, they think they'll miss making another nickel, and they don't think it's so important. But let one of them get charged with something and have to come before a jury, and they'll want to come face to face with the most qualified persons, the most educated persons, those who most understand the law. Only then will they understand the importance of serving."

Change has come about in Mississippi. Today there are women and members of minority groups in politically appointed positions where only white men once served. Still only a few nurses are a part of the change.

First Lady Hillary Clinton, speaking at the American Nurses Association PAC luncheon in 1997, said: "Nurses know what's really important in the health care system, and you can have a tremendous impact on what you care most about. You are responsible for improving lives for all of us."

That same advice can be applied to those nurses who are considering public service. Nurses must not hesitate to serve. It's too im-portant to the profession, to patients, to the public, and to each other to let someone else serve for you.

REFERENCES

American Nurses Association. (1997). *Seeking federal appointment: A guide for nurses.* Washington, DC: American Nurses Publishing.

Coalition for Women's Appointments. (1997). *A project convened by the National Women's Political Caucus.* Washington, DC: Author.

Goldwater, M., & Zusy, M. J. L. (1990). *Prescription for nurses: Effective political action.* St. Louis: Mosby.

National Women's Political Caucus. (1997). *A guide to running a winning campaign.* Washington, DC: Author.

ADDITIONAL SOURCES OF INFORMATION

Information regarding federal appointments may be obtained from the state or national party headquarters, the Internet, or the Coalition for Women's Appointments of the National Women's Political Caucus. The *Federal Yellow Book: Who's Who in Federal Departments and Agencies* is a publication available by prescription and is updated quarterly. Another source is the publication *United States Government Policy and Supporting Positions,* which is published every 4 years after the Presidential election and is for sale through the U.S. Government Printing Office.

VIGNETTE

VIGNETTE

Nurses as Appointed Leaders in State Government

Mary B. Wachter

The fourth stage of political development, the highest level, is characterized as the "leading the way" stage, according to Cohen et al. (1996). Today, more nurses than ever are reaching this level. These nursing leaders are proactive on a broad range of health and social policy issues, use language that reorders political debates, build coalitions that include interests in broad health policy issues, and are pursued for appointment to high-ranking policy-making positions on the basis of their nursing expertise and knowledge.

In 1994 two of New Jersey's nurses, Jean Marshall, MSN, RN, FAAN, and Susan C. Reinhard, RN, PhD, FAAN, who had long ago reached the fourth stage of political development, were sought by the new Republican administration in the state to fill two eminent positions in the New Jersey State Department of Health. In May 1994, Marshall became the Assistant Commissioner of Health, Division of Family Health Services. In October 1994, Reinhard was appointed as the Director of Policy and Research; 14 months later she was promoted to Senior Assistant Commissioner of Health Planning and Regulation; and in June 1996 she was appointed Deputy Commissioner of Health and Senior Services. These state government posts were granted after Republican Christine Todd Whitman upset an incumbent Democrat, Jim Florio, in the 1993 elections to become the first woman governor in New Jersey's history.

Preappointment Events

During this heated gubernatorial election, nurses became actively involved in the Whitman campaign by organizing grassroots campaign efforts, such as sponsoring newspaper advertisements and attending fund-raising events.

Susan Reinhard volunteered on Whitman's campaign to shape the campaign's health policy agenda. These political activities by nurses helped Whitman recognize the value of their support and view them as important players in state politics. However, controversy within the nursing community ensued, and Whitman's enthusiasm to appoint nurses waned after the Interested Nurses Political Action Committee, the political arm of the New Jersey State Nurses Association (NJSNA), announced its endorsement of incumbent Governor Jim Florio. Nonetheless, Susan Reinhard was appointed to Whitman's Health Transition Team immediately after the election. Reinhard was identified and moved forward by the governor-elect's advisers, including a powerful contract lobbyist and well-connected Republican with whom Reinhard worked as a lobbyist for NJSNA. For 3 months, Reinhard and other health policy experts assisted the new administration in goal setting and policy development of New Jersey's health care agenda.

Once Whitman took office, she appointed Len Fishman, JD, an attorney with an extensive background in health law, as Acting Commissioner of Health. Since, by statute, this position had to be filled by a physician, the new administration planned to amend the law in order to appoint Fishman permanently. The proposed change would broaden the requirements for the commissioner's post to be someone with a background in public health. Nursing leaders in the state seized this opportunity to bargain with the new administration: the nursing community would actively support changing the qualifications for the commissioner of health, as put forth by the governor's office, in exchange for the political appointment of nurses to high-ranking state government offices and committees. To add leverage to the negotiations, Barbara Wright, RN, MSN, a Republican New Jersey assemblywoman and past executive director of NJSNA, introduced a bill in the General Assembly that expanded the commissioner's qualifications beyond those of only a physician or a registered nurse. Shortly thereafter, Jean Marshall was appointed Assistant Commissioner of Health, Division of Family Health Services, and Susan Reinhard was appointed in May 1994 to Chair the Cost Containment Committee of the Governor's Advisory Panel on Federal Health Care Reform. Subsequently the Whitman administration successfully changed the law, and Fishman was appointed Commissioner of Health.

Reinhard's leadership and intense work on the cost-containment committee caught the attention of influential policy experts and of staff within the department of health. This newly developed network was key to her next appointment. After a nationwide search, Commissioner Fishman appointed Reinhard as Director of Policy and Research, which placed her among Fishman's cabinet members. Less than 2 years later the administration consolidated all senior services in the state under the new Department of Health and Senior Services (DHSS). Reinhard was promoted to Deputy Commissioner of Health and Senior Services to lead this consolidation and manage a $1.4 billion budget for senior services.

Past Experiences and Valuable Networks

Marshall's and Reinhard's nursing careers have taken different paths, and they have built many networks that have led ultimately to their state appointments. Marshall, like many nurses, spent most of her career in the tertiary care setting. She gained a variety of experiences as a staff nurse, in-service instructor, and enterostomal therapist before eventually finding her niche in nursing education and administration. After receiving a master of science in nursing degree, with a concentration in nursing administration from Seton Hall University, she became Assistant Vice President of Education and Con-

sumer Health at Kimball Medical Center, Lakewood, N.J. Marshall built an enduring network within Kimball and its community during her 24 years of service to this institution. Robert Singer, a Republican state senator and Vice President of Corporate Relations for Community at Kimball Medical Center, was among those in Marshall's circle who advocated her appointment to the DHSS.

Reinhard's nursing background began in public health and continued in nursing education, policy, and research. She taught in various schools of nursing throughout New Jersey and Ohio before completing her doctorate in sociology and becoming an assistant professor at Rutgers, The State University of New Jersey College of Nursing. In 1991 she was appointed as director of the community health nursing graduate program at Rutgers. Reinhard continued to develop her contacts in both academia and community health.

Reinhard's educational achievements also greatly contributed to her appointment. While working toward her doctor of philosophy degree in the 1980s, she sharpened her research skills and expanded her expert knowledge of an increasing segment of the population—elderly persons. Dr. David Mechanic, a renowned author and professor of behavioral sciences at Rutgers, became Reinhard's dissertation chairman and an important mentor. Mechanic is well respected and is connected within health policy circles. His recommendation of Reinhard for her department of health appointment carried heavy weight.

Professional association involvement has been a common denominator for both Marshall and Reinhard. Both of these nursing leaders have been members of NJSNA since the beginning of their nursing careers. Marshall held her first major office in 1986–1988 as an elected member of the American Nurses Association Congress on Practice. She then went on to become president of NJSNA in 1988–1990. These highly visible leadership positions helped to strengthen her ability to build coalitions, promote sound policy, and communicate with people from many backgrounds. Through the contacts she made as president of NJSNA, Marshall became the chairwoman of the New Jersey Department of Health Nursing Advisory Committee, which has acted as a resource to the administration on issues affecting the nursing profession. During her tenure as chair, $20 million was appropriated by a former commissioner of health, Molly Coye, to create a better work environment for nurses in New Jersey. Marshall, an extremely active member of the Black Nurses Association, has always been committed to mentoring minority nurses into leadership roles. She learned this from her mentor, Dr. Gloria Smith, vice president of the Kellogg Foundation. In June 1997, she fulfilled a dream by bringing together 135 nurses of color to discuss the role of the minority nurse in today's health care environment.

In 1983 Reinhard became a part-time nurse lobbyist for NJSNA. During the next 11 years, she worked one legislative day per week in Trenton, N.J., lobbying for nursing and public health issues. As a nurse lobbyist, Reinhard made her mark among the state capitol elites as a savvy political strategist with a keen understanding of global health policy issues. The political and policy networks that she established as a lobbyist have been boundless and invaluable to her appointments.

Postappointment Achievements

Marshall's and Reinhard's nursing backgrounds, educational experiences, and professional involvements are extensive and have produced networks and resources that encompass many circles in and around nursing, policy, and political communities. Subsequently, their current experiences have proved to be challenging and rewarding. In her role as Assistant Commissioner of Health, Marshall headed the Division of Family Health Services and controlled a $220 million budget. Some of the services in this division are the Women, Infants and Children Nutritional Program (WIC), Community Health, Maternal and Child Health Regional Program, and Early Childhood Education and Special Child Health. The assistant commissioner focused on several issues, such as

decreasing black infant mortality rates and increasing childhood immunization rates. Using a "bottom up" approach, she organized urban community groups to assume responsibility for and become stake holders in the health of their communities. Programs were implemented that meet the specified needs of culturally diverse communities.

In early March 1997 Marshall realized that the personal and professional goals she had set at the beginning of her appointment had finally been met. She remarked: "I gained a wealth of knowledge from the state level and was an effective change agent who brought new approaches to the department. It became time for me to transfer this experience back to my local communities." Marshall was offered an ideal opportunity in the private sector. In April 1997 she accepted her new position as Vice President of Government and Community Relations for Meridian Health System, a growing corporation of hospitals, ambulatory care centers, physician practices, and home care services, with corporate offices in Jersey Shore Medical Center, Neptune, N.J.

However, Marshall's experience as an appointed official did not end. Her unblemished record of service in DHSS was recognized by her colleagues, and she was appointed by Governor Whitman to the Health Care Administration Board (HCAB) in June 1997. The HCAB is housed within the DHSS and makes all policy decisions for health regulations in the state. Marshall stated: "This appointment is a great transition. I'm able to maintain ties with the DHSS and increase my knowledge of the rules and regulations that affect New Jersey's health care system while molding my new role in the private sector."

As Deputy Commissioner of Health and Senior Services, the first nurse to achieve this high rank in New Jersey's executive branch of government, Reinhard has taken a leadership role on many issues, such as drafting and adopting regulations for health maintenance organizations that recognize nurse practitioners and clinical nurse specialists as primary care providers; designing and implementing a one-stop-shopping comprehensive model for all senior services in New Jersey; and developing policy to insure uninsured children. She is also Governor Whitman's representative on the board of nursing. When asked what skills have been the most valuable in her appointed position, Reinhard responded: "My research background and lobbying experience have added unique and valuable dimensions to my role as deputy commissioner. Policy development is most successful when you operate from a substantive knowledge base and understand the negotiation process."

Lessons Learned

After serving as political appointees for 3 years, Marshall and Reinhard report that they met challenges and learned some valuable lessons from their experiences. Marshall expressed that she has closely monitored the effects of power. Throughout her career, she has witnessed how power has clouded peoples' visions. "I was very conscious of the authority that I would have as an assistant commissioner. I have made sure that I would constructively use this power to empower others," she commented. Marshall has also learned to be attentive to New Jersey as a whole community with many different needs, not just health needs, and that you cannot accept an appointed position and try to change everything. She explained, "You have to identify a few major issues and focus your attention in order to see results." She also stressed that to get appointed one must take risks. She emphasized: "You must have the ability to pick up the phone and call your legislators and other connections, make an appointment to meet with them and tell why you are valuable. Sell yourself."

Reinhard believes that her biggest challenge was assuming the change agent role of bringing together state employees from four different departments and consolidating them into one division to promote more futuristic models of support for the state's 1.2 million seniors. "It is imperative to respect the uniqueness of each corporate culture while integrating a team of over 500 people. I relied on my community nursing background to assess varying world views and find ways to achieve consensus on a shared vision," the Deputy Commissioner explained. She also understands the reality of political appointments to the highest levels of government: when the administration changes, there is a strong possibility that your appointment will end. Therefore Reinhard is intensely motivated to serve New Jersey's citizens now to her maximum potential and to produce outcomes that make a difference.

She stressed the importance of wearing many hats in different networks and stated: "People get to know you from many perspectives and contacts. They hear your name in different circles, and you get people's attention." She further explained: "Nurses who are seeking a political appointment *must* strategize. They should identify their strengths, get in position for an appointment, chair a committee, and make something important happen."

Wrapping It Up

In November 1997, Christine Todd Whitman was reelected for her second term as governor of New Jersey. She is a strong governor who has recognized the value that RNs offer to policy and politics. The New Jersey nursing community has worked hard in the past few decades to reserve permanent seats at the decision-making table. Marshall's and Reinhard's accomplishments and contributions are securing nursing's place. They are two of the many nurses who are "leading the way" of the nursing profession into the advanced stage of political development in local, state, national, and international arenas.

Reference

Cohen, S. S., Mason, D. J., Kovner, C., Leavitt, J. K., Pulcini, J., & Sochalski, J. (1996). Stages of nursing's political development: Where we've been and where we ought to go. *Nursing Outlook, 44*(6), 259–266.

Chapter *28*

POLITICAL PARTIES

CATHERINE J. DODD AND SANDRA R. SMOLEY

Registered nurses are not born Democrats or Republicans, and, like a growing number of Americans, nurses are tending toward an independent political stance. There is no fault to be found in partisan independence. However, if one wishes to have an impact on the development of public policy, especially as it is formed through the legislative process, one must join either the Republican or the Democrat party. Party affiliation is essential in our system of developing social and administrative policy and political power.

This chapter will explore party influence in policy development. We will examine why people choose (or do not choose) to affiliate with a particular party, how the role of political parties in the United States is changing, how to influence parties, and how to get involved in the party structure of the two main parties in the United States—the Democrat and the Republican parties. We will discuss third parties in the context of influencing policy development. However, because each party develops its own rules as to structure and leadership, our attention will focus on the two major parties.

ORIGINS

Parties were formed and continue to exist to elect people with shared values, beliefs, and goals. During America's growth, several parties emerged and changed as we grew from 13 colonies to 50 states. Throughout history, political parties attempted to elect candidates who would support the platforms adopted by the party. Those platforms articulated the views and values of party members. Party principles, positions, and names have changed with time. For example, the Democratic-Republicans of Thomas Jefferson's era became the Democrats of Andrew Jackson's time, and that party is today's Democratic Party (DeLaney, 1995).

In the nineteenth century, under the leadership of Abraham Lincoln, the Radical Republicans emerged as an alternative to the Democrats. That new third party worked to free the slaves and preserve the union (Zeman & Kelly, 1994). Forty years later, in the early years of the twentieth century, Theodore Roosevelt was elected as a Progressive Republican. "T.R." campaigned to protect the people from the monopolistic abuses of big business. The Progressives believed that breaking up the trusts would result in more competition and better prices for average Americans (Zeman & Kelly, 1994).

From the Civil War to Franklin Roosevelt's second term, African Americans voted Republican. Since the 1940s they have supported the Democrats. From the time women won the right to vote in 1922, until the 1980s, they were more likely to identify with the Republican Party.

During the twentieth century, the Democrat and Republican parties have dominated the political terrain. Party conventions controlled the selection of Presidential nominees until fairly recently. By 1972, however, the process of nominating the Presidential candidates had moved out of the convention and into candidate-centered, media-dominated primary elections. Indeed, many of today's candidates are packaged by public relations machines prepared to respond instantly to every public opinion poll. A primary goal is to establish a direct personal and political, albeit superficial, relationship with the voter rather than relying on the strength of the party and its platform (Skowronek, 1993).

During the twentieth century, party identification was usually heightened during Presidential election years, when Presidential candidates were selected and party platforms were adopted at national conventions. The use of mass communication tools (radio, television, and direct mail) to influence the Presidential candidate selection since 1975 has diminished the public's focus on party platforms and ideals (Skowronek, 1993).

Platforms were, at one time, an integral part of the American election process. In the days before mass media reduced a volume to a sound bite, long-winded orators would dominate the party conventions with their commentary on each and every platform plank. Newspapers routinely printed party platforms in their entirety. Candidates campaigned, more often than not, by referring to the party positions outlined in the platform. For the intelligent voter who took the time to read, the positions of the parties and their respective candidates were clear.

The situation is vastly different today. Conventions are unimportant except as vehicles to garner as much prime-time television coverage as possible. Nominations are routinely sewn up in primary elections that occur months before the conventions. Likewise, party platforms are virtually ignored by candidate and public alike. To be sure, platforms are still drafted. Occasionally a particular platform plank will provoke a fight between competing factions within the party. Though a close, controversial vote on such an issue makes good theater for columnists and pundits, the great majority of the voting public pays scant attention to these battles.

The platforms of the two parties are rarely read by anyone except those who drafted them. In recent years it seems that even the Presidential nominees of both parties have not read the platforms. If they have read them, they do not seem to acknowledge certain critical components of them.

Bob Dole never publicly addressed his party's position on abortion. Bill Clinton never embraced his party's position on welfare. The person running for office, and the image created for him or her by public relations experts, have become far more important to electability than the platform on which he or she runs.

Not only has the focus on public relations and the individual diminished the import and impact of platforms and conventions, but party factions have banded together to steer the party in a particular direction on a given issue or set of issues. The most recent example of this is the Democratic Leadership Conference (DLC). The DLC was formed in the 1980s. The founders of the group were primarily Democratic governors, mostly from the South. Among their number was Arkansas governor Bill Clinton. The overriding goal of the DLC was to elect a Democratic President—something that had occurred only once in nearly 20 years. Their belief was that the party and its platform had been too liberal for the American public in recent years.

They were determined either to move the party to the right or to gain control of the party's nominating mechanism and nominate one of their own to run for President. They succeeded on the latter score with the nomination of Bill Clinton for the Presidency. Clinton ran as a moderate, rarely referring to the party platform—which was far more liberal than he wished to be perceived. The strategy certainly proved successful; Clinton was elected president. Though his personal views may well be to the left of his actions as President, the electorate and a Republican majority in both houses of Congress have kept him much closer to the political center than many in his party seem to like.

Clinton and his DLC colleagues learned one lesson well: getting elected is far more important than strict adherence to the esoterica of a party platform. The days when either party's nominee is held hostage by platform writers are, we believe, behind us forever. At a time when a move to the center is deemed "smart politics," the often flowery statements of philosophy that appear in platform language are probably best left out of the glare of the media.

The key differences between the two major party platforms are on social issues. These differences sometimes reflect the extremes of the party philosophies and not the majority of voters who are registered within the parties. The reason that the party platforms are often more extreme than the majority of party registrants is that party machinery occasionally falls under the control of the "true believer." These are people, frequently interested in only one issue, who involve themselves in party offices and activities and advocate tirelessly for their issue.

Both parties have come under the control of the more politically active among their membership. In 1964 the Republicans were perceived to be too far to the right of the general electorate, whereas in 1972 the Democrats, controlled by the McGovernites, were viewed as too far to the left. These cycles occur in both parties from time to time and generally come to an end after a crushing election defeat.

IS IT STILL A TWO-PARTY SYSTEM?

The 1992 presidential election saw the emergence of a "third party" candidate. Multimillionaire Ross Perot was nominated by the Reform Party, a vehicle largely of Perot's creation. Nineteen percent of those who voted in that election favored his candidacy, a major showing for a third party. Many voters were disillusioned by the two major parties and their tendencies toward negative advertising and their financial obligation to either "Big Business" or "Big Labor" political action committees.

Third-party movements are common in American politics. Most are created around issues or philosophies rather than personalities. In recent years these included the Green Party, which focuses on environmental issues; the Peace and Freedom Party, which advocates a particular view of social justice; the Libertarian Party, which seeks less government; and the American

Independent Party, which calls for a return to "traditional values." To date, third parties have been unsuccessful in national elections but have won various offices at the local level in several states. Many states have election laws that discourage third parties by requiring a significant percentage of registrants in the party to sign up before the party is recognized and put on the ballot (DeLaney, 1995). John Anderson, a third-party candidate for President in 1980, was unable to get on the ballot in many states because his party could not meet those standards (Chapman-Hughes, 1985).

THE MAJORITY PARTY DETERMINES THE RULES

Most nurses are registered with one of the two major political parties. However, those not actively involved with party politics will "vote across party lines" or "split their ticket" on the basis of the qualifications of a given candidate, rather than vote the "straight ticket" of the party in which they are registered. Nurses regard themselves as independent thinkers, and most will say that they do not select candidates on the basis of their position on a single issue or adherence to the party platform.

The growth of the "independent" voter movement throughout the country has prompted many states to institute "open" primaries allowing voters to cross party lines in primary elections. In other states the primary elections for state and federal offices are "partisan" primaries, requiring voters to choose only from among those candidates of the party in which they are registered. General election ballots list all candidates, and voters are free to cross party lines. With the decline of support for the party platform, many candidates for local offices no longer rely on their party identification and "party slate" or "straight ticket" voting to help them get elected (DeLaney, 1995).

People who are *actively* involved in politics, including nurses, usually vote the "straight ticket." They rarely vote across party lines because they understand the role and power of the majority party in state legislatures and in the

U.S. Congress. Moreover, nurses involved in politics understand that politicians most often get their start in local, nonpartisan elections and then seek higher partisan office. If a Republican nurse indirectly supports a candidate for school board who is a Democrat, and 2 years later that person is elected to the legislature, that Republican nurse helped increase the numbers of Democrats in the state house. As former Speaker of the U.S. House of Representatives, Tip O'Neill observed, "All politics is local." Thus, getting involved in local party politics is essential if one seeks to make a lasting impact on the development of social policy.

For the past 130 years, either the Republican Party or the Democratic Party has held the majority in one or both houses of Congress. The majority party determines the leadership and makeup of Congressional committees. The majority party selects the Speaker of the House and the Majority Leader of the Senate. That decision is often made on a purely partisan basis. Committee chairs determine which bills are heard. The Senate Judiciary Committee confirms cabinet members and can impeach the President. If the Senate is controlled by the opposite party of the President (the Executive Officer), cabinet appointees will have to meet a more stringent "litmus" test. This process is replicated in many state governments as well.

When the chief executive (president or governor) is from the opposite party to *both* legislative houses, the majority party virtually controls what legislation is passed. Though the executive can veto legislation passed by the majority party in both houses, this may work against him or her if the public becomes frustrated with the lack of work accomplished by the government. Even if the chief executive exercises the veto power, the party controlling both houses has the opportunity to override the veto, thereby advancing its legislative and policy agendas.

Passing legislation requires cooperation. Once elected, legislators rely on their "fellow party members" to support them. If a legislator consistently demonstrates "independence" from his or her party colleagues, why should they bother to help pass his or her legislation? Third-party elected officials have little or no clout in the appointment process and in the structure of the legislature that wields power. They are important only when their vote is needed to break a tie or override a veto. Their appointment to key committees is dependent solely on the relationships they have made with the majority party leadership. Therefore, if nurses want to identify themselves as independent thinkers in the ultimate game of passing legislation, they need to remember that the party with the most "marbles" (votes) wins. That is why politically active nurses usually "vote the party ticket." If you do not like your ticket, get involved in selecting who is on the ticket by becoming involved in party politics. It is not a difficult process.

Nursing is fortunate to have party activists and leaders in both parties. Without nurses lobbying in their own party to win bipartisan support for direct reimbursement under Medicare for advanced practice nurses, that provision would not have become part of the 1997 budget reconciliation process. Without bipartisan efforts to restore funding to the Nursing Education Act in 1997, funding for graduate nursing education would have been cut by more than $50 million dollars.

During the debate on national health care reform, the DLC emerged as a moderate "middle of the road" group of Democrats to offer compromises to the extreme Democrat and Republican party leadership. Nursing's Agenda for Health Care Reform was very similar to the DLC proposal, perhaps because nursing's leadership reflects the diversity of the country and the proposals crafted reflect compromises needed to secure successful policy development.

GETTING INVOLVED IN PARTY POLITICS

First, make an informed decision. Select the party that best reflects your values. Contact the state and national committees of the Democrat and Republican parties. Ask for their platforms. Ask for the list of committee members and an organizational plan or bylaws. Search to see whether you recognize any names. In addition, check to see whether there are any registered nurses on either list.

Active membership in a political party has advantages. One can join a party simply by registering to vote with that party identification. One can become active by participating in local clubs, meetings, party activities, and political campaigns. Being involved will accomplish the following:

- Give you a more significant role in selecting the candidates who will stand in the general election because candidates seek out endorsement and support of local party leaders and activists. Candidates will be likely to ask you for advice.
- Make you confident that the candidates you support have ideals similar to yours—even if you do not know a great deal about the candidates on a personal basis.
- Allow you to help shape the issues for your party and its elected officials because your voice is louder when you belong to a group of people who share similar values.
- Create the possibility that you may be asked to serve as a political appointee on governmental bodies, which provides countless opportunities to expound on the value of nursing in the public policy arena.
- Enable you to work to restore accountability of elected officials to the party's principles.
- Give you access to elected officials and their staff. (Politically successful nurses create and maintain relationships with key staff of elected officials, thus opening doors for input on critical issues.)

The best place to get started is volunteering at the local party level either in a district caucus, a club, or a precinct. Parties are most active during even-numbered (Congressional and Presidential election) years. Nurses who become active in party politics lend the credibility of their profession to the party. Volunteer activities for a local party may include fund raising, voter registration and identification, and "get out the vote" activities. When nurses work on candidate campaigns, they are frequently asked to try to convince the "independent" voters—those not affiliated as Democrats or Republicans.

When a nurse calls a voter and says, "Hi, this is Lillian Wald, and I am a registered nurse and am calling on behalf of Lucy Stone, who is running for Congress," the voter at the other end of the line does not automatically associate this call with a political party. Lillian Wald has much more credibility than if she says, "Hi, this is Lillian Wald, and I'm calling from the Lucy Stone for Congress campaign."

Nurses are valuable party activists because they know how to get things done. Their profession requires them to assess, plan, intervene, evaluate, and report. Nurses have excellent communication skills and are willing to work hard. Most important, for political purposes, nurses have friends and colleagues they can recruit to assist.

Once you have established yourself as a credible party activist, consider running for party or political office. State and local party operations have different rules. Some local committees are elected by the voters, and others are elected in caucuses. Find out the rules and develop a strategy: assess the situation, plan your campaign, and run. You must request and receive the support of others. Support comes when you commit to doing something and you follow through. Your credibility is a reflection on both our profession and your political acumen.

Election to local committees and state party committees will present you with the opportunity to serve on the platform committee, where you can advocate the inclusion of nursing's agenda in the party principles. Most delegates to national political conventions are elected in caucuses and by direct delegate selection on primary ballots. Procedures vary from election to election and from state to state. Nevertheless, to win, you must convince people to vote for you either by attending a caucus meeting or by voting at the ballot box.

As an active Democrat, I ran for the local Democratic county committee in 1984 and was reelected in highly competitive primary elections four times. My participation through

"Nurses for Pelosi" landed me on Congresswoman Pelosi's district office staff and later an appointment to the State Democratic Executive Board Platform Committee and Rules Committee. With each campaign, I expand my network of business people and community leaders whom I can call on to support nursing and health care issues. [Catherine Dodd, MS, RN]

As a lifelong Republican, I moved from an active commitment to community volunteerism into elective politics. In 1972 I was elected to the Sacramento County Board of Supervisors, the first woman supervisor in county history. In those days I was one of just five elected women officials in a large metropolitan area. We were a small but effective group. Four of the five of us were nurses. I served as a supervisor for nearly 20 years and served as the president of both the state and national supervisors associations. Both Presidents Reagan and Bush appointed me to national task forces, where, be assured, the nursing viewpoint was heard. [Sandra Smoley, RN]

Involvement in party politics by nurses will guarantee that a nursing agenda is part of the platforms of both major parties. It will also provide access to the decision makers, and it will give public credibility to the political process. As Democrat Eleanor Roosevelt said, "You must do the things you think you cannot do." And as Republican Susan B. Anthony said, "Failure is impossible." So, get involved.

REFERENCES

Chapman-Hughes, C. (1985). Political parties and clubs. In D. J. Mason & S. W. Talbot (Eds.). *Political action handbook for nurses* (pp. 367–375). Menlo Park, CA: Addison-Wesley.

DeLaney, A. (1995). *Politics for dummies.* Foster City: IDG Books Worldwide.

Skowronek, S. (1993). *The politics presidents make.* Cambridge, MA: Belknap Press.

Zelman, A., & Kelly, K. (1994). *Everything you need to know about American history.* New York: Scholastic.

Chapter 29

LOBBYING POLICYMAKERS:
Individual and Collective Strategies

RITA WRAY, SALLY S. COHEN, AND SUSAN C. REINHARD

Responsibility for influencing health policy rests with each nurse. As an individually licensed professional, every nurse is accountable to society to promote and protect the public's health. Indeed, it is the nurse's ethical obligation to promote "community and national efforts to meet the health needs of the public" (American Nurses Association, 1995). Direct participation in developing health policy is the most effective and efficient nursing strategy to accomplish this social mandate.

As a member of a profession, however, the nurse need not—nor should not—act alone to influence public policy development. One reason is that the cumulative knowledge and collective experience of many nurses guide the most innovative recommendations for policies. Another is that influencing policy development is a political process best negotiated when colleagues work together in a coordinated fashion to effect change. Nursing's voice in shaping policy is strongest when individual or grassroots lobbying is in concert with an overall lobbying plan.

LAYING THE FOUNDATION

To communicate nursing's viewpoint effectively to policymakers, a certain amount of preparation is needed. The first task is to become a registered voter and vote regularly. Next, nurses need to learn *what* to lobby, *whom* to lobby, *how* to lobby, and *why* to lobby.

Knowing *what* to lobby entails two key aspects: understanding the general policy issue and understanding the specifics of the proposed legislation. For example, in lobbying for the rights of adolescents at a community health center, nurses should have a basic understanding of certain ethical issues, such as the need to balance patient and societal concerns with the rights of minors seeking treatment. When nurses are lobbying for specific proposals, however, legislators need to hear nurses' professional views on specific aspects of a bill, such as who should be able to prescribe a certain course of treatment, including contraception, for how long, and under what circumstances.

The best way to become informed about the history or background of a particular topic or piece of legislation is to contact the organization(s) likely to be involved with that issue. Begin by contacting your professional associations to inquire about nursing's position and involvement. Meet or speak with the government relations staff and ask what written information is available (often in the association's newsletter). Sometimes copies of written testimony can be obtained from the organization.

It is also helpful to contact other professional, industry, and consumer groups (the American Medical Association, chambers of commerce, and the National Business and Industry Association, among others) that may be involved in the particular issue. Legislators hear regularly from all these groups, and it is helpful to know the perspectives they are advancing. The Grassroots Action Information Network (GAIN) offers U.S. Chamber of Commerce members an opportunity to become real players in influencing legislation. By using state-of-the-art technology, GAIN helps to make a difference in public-policy debates and provides timely, useful information on many issues by supplying a variety of document services. They provide information such as the following:

- Backgrounders, which provide a basic understanding of the issue
- Issue updates, which report on recent significant developments to keep one "up to speed"
- Action calls, which explain the stakes associated with a specific upcoming Congressional vote and direct recipients on how to take appropriate action
- "For your information" (FYI) documents, which announce miscellaneous items of interest

If you are dealing with a specific piece of legislation, be prepared to address legislators' most common concerns. They want to know how this legislation will affect their various constituencies, the cost implications, and the implications of not making this bill a law. It is also politically astute to discuss who (or what groups) supports and who opposes the bill and reasons that the legislator should support nursing's position despite potential opposition.

Knowing *whom* to lobby is an obvious but often poorly understood necessity. Most voters know the names of their President, federal Senators, and state governor, and some know the names of their Congressional representatives. Fewer can name their state representatives, and almost none know the key staff who actually research and draft policy proposals. Often communication bypasses the legislators, thus mandating working directly with staff. It is also important to be clear about legislative jurisdictions and not write to federal legislators about issues that fall under the domain of state legislators (e.g., the licensing of health professionals).

Many books, pamphlets, journals, and newsletters provide information about policy issues and policymakers. Local organizations, such as the League of Women Voters, distribute brochures outlining the political structure and process of specific cities, counties, or states. They also publish directories of elected officials in these specific locations, which include the officials' names, addresses, telephone numbers, and other information. For some, a telephone call to one's town hall or board of elections is a simple way to begin.

The right person to talk to is the one whose influence or vote will advance your policy position. It is critical to identify who holds what power and who pulls what strings. The more information you have, the better position you will be in to influence legislation. Legislative leaders, chairs, and members of committees who will vote on the bill, your elected representative(s), and their aides need to hear nursing's view.

Once you identify the appropriate policymaker for a selected issue, it is helpful to assess that person's orientation—for example, the legislator's political background, philosophies, party affiliation, year of reelection, history of involvement with nursing and health issues, committee assignments, and key bills sponsored. This information is routinely available from the legislator's local office and can also be ascertained from local, state, or national nurses' associations or a nurses' political action committee (PAC). Those who have been endorsed by a nurses' PAC are recognized friends of nursing. It is wise to thank these legislators for their past support and to cite examples of how their actions have affected nurses and health care consumers.

Knowing *how* to lobby begins with understanding the legislative process and the current status of your issue within this process (see Box, page 395, in Chapter 22). An adage states: "Timing is everything in politics." It does little good to talk to your senators about a bill that is stuck in the other house. Furthermore, the current political climate will drive or restrain the movement of your issue through the legislative process. Therefore it is important to place your issue in the context of the larger political climate (and in alignment with the driving forces). During periods of fiscal restraint, a policy alternative that is cost-effective will receive more attention than one associated with increased allocations or unknown financial implications.

Knowing *why* to lobby is the underlying impetus for all the above. The reason to lobby is simply to shape health policy so that is will best meet the needs of patients. With the "why" in mind, commitment and planning become key ingredients. The most effective way for individual nurses to lobby is to work in concert with the profession's collective strategy. The American Nurses Association has been actively involved in many health issues and has urged a coalition-building strategy for moving nursing's policy agenda (Betts, 1996). The Nursing Organization Liaison Forum is one tangible product of a coalition-building strategy. This forum provides a vehicle for many professional nursing organizations to collaborate on a nursing policy agenda.

The danger in acting alone is that individual efforts may conflict with or jeopardize whatever lobbying has already taken place. The benefit in working together is that individual efforts can reinforce the unified message.

SPECIFIC LOBBYING STRATEGIES

Once you have the basic information, you have several specific strategies from which to choose. You can write, call, telecommunicate with, or meet with legislators. In some situations, you may be in a position to provide oral or written testimony. The guidelines offered here are classic and commonsense words of advice. They produce results.

Writing to Policymakers

In writing to a legislator, several key points will make for more effective communication. Letters should be typed if at all possible (see Box on page 484). Letters should include an inside return address, preferably indicating that you are a constituent (i.e., you live and vote in the legislator's district). Be sure to state that you are a nurse and, if pertinent, include your position, place of employment, and other relevant data (e.g., a special interest in working with youth or your leadership position in your professional association). If legislation has been assigned a bill number, refer to this number in your letter (you can get this information from your association, legislative aides, or toll-free legislative numbers). If you know that the legislator sits on a committee that is dealing with the bill, make reference to the committee as well. State your stand on the bill and give one or two examples of the significance of the legislation—either pro or con. Letters should be concise. If appropriate, offer your assistance or expertise in the event that additional information is needed.

Telephoning Policymakers

Given the demands on most nurses' time, calling often offers a more realistic way to communicate with policymakers. When time is short (such as when a bill is posted for a vote in a day or two), it is often the method of choice.

The first (and sometimes most important) point of contact is the receptionist or staff person answering the phone. These individuals are critical gatekeepers and often consciously or unconsciously influence the policymaker's views on your issue. Developing rapport with these key people is worth your time, especially when you call regularly. Make sure your message to the staff is clear and simple. For example, if you are seeking a yes vote on a specific bill that will be considered in a committee meeting that week, ask the staff person to deliver that message and include only one or two sentences. For example, say, "Please vote yes on Bill No. _____ and support the provisions for increased funding and compliance reports." Anything longer is too complex for a phone message. State your organizational affiliation, employment setting, or both whenever possible, and give your nursing credentials.

POSITIVE TIPS TO KEEP IN MIND WHEN WRITING YOUR LEGISLATORS

- Write on personal, not hospital or agency, stationery. Sign your name with "RN" after it. Be sure to include your return address on letters—envelopes are discarded.
- Open your letter by clearly stating the following:
  - Your reason for writing (include bill number and title; state your support or opposition).
  - The rationale for your position. Your personal experience is the best supporting evidence.
  - What you want the elected official to do (support, oppose, draft new approach). Vagueness will get you a vague reply.
- Be constructive, reasonable, and courteous. If a problem exists, admit it. Describe the best approach if you oppose the bill. Neither threaten nor ask the impossible.
- Be brief and write about one subject. Explain how the issue would affect you, the nursing profession, patients, and/or your community. The letter should be one page or less in length.
- Know what committees your legislators serve on and indicate in the letter whether the bill will be brought before any of those committees.
- Consider timing. Know the current status of the bill (where it is in the legislative process). Write early, before the issue becomes popular and before the elected official takes a position. Provide time to respond to the official's reply.
- Use your own words. They can make a difference! Avoid slogans or phases from newsletters and letters.
- Ask your legislator to explain his or her position on the issue in reply. As a constituent, you're entitled to know how and why they feel as they do. Keep a copy of all correspondence for your files. Send a copy of your letter, and any response from the legislator, to the appropriate staff at your professional nursing organization.
- Thank your legislator if he or she responds with a favorable vote, a good speech, or fine leadership in committee or the floor (everyone appreciates a complimentary letter). If you are displeased, don't hesitate to communicate your concerns.
- Address written correspondence as follows:

U.S. Senator	U.S. Representative
Honorable Jane Doe	Honorable Jane Doe
United States Senate	House of Representatives
Washington, DC 20510	Washington, DC 20515
Dear Senator Doe:	Dear Representative Doe:

  The same general format applies to state and local officials.
- Facsimile transmission and electronic mail offers speed and conveys a sense of urgency. If you choose this method, follow up by sending the original letter through the mail.

LAGNIAPPE (A LITTLE EXTRA)

- Don't become a constant "pen pal." Quality rather than quantity is what counts. Don't "nag" if the vote does not reflect your views every time.
- Don't overstate your case. Be practical—exaggeration will only discredit you.
- Don't be rude. A rude letter neither makes friends nor influences the legislator.
- Don't threaten. Threats are rarely effective.

Telecommunicating with Policymakers

In the age of telecommunication, both facsimile transmission and electronic mail are valuable communication tools. Depending on the issue and timing factors, these tools are able to catch your legislator's attention and expediently convey your message.

When using these tools, include only pertinent information, write concisely, stress the impact an issue will have, encourage the legislator to act, and include a return fax number or E-mail address. Fax and E-mail messages can be sent for urgent matters but should be followed with a mailed letter, even if it is identical to the original message.

Meeting with Policymakers

Meeting with legislators, appointed officials, and other policymakers may seem like a daunting challenge but is routine in the political arena.

Since nurses are experts in face-to-face interpersonal communication, they can apply these assets to political meetings.

Informal meetings provide the best opportunity to establish and maintain working relationships with officials and their staff. If you attend political events, such as campaign fundraisers and town meetings, you can introduce yourself and your interest in a casual setting. By listening to speeches and chatting with the official, the staff, and other guests, you can learn more about the official's political and friendship networks, personal and professional goals, and grasp of specific issues. These events provide a social context in which to build a personal relationship and to secure more relaxed access in the future. Check local newspapers for announcements or call your legislator's office for meeting details.

Inviting policymakers to nurses' events through nursing organizations or the workplace is another excellent way to build political relationships. With the psychological security of numbers, groups of nurses can begin to overcome their fears of unknown encounters with the political world, while at the same time, policymakers are impressed with nurses' expertise, social conscience, and commitment. For example, one nurse legislative committee invited the state assemblyperson to attend a Nurses' Day luncheon in which the legislator moved from one table of staff nurses to the next to listen to their concerns and ideas for better health care. A legislator who spent a morning with a clinical nurse specialist in neonatal intensive care told his colleagues that they needed to listen to what nurses have to say about how to reduce the infant mortality rate. Honoring political officials who have supported nursing and health care issues is another way to foster linkages.

Ongoing contacts are critical in the lobbying process, and these informal and semiformal interactions are particularly useful. The unwritten protocols for lobbying and politics follow the same conventions as other social situations. This means that before you employ a heavy-handed lobbying approach, it is necessary to develop rapport with the legislator or his staff to gain

their trust. You need to get a sense of who they are and what they already know about nursing and other key issues. This must be a part of ongoing lobbying, not just part of the initial encounter. To bypass or ignore this step can minimize the effectiveness of even the most skillful lobbyist, because the most important element, credibility, has not been established.

At various stages of advocating a particular policy position, formal meetings with legislators, appointed officials, and staff are essential. The timing of these meetings is a fundamental part of the overall political strategy for advancing nursing's agenda. Therefore nursing's political clout is strengthened when individual nurses talk with their colleagues and organizational leaders to coordinate their efforts.

Preparation is the key to a productive meeting (see Box, p. 486). Make appointments in advance by telephone, or send an introductory letter to a staff person, followed by a telephone call. Dropping in is rarely desirable. When you make the appointment, identify the bill(s) or issue(s) that you wish to discuss. At the federal level, it is customary for a staff person to meet with you unless there is a particular reason to meet the legislator in person. At the state and local levels, you should be able to schedule a meeting with the legislator, but it is helpful to include appropriate staff. At any level, find out the name of the legislative assistant who deals with health issues, meet with that person, and keep correctly spelled names, titles, and telephone numbers for future contact and follow-up.

In most cases, policymakers meet with constituents in legislative offices, although it is sometimes possible to bring the policymaker to another locale, such as a nursing organization's headquarters. This is particularly true several months before an election, when legislators are seeking endorsements and want to meet with nurses to learn their issues. In either case, it is usually best if two or three nurses meet with an official. For example, a clinical nurse specialist teamed with a nurse lobbyist or an experienced member of the nurses' association's legislation committee can lobby convincingly for prescrip-

---

ARRANGING EFFECTIVE LEGISLATOR MEETINGS

1. Call for an appointment. Don't just walk in and expect to see the legislator. Surprises can be embarrassing for everyone. Make an appointment well in advance, and specify what you'll be talking about. This lets the legislator prepare for the meeting or delegate a person on his or her staff to meet with you. Remember, if you can't meet with the legislator, spend time with the staff. It can be highly rewarding.

2. Be organized. Have an agenda to keep the meeting from going astray. Remember, the legislators and their staffs will form an opinion of you, your group, and perhaps your cause. Know your subject, don't overstate your case, and maintain a professional manner.

3. If you are going as a group, have a preliminary meeting. This will ensure a smooth presentation. Decide who will present each topic. Choose a leader to direct the conversation and see that your agenda is followed.

4. Always be a good listener. What the legislator says will provide insight into strategy for follow-up or suggest who needs to be included in another meeting. Remember, the legislator needs to have his or her point of view understood just as much as you do. Being attentive to his or her concerns and issues does not mean you have to agree or compromise your position.

5. Be on time and don't overstay your allotted time. If the legislator asks you to continue, do so. But remember that legislators run on very tight schedules. If you're well organized, you can cover the critical aspects of your case in a limited time.

6. Don't let the legislator evade the issue. And don't be afraid to ask for a commitment. Ask how he or she stands on the issue or on specific aspects of a bill. Be tactful! Hostility will only ensure that the legislator will be "unavailable" when you want his or her ear again. Rely on your agenda to keep on the subject. Pay close attention to the legislator's arguments if he or she is against your position; they will provide fuel for further issue strategy.

7. Don't be awed. Sure, it's an important job, but legislators are people, just like you. It's highly likely they won't understand your issue as well as you do—not because they're dumb or don't care, but because legislators must be "generalists" on a wide range of issues. Discuss the issue. Don't lecture. Don't get defensive.

8. Leave fact sheets—short ones. Emphasize the impact of programs or legislation on the legislator's constituents. Make sure your facts can be verified; if you quote numbers, be able to back then up. Offer to provide more information as requested.

---

tive rights. While the former concentrates on the clinical questions, professional experiences, and proposed benefits for consumers, the latter focuses on the political process and climate. It is important to identify one nurse as the lead spokesperson so that the discussion will have continuity. That person should be responsible for introductions, handouts, moving the agenda, and the follow-up communication(s). Another person can take notes and be sure to get details, such as staff names and other references.

Be prepared to discuss the one or two issues you identified as the focus for your meeting. The impact of advocating a specific policy position is diluted when too many issues are discussed at one time. If possible, provide a one-page written summary of the information you want the legislator to have. Fact sheets from a nursing organization, data you have collected, pertinent articles, or brochures describing your organization are some examples of instructional material. Since visits are sometimes limited to 10 to 20 minutes (more at the state and local levels), leaving handouts that summarize information that you could not cover is a good strategy. Leave your business card if you have one, or write your name and contact information ahead of time so that you can leave it with the official or staff person.

Providing Formal Testimony

Nurses often have the opportunity to present their views on legislative, regulatory, and budget matters to policymaking groups, such as legislative and appropriations committees, task forces, and regulatory boards. This is a powerful way to advance nursing's agenda. Presenting testimony to those political bodies provides a formal mechanism for communicating directly with key policymakers and articulating nursing's view for the public record.

Presenting testimony requires skills that can make the difference between merely going through the motions of testifying and being a successful political player. Public hearings provide an important opportunity for nurses to explain their concerns. It is essential that expert testimony be delivered smoothly in order to convey a positive image of nurses to the public and to the political body holding the hearings.

Whenever possible, consult the professional nurses' association to ask whether it has prepared testimony on the particular topic, to determine its official stand on an issue, and to review actions taken or planned. If you need to prepare testimony on your own, you will find the resources of the professional organization useful. If more than one nursing organization plans to testify, consider preparing a joint statement or having one witness from each organization submit a written statement. A public display of unity on behalf of nursing is beneficial in promoting the adoption of public policies advocated by the profession.

INITIAL STEPS

Getting information about planned hearings is the first step. It is nursing's responsibility to keep informed of hearing dates and topics. The professional association is a central source for this information. Staff members review the agendas and special announcements that are sent regularly by governmental offices and agencies. They are in close contact with committee chairs and key staff, who alert them to future hearings. Organizations and individuals can also write to designated officials, asking to be notified when particular hearings will be scheduled.

The opportunities to testify are far greater than any nurse's or organization's capacity to participate. Priorities determine the choices. There are times when a written statement inserted into the printed record will suffice. At other times, oral testimony is warranted.

Once notified of the hearing, follow the instructions for submitting testimony. They can vary markedly for each committee and for each hearing. Some committees require an outline summarizing major points of the testimony. Others prefer to review the applications for presenting testimony or the actual testimony itself before making the final decisions as to which organizations will be invited to testify. Committees have varying formats for length and number of copies to be submitted in advance. Being familiar with these guidelines can help you avoid problems or surprises.

WRITING THE TESTIMONY

Draft the written testimony and then excerpt the key points you will include in the oral statement on the day of the hearing. Before writing the testimony, be clear about the intent of the hearing. Often hearings are held on a specific bill that is being drafted or has already been introduced. In such cases, be familiar with the bill and state your views for or against it. In other instances, hearings are held on a general legislative issue, not necessarily in bill form. This situation is usually more difficult because the parameters of the hearing are less clearly defined.

The intent of the hearings will also influence the style used in writing the testimony. Fact-finding hearings differ from hearings on specific bills. The former requires a more objective approach, focusing on what has transpired in relationship to an issue. In the case of a specific bill, a convincing pro or con case should be made. The language and tone used may need to be different in order to convey a certain point of view. Always try to be as logical and concrete as possible. Hearings are not the place to air personal gripes and complaints.

In writing testimony, several points are important:

- Whenever possible, include recent statistical data and cite specific examples to substantiate major points. Rhetoric without documentation is ineffective.
- Discuss the issue with nurses and other health professionals, as appropriate, to ensure that you have a full grasp of the topic. If possible, review previous testimony on the same issues.
- Consult with key constituents of your organization to be sure your testimony agrees with organizational priorities and current thinking.
- Include in the first part of the testimony a description of your organization, its membership, and why the hearings are important to your organization's activities.
- Adhere to every instruction regarding format and include a title page identifying the hearings, committee, date, and your name.

SELECTING A WITNESS

For organizations, the person writing the testimony often is not the person who will testify. Whenever possible, select a witness who is from the district represented by the chair or another member of the committee. The organization's president or an expert on the issue is frequently selected. Always select a witness knowledgeable in the subject area who is a good public speaker. The witness's familiarity with the subject will strengthen the delivery and ensure accurate responses to impromptu questions. All witnesses, no matter how seasoned, should be briefed about the legislation and the committee's record on the issue. If you are selected as a witness,

notify your elected representative of your appearance, especially if he or she serves on the committee holding the hearings.

PRESENTING TESTIMONY

Presenting testimony is like staging a theatrical production. It requires setting the stage (writing the testimony), selecting the actors (choosing a witness), and rehearsing the script (briefing the witness). The quality of the final production is dependent on the director (the committee chair), the preparation of the actors (the witnesses and committee members), and how well they relate to each other. A few suggestions can make for a smoother production:

1. Be prepared to wait well beyond the time you were told you would testify. Meetings often begin late, and committee members' questions can lengthen the proceedings. If the chair indicates that there are enough votes to support your position and requests that you submit your testimony but not make an oral presentation, comply without objection. There is no need to speak if you have already won.

2. If you speak, be sure that the oral statement is succinct, outlines the key features of the written testimony, and can be presented within the time frame specified by the committee guidelines. Although it is helpful to have a prepared statement, the most effective witnesses speak spontaneously and do not read word for word from a prepared text. If a prepared statement is read, try to interject spontaneous comments, such as a personal anecdote or a summary statement. Rehearse the statement in advance to be sure you are within the allotted time.

3. Establish eye contact with committee members, especially the chair. Hearings can be tedious proceedings for members, and efforts to ease the routine are appreciated and make the presentation more effective. The more natural and relaxed the presentation is, the greater the impact it will have.

4. Relate a personal story. Stories such as those of patients needing dialysis who told their stories to Congress when Congress was deliberating on Medicare or those of persons with acquired immunodeficiency syndrome when funding for medication was threatened are powerful approaches to presenting testimony.

5. Prepare answers for potential questions. Try to contact a committee staff person when submitting the written statement to see whether you can suggest or submit certain questions or whether you can review the questions in advance of the hearings. Knowing the questions beforehand helps alleviate anxiety. If you are not prepared to answer a question, do not guess. It is perfectly acceptable to say that you are not familiar with an issue or detail but will look into the matter and submit a written statement for the record. After the hearing, ask the committee staff person what procedure you need to follow to fulfill this promise.

6. Circulate copies of the written statement to persons interested in the topic, including the press, other legislators, and other organizations. You may find important allies for future coalition building.

FOLLOWING UP

Follow up on all communications—letters, personal meetings, or testimony—preferably by letter. Thank the person for his or her time and attention to your concerns and include any additional information that you promised. To develop a reciprocal relationship, maintain contact with staff or legislators periodically (about every 6 months). Regular communication is more effective than crisis communication.

Inform your professional nursing organization and other nurses about the hearing's proceeding and action. Offer your continued expertise and involvement as the issue moves through the political process.

SUMMARY

Because the political process is continuous, communicating with policymakers should be an ongoing endeavor. Remember that legislators respond well to considerate, thoughtful communication. With nurses' skill in interpersonal relationships, we have the potential to shape health policy through influencing legislators.

Not every nurse is ready to testify before a committee of the U.S. Senate. We are all at different personal, professional, and political stages of development (Cohen et al., 1996). However, all nurses can take the first steps: voting for identified supporters of the nursing agenda and writing to legislators about nursing's position on matters of importance to nurses and patients. Accepting the challenge to lobby policymakers is a fundamental part of the advocacy role—a role that is the core of our profession's promise to society.

REFERENCES

American Nurses Association. (1995). *Code for nurses with interpretive statements*. Kansas City, MO: Author.

Betts, V. (1996). Nursing's agenda for health care reform: Policy, politics and power through professional leadership. *Nursing Administration Quarterly, 20*(3), 1–8.

Cohen, S., Mason, D., Kovner, C., Leavitt, J., Pulcini, J., & Sochalski, J. (1996). Stages of nursing's political development: Where we've been and where we ought to go. *Nursing Outlook, 44,* 259–266.

Joel, L. (1991). Nursing's agenda: The challenge of process. *American Nurse, 23*(6), 5.

Kelly, L., & Joel, L. (1995). *Dimensions in nursing.* 7th ed. New York: McGraw-Hill.

MacPherson, K. (1987). Health care policy, values, and nursing. *Advances in Nursing Science, 9*(3), 1–11.

U.S. Chamber of Commerce. (1996). *Building an effective government affairs program*. Washington, DC: Author.

Wakefield, M. K. (1990). Political involvement: A nursing necessity. *Nursing Economics, 8*(5), 352–353.

Chapter *30*

THE AMERICAN VOTER: Political Campaigns and Nursing's Leadership

CANDY DATO AND PATRICIA FORD-ROEGNER

American voters are courted relentlessly by a stream of media messages even as their very audiences scorn them. Americans are not voting as they have in the past, and the degree of cynicism has risen. Yet the process continues, and nurses have become more involved than ever in campaigns and in getting elected to office.

Political campaigns have become fraught with issues of concern to the voting public. Internally they paradoxically combine organization and chaos in the attempt to meet the many challenges and demands presented. Nurses as campaign volunteers or staff are highly sought because of their experience in creating order out of chaos. Nurses are addressing both the internal organization and the complex questions about campaigning.

CURRENT ISSUES AND TRENDS

Voting Patterns

The most political act every nurse, indeed every citizen, can perform is to register and vote. We can also make certain that our family, close friends, colleagues, and students are also registered to vote and do vote.

For many years government relations professionals and political scientists have sounded the alarm about national trends of limited and declining participation in electoral politics in the United States. Though Americans clearly love patriotic symbols, fireworks, and parades, too few are motivated to vote for the most powerful position in the world, President of the United States. As nation after nation has launched protests for democracy and the right to vote, Americans are not exercising that most precious freedom.

Voter turnout in the United States has been declining since it reached its highest level of 63% of the voting age population in the 1960 presidential election. Presidents have been elected with barely half of the eligible electorate participating in national elections. Midterm elections fare worse with one third, and local elections may only draw one fourth of the electorate. Between 1976 and 1988, the levels did not exceed 54% in any presidential election year. There was an increase in the 1992 election, reaching 55% and causing many to question whether this was a sign of a shift in behavior. The 1996 elections demonstrated that there had been no such shift—the 49% turnout representing a decline in both percentage and actual numbers of voters from 1992 (Federal Election Commission, 1997). It was the lowest voter turnout in an election year since 1924, when women were first franchised and were unfamiliar with voting, and laws discriminated against the registration of immigrants. The U.S. Government gives legitimacy to countries that have elected governments, but the United States itself rates low, number 17, in comparison with other Western industrial nations in turnout figures (Solop & Wonders, 1995).

Another cause for concern is the demographics of those who do vote. Nonvoting is disproportionately more common among those of lower socioeconomic status and people of color. In 1992, 64% of whites voted, whereas only 54% of African Americans and 48% of Hispanics voted. Additionally the entire electorate is older, with only 38% of the 18- to 20-year-olds voting in 1992, in comparison with 46% of the 21- to 24-year-olds and 70% of those more than age 45 years. "The data are unambiguous in portraying an electoral system in which older, affluent, majority-culture citizens are much more likely to participate in electoral politics than younger, less affluent individuals and people of color" (Solop & Wonders, 1995, p. 70).

The reasons for this phenomenon among all groups have been attributed to both personal reactions and structural problems in the voting process. Cynicism, alienation, social disconnection, boredom, satisfaction with the status quo, and a lack of a sense of political responsibility have been viewed as reasons for nonvoting. Political action committees, negative campaigns, lackluster candidates, political media, television, the educational system, and the "me generation" have all been mentioned as possible contributors to this low turnout. The League of Women Voters (1996) found in a survey that nonvoters are less likely to grasp the impact of elections on issues that concern them, discuss political issues less often than voters, believe that they lack sufficient information on which to base their votes, and find the voting process difficult and cumbersome. In addition, they are less likely to be contacted by organizations that encourage voting, and they attach less importance to voting than to other daily activities. The researchers also found that contact and connections such as encouragement by family and friends were instrumental in changing voting behavior.

It has been posited that this knowledge gap effects Americans' views on politics and their voting behavior. "Whether uninterested, uninformed or simply ignorant, millions of Americans cannot answer even basic question about American politics, according to a survey by the *Washington Post,* the Kaiser Family Foundation and Harvard University" (Morin, 1996, p. A1). Theories regarding why Americans don't know more about government include less basic education about government, less time to keep informed, and the use of television as the primary source of information. In a random sample of 1,514 adults, those with more knowledge were compared to those with less. The adults with more knowledge were more mistrustful of government while also having more faith in the political system. They saw their vote as a remedy and were twice as likely to have voted (Morin, 1996). "The information gap is affecting how politics is practiced, dumbing down democracy and making political campaigns increasingly negative and character based" (Morin, 1996, p. A7).

Another gap in voting, the gender gap, reached its peak in the 1996 elections, causing one author to refer to 1996 as the "Year of Women Voters" (Dodson, 1997). Men were evenly divided in voting for Clinton (44%) and Dole (43%), whereas women voters' support for Clinton was considerable (54% versus 38%) (Dodson, 1997). This large gender gap grew out of a full-scale effort to win women's votes by "connect[ing] private concerns of home and family to the political as never before" (Dodson, 1997, p. 27). Women have been found to differ from men in their views on government, with women viewing government as being able to help solve problems and men more likely to see government as the problem. Women are also less likely to support spending cuts on social programs because they are more supportive of the social safety net and the human impact of public policies in general. Furthermore, women are more tolerant of gay rights, are more concerned about the environment, and place a higher value on the notion of community (Dodson, 1997).

The National Voter Registration Act

Another view of low voter turnout is that it is reflective of a structural problem, access to the voting process. Starting in the 1980s, several groups (Project VOTE, Human SERVE, National Coalition of Black Voter Registration, and others) were mobilizing local groups to change the power structure. Grassroots efforts for inclusion were begun to challenge the prevailing political system, which was seen as victimizing the poor and disadvantaged. Past social movements had successfully created more inclusion by expanding the franchise to women (1920), people of color (1965), youth (1971), and the differently able (1984). The elimination of poll taxes (1964) and literacy tests (1965) also expanded the franchise.

Local barriers were initially targeted until it became evident that it was more efficient to join together to work on the problem nationally in order to bring sweeping reforms of voter registration to the struggle for the disenfranchised. The League of Women Voters of the United States was a major leader in the coalition to support the passage of legislation designed to reform our current system and make it easier to register. Its 1991 *Fact Sheet* states:

> National voter registration reform is not a panacea but it is an important and necessary first step to encourage voter participation. At least one-third of all eligible voters—70 million people—are not even registered to vote. One-third of the adult population moves every two years. The confusing array of state and local registration practices nationwide constitutes a significant barrier to voter participation.

In the late 1980s, voter registration reform was seen as a partisan issue that the Democratic Party supported and the Republicans did not. President Clinton came into office with the expansion of voter registration as part of his platform. The goal was to empower those without money to have access to government. He signed the National Voter Registration Act (NVRA) into law on May 20, 1993, and it went into effect January 1, 1995. Clinton's success is the success of a broad and influential political struggle and social movement, an appealing attempt to engage the masses. It was hoped that through the expansion of the population regis-

tered to vote, the NVRA would create the possibility of destabilizing the status quo and lead to a reconstitution of power relations (Solop & Wonders, 1995).

The NVRA provides for the establishment of several mechanisms, the key of which is the "motor voter" registration. Any application, renewal, or change of address for a driver's license or nondriver's identification card also serves as an application for voter registration. Agency registration established distribution of voter registration application forms and assistance at a variety of governmental and nongovernmental agencies, including libraries and unemployment, public assistance, vocational rehabilitation, and Social Security agencies. Mail-in registration was also established in those states where it did not already exist. Additionally, the NVRA eliminated the purging of nonvoting registrants from voter registration lists and required election officials to send all applicants a notice informing them of their voter registration status.

Human SERVE (1996) and the League of Women Voters (Duskin, 1997a) reported that the NVRA brought about the largest expansion of voter registration in a 2-year period in the history of the United States, an estimated 12 million new voters. Some states such as Georgia had phenomenal increases (from 85,000 registering in 1994 to 181,000 in the first 3 months of 1995). Although it had been projected that nearly half of the added registrants would actually vote, the numbers were much lower in the 1996 presidential election, suggesting that structural issues are not the only reasons for low voter turnout.

CANDIDATES

Women Candidates

Elected officials at all levels of government do not reflect the gender diversity in the United States. Women have largely been restricted in their journey to the heart of political power in this country. In 1992, the "Year of the Woman," that pattern was altered somewhat when women moved into national and statewide elected offices in greater numbers than ever before. The number of women candidates for the Congress, Senate, statewide elective executives, and state legislatures has been climbing steadily for the past 20 years. In 1976 there was one woman candidate for the U.S. Senate, five for Congress, two for governorships, and 1,258 for state legislatures. Records were set in 1992 with 11 for the U.S. Senate; in 1994 with 10 for governorships and 2,285 for state legislatures; and in 1996 with 120 for Congress. The numbers of women candidates declined for some offices in 1996, with nine candidates for the Senate, six for governorships, and 2,273 for state legislatures (Center for the American Woman and Politics, 1996).

In 1997 the number of women in elected office reached record levels, with 60 (11.2% of the 535 seats) in Congress and 9 (9%) in the Senate. The number of women in statewide elective executive posts, such as governor or comptroller, dropped from the 1995 record of 85 to 81 in 1997, representing 25.1% of the available positions. In 1997 women legislators held 1,588 seats (21.4% of the available seats). This represents an increase five times that of the 4% held in 1969 (Center for the American Woman and Politics, 1997). The number of women of color remains a particular concern; for example, only 21 have ever served in Congress (Duskin, 1997b).

Increasing the numbers of elected and appointed women is more than an issue of justice and equality. The Center for the American Woman and Politics studied the impact of women in state legislatures and found that female elected officials differed from their male counterparts in terms of their attitudes and their top-priority bills. The women were more likely to emphasize women's rights and bills dealing with "women's traditional areas of interest— health care, the welfare of children, the family and the elderly, housing, the environment and education—that stem from women's roles as caregivers in the family and in society more generally" (Carroll, Dodson, & Mandel, 1991, p. 7). Women legislators from both parties were more likely to support feminist and liberal policy positions than their male colleagues. They found "compelling evidence that women are having a distinctive impact on public policy and the political process" (Carroll et al., 1991, p. 3). They also found that the commitment to represent the interests and issues of women does not diminish as women legislators move into leadership positions.

Women legislators differ from men in their leadership styles and are changing political processes and institutions as well as influencing public policy. Women legislators involve citizens more, finding their input helpful. They are more likely to bring government into the public view. They are more responsive to the economically disadvantaged, working to bring them greater access (Carroll et al., 1991).

Congresswoman Carolyn McCarthy embodies many of the characteristics of a woman/nurse candidate coming up against a male incumbent. She overcame many obstacles and is seen as a heroine to many. Like many other women, she was not considered to be a serious contender and was thought of as a one-issue candidate. What mobilized people to support her was her media exposure and her commonsense approach to a variety of issues.

There are many factors relating to the movement of women into political office. The ratio of male to female candidates still remains two to one (Duskin, 1997b). Many women candidates belong to or receive formal and informal campaign support from women's organizations, women's political action committees (PACs), and professional associations like the American Nurses Association (ANA), whose members are mostly women (Carroll et al., 1991). Women continue to juggle their home and work responsibilities, and they are concerned about the tenor of political races (Duskin, 1997b). Incumbents, who are largely men, win elections 95% of the time (Duskin, 1997b). The current campaign finance laws favor incumbents. Women have the same problems as incumbents in general; they are lacking in money, name recognition, and the built-in advantages that incumbency offers. For example, incumbents receive seven times more

PAC money than challengers (Duskin, 1997b), and expensive campaigns rely on media coverage. Women challengers do, however, win as often as male challengers. The dual, and often related, concerns about the power of the media and the exorbitant cost of campaigns, geared to short television spots without substantive discussions of issues, plague American voters.

Ethnic Diversity

The lack of ethnic representation in campaigns and hence in public office is another concern to nurses. As with women candidates, incumbency is a major obstacle. A single issue, such as ethnicity, however, is no longer sufficient for a candidate to win. Candidates must encompass other concerns and form alliances with other groups.

Redistricting, which was based on ethnic criteria, has enabled more women and minority candidates to come into office by opening up seats (Duskin, 1997b). Redistricting itself has been undone by the courts (1997) and will be a limited strategy for increasing ethnic representation in legislatures. It was surely not the answer to the lack of diversity in public office, but it is one means by which women and minorities have been able to run for office successfully. It often, conversely, protected incumbents and has been considered both gerrymandering and unconstitutional. It was thought that the creation of majority-minority districts through redistricting would increase voter turnout in those areas. Preliminary studies have not upheld this belief. "Empowerment, in the sense of having a much greater chance of electing a legislative candidate of one's choice (frequently equated with of *one's own group*), does not invariably lead to greater participation" (Brace, Handley, Niemi, & Stanley, 1995, p. 201). Pennsylvania is additionally protecting incumbents through restrictive measures that require candidates to get thousands of signatures within a short period in order to have their name placed on the ballot.

Term limits was viewed as a potential reform measure against incumbency by those who view career politicians as inherently dangerous. This popular reform was brought to a halt by the U.S. Supreme Court ruling that invalidated state laws limiting terms. Thus the future of term limits was left in the hands of Congress. Many believe that the members will not support term limits because of their own self-interest.

There are numerous efforts of underrepresented populations to be organized into voting blocks. Witness the Million Man March; the election of a Hispanic woman in conservative Orange County, California; and the increasing organization of large immigrant communities.

Recruiting Candidates

Recruiting candidates to run for office is routinely done by political parties, activists, and interest groups. Incumbents leaving political life often endorse a successor, but those who are not in the "old-boy network," namely women and minorities, are unlikely to be considered.

Politically active nurses are beginning to recruit candidates. These candidates are both nurses and nonnurses who support important issues in nursing. There are responsibilities associated with the recruitment of candidates. Campaigns need time, money, and volunteers. Nurses encouraging someone to run for office must deliver some of each of these commodities. If the recruited candidate then wins, nurses now have influence with this new member of a particular political body. They may also have accomplished another goal of delivering a clear message to the opposition, who may, in fact, have been one of nursing's opponents. If nurses can affect just one election, they already have political power, and for politicians whose main goal is getting elected and reelected, the political power of nurses will not only be acknowledged but also sought after.

Nurses have developed long-range plans for grooming nurse leaders who will take on increasingly advanced leadership roles in electoral politics, including running for office. This type of visionary planning will ensure nursing's rightful place at the policy levels of health care. It will also help increase the number of women and minority-group members in public office. Nurses are challenged by the power of incumbency and the barriers it presents to diversity.

Choosing a Candidate

Nurses are interested in choosing candidates whose values and beliefs are closely aligned with their own. Nurses work on campaigns through their affiliation with organized nursing efforts such as ANA-PAC, state nursing associations' PACs, and specialty nursing organizations. They also join local groups of nurses working with a particular candidate or groups of nurse friends. Many work on campaigns of candidates they support as individual citizens and nurses. Whatever the situation, deciding whom to chose is important because nurses have a positive public image to uphold and want to use their time wisely and effectively. Nurses choosing candidates as part of an organized group such as a PAC have more political factors to weigh in making these decisions. They may not choose candidates in every race they look at after balancing the considerations involved.

What does one look for in a candidate or campaign? Candidates may be known by their previous legislative work either in the office for which they are again running or in a different office. Nurses may know candidates as a result of their political party activities or their participation in community organizations, or from the neighborhood. PACs often have a structured format for interviewing potential candidates to determine their position on issues of concern to the nursing community.

When deciding on a candidate to support, consider the person's position on issues, voting records, qualifications, and electability. Many factors that have an impact on a candidate should be taken into account (see Box on p. 498). Nurses bring valuable personal interaction skills to a campaign and should use these skills in evaluating candidates.

CASE EXAMPLE   Carolyn McCarthy's Story

The story of Congresswoman Carolyn McCarthy embodies many of the issues and concerns of women candidates, nurse candidates, and voters. Carolyn McCarthy was an American citizen—a wife, mother, housewife, and licensed practical nurse—and had lived in Nassau County, Long Island, her entire life. The chronicle of her move from a comfortable suburban lifestyle to horror and grief, and finally to public service, is moving.

On December 7, 1993, a Long Island Railroad train with rush-hour passengers was traveling east and headed for disaster. When the train reached the Merillon Avenue Station, Colin Ferguson had opened fire, wounding 25 people and killing six with a 9-millimeter semiautomatic weapon. Carolyn McCarthy's husband, Dennis, was among the dead, and her son, Kevin, was severely wounded. During the months that followed, Carolyn McCarthy became the spokesperson for the families of the victims, while caring for her son in his struggle to regain his health and his life. Her face, her voice, and her words came to symbolize the struggle for gun control legislation. Three years later that battle propelled her into Congress, aided by a community outraged about an incumbent legislator who opposed gun control.

The Fourth Congressional District of New York is largely Republican, filled with commuters who take the Long Island Railroad and share the sadness and outrage of the McCarthy family. When their Republican Congressman, Daniel Frisa, voted to repeal a ban on 19 specific types of assault weapons, Carolyn McCarthy resolved to run against him for Congress (Barry, 1996). Her anger and indignation reflected the feelings of many of his constituents. She approached the Republican Party with her concerns; her bid to run against Frisa in the primary was rejected by them. The Democrat Party reached out to her, and she accepted their support, crossing party lines to act on her conscience and with her heart.

Carolyn McCarthy was an unknown candidate who had never sought public office, never been involved in any political activities, and never dreamed she would be running for the U.S. Congress. She was not, however, unknown to the public. She was well known for her work on gun control and her family tragedy. She had already been in the limelight and continued to get media coverage throughout her campaign. Her story is also the story of a citizen going to Washington, a story that warms the hearts of many cynical Americans tired of career politicians. She was an attractive candidate who had credibility as a nurse and a clear personal passion with which others identified. She stepped forth to challenge an incumbent who had voted with his party, showing particular insensitivity to the wishes of a community wracked by a tragic massacre.

Her opponents used negative campaigning by portraying her as a one-issue candidate without the talent and experience that would qualify her for public office. She herself ran a campaign that focused on issues—issues that she knew from her experience as a citizen, community member, woman, and nurse. She rapidly expanded her platform to include health care reform and environmental protection and targeted tax cuts for working families. On November 6, 1997, she was elected, strongly defeating the incumbent. On election night she wore buttons on her red suit, one of which read, "When women vote, women win" (Barry, 1996).

NURSES AS VOTERS AND CAMPAIGNERS

Nurses affect the political process by their individual and collective support of candidates. Nurses and other health care workers can also have a considerable impact on those with whom they come into contact by explaining the importance of voting and its effect on their daily lives. Health care issues are tied to public policy and are thus dependent on the votes of elected officials. Pushing for the passage of health care legislation is one way nurses can show the public and consumers that patient advocacy does not stop at the health facility door. Imagine 2.2 million nurses with buttons saying: "I am a nurse. I vote—do you?"

Voter registration drives provide an excellent opportunity for nursing students or nurses new to political activities to get involved. At university settings it is an opportunity to reach the younger population who are eligible to vote but may not have been exercising that right. Such drives can also provide a public relations opportunity by enabling nurses to be visible in large educational, health care, and other facilities, thus receiving credit for promoting community involvement. Increasingly, nursing has built

stronger ties with consumers in order to gain support for nursing's health care agenda. Nurses can get specific details about organizing and conducting a voter registration drive from organizations such as the National Women's Political Caucus, the Women's Campaign Fund, and the League of Women Voters.

Voter registration efforts have been targeted to both the general public and more specifically to nurses. The ANA and state nurses associations (SNAs) increased efforts to register nurses in 1996 in their "Registered Nurse/Registered Voter" campaign, launched during ANA's centennial, which reached almost 200,000 nurses. The potential power of the nurses' vote is great: 1 in 44 women voters in the United States is a nurse. The ANA and SNAs sent out colorful posters featuring a photo of Isabel Hampton Robb with the title "This nurse couldn't vote." Literature regarding the importance of both registering and voting was disseminated broadly through the Internet (American Nurses Association, 1996), including the following phrases:

- The truth is, the voices of nursing can be heard louder than ever this next election day, November 5.
- Four-years ago, the potential voting power of registered nurses approximated the combined votes received by Clinton, Bush, and Perot in Tennessee, Washington, South Carolina, Minnesota, and Indiana, and exceeded Presidential vote totals in 29 other states. Indeed, if all 2.2 million registered nurses had voted in the 1992 Presidential election, they would have equaled more than 2% of the entire popular vote for President nationally.
- Without a doubt, 2.2 million is a big number to politicians eyeing offices in the fall who need to respect mandates from you and other registered nurses.
- Maybe you agree that the potential voting power of the country's largest health care profession on November 5, Election Day, is awesome. But the potential won't be realized unless you take steps today to register to vote.

Until the early 1980s, few nurses had political campaign experience. The number of nurses who now campaign has increased tremendously because they followed the lead of those nurses who plunged into political campaigns. Nurses were encouraged to take advantage of a variety of political training workshops offered by the National Women's Political Caucus, the Women's Campaign Fund, the Democratic Party, the ANA, and others. Political and legislative workshops sponsored by the ANA and SNAs became popular. Specialty nursing organizations and major unions followed. Nurse campaigners are now a part of the cadre of experienced volunteers and paid staff available to potential candidates and campaigns of both political parties. Elected officials regularly recommend nurse campaigners to their colleagues. With more nurses serving as lobbyists and public policy staff at the national and state levels, as well as an increasing number of nurses who receive political appointments, nursing has become a serious player in the American political process.

Campaign experiences provided nurses with the understanding and experience needed to become candidates themselves. An ever-increasing number of nurse candidates run for and win state legislative and county races. In 1997, approximately 80 nurses held seats in state legislatures. In 1992 Eddie Bernice Johnson, of Texas, became the first nurse elected to Congress, followed by Carolyn McCarthy in 1996, and Lois Capps from California in 1998. More will follow. Voters are looking for candidates who offer a credible and fresh approach to problem solving. Nurse candidates fill that vacuum.*

Nurses must make sure that the campaign staff knows they are nurses. Being a nurse is a professional identity and can add to political identity. Nurses already have numerous skills that are invaluable in a campaign, so they should make their talents known. As volunteers, nurses must take the initiative to make sure their worth is recognized. Nurses considering volunteering for a political campaign should assess campaign needs and their own availability, interests, talents, and experiences. By ascertaining who the leaders of a campaign are, nurses can then tell these leaders about themselves, how much their time is worth, and what they are doing or would like to do in the campaign. To get what they want, nurses will have to use both communication and negotiation skills and can make a place for themselves in the campaign in areas of responsibility, such as scheduling and coordinating other volunteers or running the whole campaign. High visibility in a campaign can earn nurses enormous political credit.

NUTS AND BOLTS OF CAMPAIGNS

Before getting involved in a political campaign, consider the goal. Is it to help a particular candidate who is a friend of nursing or who shares values and priorities with nurses? Is it to develop your relationship with a particular political party? Does interest in organizing local nurses into a political power group warrant becoming involved in a campaign? Is the possibility of a staff position appealing? Will involvement in this campaign further a personal political career? (See Box, p. 498.)

Recruiting and choosing a candidate, knowing precisely what to offer personally to the campaign, understanding how dedication of time and effort to the campaign may affect one's own career, and being aware of the importance of campaign planning might result in an offer or request to become part of a yet-undeclared candidate's exploratory committee.

Exploratory Committees

An exploratory committee enables a candidate to test the political waters. Before the campaign begins, a candidate must determine which

---

*There are restrictions on the political activity of nurses who work for the federal government in Veterans Administration hospitals, the public health service, and the military. Appendix B provides a discussion of the do's and don'ts for these nurses, as dictated by the Hatch Act. Nurses working for the federal government need to monitor changes in the Hatch Act. Nurses working in state facilities should check state laws governing political participation.

QUESTIONS TO ASK WHEN CONSIDERING SUPPORT OF A CANDIDATE

The Candidate

- What kinds of experiences would the candidate bring to the office?
- Is the candidate's political knowledge and skill respected by his or her peers?
- What is the candidate's voting record in the office for which he or she is running or in a different previous office?
- What committees and positions of leadership has the candidate had while in office?

The Campaign Staff and Plan

- Has the staff researched the political unit where the candidate is running?
  (A campaign needs an up-to-date profile of the district to develop a winning campaign plan.)
- Does the campaign have an overall plan and component parts?
  (One can consider his or her own professional skills in planning and organizing and ask whether these plans seem realistic. For example, a campaign that has a projected budget, but no plan regarding how it intends to raise funds, is deficient.)
- Is the campaign managed in a professional manner?
- Are schedules adhered to and tasks completed on time?
- Do the candidate and campaign manager work well together?
- Do they recognize that in areas such as polling, public relations, and fund raising, hiring political professionals may be well worth the cost?
- Are there creative plans to combine professional and volunteer help?
- Is the volunteer coordinator personable and capable of planning and staffing key events?
- How well will the candidate and his or her team work together?

Electability

- What is the likelihood of the candidate's being elected?

- Do polls show a high positive or negative rating for the incumbent?
- Does the voting public recognize the challenger's name?
- Does the candidate have his or her party's backing?
- If not, why not?
  (Women candidates who enter politics as a result of their concern over local issues are often unable to obtain party support, but this should not preclude their becoming viable candidates.)
- Is the candidate a good public speaker and one who appears to enjoy campaigning?
- How much does the candidate want to win?
- Is this an open seat because of the incumbent's retirement, or is it a new seat created as a result of redistricting?
- Is this candidate challenging an incumbent?
- What is the political makeup of the district?
- Is the district heavily Democrat or Republican?
- Is there a large independent vote?
- In the previous election, what percentage of registered voters voted?
- Is this a Presidential election year, in which one can expect a higher voter turnout?
- What was the incumbent's margin of victory in the previous election?
  (If the incumbent is popular with the voters and received, say, 78% of the vote in the last election, the challenger's chances are slim.)
- Who lives in this election district?
- Where do people work?
- What are the major media sources?

Risk/Benefit Ratio

- What is the potential damage if the candidate is supported and loses?
- Does this potential damage outweigh the benefits of supporting the candidate?

of the people encouraging him or her to run for office is ready to commit time and money. It is a time for a candidate to assess his or her relationship with the political party and gauge the amount of support, financial and otherwise, available for a campaign. A candidate uses this period to determine what sections of the registered voter population will be in his or her corner and how to reach those who are swing voters or independents. It is a time to develop relationships with both individuals and groups and is invaluable to a campaign.

The exploratory committee may be formal, with a long list of prominent names on a raised letterhead, or small and informal. Seats on these committees are often prestigious, with membership a sign of having "arrived" as a valued political participant. The significance of these committees increases with the level of office sought. The legalities surrounding the formation of an exploratory committee for fund-raising purposes is regulated by the Federal Election Commission or by state election commissions.

Campaign Managers

An important early step for a candidate is choosing a campaign manager. This important decision may be influenced by the political party as well as the candidate and those working closely with him or her. The political network of former candidates and current activists will supply a candidate with suggestions for a manager. Politics involves getting to know who knows what and whom and keeping in touch.

Experience, especially if it has been successful, is important. Campaigns for higher public office often require an experienced campaign manager. Nevertheless, enthusiastic, energetic, and talented organizers successfully manage their first campaigns.

Since the early 1980s, the hard work of political women has produced an explosion of women campaign managers, including the major adviser of Senator Dole's presidential campaign (see Chapter 26 Vignette). This was not unplanned. For years, political women in Washington, D.C., and across the country, have donated time, money, and expertise to serve as mentors to each other. Women's political organizations, such as the National Women's Political Caucus, and numerous women's organizations have provided training in campaign management as part of their effort to reach out to women and increase their involvement in the political process. It is real revolution. Nurses are increasingly moving

into these positions, where they use skills developed in nursing.

From the beginning, the candidate and the manager must understand each other's roles. A campaign can begin to fall apart if the candidate, instead of the person hired to do so, is managing the campaign. A trusting relationship is essential.

Campaign Calendar

A campaign calendar is a critical part of campaign planning. It is a tool used to divide the numerous campaign activities into manageable pieces. A good campaign will have carefully thought-out goals, priorities, and phases that are meticulously scheduled throughout the campaign period.

The calendar outlines a time schedule for the campaign, supports the staff's focus on details, and helps to prevent internal crises. For example, planning "get out the vote" telephone banking before election day involves knowledge that the telephone company needs 3 weeks' notice to install additional lines and that a friendly union will be scheduling its phones for several candidates. Building this requirement into the plan ensures that the telephones will be in place on schedule. Without such planning, the campaign might have no telephones but would have many angry and frustrated volunteers, and additional expenses as a result of the effort to obtain telephones on short notice.

Recruitment and Training of Volunteers

Volunteers are the core of any political campaign. In a low-budget campaign, they can be *the* campaign. They should be treated with respect; their time should be well used, accounted for, much appreciated, and recognized. Volunteers can enjoy the time they spend working together. The team of volunteers in a campaign should feel as though they are an integral part of that effort, and they should be thanked and thanked—and thanked again.

First, volunteers must be recruited. Active, enthusiastic nurses can be drawn from all health-related areas: hospitals, clinics, doctors' offices, temporary agencies, community health agencies, and others. If enough volunteers are recruited, no one will be overburdened.

An ideal way to recruit volunteers is to schedule an event that will involve one or more candidates—perhaps a coffee in someone's home or at a public meeting place. Candidates should make opening remarks, respond to questions, and ask for the support of nurses. The following are steps to take when recruiting potential volunteers through a "candidates' night" to which all candidates for particular office are invited.

1. Ask candidates for their schedules (well in advance) and select a date when all will be available. Advertise the event as a special reception for nurses.
2. Work backward from the date of the event and plan every detail. Create a flyer and distribute copies to area nurses; arrange other publicity; contract for a meeting place; order refreshments; and decide who will introduce the candidates and determine the format, including how long each is to speak and whether there is to be a question-and-answer period. Then delegate the tasks to get the job done.
3. At the event itself, have an attendance sheet at the entrance, requesting name, address, and telephone number. If it is feasible, spend time with each guest and ask if he or she is interested in volunteering for upcoming political activities. Take notes (name, address, and telephone number), and follow up with a telephone call to confirm the volunteer's commitment. For larger crowds, distribute volunteer cards and make a strong pitch for volunteers.

There are other ways to recruit volunteers:

- Host a social event with a political theme for area nurses. Make it festive and fun. Invite several local political personalities to attend.
- Cosponsor an all-day political skills seminar in conjunction with your local political par-

ties. At the conclusion, sign people up for jobs that appeal to them.
- Call a meeting to discuss upcoming political projects. Encourage each member of the core group to bring two friends. Then involve guests in the conversation, planning, and strategy. By evening's end, they will be ready to help.
- Organize informal get-togethers, such as brown bag lunches, at or near nurses' workplaces. Invite a local campaign manager or politically active nurse to speak; then sign up volunteers.

Volunteers must be carefully cultivated, cared for, trained, appreciated, and thanked. Here are some tips:

- Volunteers are just that: they do not get paid. They must feel needed and appreciated, or they will play tennis or watch television instead.
- Nothing is more frustrating than volunteering and then not being called on. If someone offers to tackle a job, put her or him to work immediately.
- Do not leave anything to chance. Volunteers benefit from clear, detailed instructions; campaigns do, too.
- Do not try to pull the wool over a volunteer's eyes. If you convince someone to do a 2-hour job that grows into 20 hours, she or he has every right to quit in the middle.
- Everyone has strengths and weaknesses. Most people will be honest in assessing whether their talents lie in answering the telephone or writing a speech. Enlist the volunteer's help in making good assignments from the outset. Underutilized and overwhelmed volunteers become frustrated, and then they quit.
- Keep records of jobs that volunteers have done, so you or someone else may call on them again.

Local community issue groups can provide additional information on volunteer recruitment. Handbooks are developed on a regular basis by a broad range of organizations such as the American Association of Retired Persons and the League of Women Voters.

Fund Raising

A candidate's war chest and his or her ability to raise money demonstrates the seriousness of the candidate. One must raise money to get money. Major contributors who give large donations to a campaign want to know how much money a candidate has raised before they will contribute. It is also the first question asked by PAC directors. A volunteer or group that successfully raises money will definitely be appreciated.

Fund raising is both an art and a skill. Most organizations see the value of contracting with professional fundraisers and find that it is worth the initial outlay. The manner in which a fund-raising appeal is conducted is vital. An error-free, attractive, and creative appeal for donations is worth the effort. An expert fundraiser knows how to do it and how to get the best price.

As a candidate or volunteer fundraiser, start with family, friends, and colleagues. If time and money permit, target messages to specific groups in order to get the most from the appeal.

Much can and should be explored with respect to fund raising. Additional tips are provided in Chapter 33.

Individual Voter Contact

Everyone involved in a campaign—the candidate, staff, and volunteers—is in the campaign to win, which means garnering more support than the opponent does. This is accomplished with a plan that is based on knowledge of the district voters, who will support the candidate, who will not support the candidate, and undecided voters. Once voters have been identified, they must be contacted personally. One important fact here that often surprises those new to politics: campaigners do not want to contact all voters—just those who will or might vote for one's candidate.

An effective campaign gets the voters' attention. Voters are bombarded by information during a campaign. The goal is to get voters to notice one's candidate, think about his or her commercial, and open mailed advertising pieces. Candidates are noticed when their messages are presented clearly and creatively, and repeated over and over. Repetitive contact and follow-up are essential to persuading voters.

The three most traditional ways to contact individual voters are through telephone banks, canvassing, and direct mail. Telephone banks and door-to-door canvassing are labor intensive, so a large number of volunteers must be recruited. They will also be needed to make follow-up contacts. Telephone banks, if well organized, can reach more voters in a shorter amount of time than canvassing. For telephone banks, a well-prepared script for volunteers is necessary. The numerous details involved in these efforts necessitate good planning. For example, 2 or 3 hours of telephoning a night is all a volunteer can usually do, so you must consider a number of variables when planning a telephone bank project: the hours, the number of telephones, the number of calls to be made, and so on. Telephone lists must be obtained, or numbers will have to be looked up before the telephoning can be done. In some areas, electronic dialing is available, utilizing names or numbers of members of political parties or organizations. Nurses, and other volunteers new to phone banking, may welcome coming in as a small group. Organizing groups of nurses from a particular hospital may be a way to bring in new volunteers.

A campaign kit is essential for canvassing. This kit can include information about the candidate, his or her position on issues of interest to the target group, volunteer cards for interested individuals to complete, campaign buttons, maps of the area, and sample outlines of what to say to the voters. It is necessary to avoid planning telephone or canvassing events that will conflict with popular events such as the World Series.

Direct mail should be well designed, attractive, and personalized. If possible, a specific message should be directed to the concerns of particular voters, such as nurses, senior citizens, parents, or teachers. Such targeted messages are known to be among the most effective. Many campaign managers believe it is worth the expense to obtain professional help in writing direct mail pieces.

New approaches to voter contact include organized efforts through churches and social organizations. Technology is expanding the horizon, as well, with web pages and E-mail messages abounding.

Media

Successful campaigns combine a well-funded and strategic media plan with a well-funded and carefully targeted voter contact program and field operation. The media plan should complement efforts to contact the individuals. Next to personal contact, television and radio are the most persuasive methods. Advertisements or articles that appear in local newspapers are often useful in local races, especially when money is tight. Television time is expensive, although creative campaigners can get free coverage as a result of innovative campaign techniques. For example, a candidate can schedule "work days," such as spending a day in a clinic with a nurse or with a teacher in an elementary school, and obtain coverage for the experience. (See Chapter 13 for a discussion of gaining access to and using media.)

Getting Out the Vote on Election Day

The final campaign step is getting people to vote on election day. Volunteers will be needed to telephone people, reminding them to vote. The intensity of the whole campaign heightens in the last few days. Voters may need babysitters or a ride to the polls. It is important to assist voters in many ways. Besides poll watchers, you will need volunteers to circulate near the voting place to persuade as-yet-undecided voters.

Thank-yous

Not enough can be said about thank-yous. Whether the campaign is successful or not, people who gave their time to the campaign should be recognized and appropriately thanked.

After Your Candidate Wins

After the glow of the victory celebration has worn off, it is important to build on one's relationship with the candidate, who is now an elected official. Most elected officials take their role in representing their constituencies seriously and need to hear from a broad range of voters. Nurses can continue to offer these officials a wealth of information about issues affecting the health and welfare of the community. Nurses interested in paid or appointed positions can now campaign for themselves, using the same skills that were successful in electing their candidate (see Chapter 26). Nurses frequently take on volunteer advisory roles on health issues. Those seeking staff positions may have assumed considerable responsibility during the campaign. They may continue to do so—for example, by creating events that help the newly elected official have access to a greater number of constituents. They may ask other supporters to recommend them to the elected official.

Grassroots Politics and Legislative Networks

In his significant work, *Why Americans Hate Politics*, E. J. Dionne, Jr., makes this important point:

> In our efforts to find a new world role, we would do well to revive what made us a special nation long before we became the world's leading military and economic power—our republican tradition that nurtured free citizens who eagerly embrace the responsibilities and pleasure of self-government. With democracy on the march outside our borders, our first responsibility is to ensure that the United States becomes a model for what self-government should be and not an example of what happens when they lose interest in public life. A nation that hates politics will not long survive as a democracy. [1991, p. 355]

All politics is local. Grassroots politics, legislative networks, and coalitions are vital to the development of public policy. Much has been said and written about Americans and our search for community as the nation's population becomes more diverse, and racial and economic groups grow further apart. For example, women ask why male politicians "don't get" their concerns about child care, housing, sexual harassment, or health care issues.

Grassroots political and legislative networks can provide a meaningful and useful service. More and more organizations, large and small, have come to realize that "back to the basics" in politics is a good idea. Worksite and school-based citizens' projects need to be developed so that citizens' needs can be defined and communicated to legislators and appointed officials. Women officeholders are more likely than men to acknowledge and use citizens and citizen groups and are more responsive to disadvantaged groups (Carroll et al., 1991).

Since the creation of the Congressional and Senate district coordinators network at the ANA more than 15 years ago, there has been a dramatic shift in the acceptance and appreciation of grassroots networks and voter contact programs. Handbooks on network building are widely used by major unions, consumer organizations, professional nursing organizations, hospitals, and small businesses. The ANA has expanded its grassroots network to include thousands of nurses around the country through the development of the Nursing Strategic Action Team (N-STAT).

Coalition politics is on the rise as well. The debate around national health reform brought together traditional and nontraditional allies to tackle the economic and social crisis. Nursing organizations are increasingly working together to present a unified force while simultaneously building coalitions around issues of concern to other groups interested in health and social welfare—for example, the ongoing issues of health care financing, women's health concerns, and professional deregulation. Nursing has also expanded its connections and liaisons with consumers themselves and the advocacy groups that represent them.

NURSING'S POLITICAL FUTURE

Nursing's political future remains bright because an increasing number of nurses are involved in all aspects of politics and health-policy decision making. For nursing as a profession to take its place as a serious political and policy player, we need more risk taking, more coalition building outside nursing, and more inclusiveness of all who provide nursing care and expertise.

REFERENCES

American Nurses Association. (1990). *Political and legislative handbook.* Washington, DC: Author.

American Nurses Association. (1996). Be an RN voter, register to vote [on-line]. Available from *http://www.nursingworld.org/gova/votenews.htm.*

Barry, D. (1996, November 7). An L.I. story: Next stop Washington. *The New York Times,* pp. A1, B14.

Barry, D. (1997, June 22). An icon goes to Washington. *The New York Times Magazine,* pp. 21–23.

Brace, K., Handley, L., Niemi, R. G., & Stanley, H. W. (1995). Minority turnout and the creation of majority-minority districts. *American Politics Quarterly, 23*(2), 190–202.

Carroll, S. J., Dodson, D. L., & Mandel, R. B. (1991). *The impact of women in public office: An overview,* New Brunswick, NJ: Center for the American Woman and Politics (CAWP), Eagleton Institute of Politics, Rutgers—The State University of New Jersey.

Center for the American Woman and Politics. (1996). *Fact sheet: Summary of women candidates for selected offices, 1968–1996.* New Brunswick, NJ: National Information Bank on Women in Public Office, Eagleton Institute of Politics, Rutgers—The State University of New Jersey.

Center for the American Woman and Politics. (1997). *Fact sheet: Women in elective office 1997.* New Brunswick, NJ: National Information Bank on Women in Public Office, Eagleton Institute of Politics, Rutgers—The State University of New Jersey.

Congress of the United States (1996). U.S. Representative Carolyn McCarthy (NY-04): Biography. Washington, DC: U.S. House of Representatives.

Dionne, E. J., Jr. (1991). *Why Americans hate politics.* New York: Simon & Schuster.

Dodson, D. (1997). Women voters and the gender gap. Center for the American Woman and Politics: *News and Notes, 2*(2). New Brunswick, NJ: Center for the American Woman and Politics (CAWP), Eagleton Institute of Politics, Rutgers—The State University of New Jersey.

Duskin, M. S. (1997a). League reaches out to push participation. *The National Voter, 46*(2), 4–7.

Duskin, M. S. (1997b). Number of women office-holders edges upward. *The National Voter, 46*(2), 11–12.

Federal Election Commission. (1997). National voter turnout in federal elections: 1960–1996 [on-line]. Available FTP: *http://www.fec.gov/pages/htmlto5.htm.*

Human SERVE. (1996). *The impact of the National Voter Registration Act (NVRA) January 1995–June 1996: The first eighteen months.* New York: National Motor Voter Coalition.

League of Women Voters. (1991). *Fact sheet.* Washington, DC: Author.

League of Women Voters. (1996). *League of Women Voters* [on-line]. Available FTP: *http://www.1wv.org.*

Morin, R. (1996, January 29). Who's in control? Many don't know or care. *The Washington Post,* pp. A1, A6, A7.

Schmitt, E. (1996, November 7 [Late Edition—Final]). The 1996 elections: The presidency—the voters. *The New York Times,* p. B6.

Solop, F. I., & Wonders, N. A. (1995). The politics of inclusion: Private voting rights under the Clinton Administration. *Social Justice, 22*(2), 67–87.

U. S. Bureau of the Census. (1996). *Statistical Abstract of the U.S.: 1996* (116th ed.). Washington, DC: Author.

Woodwell, W. (1997). Talking about turnout. *The National Voter, 45*(2), 9–10.

VIGNETTE
Managing a Campaign
Joanne W. Rains

Electoral politics is not for the timid or the weary. It is not for passive spectators who view life from the periphery. Electoral politics is designed for those who are energized by involvement, who are sincerely committed to building a better world, and who are convinced that their individual and collective actions do make a difference. Electoral politics is also one valid strategy for promoting health.

I jumped headlong into the campaign arena, propelled more by enthusiasm than knowledge. When I first consented to manage the campaign of the man running to be my state representative, my political credentials made a short list: a record as a consistent voter, and clarity in my political ideology and partisan commitment. I brought, however, the organizational and interpersonal skills acquired within my nursing profession. Since then, I have managed four successful state races, consulted on an unsuccessful state bid, attended four sessions of a national campaign management school, hosted fundrais-ers, and earned a reputation as an intrepid political activist.

Lessons can be learned from both election-day victories and defeats. This vignette chronicles the details of the successful races, including the strategies and tactics employed to win, followed by a brief analysis of an unsuccessful race in the same district. A final section reflects on these experiences and lessons as they apply to other situations requiring nursing leadership in group communication, persuasion, and social change.

Electoral Successes

Being asked by Doug Kinser to manage his campaign involved being in the right place at the right time. Doug was a family friend and fellowQuaker. He was challenging a seven-term incumbent and didn't have the seasoned campaign staff enjoyed by most incumbents. As a hospital administrator, he saw the health care industry from the inside and was a health advocate. The Democratic Caucus projected that his election would tip partisan control in the House to the Democrats. These diverse factors characterizing his candidacy meant an opportunity to focus my personal, political, and professional skills in one direction and help him be elected.

The size of our district and the scope of our campaign made it possible for me, as manager, to both devise strategy and execute tactics. The campaign was significant enough on the local and state levels to include all the diverse components inherent in larger campaigns, and yet small enough for me to experience each part. House District 54 includes approximately 26,500 registered voters living in almost 400 square miles of rural Indiana farmland. A drive across the district takes about 30 minutes, but almost half of the voters live in one centrally located city.

In the first campaign I sought consultation from the State Democratic Caucus, but during the three subsequent campaigns I relied more on myself, Doug, and our combined wisdom. I had acquired essential skills through campaign management education and could therefore make a more independent contribution. The following, an amalgamation of four campaign cycles, discusses campaign strategy, tactics, and reflections.

The Strategy: A Campaign Blueprint

A good campaign is based on sound strategy; good managers develop the strategy early, build it from accurate data, and use it as an anchor amid any campaign chaos. Strategy includes a clear statement of campaign goals and how they will be achieved. My job began with the creation of this strategy.

The first step involves a quantitative research process called "targeting." I retrieved past voting records of the district by precinct from old newspapers in our public library. The courthouse also housed the information, but papers were stored in heavy boxes stacked high on shelves. Past voting behavior provides the best predictor of future votes. For each precinct, I calculated the projected voter turnout (how many voters will actually cast a ballot), partisan performance (how many vote primarily for Democrats and how many for Republicans), and persuadability (how volatile or firm is their voting pattern, and can they be persuaded to alter past loyalty to one party or another). This enabled me to calculate how many votes we needed to win and to determine who and where those voters were. By ranking the precincts in the order of their importance to our campaign, I was "targeting" the voters whose votes we needed to win. Identifying the relative importance of each precinct also helped me allocate our finite resources of time, people, and money to the most important locations and voters.

As a nurse scientist, basing our campaign on research data was logical and sound. Not leaving the election to sheer chance or hard work, I had quantified our goal and understood where to find our "party loyals" and our "persuadables."

After identifying the voters whom we wanted to persuade to vote for our candidate (the "who" and the "where"), we needed to know "what" to say to them. The overall success of the campaign depended on communicating a clear theme that would capture voter attention and motivate them to vote for Kinser. Our theme could not, however, be derived in a vacuum. We needed survey research in three areas: (1) on the voters, (2) on the nature and propensities of the district, and (3) on the opponent. Each component was essential in the brainstorming that created the campaign theme.

Our first survey research, called a benchmark poll, gave us the point of reference in the campaign, a baseline. It revealed what the voters were thinking, as well as important information on name recognition and approval ratings. A consultant helped write our telephone survey form. I secured a location, recruited and trained volunteers, and supervised the telephone survey, which we held on three successive evenings. (Volunteers as a resource in our campaign will be discussed later.) I ensured that our completed calls matched the geographic distribution and gender balance of likely voters. The poll results were used to develop a campaign theme that was concise, compelling, and connected to the voters' agendas.

In subsequent races, when campaign funds were more available, we hired a consultant to conduct the poll and statistically analyze the results. We always, however, played an active role in devising survey questions and making sense of survey results.

Other needed information was acquired through "opposition research." Using informal and formal sources, we investigated the opponent's strengths and weaknesses, and compared and contrasted them with Kinser's credentials. We considered the current political environment and projected how each candidate would or would not be aided by the conditions. To make the best use of this information, we considered it all in relationship to the district: its norms, rituals, beliefs, and values.

As an example, we used opposition research data to devise the campaign theme "Committed to the Community." It contrasted the opponent's superficial community ties with Kinser's lifelong link to multiple aspects of the community. The meaning of the contrast is heightened by the strong local emphasis on "community."

How important are issues in relationship to the development of strategy? As a scientist I prefer to accord issues a primary role, but as a politician I know that the personal image of the candidate is more important to the voters. They care about character traits like honesty, intelligence, and commitment. We did not discount or ignore issues, but in the development of the campaign strategy, issues were used to convey image and character. The substantive elements of issues were utilized in the policymaking that occurred as Kinser served as our state representative.

The development of campaign strategy is not a public process. It is done early, before most of the public realizes it is an election year. It is created by a small, inner circle of trusted people: the "kitchen cabinet," or those who brainstorm at the kitchen table. For me, the exciting part

was distilling the research findings and creating a succinct and relevant theme. For this challenge, an appreciation of words and a talent for turning just the right phrase serve well. I also enjoyed the assurance that a thoughtful, data-based foundation for the campaign had been laid. In weeks remote to that calm time, when fatigue, deadlines, and unpredictable media events enveloped us, the carefully derived theme (what to say) and campaign strategy (who and where those voters were) served as unchanging guides.

The Tactics: Carrying Out the Plan

In contrast to an unchanging strategy, tactics are the flexible "hows" and "whens" used to implement the strategy. Tactics are altered as new developments, positive or negative, stir the political waters.

Volunteers are key to the implementation of tactics, and their recruitment, training, management, and retention consume much time and energy. Doug and I kept a list of any person who said, "I'm supportive; just let me know when there is something to do." A note was made of the volunteer's abilities, including phone skills, physical stamina for walking, image and interpersonal skills, clerical abilities, and, very important, dependability. A good manager matches skills to tasks and will effectively translate volunteers' stated willingness into campaign action.

Recruiting volunteers is much like fund raising: the first tenet is that you simply must ask. No one is exempt from being asked. I grew to appreciate *lists* of people: district nursing lists, hospital employee lists, political-action-committee member lists, and precinct committee lists. The names of people who had previously volunteered made a valuable list. I found that those who state their interest are more abundant than those who will actually follow through.

We trained volunteers to make personal voter contact and sometimes used their numbers to generate a sense of momentum and enthusiastic support. Specifically, our volunteers were crucial during phone bank sessions, voter registration drives, yard sign distribution projects, door-to-door canvassing, and election day activities.

Our first phone banks involved polling. Our polls were conducted for three consecutive evenings from 6 to 9 PM. With 10 phone lines available, I recruited 12 to 15 volunteers for each night. Recruiting more than I needed proved to be prudent because there were always those with last-minute conflicts or who forgot altogether. Our volunteers completed between 250 and 400 calls to registered voters.

Voter registration was enthusiastic; besides expanding the base of voters, it was the initial mobilization of volunteers who would walk door to door. In Indiana, voters are purged from the registration list if they fail to vote within a certain span of time, currently 48 months. Know the voter registration laws and procedures in your state. In registering voters, I believed that I was enabling someone whose address or name had changed to update easily, or was empowering citizens who had previously been uninterested in or incapable of being a part of the process. Another benefit of this door-to-door effort was leaving our campaign literature at each door.

Not every campaign needs yard signs. We employed this tactic for two reasons: it was an expected local tradition, and it fostered name recognition. We made sure the signs were distinctive enough to be understood at 55 mph. I orchestrated a "yard-sign weekend" in mid-October to create the effect that overnight hundreds of signs had sprung up. To create the most impressive effect, we concentrated first on the main traffic arteries of the largest town. We relied on strong volunteers, adept with a hammer, and those who had pickup trucks to carry the signs. Care was given to the ongoing maintenance of the signs, because some vandalism is to be expected.

Our schedule of door-to-door canvassing was in harmony with our strategy: areas were covered in the order of our priority ranking. Afternoons from 4 to 6 PM worked well for small

groups and Kinser, but Saturday mornings were the most productive. A master schedule of approximately 2 months was prepared and distributed to potential walkers. We would meet at a restaurant at 9 AM to eat, enjoy each other, and create energy. I distributed assignments, maps, scripts, literature, and buttons. Working in pairs, usually covering opposite sides of the street, gave support and safety.

Another tactic was our "get out the vote" phone bank. One week before the election, we began to call voters who had been identified as supportive and reminded them of the upcoming election. We asked: Do you know where to vote? Do you need a ride to the polls? Do you know how important it is to vote? These calls were intended not to persuade but to turn voters out.

Election days are rich with volunteer opportunities. Early risers put up signs at each poll across the district; we coordinated this job with other campaigns running on the Democratic ticket to avoid duplication in driving across the district. Poll workers outside each polling place had a small card available to hand out to voters, but more important they personally communicated their support for Kinser and his interest and attentiveness to these voters. Assignment of volunteers to each polling place was based on targeting data. The most crucial and "persuadable" precincts were staffed by the most dependable and influential volunteers, such as the candidate's wife, other family members, and the most loyal volunteers, including high school students. An attempt was made to orient each group of students so that they could have a broad vision of campaign strategy and could view elections as more substantial than merely soliciting votes at the polls.

Other, less volunteer-intensive tactical components involved the media, receptions, and targeted mailings. Our media involved radio, daily and weekly newspapers, and cable television. Our media "buys" were determined by the audience we wanted to reach. We wrote or approved scripts that reiterated our theme overtly and subliminally.

We knew that successfully generating media coverage required the cultivation of relationships with editors and reporters. What used to be called "free media" has been renamed "earned media." *Free* refers to the fact that the campaign does not buy the space—for example, for a newspaper article on a debate; *earned* refers to the effort expended in cultivating a relationship with the news media that will influence the slant of the coverage, or whether coverage is even given. I made a point of knowing the news people and maintaining an amiable rapport. What was more important in our community was the relationship between Kinser himself and the media. Early in the campaign, he established a reputation with them as an honest and approachable person. Later, when some philosophical differences emerged, there remained a personal foundation of respect that influenced their reporting.

We devised targeted mail, tailoring the message to the audience. Among the targeted groups were partisan supporters, "undecideds," labor union members, and those sensitive to specific issues. The important feature was identifying the unique point of persuasion for that particular audience and then crafting appropriate rhetoric. Friends at the local post office proved helpful in expediting the delivery of bulk mail.

Receptions served many purposes. Each reception focused on a specific community group or members of a specific profession. Each invitation was sent by direct mail, enhancing name recognition and informing voters. Each reception expanded the candidate's personal voter contact and broadened our volunteer participation. To each reception we invited a special guest, such as an important legislator or a distinguished speaker. This generated "earned media" coverage and fostered relationships with the special guests. Each invitation had a fund-raising component, suggesting a contribution amount.

Our first reception targeted nurses and was held at my home from 3 to 5 PM on a Sunday afternoon in August. Eight nurses cohosted the reception. We invited nurses employed in the local hospital, nursing homes, physician offices, schools, and public health agencies. We requested a $15 minimum contribution to the campaign. Besides the benefits to the campaign, the reception promoted the socialization of local nurses and heightened awareness of the significance of electoral politics in the promotion of health.

Another component of the manager job is to evaluate and promote candidate morale. The personal strain for candidates and their family is significant, even when the commitment is total. Positive feedback and encouragement were minor expenditures on my part but were valuable boosts to the person who ultimately stands alone at the microphone.

The implementation of campaign tactics varies with the available resources: time, money, technology, and people. The most important issue is that the carefully developed strategy, through persistent and thorough work, actually becomes reality.

Electoral Defeat Analyzed

After four successful elections and a productive time as a policymaker, Doug Kinser resigned at mid term from the Indiana House of Representatives. The change was prompted by a desire to return to school and earn a law degree. His replacement, Dave Copenhaver, was elected by precinct committee men and women and served well for the remaining legislative session. Early in his tenure he recruited me to serve as his campaign manager, and we eagerly began raising funds and establishing networks for the campaign ahead. A change in employment brought new demands on my time and priorities, and as these realities became clear, I scaled back to a consultant role. From that periphery, I make several observations of this electoral defeat.

Campaign strategy, as described earlier in this chapter, is the fundamental coherence and guide for every campaign activity. With a well-conceived strategy, a campaign has the blueprint to communicate with, connect with, and convince a majority of voters. Without that coherence, the campaign risks the opponent's setting the agenda, defining each candidate, and controlling the media messages. The campaign reacts instead of acts.

The Copenhaver strategy lacked a compelling theme that defined his candidacy and connected with constituents. It lacked the research that told where the voters were and what messages would resonate with their concerns. Without that guidance, the opponent could attack through well-timed media and could orchestrate his own messages for those crucial few days before the election. Without the direction of a well-researched strategy, the candidate's efforts lacked focus—for example, walking door to door in precincts that would not yield partisan or persuadable voters. Though other factors contributed to a defeat at the polls, an insufficient strategy earns primary credit.

Secondary factors include issues that the candidate or campaign manager could control. One was desire for the office. Copenhaver lacked an intense, encompassing, or even visceral drive for this electoral success. Despite his superior credentials and preparation for office, the campaign lacked a spirit of energy. Further, an attack ad placed late by the opponent was problematic. A proactive monitoring of the opponent's ads in the county papers could have eliminated some last-minute responding, and perhaps a better relationship with the editor could have been beneficial.

Other factors are beyond the purview of the campaign. Examples include the mood of the electorate, voter turnout, the influence of other campaigns (like Presidential or Congressional), and partisan activities at all levels. Though voter turnout was high in this district, a stronger showing was needed by the party faithful. It is important to note these factors, because even issues outside your control can be integrated into a well-constructed strategy.

The merit of this brief analysis of defeat is its juxtaposition to the preceding description of winning strategies and well-executed tactics in the same political district. Certainly, election years vary in ways that make each race a unique situation, but there remain some consistent elements. Each point raised in the defeat analysis has a recommended antidote in the winning scenario. This section, therefore, affirms the positive contribution of activities discussed with electoral success and makes the point that the omission of any central element can provide the opponent with a winning edge.

Reflections: Growth and Other Applications

Personal and professional growth through political involvement will come as surely as election day. Because of my experience as campaign manager, my life is richer and my sense of potency in some spheres is unquenchable. I gained friends who share values and the willingness to put them into action. I've given my two sons of high-school age political experiences and interesting dinner conversations. The following reflections emerge from these experiences:

- Manage a campaign only if you are convinced that what you are doing will make the world a better place. The thrill of rubbing shoulders with dignitaries or the lift derived from making a new friend won't be enough to sustain you during hectic days full of deadlines and nights in which even your dreams are political. What sustains you is the commitment that parallels your commitment to nursing and health and caring about society. For me, being a campaign manager enables me to promote health and improve society.

- Enthusiasm and commitment surpass prior experience as a prerequisite for any political involvement. The mentoring of novices is standard in the political culture. Seize that first opportunity to contribute. If you are more than a novice, challenge yourself to become politically competent and even expert.

- Good interpersonal and group dynamics can propel a mediocre campaign to success; ignored interpersonal issues can destroy the most brilliant and deserving campaign. Don't ignore the interpersonal. Campaign management is the management of people in their pursuit of identity and contribution. What better background to meet this need than nursing education and experience!

- As a political novice, I viewed politics as flimsy and shallow in comparison to the rigors of scientific inquiry and the standards of scientific protocol. I grew, however, to see the two as distinct arenas with unique rules, not the least of which is the definition of truth. In the political arena, truth is what people will believe; it is negotiated. In the scientific arena, truth is discovered and is replicable; it is researched. Not until I saw this distinction could I embrace the political arena as substantive enough for my standards as a nurse. I grew through this in the early months of the first campaign and see it now as a valuable distinction for nurses and other scientists to make as they pass between arenas with such diverse ground rules. Frustration and ineffectiveness result when rules and arenas are inappropriately mixed.

- One of the most fundamental ways to influence policy is to influence the makeup of the body of policymakers. Elections give birth to the body of legislators who shape our society and future. Our influence as citizens begins in the election cycle: seeking out those who are equipped for elected office, encouraging and empowering them, and working to elect them. Specifically needed are legislators sensitive to the complexities of health care and the multifaceted determinants of health. Once they are in office, you will understand their values and biases, have access for input and continued contact, and learn more about the process through their inside stories. In this regard, I see campaigns and elections as the "primary prevention" of policymaking.

- The thought processes and concepts of campaign management are applicable in a multitude of situations involving group communication, persuasion, and social change. I've pulled from my campaign experiences as I've led more than 200 faculty through a curriculum revision process. In public health, I've applied some of these processes to promote health behavior changes in populations at risk. There is use for campaign strategies and tactics in organizing coalitions in order to pass legislation. In fact, any situation that involves orchestrating change among a group of people will be a likely arena to apply campaign management skills. The professional skills I now possess and use to promote health are a wonderful blend of nursing science and political science, with only a vague, fuzzy distinction between the two.

The Intersection of Health and Campaigns

The health of our world is influenced by public policies, and those policies are created by individuals who win elections. When nurses participate and provide leadership on the campaign trail, we create opportunities to share nursing's values and priorities and to elect people who see the connections between sociopolitical and economic policies and the health of people. In my practice, campaign management is a profoundly far-reaching strategy for health promotion.

UNIT IV CASE STUDY

Pilgrim in Politics

Eve Franklin

HOME ON THE RANGE—AGAIN

The Missouri River is running just below flood stage. The early June warmth is melting the unusually heavy snowpack high in the Rocky Mountains. The snowmelt combined with the heavy spring rains has put much of north-central Montana at risk of serious flooding. The Sun River, the waters the Blackfeet called the Medicine River, originating from springs at the continental divide, was rising over its banks. Trotting along the river trail with a few other early-morning joggers, on such a clear and promising day, it was difficult to perceive the danger in the water spilling over Black Eagle Dam. But the thunderous pounding of 30,000 cubic feet of water per second crashing over the concrete dam structure built in the 1890s and the uncharacteristic whitecaps on the Missouri were unmistakable signs of a river system poised to create chaos and damage along its banks.

I was home from the state capital, Helena, at the close of the 1997 legislative session. In budget language, I was a "vacancy savings" during my 90-day stint as a full-time legislator in the Montana State Senate. In layman's terms, I take a leave of absence without pay from my "day job" on the faculty of Montana State University College of Nursing. While the college cobbles together a jigsaw arrangement of faculty assignments during my absence, I relinquish my faculty salary and instead collect the grand sum of $58.60 per day for my legislative service. Montana is a rural state with a strong agricultural economy, and we meet on a biannual schedule stretching from January to April. During the period between full-time sessions, we have responsibilities to serve on interim legislative committees and a moral obligation to engage in necessary constituent service.

The service may include such varied activities as following up on delinquent child support, assisting an individual to understand the state contract bidding process, advocating a small business loan, unearthing the details of a bungled pension application or worker compensation claim, and perhaps, though no particular grievance may be identified, meeting a generally dissatisfied constituent for coffee. This service is an expected portion of our role, and the legislator receives no remuneration for the hours of essentially volunteer work accomplished without the luxury of staff or material resources.

I am always struck with what a good background nursing is for the role of a citizen legislator—we learn to accomplish a great deal without the benefit of very much institutional support.

The 4-month January-to-April schedule was originally designed to make it possible for legislators who were primarily engaged in farming and ranching to attend to the details of state government during the slack times on the ranch. In 1997 we still had more farmers and ranchers serving in the legislature than representatives of any other one single vocation. We certainly had more ranchers than lawyers, which probably set us apart from the majority of other state legislatures.

As I work my way along the trail, the tumultuous waters are a curious contrast to the peace I feel at being at home on the high plains of Montana. The peace of mind has been a long time coming—years, in fact. This sense of peace has a great deal to do with a grateful entry into my middle years, where I have achieved a more grace-filled relationship with myself, my family, my friends, and my professional life. I almost don't recognize it for what it is at first. It can be easier to cling to the more familiar anxiety, the tension of a pressured existence, than to learn the skills of living a more integrated life. I have often described myself as a relatively low-key person functioning in a "type A" life.

Six years of serving in the state senate, two campaigns of my own, multiple campaigning for others, a full-time job teaching nursing, multiple board responsibilities, community involvements, and marriage have challenged this basically slow-paced personality to perform at a level I never would have imagined possible even 10 years ago.

"I don't remember how to relax," I confessed to a friend during my first week back in Great Falls. On the ninetieth day, the president of the state senate dropped the gavel, announcing the Latin, *sine die,* to mark the end of the fifty-fifth session of the Montana legislature. I had made a decision shortly after that moment to take a summer hiatus, which meant making an effort to act like "normal" people and (1) work in the garden, (2) read mystery novels, (3) not accept a summer job in order to make up for my lost salary during the legislature, and (4) put a few limits on my legislative activity and enjoy the brief Montana summer. Yet I felt like I was in an odd type of purgatory between work and play: not wanting to do the first and not knowing how to do the latter.

"Run," advised my friend Barbara. "Every morning, get up and do some vigorous exercise." Not surprising advice from a woman who at 57 regularly ranked at the top of her age class in competitive runs. I did, however, follow her guidance—not out of any particular commitment to physical fitness but out of desperation. I had to find a way to join the rest of the world. The chafing of role demands and personal need has a good deal to do with the realities of being a state senator in a rural state, in a close-knit community that expects a very personal relationship with the legislators, whose home telephone numbers are in the directory and who assume they will be contacted—and we are. We would be considered irresponsible and unresponsive if we did not make ourselves readily available to several thousand constituents or, for that matter, anyone else in the state who might have something to say. In a state whose political history is deeply rooted in the concept of an accessible citizen legislature, where your state senator or representative might also be your son's math teacher or might work the neighboring farm, there is a strong connection to the individual who is elected to serve in state government. There is an instant intimacy that is very much a parallel of the relationship that nurses have with patients. We come in contact at times of crisis in an individual's life and share an intensity of thought and feeling, share his or her most precious concerns and needs, and go about trying to solve the individual's problems.

I was first elected to the Montana State Senate in 1990 after having lived in Great Falls for less than 3 years. At 32 years of age, I came to make a life different from what I'd known as a "genetic New Yorker." Despite the style differences, I found life oddly familiar to my soul and a profoundly good fit for the adult I'd become and the person I still hoped to be. A geographic transplant, I came west to Montana a few years before the wave of "nouveau Montanans" flooded the western part of the state. These refugees from southern California, New York, and Portland, who had escaped to purchase a 20-acre Montana "ranchette," generally arrived with little regard for Montana history, culture, or community.

One of the sweetest comments I heard during my first years here was made to me by a friend who had grown up in Anaconda, Montana, in the 1950s (pronounced *Anda*-conda by the local folk, but no one seems to know why). Anaconda, then a bustling company town, was dominated by the Anaconda Copper Company. It was a rough-and-tumble society that is the legacy of the Copper Kings and the Railroad Barons, with a fiercely close-knit ethnic population of Irish, Slavs, and Italians. Along with Butte, it has been the beating heart of the Montana labor movement.

"A lot of people move to Montana, and they don't *get* it, Eve," confided my Anaconda friend. "You get it." This was a balm to the soul of a "new girl" who wanted very much to belong in her new home. But exactly what was it that I seemed to "get"? Through the years, as I developed a deeper sense of the social and political context of Montana society, this passing comment assumed importance to me on different levels. A comment made in a casual conversation became more than a compliment about my ability to get along. It was a trigger for thoughts about community, class, and political context. Why did this eastern urbanite feel so much at home in rural Montana?

What has become clear to me is that what we define as community has a great deal to do with a transcendent appreciation that grows from the mutual need of neighbors, be they rural or urban. Montana homesteaders knew they couldn't get through a harsh winter without their neighbors; growing up in a working class neighborhood in New York City, I knew that neighbors counted on neighbors to help them through a multitude of situational crises of daily living. This often involved borrowing a needed household item, a small loan for a quart of milk, and, of course, sound advice on the trials and tribulations of life that was passed down through generations of Sicilian and Jewish women. What I shared with my Montana neighbors was a traditional sense of community, not based on the unique idiosyncracies of rural or urban life style, but instead grounded in an economic reality that was fertile soil for a real connection between neighbors: interdependence, necessity, and, ultimately, friendship.

The "nouveau Montanans," who identified strongly with right-wing political thought, came to Montana with a romantic notion of the "independent West" based on John Wayne movies and Merle Haggard songs. "Take your retirement and take your so-called social security," Merle sang in the 1980s. "Set me free somewhere in the Middle of Montana."

I'm not sure how Merle planned for these folks to take care of themselves in their old age. We in public policy suspect that it would have something to do with tax dollars contributed by other citizens—neighbors—who did not entertain the luxury of feeling quite so "free" of the constraints of civic responsibility.

The "nouveau Montanans" brought with them a desire for 20 acres of land designated "agricultural" for tax purposes, a Rottweiler, and a no-trespassing sign. These folks were a part of the electorate that begrudged funding for public schools and public services and rejected the use of federal funds (except for road construction, because that money is miraculously cleansed, unlike the "tainted" federal money that would be channeled for Head Start, Educational Goals 2000, or health care). This self-involved attitude is actually the antithesis of historic Montana attitudes. Although Montana culture has always valued independence and self-sufficiency, these qualities are seen in the context of community.

This morality play is not unique to Montana. We are a microcosm of the political and social struggles for community throughout the country. We all have a stake in the collective fate of our community—whether it's New York, California, Milwaukee, Terre Haute, or Montana. A no-trespassing sign does not release us from our shared destiny.

THE LADY WITH THE LAMP—AND THE GAVEL

Most of us who enrolled in nursing school were affected by an altruistic notion of ministering to a pained world, healing bodies and spirits one at a time. I recall drinking in the stories about visionary nursing pioneers: Mary Breckenridge, founder of the Frontier Nursing

Service, who traveled on horseback from "holler" to "holler" in rural Kentucky; Lillian Wald, who climbed tenement steps and negotiated rooftops on the lower east side of Manhattan to reach her patients; Dorothea Dix, who made great strides in humanizing mental health care; Margaret Sanger, who educated poor women about their ability to control their reproductive lives, ultimately enduring prison and exile for violating the Comstock Laws; and, of course. Florence Nightingale, who revolutionized modern hospital care. Many of my classmates in 1974 came from a traditional model of nursing, religion, and womanhood. When St. Ursula's School in the Bronx released its senior class of girls, an overwhelming percentage of this high school graduating class ran across the Grand Concourse, a wide boulevard lined with prewar brick apartment buildings, and registered for the nursing curriculum at Lehman College. Not being a member of that comfortable enclave of parochial-school girls who had been putting Band-Aid strips on their cats since childhood, I came to the nursing program with an as-yet-unformed jumble of ideas about nursing and my relationship to it. I knew it had something to do with implementing social justice and good works, about choosing meaningful work in a superficial world. I also knew it was how I could make sense of personal and familial history and my integration with the larger world: pioneering Zionism meets rural Kentucky, the labor union activist meets Mother Teresa, the action of the young anti-Nazi partisan Chana Senesh meets the abstraction of feminist historian Barbara Erenreich. Nursing provided a way for me to give personal voice to social action and form to feminism. It seemed that there was nothing more radical, more challenging, more "womanly," than to be a strong woman in traditional woman's work. We novice nurses did not have the luxury of assuming the male vestments of power used by women who entered traditionally male fields of law, medicine, and business. Feminist nurses

would meet the challenge of health care with the inspiration of our foremothers, our wits, and a darned good baccalaureate education.

Adult developmental theory suggests that both personal and professional growth follows a path that has recognizable patterns and dynamics. The making of a nurse legislator includes a personal journey as well as professional growth. To become an effective nurse and advocate, one must not allow the idealism of youth to be lost in fact; rather, the idealism becomes strengthened by the intimate knowledge of work that has to be done and the wisdom of having "been around the block a few times," as the idiom goes. In the 1980s a social observer described the "imposter" complex. This syndrome particularly hounded young professional women in their thirties, who found themselves acknowledged as experts on the job and as functioning well in roles with significant responsibility, and yet who lived with the "dirty little secret" that they felt somehow they were play-acting—acting as though they had expertise and power—as though they were "imposters." A wonderful epiphany occurs when we are able to shed the fears of being a professional play actor, a big kid in grownup clothes, and accept on a visceral level that we do, indeed, have expertise to offer clients and colleagues. We have learned our trade through intellectual inquiry, curiosity, and perseverance.

I recall being asked in 1991, at the start of my first legislative session, "Who do you work for?" The assumption being that a "thirtyish" woman with a relatively unpretentious style and in tailored clothing was likely someone's secretary ("and lucky to have her, I might add"). Or someone would ask, "Who is your husband?" assuming I was a legislative spouse. Since I hadn't yet acquired a husband, nor could I word-process very well, I was bemused by these assumptions and corrected them: "I'm Senator Franklin." My delight was the embarrassment of lobbyists who knew they would have to redeem themselves after this faux pas. But the identity errors made during the first few weeks of Senator Franklin's first legislative session because of her newness to the political scene soon evaporated. My imposter struggles were dissipating as I reached new levels of confidence.

Despite having spent all my adult professional life tending to the feelings and needs of others, I was not at all confused about where the desire to care needed to change to a commitment to battle and, in the political context, an absolute requirement to fight. In politics, as in nursing, caring means little if you can't deliver; compassion is limited if you don't have the gumption to fight for good outcomes; and being kind is as vacuous as being "nice" if it doesn't mean beneficent action and advocacy.

Our foremothers knew this: Florence, Dorothea, Mary, Margaret, Lillian, and so many others who effected change. They were nurses and they were expert politicians. They worked the system in order to create change, and they changed the system when it didn't serve human need. They tapped into power, influence, and money when it helped the cause. They knew that without connecting to powerful forces in our culture—either the power of the elite or the power of the "masses"—their work simply could not be done.

By the end of the 1991 session, I had gained a reputation as a nurse legislator who had passion for and knowledge about health care issues. I had sponsored a bill requiring insurance companies to cover the cost of mammography on a preventive model. This was a contentious requirement, known in insurance lingo as a "mandated benefit." It was a public policy demand that private and public insurers make mammography as an early screening tool available to their customers without their having a diagnosis of breast disease.

The health care and consumer advocates argued for the bill, using the adage that an "ounce of prevention is worth a pound of cure."

Wouldn't we be saving great sums of money and oceans of human misery if we could spend a little money up front for preventive measures instead of paying such a high price at the other end? The insurance companies bared their fangs and fought back relentlessly. Of course, we have sympathy for the poor victims of breast cancer, they intoned when testifying at committee hearings, but we can't possibly cover mammograms—it will raise rates for all our customers. They could report to the penny how much it would raise monthly premiums to "cover" the cost of this screening tool, but they simply couldn't grasp the concept that prevention is less costly than tertiary care. Those of us who had been around this block before knew the dark reality that the acute care paradigm drives the system. Whether or not the insurance guys and gals could "get" this concept was not the real issue. They didn't want to get it because a paradigm based on prevention would irrevocably alter life and business as they knew it.

Finally, the bill passed—not necessarily because of my fine legislative prowess, but because several legislators on the health committee who were generally most sympathetic to insurance industry positions had been touched by great personal sadness in their own lives, having lost a wife or another beloved relative to breast cancer. These were the humanizing moments, when even the most hard-core apologists for the insurance industry's position blushed with embarrassment while they held tenaciously to the "bottom line" theory of financing for the delivery of health care services.

MODERN HEALTH CARE REFORM, OR THE RED MENACE IN WHITE SHOES

In the interim period between legislative sessions, I was asked by our senior U.S. Senator Max Baucus to participate in a citizen's effort to explore options and recommend changes in the health care system at the state level. Max (Montana citizens like the familiarity of being on a first-name basis with their legislative delegation except in the most formal settings) had the vision and savvy to see that, although the Clintons were beginning to examine health care reform at the federal level, the action had been at the state level throughout the early 1990s. Minnesota, Vermont, Oregon, and North Dakota, to name a few, had undertaken serious reform efforts spurred on largely by the escalating cost of health care and the explosive effect on state Medicaid budgets. Max wanted to ensure that Montana was not left behind in the rapidly changing health care scene. He and his staff assembled a variety of folks representing business, labor, agriculture, seniors, Indian nations, and consumers, as well as the dean of the Montana State University College of Nursing—and one nurse legislator. The senator supported this exciting effort with staff and resources from his Montana office. With breakneck speed and intensity, the committee met to develop what we hoped would be the basis for legislation that would address the unique health care needs of Montana.

The vast geography of Montana defines many of our important policy issues. Our geography defines the history of settlement, economic development, and health care beliefs. Rural health care theory is accepted throughout academia as a legitimate theoretical framework in which to view the health needs of rural people and to find relevant responses. No one anecdote summarizes classic rural stoicism, which has been documented by theorists, as succinctly as the conversation I had with a family during a 3-day countrywide telephone outage during the first month after my arrival in Montana. Opal's husband had chronic heart disease and had experienced episodic acute symptoms that required medical attention. They were both in their mid-seventies and lived on a small ranch about 35 miles from town.

"Are you concerned about being without your telephone?" I explored sincerely.

Opal gazed at me a bit quizzically. "Well, now," she responded rather matter-of-factly, "I just load 'im in the pickup and drive to town." Silly me, but of course I'd just come from a health care environment where some of my patients would call 911 for a hangnail. Seriously.

"Health" as a concept in rural theory has been defined by some as the "ability to do one's work." Tom T. Hall, a popular country music singer in the 1970s, recorded a song with a poetic title: "Whose Gonna Feed Them Hogs." This 4-minute song describes an incident in which the musical narrator is briefly hospitalized and finds himself sharing a hospital room with a very ill hog farmer. The clever ditty goes on to say that, in his delirium, worrying desperately about his farm chores, the old farmer calls out repeatedly, *"Whose gonna feed them hogs?"* Finally, in the last musical bar, the farmer shakes off his delerium, puts on his overalls, and leaves the hospital to slop his livestock. Congruent with perceptions of health described in rural health theory, this fictional character had recovered his health. Where there's work, there's health.

I use this song as a teaching tool in the classroom with nursing students to illustrate the very poignant and real aspects of health care beliefs and behaviors.

The vastness and isolation of Montana have also led to a health care system with huge gaps in service, resulting in innovation and sometimes quirky practices designed to respond to community need. Anecdotally there are many examples that highlight the realities of health care and the challenges for reform of health care delivery in a rural state. One afternoon a legislator from Wibaux (pronounced Wee-bow), a community so far to the eastern part of the state that it is 700 miles from the western border, stopped me in the senate cloakroom for a little consult. The cloakroom is a narrow vestibule that is a pivotal part of legislative culture, a place out of the public eye where for a few moments legislators can shed the armor, chuckle over events of the day, share a cigarette in the "smoking corner" (not me, of course), or do a little insider horse trading.

"What do you know about pharmacy law?" she asked, showing real concern. It had come to her attention that a well-used custom in the health care delivery system of that community could potentially be a violation of state law. Wibaux does not have a pharmacy. For the citizens of Wibaux to have prescriptions filled, the bus driver for InterMountain Bus Line would pick up a prescription in a larger community 70 miles away and would transfer the needed medication to the interested party at the crossroads of Highway 94 and Highway 7. A question apparently came up as to whether or not this was a violation of state pharmacy law—the "dispensing" of medication not by a licensed pharmacist but by a bus driver. This legislator was feeling considerable consternation that an integral part of the health care delivery system in that isolated community was threatened.

The parking lot at the local Great Falls hospital center has electrical plug-ins for recreational vehicles. It is not unusual for families to camp out in their RVs when traveling with an ill family member seeking care. As a mental health nurse, I became particularly aware that many folks who needed mental health services received it only in the form of a trip to a general practitioner's office—and may have to travel a considerable distance at that.

The vastness and isolation of the region have also been a deterrent to recruiting and retaining health care providers to rural areas. Health care professionals may have been drawn to the beauty of the place but often succumb to the strain of professional isolation and the rigors of being the only provider in a vast area—no one with whom to share calls, and no one to consult with on a regular basis over a cup of coffee. I have a professional acquaintance, a psychiatric nurse who was for many years the only mental

health resource in a small city in eastern Montana. The only way she could take a vacation was to leave town, because everyone knew where she was and when to reach her in the most informal of ways: "Oh, you need to talk to Marge? I just saw her at the grocery store, and she should be home in a few minutes."

As we moved into an era of serious discussion of health care reform at the federal level, these rural characteristics only highlighted for me the need for a state-driven effort to examine our health care needs and define the kind of delivery system best suited to respond to those needs. If even the state's regulatory practice, as in the case of the pharmacy issue, didn't always acknowledge the realities of health care delivery in a rural context, we had reason to be concerned about the implementation of aspects of a system designed at the federal level or by private industry headquartered in another part of the country. With a heightened awareness of issues affecting rural health care delivery, our Montana Citizen's Health Care Advisory Group worked with a great sense of purpose.

In 1993, Hillary Clinton visited Great Falls, Montana, at the invitation of Senator Baucus after we had passed our health care reform bill. Participating with Mrs. Clinton on a panel before 500 local people was an exciting experience, indeed. She charmed us all with her warmth and straightforward manner, but I watched her win the heart of the audience when she said, "I've traveled all over this country, exploring health care. I've seen rural in Tennessee, I've seen rural in North Carolina and Georgia—but this, this is mega-rural." Hillary was right on target—any changes in our health care delivery system had to be sensitive to our "mega-rural" nature.

As our citizens committee evolved, our lively discussion and research made some things clear. We agreed on certain principles of improved access, quality, and attempts at cost containment. We also agreed on solid support for advanced practice nurses as a way to improve access and quality. However, the disagreement between the activists who wished to formally recommend a single-payer system and those who wished to follow a more familiar regulated, multipayer model could not be resolved. In October 1992 the committee completed a document that we described as a "principled framework" that could act as a model for either payment system.

Major provisions of the framework included a commitment to guaranteed health benefits for all Montana citizens, a data collection process to serve as a tool for future policy research, insurance reform that would deal with the onerous practice of establishing the preexisting-condition exclusion and provide for guaranteed cost-control mechanisms, and a network of regional planning boards that would focus on community involvement and planning. A high-level "blue ribbon" panel was created—the Montana Health Care Authority, whose mission would be to study and steer the health care reform efforts of the state. Appointed by the governor with bipartisan input, the five members of the authority would become our policy experts and sages on the matter of reform. One of the most exciting aspects of the model was an ambitious plan for public input in the form of town meetings and public hearings to be conducted all over the state.

We expected that the document would become a bill that, if passed in the 1993 session, would legislatively empower this panel of trusted Montana citizens to put the full resources of the state behind a deliberate process of reform spelled out in our recommendations. It was a time of great enthusiasm and hope for nurses and other consumer advocates who had devoted themselves to improving health care. I was proud that our document and eventually our bill would parallel so closely many aspects of the American Nurses Association's policy statement, Nursing's Agenda for Health Care Reform.

During the 1993 session I ate, drank, and dreamed health care reform legislation. I was the chief sponsor of the bill, and we glibly tried to dub it *HealthMontana*. But the pedestrian practice of referring to bills by number prevailed, and no one, including me, could use that catchy name. We all referred to the legislation by its computer tracking number, Senate Bill 285. Taking on sponsorship of a weighty bill means that you are head shepherd, facilitator, negotiator, cajoler, counselor, conniver, compromiser, peacemaker, and sometimes, when you simply must, capitulator. It was a tough, exhilarating time. I stretched every muscle and fired every synapse that I could muster in my sophomore legislative session. I was playing with the big kids, and it was a very, very serious sandbox with real-world implications for our health care future. This was the embodiment of everything I held dear in nursing.

The bill received support from our Republican governor, logistic assistance from our Democratic insurance commissioner, and enthusiastic support from groups as varied as the Montana Cattlewomen's Association and the AFL-CIO. The bill passed the Senate 49 to 0 and sailed through the House. I had done everything in my power to keep from politicizing the effort or exploiting it as a divisive partisan issue. I argued that this issue was bigger than all of us and that if we stayed true to our task, partisan politics could not destroy our sincere desire to improve health care delivery. Exhausted and driven, I returned home after the session, ready to face the challenge of reforming health care through Senate Bill 285—Lillian, Florence, and me.

Admittedly, the legislative approach in Senate Bill 285 represented a big change in thinking in relation to health care. But the progressive 6-year process of benchmarked activities set forth in the bill allowed for much intellectual and philosophical freedom. I felt secure in the knowledge that we were embarking on the first 2-year phase of health care reform—that reason and sincere concern for the welfare of our citizenry would win against resistance borne of narrow industry interests.

By the summer of 1993, the Montana Health Care Authority members were appointed, and a brilliant, nationally recognized health policy consultant was engaged to facilitate the education of authority members, as well as the public, regarding the options available to us in the structuring, organizing, and financing of health care services. The Montana Health Care Authority, made up of some of the state's most illustrious citizens, set out on the road in a dizzying schedule of open public work sessions, engaging citizen groups from Libby in the northwest corner to Miles City in the southeast in this public conversation. As they began this larger-than-life task, the seeds of fear and distrust were being sown by detractors emerging from the shadows. Some detractors among those resistant to any change called it a million-dollar "study" bill, and other naysayers found no comfort in the deliberate data gathering and study aspects of the legislation, calling it much too radical.

Ah, but it was a brief moment in the garden. An unholy alliance of right-wing ideologues, fringe insurance peddlers, and, sadly, a large number of Montana physicians was formed to discredit the effort before it had barely begun. Within 9 months of the governor's putting his signature on Senate Bill 285, and after the hope-filled inauguration of the Montana Health Care Authority, the threads were beginning to unravel. It was January 1994 when a leader of a right-wing tax protest group held a press conference in conjunction with half a dozen other professional obstructionists, including the Christian Coalition and Montana Right to Life, and Montana's Republican junior U.S. Senator to announce their vigorous opposition to the direction of the Montana Health Care Authority. Their agenda included an effort to wholly discredit the health care reform effort

and to embarrass our moderate Republican governor, whose presence was requested at the press conference.

Essentially they called the plan "perverted," insisting that our true intent was to deny health care to old people, euthanize the terminally ill, and promote "abortion on demand." It was labeled a plan that undermined everything American, good, and true. It was almost laughable to make such accusations, but they were deadly serious and I was having a little trouble maintaining a sense of humor.

Thus the assault on health care reform began in earnest, and it did not stop until the demonization of Montana health care reform was complete. Although largely quiet during the legislative discussion, the right wing of the Republican party, pivotal supporters of the governor's party, became wild-eyed in their accusations about the unwholesome nature of the provisions of Senate Bill 285 on its implementation. The popular governor who had so vocally supported health care reform, even including it in his State of the State address in 1993, distanced himself from the Montana Health Care Authority. His withdrawal of active support paralleled the rise of the radical and religious right in our state's political power dynamic. Though the Montana Health Care Authority continued its phase-one mandate, which included 18 months of planning and study and the implementation of small-group insurance reform, the seeds of fear and distrust were being sown by an effective alliance of the industry status quo operatives and the religous right.

Later, in the spring of 1994, a nurse colleague of mine in another city reported to me with some distress a comment that had been made during public testimony at a Montana Health Care Authority town meeting. A physician vehemently opposed to the health care reform effort had alerted the assembled citizens to the potential dangers ahead: "Remember what happened the last time we listened to someone named Eve!" he warned. My, my—state health care reform and my championing of it had reached biblical proportions deserving of Old Testament wrath. Eve in the garden had eaten of the apple of health care equity. Could she ever again be an innocent, or had she been changed forever by the no-holds-barred rules of health care politics? Answer: she would be forever changed.

Part of my tenacity in fighting the fight that lay ahead was fueled by my recognition that the dynamics of this struggle was a parallel of every struggle nurses have ever had with physicians at the bedside over patient care. It was archetypal that one of the state's most visible champions of health care and one of the most publicly vocal opponents were physicians.

I had completed my first 4-year term in the state senate and had stood for reelection. A statewide militantly anti-health-care-reform group based in Great Falls, made up largely of obstructionist physicians and a few of their disciples, made my involvement in health care reform a major rallying point in their efforts to defeat me for a second term. Their one issue was the establishment of a health care system based solely on medical savings accounts (MSAs). No deviation from the dogma of total devotion to MSAs would be tolerated. They backed my opponent, footing the bill for a fund-raising letter mailed widely in conjunction with the local chapter of a nationally organized right-wing religious extremist group. Never was that adage "Politics makes strange bedfellows" more apt. To torture myself, I would multiply the membership of the physician group—approximately 75—by $500, the maximum legal contribution for one physician and one spouse. My arithmetic told me they had the potential to raise $37,500 to defeat me—three times the budget for a typical Montana legislative race. That was a war chest so opulent that it made me break into a metaphorical fund-raising sweat. In retrospect, this was just the motivator I needed. My

competitive urges were on overdrive, and I'd be damned if I'd allow an honest desire to improve health care to be distorted into something unrecognizable. The antireformers' extreme and one-dimensional focus on "patient responsibility" left me furious. It mimicked the sociological concept of "blaming the victim." When in this whole process did it become the patient's fault that the health care system wasn't working? I raised more money, knocked on more doors, built more yard signs, talked to more voters, and smiled beatifically. I chose to think that the credibility of nursing's commitment to health care was vindicated when I won the reelection campaign by 61% of my district's vote.

THE PEGGY LEE HEALTH CARE REFORM PLAN: IS THAT ALL THERE IS?

What I came to understand was, though I had survived politically, the work of the Montana Health Care Authority had been irreparably damaged by campaigns of innuendo and policy bashing. The authority had generated a huge body of work but, because of unbearable political pressure, was not permitted to continue past the first phase set forth in the provisions of Senate Bill 285.

As a member of the Montana Health Care Authority would say to me later, "I was afforded a million-dollar education in health care that I am not being permitted to use." The governor withdrew his support, feeling, I can only assume, that he had spent just about all the political capital he wished to spend on this whole affair. After the failure of the Clinton health care plan, most were in a duck-and-cover mode when it came to health care. The 1995 legislative session, with a new Republican majority that owed much to the right wing, passed a bill nullifying Senate Bill 285 and putting in its place an ineffectual poor-cousin-of-a-committee, with little stature and minimal resources. The legislature passed a few bills touted as moderate health care reform. In fact, they were in large part a codification of insurance custom, with the modification of a few of the more onerous measures related to preexisting conditions. Tweaking of insurance law passed for "incremental reform," and I couldn't get an honest hearing for a retooling of the Montana Health Care Authority in the Republican-controlled committee. Moderate Republicans were on the run from the right wing of their party and wouldn't seriously touch health care with a 10-foot pole. The die was cast in the world of power politics, and I would be a persona non grata in the legislative health care scene for one session. I became a Leadership Circle contributor, pledging $250 dollars to the American Nurses Association's political action committee, and prepared for the next round.

Occasionally people would ask, "Are you discouraged that the work of the Montana Health Care Authority wasn't followed through?" My answer is always the same: "I'm a nurse. I've worked with chronically ill patients for years. I don't get discouraged in the face of chronicity." You take pleasure in the small triumphs and the increments of progress and acknowledge that you're in it for the long haul.

Though the Republican majority played bait-and-switch with public opinion and the Montana Health Care Authority was being discarded in the legislative scrap heap, Montana was being alerted to the new reality of the health care industry. In 1993, when Senate Bill 285 was passed, the rest of the big markets in the country were becoming battlegrounds for big managed care companies. At that time we had one fledgling health maintenance organization network operated by Blue Cross–Blue Shield of Montana. But Montana's attitude toward health care reform was about to come of age. In the period between 1995 and 1997, our insurance commissioner and the Montana Department of Public Health and Human Services went to work to create a body of state law that would

provide oversight for the managed care industry, which was knocking on the regulatory doors of our state. The big managed care companies had eaten California, and rumor had it that they were heading our way.

"You thought government involvement in health care was bad," I'd say to anyone who would listen. "Wait until private industry takes the market share. Everything you worried about in relation to government—bureaucracy, lack of choice of provider, and even high cost—will occur under the auspices of private industry. But industry control will be a lot less benign than government control."

Ironically, though I was perceived by the health care foes as being some kind of Nurse Ratchet of big government, I've never been a proponent of a so-called government-sponsored system. Nevertheless, I have the deepest reservation about the concept of the free market at work in health care. There is big money to be made from the vulnerability of others, but I suspect it has more to do with the strict application of the corporate bottom line than with "healthy competition." Whoever said it was acceptable for corporations to get rich from the misery of others? Certainly not Lillian, certainly not I.

THE YEAR OF THE BLACK HELICOPTERS

In 1997, in a surprise move during a Democratic Party caucus, I was drafted to be minority whip for our merry band of partisans. This position is second in command to that of the minority leader, who is the chosen leader of the senate Democrats. I was honored, pleased, and a little horrified. At 42 years of age, I have mercifully been released from an imposter complex. Now, instead of saying, "Who, me?" my innards say "Why not me?" Once again, my belief that a good nurse is prepared to meet any challenge is confirmed by events. The whip role is curiously familiar, reminding me of a combination of my days as a hospital administrator and the hours worked in a psychiatric emergency room.

The 1997 session came on the heels of the infamous Jordan, Montana, stand-off, where members of the Montana militia movement holed up on a remote ranch, keeping both local law enforcement and the Federal Bureau of Investigation at bay. This was the atmosphere that preceded our return to Helena to do the business of the state.

My beloved citizen legislature, of the state that sent great humanists like Mike Mansfield and Pat Williams to Congress, was undergoing a seizure that gripped other parts of our nation as well. The 1997 legislature was heavily influenced by right-wing thought. We debated and in some cases passed bills that dealt with these issues: public bare-butt paddling, reintroduction of corporal punishment in the public schools, new censorship laws that included libraries and schools, and acquired immunodeficiency syndrome, to name a few. We passed a resolution or two condemning the United Nations and the federal government. My colleague and seatmate, in an attempt at satire, drew up an amendment to one of these resolutions, condemning the use of black helicopters to monitor citizen activity. Black helicopter surveillance is a favorite paranoic fantasy of militia sympathizers. If he had actually followed through and presented it on the senate floor, it might have passed.

In this environment, health care issues were dealt with by the passage of a managed care regulatory bill and state codification of the Kennedy-Kassebaum insurance reform bill. In an atmosphere where insurance interests ruled supreme, I was publicly accused by another legislator, with whom I regularly did ideologic health care battle, of being a member of a dark, unnamed "special interest group." I took great pleasure in owning up to that membership in a letter to the editor of a major daily newspaper. "Yes," I declared, "I belong to the Montana Nurses Association, a group of 1400 nurses dedicated to improving health care. Our special interests are quality health care, consumers, and supporting the professionalism of nursing."

A FEW THOUGHTS ON WHAT I HAVE LEARNED

I have often extolled the virtues of nursing education and nursing practice as fine preparation for being a legislator. We are well grounded in the use of assessment skills at every level, we know how to construct an action plan, we are outcome oriented, and we posses the skills to evaluate our actions. We practice stick-to-it-iveness and commitment to follow through, and we are in touch with many of the existential issues of the human condition. There are, however, some inherent dichotomies in being both a nurse and a legislator. So much of our professional socialization in nursing prepares us to support the needs of others, deflect attention from ourselves, and avoid conflict. We seldom think of political animals as deferring to others, smoothing troubled waters, or taking a back seat in a public arena.

My observation is that, for nurse activists to be successful, we must develop a set of skills that have not been reinforced through nursing education: a mature comfort with our own skills and an understanding of how to use the power of our personalities. We must shed the albatross of nursing, the need to be "liked." It is in learning these new dimensions of our role, in fact, of our personhood, that we become effective in more than one style of advocacy.

Blending conventional political skills with nursing consciousness creates a synergistic power cell. We are living out a new model of political action, transforming both ourselves and the political arena in the process. The behaviors that are traditionally associated with altruism are powerful medicine in a society that needs social, political, and economic healing. The ethic of professional nursing has provided the way to meet the challenge of meaningful social involvement and political action.

Unit V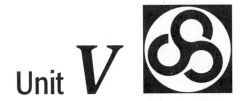

CONTEMPORARY ISSUES IN PROFESSIONAL ORGANIZATIONS

Unit V

describes policy and politics related to nursing organizations. Although these organizations have their own internal policies, they use political strategies to influence public policies that support nursing and promote the health of individuals, families, and communities.

Chapter 31 discusses current issues and trends related to professional organizations and challenges readers to think creatively about the purpose, structure, and activities of these organizations. Chapter 32 describes how nurses can influence their professional organizations to shape their goals and priorities. This chapter is followed by a vignette on the efforts of two nurse leaders who transformed the National Black Nurses Association into a grassroots organization that is influencing health policy and health care through local and national action.

Health care financing continues to be controversial, but nurses have recognized that political action committees, or PACs, provide an important vehicle for individuals to pool their financial resources to back up their organization's endorsement of candidates for public office who are supportive of nursing and quality, accessible health care. Chapter 33 describes the purpose, role, and functioning of nursing PACs and discusses fund-raising strategies.

This unit concludes with a cast study that is actually a collection of stories from national nursing organizations. Their stories show the organizations in action, influencing health policies, primarily at the national level. Although these organizations do not endorse or financially support candidates for political office, they do use "political" strategies to bring nursing's perspective on health matters to policy arenas.

Chapter *31*

CONTEMPORARY ISSUES IN PROFESSIONAL ORGANIZATIONS

Linda J. Shinn

Each day countless Americans act on the notion that there is strength in numbers and that by joining together they can effect change or accomplish a goal. This coming together for a common purpose is usually formalized by the creation of an organization, often called an association, that people join or participate in to further mutual interests.

> The Book of Genesis mentions that members of the same trade or craft tended to congregate geographically. Historians believe that associations existed in ancient Egypt and China, and in Roman times the trades maintained apprentice training agreements and protective regulations. Merchants of ancient Phoenicia who plied the seas often banded together to form mutual-aid societies. [Ernstthal & Jones, 1996, p. 1]

Today, associations exist for such diverse purposes as protecting the interests of elderly persons, advocating child nutrition, representing teachers in the workplace, and preserving the wilderness. Seven of ten adults belong to at least one association; one of four adults belong to four or more associations (Ernstthal & Jones, 1996).

Nurses, too, have created organizations to act as advocates for their unique interests and causes and to control their destiny. For example, the American Nurses Association was formed in 1897 to improve educational standards and to achieve licensure and registration for nurses. The American Radiological Nurses Association was founded in 1981 to promote the interests of radiological nurses (Kelly & Joel, 1995). Though computations vary, it is believed that there are more than 75 nursing organizations in the United States focused on a clinical or functional area of nursing practice. It is estimated that more than 1 million of the nation's nurses belong to an organization or association.

Not unlike the health care industry, associations are big business in today's world. Associations, including nursing organizations, are faced with competition in the marketplace; demands for improved service; and the need to operate ever more efficiently and effectively and to provide member stake holders with a tangible return for their investment of dues dollars.

This chapter will explore the changing environment faced by all associations, the influence of the changing environment on association functions, and implications for nursing organizations.

ASSOCIATION FUNCTIONS

Associations are created for a specific purpose or mission. Associations work in the following functional areas to achieve their missions:

- Programs and services
- Image and identity
- Human resources
  - Members
  - Leaders
  - Staff

- Fiscal resources
  - Dues and nondues revenue
  - Reserves
- Structure and governance

Programs and Services

Associations have historically provided members with a "generic," one-size-fits-all set of programs and services. Information and advocacy have been the mainstay of the programs and services of most associations, including nursing associations. Information and advocacy are often delivered through education programs, newsletters and journals, credentialing mechanisms, and public policy initiatives. Significant challenges face associations in these areas.

INFORMATION

The *raison d'être* of most associations has been the information business. Associations have often been the best source of information for the trade or profession it represents, packaging and delivering information through scholarly journals, newsletters, or educational programs.

The advent of computers, the World Wide Web, and a myriad of places where every member of a profession can shop for information (in many instances, free information) makes it increasingly difficult for the association to serve as a single source of information for a profession.

At the same time, consumers (association members are consummate consumers) want products and services customized to fit their unique needs and wants. For example, the Levi Company makes it possible for the customer to have a pair of jeans customized to fit his or her figure for only $10 more than the usual retail price. The wild success of the Cable News Network demonstrates that people want information when they want it and when they need it.

The emerging role of associations is to help members figure out how to take the information coming their way, sort it, make sense out of it, and use it to add value to their business or profession. Associations might become the "middle-men" between information producers and information users, helping members decide what information is relevant, useful, and meaningful. Not only will this information have to be customized to member needs and wants, but it will have to be delivered when the member needs it and wants it, in either a print or electronic format, not when the association wants to provide it. Large tomes of information will have to be synthesized by the association and provided to members in "bites." The desire for information in "bite-sized, easily digested chunks" provides a great challenge for nursing associations that have long published scholarly journals and treatises on professional issues.

Education programs have been a prevalent strategy for delivering information to members. The increased necessity for lifelong learning to survive in today's job market can be a boon for association continuing education programs. However, content, delivery mechanisms, and prices must be suited to the needs and wants of customers.

A focus on lifelong learning augurs for a greater partnership between nursing organizations. This could include the opportunity for members to take advantage of education offered by another association to assist them if they decide to change specialties or prepare for work in a new practice setting.

The level of customization and attention to individualized needs demanded by consumers in all marketplaces will become increasingly prevalent in nursing organizations. Nurses' expectations may demand a much greater partnership between nursing organizations so that an array of customized products and services can be provided. The nursing consumer market may call for a kind of "nursing association mall," where the nurse can stop once and shop. In other words, associations might better serve their members and the profession by joining together to provide a centralized access point where nurses can view and order the array of products and services available from nursing organizations. For example, information about standards, continuing education offerings, certification, position statements, and practice guidelines could be included in a nursing association "mall."

ADVOCACY

Public policy is another key program for many associations. There are a number of trends that influence association advocacy programs. Trends and related implications include the following:

- Mistrust and cynicism about government at all levels may manifest itself in increased mistrust or lack of support for association governmental affairs programs.
- Concerns over political fund raising may result in increasing difficulties for fund raising by nurses' political action committees (PACs).
- The shift of federal responsibilities to state and local levels of government will necessitate a shift of national resources, including personnel and money, to state and local levels of an association.
- The interest in "reinventing government at all levels," including greater public-private partnerships in doing work historically in the domain of government, requires associations to remain vigilant to "reinvention" schemes and to partner with government in the association's area of expertise.
- Legislators are now tapped into cyberspace and are urging their constituents to provide immediate opinions or views through E-mail or chat rooms. The role of the association as intermediary between member and legislator may shift to helping members learn how to be advocates for various causes in cyberspace. In addition, the role of a "grassroots" network that can be influential and persuasive at the local level has become more critical.

The increasing shift of federal responsibilities to the states will have an impact on how nurses influence public policy. Nurses have built a formidable national mechanism to influence health policy through development of "grassroots networks" that can be relied on to relay nursing's views to Congress; through building a well-funded PAC to help elect members of Congress favorable to nursing; and through grooming nurses to be spokespersons, lobbyists, and office holders. With few exceptions, state and local nursing systems for influencing public policy are not as successful or as sophisticated as the national system. Though it is important to fortify national mechanisms to influence public policy, a foundation of human and fiscal resources must be built state by state and community by community if nursing is to continue to influence public policy. More attention to influencing the views of local office holders on health-related matters, contributing to local candidate coffers, and supporting nurse candidates for local office will increase nursing's strength and influence in public policy. Strengthening state and local resources necessitates more collaboration and alliances among nursing associations at state, chapter, district, and local levels.

Nurses have historically partnered with government to improve the nation's health. Immunization programs, acquired immunodeficiency (AIDS) awareness activities, and health screening initiatives are good examples. In an age of greater interest in public-private partnerships, nursing has an opportunity to get even more done through local government. Jarrat, Coates, Mahaffie, and Hines (1994) suggest that associations might:

- Offer training programs for local elected officials
- Channel issues, ideas, and know-how into the process of reinventing government
- Set up voluntary teams to help state and local governments develop public policy

Nursing is well suited for each of these roles. For example, a district nurses association might conduct a seminar for a county council on Medicaid cost savings achieved by publicly supported prenatal care programs, an organization of nurse executives might provide expertise on organizational restructuring, or a chapter of occupational health nurses might offer policy consultation on workplace safety standards.

The media have become the most significant "influentials" in shaping public policy. "At the same time, government shapes public opinion by using more showmanship, such as televised town meetings" (Jarrat et al., 1994, p. 122). Refocusing nursing's "grassroots network" on state and local initiatives is important, but greater attention must also be given to grooming and supporting a cadre of media-savvy nursing influentials to help shape public opinion in every community.

Image and Identity

Image is the *perception* of what an association "is" and "does." Identity is *what* the organization "is" and "does." Organizations must be concerned about an external and an internal image and identity. Legislators, regulators, media, other organizations, and the public-at-large compose an association's external audience. Members and member prospects are the internal patrons of an association.

Futurists note that, as the twentieth century ends, the era in which people defined themselves (and were defined by others) in terms of their institutional affiliations—for example, as a nurse and member of the American Nurses Association, as a dean and member of the American Association of Colleges of Nursing, or as an advanced nurse practitioner certified by the American Nurses Credentialing Center—may be ending. Futurists suggest that we are moving from the "individual" to the "dividual." The concept of the "individual," connoting a unified single person, may no longer be relevant. Rather, the concept of the "dividual," understood as the many connections and affinities that one person has to multiple aspects of personality and need, is more pertinent. Thus the association marketers and the public relations and communications specialists will be challenged to capture and portray the multifaceted nature of a trade or profession and the individuals in them.

The concept of the "dividual" is emerging in nursing as nurses assume the role of home health nurse, oncology nurse, hospice nurse, and AIDS nurse, often all in one day. The ability to portray the diversity of the profession and to appeal to the "dividual" will necessitate more strategic partnerships between and among associations.

Associations will have to think about appealing to members and prospects by personalizing the association to the multiple aspects of people's interests. For example, a nurse might be an inveterate international traveler, a budding archaeologist, or an author and consultant. An association interested in getting and keeping this nurse as a member will have to package its products and services to meet the many aspects of this nurse's personality: matching the association's travel program, providing opportunities to write for publication, and offering an individual health insurance program to meet this person's interests and needs. In fact, the association's regular publication might carry a cover individualized to the nurse's interest in order to capture the nurse's attention and allegiance. Today's technology makes it possible for the association to track member demographics and member needs, wants, and buying habits and to respond to them.

An association's internal image, to its members, member prospects, and other stake holders, is as important as an external image. Associations, including nursing organizations, are going to have to rid themselves of practices that yield images of slow decision making by elitist decision makers who spend association resources on activities that are not perceived by members as tangible benefits. For nursing organizations, the internal image can be improved through continuous assessment of member needs, wants, and opinion at every level of the organization. Subsequent follow-up with an array of customized products and services that meet member needs and that are delivered locally will also help improve the organizational images. Moreover, in an era in which the packaging of the product is almost as important as the product itself, nursing organizations are going to have to package themselves to be more appealing. Groups such as the National League for Nursing and the American Nurses Association must not only be "new and improved" but must have a contemporary styling that *conveys* "new and improved."

Association marketers and public relations and communications specialists will be challenged to capture and portray the multifaceted nature of a trade or profession for external publics as well. Representing the diversity and interests of an association's members presents a particular challenge in the public policy arena. Associations have long prided themselves in representing a profession and speaking with one voice before the makers of public policy and the public at large. The diverse interests of members may mean that speaking with a single voice on every issue is a thing of the past.

Associations might better serve their constituency by representing an array of viewpoints and by serving as a single source of credible information about those viewpoints. Speaking with one voice, particularly in the policy and political arenas, would be saved for those matters that are highly important and have strong potential for impact on the profession. It would then be essential for associations and groups of associations, such as the Tri Council for Nursing and the Nursing Organization Liaison Forum, to have in place the ability to respond in a strong voice and timely manner when there is a likelihood of having an impact on and success in influencing policy.

When associations serve as a credible source of information for an array of viewpoints, they can provide members or member segments with the tools to represent themselves or, on some issues, a smaller constituency. Such strategies may provide one option through which various interests in an association speak about controversial and often divisive issues, such as end-of-life decisions or right-to-life matters.

Human Resources

MEMBERS

Peppers and Rogers (1993) suggest that businesses no longer will sell a single product to many customers; rather, businesses will sell as many products as possible to a single customer—in other words, will aim for "share of customer" rather than "share of market." Translated into association speak, associations may need to quit worrying about capturing more and more of the potential member market and worry about getting those "already on board" to buy more of the association's products and services and to give more to association foundations, PACs, or fundraisers. Stated another way, associations will need to focus more on retention than on recruitment. Providing an array of products to one particular customer might also mean looking at customers "who are not members" and, rather than convincing them to be members, keep them attached to the association in a product-buyer status.

Nursing organizations will increasingly compete with each other for the time, attention, and dollars of nurses. Members today are asking: "How will membership help me? How will membership 'put money in my jeans'?" Members and prospects will gravitate to associations that can answer these questions—and it is likely not to matter whether the organizations are nursing organizations. The days of joining an organization for altruistic reasons are over. The association that will fare the best in the future is the one that focuses on "what we can give to the member" rather than "what we can take from the member."

The changing demographics of the population of the United States is an important consideration for association membership. Hispanics are the fastest-growing segment of the U.S. population, particularly in the West, Southwest, and Southeast. Jarratt et al. (1994) report that Hispanics present an opportunity and a challenge for associations. Although Hispanics and other minority groups are likely to be a huge pool of potential members, associations are shaped and operate in a culture that has been largely fashioned by white North Americans. The demographic trends require that nursing organizations representing a variety of cultures and ethnic groups think about how to work together. Such collaboration might include joint memberships and sharing of culturally specific programs, products, and materials.

LEADERS

Association executives participating in an American Society of Association Executives (ASAE) Foundation trends panel identified accountability to members and other key stake holders as one of the greatest challenges facing association leaders at the turn of the century (Foundation of ASAE, 1996). Leaders will be held increasingly responsible for the outcomes achieved with the association's resources.

Association leaders need to be much more comfortable with ambiguity in the face of constant change. Association leaders must shape their capacity to know what members' needs will be in the future. This will necessitate spending more time thinking about and planning for the future and communicating with members and other key association stake holders such as vendors and funders. Association leaders will have to strike a balance between leading members and not being too far out in front.

Leaders must have help in striking this balance. Few association leaders come to the role of board member or to the committee table with preparation, training, education, or practical experience (i.e., "Association 101"). Constant investment in leader education and training, including strategic thinking, facilitation, and consensus-building skills, will be required for leaders to meet the challenges in the days ahead.

Many organizations report that members have less time to serve in volunteer roles within associations. Members today want to work for an association by doing a job, using their brains, achieving something meaningful, and either signing up for another job or moving on to another aspect of their lives. Care will need to be taken to provide opportunities for those who want to serve and then move on.

Almost all associations are "graying," particularly at the leadership table. The majority of associations are filled with baby boomers who may give up leadership responsibilities during the next twenty years or want to contribute smaller chunks of time and effort. On the other hand, there are predictions that the boomers will work longer and many will prefer part-time

work. This inclination has implications for managing multiple generations of members and volunteers in one organization. Associations will be challenged to develop and implement succession plans to groom and train future leaders, plans that provide for a mix of seasoned and fresh leaders for the association. Association nominating committees must begin to serve as search committees and work year around to identify and develop talent for the association. Limited human resources to lead nursing's professional organizations necessitate attention to grooming leaders for the future, profession wide, not just organization by organization.

In addition, nursing leaders must sharpen their capacity to forecast the future, including changes in the marketplace that will demand nurses in differing numbers and with differing skill sets for different practice sites. Nursing leaders are also going to have to sharpen their ability to learn from events, mistakes, and miscalculations. For example, the profession missed the mark in not anticipating the restructuring that would take place in health care institutions and the subsequent consequences for nurses. At this time, nursing's leaders should be anticipating what will happen after "managed care" and should be readying the profession to meet the next wave of change and challenge. Nursing's leaders must strive to unite the profession around a common agenda. Too often, nursing's professional organizations have been successful only in uniting the profession around a common enemy—for example, the registered care technologist.

STAFF

Associations must select competent, seasoned association executives to lead staff teams and to partner with leaders. Historically, professional associations have selected a member of the profession to serve as the chief staff executive of the association. Association management involves a special set of skills and competencies that Tecker and Fidler (1993) describe as "relationships among people, relationships among actions, relationships among resources and effectively converting information into the knowledge required to support these relationships." ASAE has recently described the body of knowledge necessary for association executives and offers a certification program leading to the certified association executive (CAE) credential to attest that an individual is competent in this body of knowledge.

Professional associations including nursing organizations must begin to select association executives for their expertise in association management, recognizing that leaders of the profession may not always possess these proficiencies. The CAE credential should also be a requirement for hiring future chief staff executives, and executive compensation should be tied to association performance.

Nursing associations should consider sharing staff resources, particularly those one-of-a-kind experts such as nurse economists. Nursing groups should also consider cross-training staff, particularly nursing staff, in each other's organizations to ensure a pool of talented association executives for the future. Adequate staff resources at the state and local levels are the challenge ahead for many nursing groups. One way to meet this challenge is through a partnership among national nursing organizations in funding state and local staff resources to achieve an agreed-on agenda.

Fiscal Resources

DUES AND NONDUES REVENUE

Associations have allowed their dues/nondues revenue ratios to become disproportionate. On average, dues comprise about 37% of total income for individual member associations and about 41% of total income for health care/medical individual member associations (ASAE, 1997). Associations have built nondues revenue streams, such as advertising in publications, presenting conference exhibitions, and offering affinity programs (i.e., credit cards and insurance), to keep member dues low. These nondues revenue streams are jeopardized as businesses cut back on expenses, such as advertising

dollars, or determine that the return on dollars given to associations is not worth the investment.

When nondues revenues become increasingly harder to raise, association dues rise. Some associations are raising dues for the first time in 10 years and are asking members for large amounts of money. Simultaneously, many employers are saying, "We cannot continue to pay dues to so many associations—many that have the same mission or purpose and provide few, if any, tangible, measurable outcomes."

A number of associations, including nursing associations, have established for-profit subsidiaries for generating nondues revenue. This strategy must be examined carefully because competition for the same dollars from nurses is likely to become keener. Nursing organizations often tap the same vendor, funder, advertiser, or exhibitor for contributions. These contributors are looking more critically at the dollars spent and outcomes received. Of equal concern is the question of whether getting into the retail business is in keeping with the association's mission. The more important consideration is the control, viability, and longevity of an association when it is resourced primarily by nondues revenue rather than member money.

DUES EQUITY

While associations are faced with members' wanting customized products and services, members will also want their association payments tailored to their usage. For example, a member of the Oncology Nurses Association (ONS) may want only the ONS Career Resource Kit and 12 issues of the *ONS News* but *not* the *Oncology Nursing Forum,* which is a part of the member benefit.

Nursing associations will be faced with developing a core package of member benefits for all members plus a menu of services from which members can select and pay for additional programs or products that meet their needs. This will necessitate paying constant attention to member needs and wants and discarding some of those programs that have served altruistic purposes but have had few tangible advantages for members.

Structure and Governance

DECISION MAKING

Few associations are structured in terms of their mission and goals. Perlov (1995) notes that associations are trying to operate in a twenty-first-century milieu with a nineteenth-century structure. Many association structures were fashioned around the hierarchical, industrial model. In addition, history, personalities, and politics, rather than the mission, goals, or plan of work, drive the structure and governance of most associations. This driver of many association structures and governance systems can be labeled culture.

Many associations are saddled with decision-making structures that make it almost impossible to arrive at a policy stance or take advantage of any opportunity without engaging a large decision tree, such as consulting a myriad of committees or lots of chapters, or waiting for a house of delegates to meet. Such modes of doing business must give way to a cadre of leaders who have an eye on the mission, a finger on the member pulse, an ear to the ground, and the confidence, trust, and backing of those who elected or appointed them to make the necessary decisions. Members are also going to have to permit leaders to take risks and make mistakes. The consequences will have to become learning and forward movement, rather than the stasis of ever more layers of decision-making, cross-checking, and second-guessing leaders.

Trends in structure and governance include smaller boards, fewer committees, and an ad hoc approach to getting business done. For example, some associations select a committee structure once the association's strategic plan is in place. A committee is created on the basis of the work identified in the plan, an assignment to carry out, and the tools and resources to complete the job and is disbanded when the job is done.

Technology has done away with the need for an association executive committee, historically created to act on behalf of a board of directors between meetings. Today, all board members can be convened to act on behalf of an association at almost any time. Increased use of technology, such as audio and video conferencing, requires training of association leaders in using these tools for decision making.

Each and every nursing organization must ensure that decision-making mechanisms are built for action. Each organization must guarantee that it is mission driven, that it is member and market sensitive in its work, and that structure and governance evolve from the strategic plan.

PARTNERSHIPS

The forging of new partnerships, strategic alliances, or coalitions is a strategy under consideration by an increasing number of associations. Partnerships within organizations, among competing associations, and with vendors are used to enhance the product mix associations have to offer. With increasing frequency, association leaders are considering merger or consolidation strategies. Members are asking, Do we need 9 local realtor organizations, 4 industrial hygiene organizations, 23 medical specialty societies, and 6 beef-cattle organizations? Nurses are also asking, Do we need 75 nursing organizations? The most significant challenge for nursing organizations is to figure out how to come together to maximize what each is good at and to share resources and expertise in order to strengthen the profession and strengthen the bonds among nursing's organizations.

ARE PROFESSIONAL ORGANIZATIONS HELPING NURSING?

Nursing associations are an integral part of the association marketplace. It is estimated that about 1 million nurses belong to some 75-plus associations ranging from the American Nurses Association to the Association for Nurses in AIDS

Care. Nursing associations are organized around protecting and advancing the interests of the profession, such as the American Nurses Association; around practice areas, such as the Association of Operating Room Nurses; around ethnic interests, such as the Philippine Nurses Association of America; and around scholarly interests, such as the Council on Graduate Education for Administration in Nursing.

Nursing's clinical and functional interests have been developed and championed by specialty organizations. Nursing's economic and political interests have been championed by the American Nurses Association. From a historical perspective, nursing's successes have been legion. Licensure, certification, advocacy, standards, expansion of practice, and improved economic well-being are among the achievements. Most of these successes have come through partnerships between and among nursing organizations.

Many nursing organizations have moved from focus on education and information about a specialty to public policy work, development of specialty standards, annual conferences, and exhibitions. There is duplication of effort in many instances—in a marketplace in which the competition with the private sector to provide goods and services to members is ever keener. The profession also must question the value of contributing millions of the profession's scarce dollars to duplicative endeavors, such as support of boards of directors, committees, conventions, conferences, and publications.

As members, vendors, and funders demand more accountability for dollars spent, the onus will be on nursing leaders to answer the following questions:

1. Is the profession better off because it has some 75-plus professional organizations?
2. Can and should the profession sustain this level of organization?
3. How can the profession ensure that the outcomes of all the organizations' efforts are appropriate to the practitioner and to the profession?

The following are related questions for leaders:

1. What is known about the needs of the profession?
2. What is known about the needs and wants of nursing association members?
3. What is known about the external environment, and what are the profession's assumptions about the future?
4. What are the capacities of nursing organizations to respond on behalf of the profession, in the interests of members, and to face the challenges in the days ahead?

Organized nursing must answer these questions to determine whether the profession's many nursing associations are helping or hindering the profession. The profession's leaders must also consider some organizational options for the future.

Options
MERGERS OR CONSOLIDATIONS

The option of merger or consolidation of organizations must be considered by nursing organizations. Other industries and professional groups (e.g., beef, industrial hygiene, real estate) are debating the merits of merging organizations. Some have put mechanisms in place to facilitate consolidation of associations. Other groups are considering a corporate structure that gives each group corporate autonomy while staff services and headquarters are shared.

JOINT MEMBERSHIPS

Another option for making the most out of associations' human and fiscal resources and expanding organizational capacity to respond to members and the marketplace is joint memberships. Some nursing associations are exploring linkages with like organizations through purchase of memberships in related organizations at a reduced rate.

Consideration should also be given to franchising an association's products and services to other associations in order to deliver a greater array of customized products and services to members.

ANOTHER NURSING ORGANIZATION

Given the history of organized nursing's inability to respond to special interests within organizations or to be responsive to member needs and wants, the genesis of yet more nursing organizations is a possibility. In the broader association world, it is estimated that some 1,000 new associations are started every year. The nursing profession is not immune from this trend.

DO NOTHING

This option is a maintenance of the status quo. In other words, the profession's organizations continue to evolve in an unplanned way.

CONCLUSION

The challenges and changes facing all associations at the turn of the century are innumerable. The collective challenge of organized nursing is fourfold:

- To strengthen the bond within the profession
- To strengthen the skills and abilities of the people of the profession: the leaders and followers
- To strengthen the profession's infrastructure, its professional societies, locally and nationally
- To strengthen the profession's fiscal resources

The trends that will influence contemporary nursing organizations are many—and the possibilities for contemporary nursing organizations to reinvent themselves are endless.

REFERENCES

American Society of Association Executives. (1997). *ASAE operating ratio report.* Washington, DC: Author.

Ernstthal, H. L., & Jones, B. (1996). *Principles of association management.* Washington, DC: American Society of Association Executives.

The Foundation of the American Society of Association Executives. (1996). *Executive summary trend analysis panels on governance.* Washington, DC: Author.

Jarrat, J., Coates, J. F., Mahaffie, J. B., & Hines, A. (1994). *Managing your future as an association.* Washington, DC: The Foundation of the American Society of Association Executives.

Kelly, L., & Joel, L. (1995). *Dimensions of professional nursing.* New York: McGraw-Hill.

Peppers, D., & Rogers, M., (1993). *The one to one future: Building relationships one customer at a time.* New York: Currency Doubleday.

Perlov, D. (1995). Personal papers. New York.

Tecker, G., & Fidler, M. (1993). *Successful association leadership: Dimensions of 21st-century competency for the CEO.* Washington, DC: The Foundation of the American Society of Association Executives.

Chapter 32

YOU AND YOUR PROFESSIONAL ORGANIZATION

Betty J. Skaggs and Christine M. deVries

To leave the world a bit better, whether by a healthy child, a garden patch or a redeemed social condition; to know even one life has breathed easier because you have lived. This is to have succeeded. — Ralph Waldo Emerson

In the simplest terms, a professional association is a gathering of people in a common industry or occupation who share ideas, promote their discipline, and advocate their beliefs. In our more complex world, however, modern associations are multitiered organizations professing a mission statement and multiple goals addressing legal, legislative, and regulatory issues; defining social and cultural factors; competing with other groups; and coping with modern technology. At the core of these associations, whether large or small, are groups of people coming together for the purpose of fostering their chosen profession. At best, professional associations provide vehicles through which individuals in a profession might realize the basic life goal to which Emerson refers in the quotation above. "A volunteer position may be the only avenue offering you the latitude to experiment with new ideas and techniques without risking failure [in a job situation]" (Klein, 1993, p. 63). Therefore the professional association can be the catalyst for creating the passion, providing the opportunities, and justifying the desire to make conditions better for patients and the profession. We have both experienced this appetite for a cause and have

focused the realization of that cause through our work with our professional association(s).

In this chapter, the development of associations, specifically nursing associations, will be explored with a discussion focused on the structure and functions of a voluntary, professional membership association. How an association develops a political agenda and translates that action into a position of strength in policy development are examined in detail. Finally, strategies for influencing an organization are suggested. Although the American Nurses Association (ANA) and its constituent organizations are used as examples, the principles and strategies explained in this chapter could be applied to any association.

INVOLVEMENT IN ORGANIZATIONS

Today, organizational membership is identified as a vital part of one's personal and professional life. Membership in one's professional association is seen as an essential activity for career growth and mobility, as well as an activity that ensures the delivery of safe, competent nursing care. Typically the active professional nurse holds membership in numerous professional and social organizations, taking an active leadership role in a select few and being a follower in others. For example, the individual nurse identifies organizations with goals that parallel her own and participates in them at a level dictated by her personal commitment and her time constraints. By way of illustration, Anne Hall, MSN, RNC, PNP, works in the OurTown Hospital's pediatric emergency department and has developed expertise in and a special passion concerning the prevention of child abuse. In addition to following practice issues on the topic of child abuse in various ANA forums and publications, she is also involved in her hospital's practice committee, the state nurses association, and the Emergency Nurses Association. Furthermore, she has found that membership in her state Women's Political Caucus chapter and the OurTown Hospital's Children's Health Coalition has been instrumental in building local networks with members of other disciplines who work with children. Anne Hall is persuaded that her involvement in all these associations is vital to maintaining her practice competencies and to providing avenues to act on her passion. Anne's level of involvement in these organizations is varied. For example, she is on the legislative committee of her state nurses association and has served as a delegate to the national house of delegates on behalf of her state association for the past 4 years. She does not have the time to serve in a volunteer or elected leadership position with the state political caucus, but she does respond to legislative alerts and other calls to action. Anne Hall understands that her level of commitment can differ from one association to another. She realizes that support demonstrated through membership is important, even when one cannot participate in a more active role.

Similarly, continuous membership in nursing organizations throughout a career provides an important source of support for one's colleagues and the organization. For example, a nurse may choose to retire from active practice for a time to focus on family responsibilities, but it is still important for that nurse to maintain membership in the professional organization. "Inactive" members read association publications, keep in touch with colleagues, write letters to the editor, and attend meetings—all of which are necessary to make reentry into practice a smoother process.

STRUCTURE AND FUNCTION OF AN ASSOCIATION

An association can have any type of structure—from an ad hoc assembly of individuals to a formal board of directors and bylaws dictating the rules of governance. Middle-sized to large professional membership organizations usually have several common activities: government relations, membership services, communications and public relations, educational programs, certification of products and/or services, professional activities, policy development, and a lobbying program. All of these activities must emanate from the mission statement. The most effective association is one in which every individual in the association, from the office assistant in the copy center to the chief executive officer (CEO) understands how her or his job directly relates to the goals and mission of that association.

Associations are usually formalized by articles of incorporation, a legal document that defines the scope of the association, establishes it as an entity, and sets out its tax structure. Although an organization is not required to incorporate in order to operate, most associations take this course of action to define limits of liability for its members, permit entry into contracts, and secure the appropriate tax status. The ANA papers of incorporation, filed in 1917, state:

> The purposes of this corporation are and shall be to promote the professional and educational advancement of nurses in every proper way; to elevate the standards of nursing education; to establish and maintain a code of ethics among nurses; to distribute relief among such nurses as may become ill, disabled, or destitute; to disseminate information on the subject of nursing by publication in official periodicals or otherwise; to bring into communication with each other various nurses and associations and federations of nurses throughout the United States of America; and to all rights and property held by the American Nurses' Association as a corporation duly incorporated under and by virtue of the laws of the State of New York.

Articles of incorporation, a legal document defining the scope of an association, is a broad, sweeping, general statement of an association's purposes. For the specific rules defining the governance of an association, one would need to study its bylaws. Bylaws describe the details of how any organization functions. For example, Article VI of the ANA Bylaws defines the board of directors: its composition, authority, accountability, and responsibility. Although bylaws are more flexible than articles of incorporation, it is important to note that bylaws constitute a legal document by which the association is run. Bylaws state the rules of the game, including reporting relationships, responsibilities and accountability, and election and terms of officers. The organization's bylaws are "owned" by the members of the highest governing body who are either the entire membership or duly elected representatives of the membership. Bylaws may be changed but only by a vote of the membership or the representative body, following a prescribed amendment procedure. Bylaws may seem boring to some, but they can be an important strategy in defining power bases.

Bylaws define organizations of all sizes, from a small organization with a board of directors elected directly by a membership of a few hundred individuals to an association as large as the American Association of Retired Persons, with 30 million members. In fact, bylaws define our highest legislative body, the U.S. Congress. They define the structure and function of an organization and establish the agreement among its members as to their common mission and goals and the relationships that will be established among the members and leaders.

The ANA is a good example of a representative structure. The house of delegates—the policymaking body of the association—consists of proportional representation from the member states. The house of delegates, under current bylaws, cannot be larger than 615 individuals elected by the members of their state nurses associations. Although the house of delegates is the highest governing body in the ANA, the day-to-day activities of the organization and the details of the implementation of policy are determined by a board of directors elected by the house of delegates.

Beyond these primary structural components, a professional organization is designed so that authority and responsibility are assigned to various bodies of experts. The bylaws provide a structure in which the functions of the organization are smoothly carried out. The structure should empower the membership to achieve its ends but not paralyze the organization. It is important that the structure be flexible enough to meet the changing needs of the association but also be clear in the assignment of responsibilities to various entities. Finally, it is necessary to define which structures to maintain as permanent committees, such as a bylaws committee, a reference committee, and a nominations committee, and which structures are to be allowed an ad hoc philosophy to promote flexibility.

It is important for an organization to maintain a body of experts to advise the board of directors on matters pertaining to that profession. For example, the ANA has two entities, a Congress on Nursing Practice and a Congress on Nursing Economics, that are responsible for developing long-range policy around these issues. Furthermore, the ANA maintains an Institute of Constituent Members Collective Bargaining Programs to deal specifically with matters and strategies related to collective bargaining.

One factor, unique to voluntary organizations, that makes the structure of the professional association more complex is that the organization contains two distinct lines of command—the members, or the volunteers, and the staff, under the direction of the CEO. In most cases the CEO is hired by the board of directors and the staff is hired by the CEO. The staff's primary purpose is to implement the programs and policies adopted by the house of delegates or the board of directors acting for the house. The chain of authority and responsibility originates in the elected board of directors, then proceeds to the CEO, and then goes on down through the paid staff. However, there are also cadres of volunteers who work with the staff for the purpose of implementing the policies. Some experts in association management argue that two lines of formal authority and responsibility—one for staff and one for volunteers—must be kept separate if the association's work is to be successful. Others advocate an informal relationship between staff and volunteers to promote the work of the association. However, in large, complex organizations, this may be difficult to manage. One way to delineate the different levels of accountability is to recall that the staff has the final accountability for implementation of strategies and products stemming from the original policy, whereas the volunteer component has the final accountability for developing, refining, or interpreting the major policy decisions. As a case in point, the house of delegates adopted a resolution to increase nursing's legislative presence and allocated funds to develop appropriate programs to carry out this mission. The political action committee identified three strategies to implement this directive of the house, one of which was a conference. The committee members (the volunteers), after defining the purpose of the conference, outlining the objectives, identifying potential speakers, and creating a general overview of how the conference should be carried out, turned the project over to staff who would contract with the hotel for meeting space, arrange for the speakers, and market the event. The volunteers interpreted the directive and created the content for the conference. Staff actually produced the conference, implementing the wishes of the membership.

In small organizations with limited resources, the differentiation between volunteer and staff roles may be less clear and the need for the division of responsibilities less critical. For instance, in many small organizations a volunteer "takes on" the responsibility of producing a newsletter, whereas in a large association there is usually a newsletter or newspaper staff. However, in both cases, the contents reflect the philosophy and programs of the membership.

As organizations become more complex, the level of hierarchy increases. In fact, large organizations usually have regional, state, and local structures to complement the national structure. Regardless of size and complexity, it is critical that lines of accountability and communication among the structural units are clear to every member of the association.

ESTABLISHING AN ASSOCIATION AS A PLAYER IN THE HEALTH CARE POLICY ARENA

One of the primary purposes of an association is to influence public policy on behalf of the constituents of that association. "Interest groups," as they have become known, exist for every single pursuit of humankind. It is unfortunate that interest groups have become synonymous with "dirty politics" in recent years, because the very purpose of an interest group is to educate around, and to promote a cause for, the betterment of people.

To become a recognized and established policy expert in any given field, an association must develop those policies it wants to promote. Policies are broad guidelines that reflect the values of the individuals making the statement. Policies are usually established by a voting body—a house of delegates—or by elected officials in collaboration with a CEO. Policy statements established by a voting body can take the form of resolutions, main motions, statements of goals and priorities, legislative platforms, and similar documents. For example, a policy statement or resolution may direct the association to join a coalition to participate in promoting increased access for children to comprehensive health care services. The board and staff of an association would be directed to allocate financial and staff resources to that end.

On the other hand, procedures designed by staff outline methods or steps to implement a policy or legislative platform. For example, a statement in a policy agenda might read: Ensure full funding of the Nurse Education Act. Procedures designed by staff to implement this policy might look like the following:

1. Write letters to Congress on behalf of the association, urging full funding.

2. Testify before appropriate Congressional committees to advocate funding.
3. Activate grassroots network to urge nurses to contact their members of Congress regarding funding for nurse education.
4. Promote editorials in targeted newspapers from nurses touting the benefit of funding nurse education.

In summary, a policy agenda comprising policy statements provide general guidelines and procedures that direct the day-to-day operation of the association and the staff.

To effectively accomplish the realization of a policy agenda, an association must have a process to adopt such an agenda. It is the responsibility of the governing members of an association to approve that agenda, but it is the primary function of the organization's staff to advance it. Depending on the size and type of group, the procedural steps involved in developing an agenda will vary. In a large organization, such as the ANA, many people are involved in perfecting an agenda. In a small group, consensus can be reached more easily.

When an association is designing a policy agenda, it is important to ensure that the proposals are politically viable. It benefits the membership to promote both a short-term agenda and one that defines far-reaching goals. In this manner, members can observe immediate success but also be cognizant of the overall mission of the association. It is important to define whether the association will have a narrow agenda, such as lobbying for the establishment of a demonstration program, or an expansive agenda, such as advocating health care reform. This decision will have an impact on the resources needed to achieve the stated agenda.

The most effective advocacy organizations have three distinct components to their operation that contribute to their political strength: lobbyists who directly lobby members of Congress or state or local officials; grassroots program that mobilizes individual nurses to communicate with their members of Congress "back home"; and a political action committee and

program. These three programs are necessary for a visible and credible association because they advance the mission of the association and hence the profession. Each of these programs and avenues of advocacy is described elsewhere in this book, but it is important to note that nursing established itself as a leader during the health care reform debate of the mid-1990s because these three elements were combined with excellent policy development, savvy media strategies, and intense coalition building among nurses, health care professionals, labor unions, and consumer representatives. Although the overall goal of universal health care failed, nursing is still reaping the rewards of those labors through continued involvement in the establishment of government policies and practices, at both the federal and state levels of government, that promote the role of the nurse in the evolving health care delivery system.

INFLUENCING YOUR PROFESSIONAL ASSOCIATION

The basic way to influence the association is to join—become a part of it! Simple support through payment of dues provides a necessary financial base to run the day-to-day operations—pay the rent, publish the newsletter, and pay the staff. Membership dues also provide programs designed to meet the fundamental purposes of the organization. Of course, more active involvement is necessary to learn about an organization, to make a significant impact on an organization, or in some instances to make involvement in the association personally satisfying.

For the nursing student, the National Student Nurses Association (NSNA) is a perfect place to begin learning about professional associations. Many registered nurses had their first experiences with organized nursing through participation in school NSNA chapters. One of the contributors to this book, Mary Foley, served as NSNA president, and Sheila Burke (former staff director for Senator Robert Dole and current executive director of the John F. Kennedy School at Harvard [see Chapter 26 vignette]) was president of the California Student Nurses Association.

Another excellent way to expand your knowledge of an organization and to express your commitment to an idea or cause is to volunteer to serve on a local committee. Most local organizations are always looking for new recruits. The work you do with the committee, the knowledge you acquire, and the reputation you build will carry your name to other nurses in the local organization and, before you know it, to the state organization. The benefits of this involvement will continue to grow throughout your career.

After nurses become involved with their professional association, they may want to influence it. There are degrees of influence, ranging from simple projects, such as persuading the board to approve the use of the association's name as a sponsor of a symposium on a local health care problem, to a long-range plan to improve the management of the association.

Efforts to influence an association will not always succeed the first time. For example, members are often not elected to volunteer bodies the first time they run; however, persistence in this realm usually pays off. To be elected to a board of directors usually requires earning name recognition among members, getting to know some of the existing board members so that they may advocate on your behalf, taking on projects that earn for you the respect of the current board, and taking on some lesser roles in the association before heading to the top. Remember, matters rarely move fast in volunteer organizations, where democratic principles guide the actions of the board and the committees.

If you have a good idea or plan that you think the association should adopt or promote, you can present it in a variety of ways. For example, a nurse who had been involved with issues related to violence in the workplace wanted her colleagues in the state association to become informed on the issue and to join with her in implementing a program for hospital education departments. She wrote an article about her success in setting up a multidisciplinary committee on workplace violence in her hospital and described some of the relevant issues. She included her name and address so that interested nurses were able to contact her. The following year at the annual convention, a group of nurses proposed a resolution to the house of delegates, asking the board of directors to form a task force to develop guidelines regarding violence for adoption by hospitals.

As these nurses realized, to encourage an association to take a public stand on issues, one must write a position statement or resolution for submission to the association board or house of delegates. The same end might be accomplished by asking the board of directors or a committee to send a letter that you compose with the signature of the association's president. Understand that such a request, unless it fits within a previously adopted position of the membership, would have to go through the association's policymaking procedure. This procedure might take a while.

Another useful lobbying technique to have an impact on public policy is to lobby other associations in addition to your own. Their subsequent endorsement will provide evidence of a broad power base and show extensive support. For example, the ANA could advocate third-party reimbursement at 100% of a physician's rate under Medicare for advanced practice nurses, in concert with associations such as the Older Women's League, which could argue that full reimbursement for advanced practice nurses will increase access to health care services for elderly women. This coordinated advocacy is very powerful in persuading legislators on a particular point of view.

Each year, during the ANA's house of delegates session, at state nurses association conventions across the country and at meetings of specialty nursing organizations, dozens of resolutions are presented for adoption by the respective voting bodies. Many of these resolutions have been written by individual nurses who want to effect change in the organization or to obtain formal organizational support for an idea or action. If you have an idea that you think should be presented as a resolution, check with the association's parliamentarian or a colleague conversant with the topic of parliamentary procedure. Then write your resolution and plan your strategy for adoption.

Professional associations are logical places to which nurses can take concerns regarding critical issues. Expressing one's concerns and questions will both inform other nurses of the situation and garner suggestions and support for a prompt solution. Issues can vary from an immediate need for relief in a disaster area caused by hurricane or flood to a problem that needs a longer time for a response, such as health care reform.

An association board or committee might be persuaded to appoint a task force to investigate a particular issue or carry out a project. A task force has a defined charge and limited time frame in which to complete its work. It ceases to exist after completing its assigned task. For example, the ANA brought together a representative body of the entire association to reach a consensus on the issue of regulation of unlicensed assistive personnel. Many of the state nurses associations were divided on how to proceed with this issue, and the ANA Board of Directors believed it was necessary to bring people with varied opinions on this issue into one room to reach compromise and agreement. After 2 days, the task force drafted a consensus proposal for presentation at the house of delegates. With the presentation of the final report, the task force was disbanded.

Task forces may be formed around specific tasks as well as specific policy questions. For example, when the ANA decided to relocate its headquarters from Kansas City, Mo., to Washington, D.C., a task force was appointed to examine the feasibility of such a move. The task force reported to the board of directors the pros and cons of such a move before the board and the house of delegates made a final decision. The work of the task force enabled the board of directors to prepare a background paper that responded to questions of members from all state nurses associations. In addition, the task force's work streamlined the discussion held in the house of delegates and led to a unanimous decision to move the headquarters.

Nurses committed to their professional associations sometimes seek elective office. Nurses who want to run for an elected position should have prior experience serving on association committees, including in leadership roles.

Nurses who want to run for an elected leadership position of an organization should consider these questions:

- What are the rules relating to nomination and election as spelled out by the bylaws of the association?
- What offices are open, and what are the qualifications for each office? Do my skills match those required by the office I will seek?
- Why do I want to run? What are my motives? What are my goals for the association and myself? If I am elected, how will the position fit into my professional and personal life? Do I have the time and energy to devote to the position and the association?
- Who will support my candidacy? Do I need to campaign? If so, who will help me? Do I need a formal campaign committee? How much money will it cost? How will I market myself? What are my strengths and weaknesses? What are my stands on current professional and association issues?

Regardless of whether one accepts the challenge of a major leadership position in a state or national professional organization, participating at any level will contribute much to one's repertoire of skills. "You can grow as an individual, hone your business and communication skills, contribute to your self-esteem, and receive credit and peer recognition" (Klein, 1993, p. 78). Certainly one must recognize the powerful network one builds when working with colleagues across a state and nation (Daily, 1992). The individual benefits gleaned from involvement in a professional organization are significant, but also know that the association, the profession, and fellow nurses benefit from your work. It is truly a win-win situation.

CONCLUSION

Our professional associations have the potential to influence the nursing profession, health policy, and patient care. Too often, nursing associations have not achieved that potential because too few of us participate. Associations need energy, expertise, and the vision of all nurses—from the student to the renowned leader. Step up, accept your responsibilities, and contribute your time, talents, and treasures. You will be richly rewarded.

REFERENCES

Daily, L. (1992). Volunteers' reward. In *Leadership: An association management supplement for volunteer leaders 1992* (pp. 43–48). Washington, DC: American Society of Association Executives.

Klein, K. (1992). Apprehension of opportunity? In *Leadership: An association management supplement for volunteer leaders 1992* (pp. 63–66, 78). Washington, DC: American Society of Association Executives.

VIGNETTE

Transforming a Nursing Organization to Influence Public Policy: National Black Nurses Association

C. Alicia Georges and Linda Burnes Bolton

Goals of the National Black Nurses Association

The National Black Nurses Association was founded in 1971 by Dr. Lauranne Sams, dean emeritus of Tuskegee University. The goals of the Association are as follows:

1. To investigate, define, and advocate for health care.
2. To educate and mentor registered and licensed practical, vocational, and student nurses.
3. To promote the economic development of nurses through entrepreneurial and other business initiatives.
4. To build consumer knowledge and understanding of health care issues.
5. To implement strategies that ensure access to health care equal to or above health care standards of the larger U.S. society.
6. To facilitate the professional development and career advancement of nurses in the emerging health care system.

Vision and Values

In 1996 the National Black Nurses Association celebrated its twenty-fifth anniversary as a national organization. The vision of the organization remains as it was in 1971. As we approach the next millennium, we will continue to work to improve the quality of life of persons of African heritage and the general public. The association's core values guide us as we plan our programmatic and community health activities. The core values serve as guideposts to fulfilling our mission and achieving our objectives. These values are as follows:

- We are health-consumer and provider focused.
- We are committed to excellence and improvement of health services.
- We value teamwork, collaboration, networks, and strategic alliances as the framework for our actions.
- We value our members as key resources for goal attainment.

- We aspire to the highest standards of personal and ethical behavior.
- We value the principles of justice, equity, integrity, and dignity.
- Leadership and accountability are critical to the governance of our organization.
- We value creativity, innovation, and research improvement.
- Our African heritage and the value of fellowship and caring guide our work.

Role of the National Black Nurses Foundation

The National Black Nurses Foundation, formed in 1991, is a separate 501(c)3 organization with its own board of directors. Its president serves on the board of the National Black Nurses Association in an ex officio capacity. Members of the National Black Nurses Association serve on the board of the Foundation along with persons from other professions and business. The mission of the Foundation is as follows:

- To alleviate the staggering health problems in the African American community by facilitating nursing research focused on the health needs of African Americans.
- To conduct critical analyses of how health policy meets or fails to meet the health needs of African Americans and to offer a forum for the study of health policy.
- To widen opportunities for African Americans to enter the healthcare professions.

We have worked diligently with our chapters and community partners to build coalitions committed to improving community health. The health care reform debates provided an opportunity for us to operationalize some of the strategies we have developed to influence policymaking decisions during the past 25 years.

National Black Nurses Day

In the quest of the National Black Nurses Association to increase the visibility of the organization and to assist association members and our community partners in working effectively with Washington policymakers and members of Congress, National Black Nurses Day was established during the presidency of C. Alicia Georges.

Our health policy committee, which is charged to educate and inform our chapters about pending legislation that would adversely or positively affect our profession and the delivery of services to African American communities, was responsible for planning the activities on Capitol Hill for the celebration. We use the National Black Nurses Day (first Friday in February) celebration to stimulate and motivate our chapters as they initiate or continue legislative activities in their communities.

We meet with the chapters before the press conference and National Black Nurses Day celebration at the Capitol and brief them on the legislation and issues that are most critical to our profession and communities. Members are given the opportunity to practice their presentations and are taught the do's and don'ts of meeting with elected officials. The guidelines we use have been developed through years of working with the Congressional Black Caucus, particularly the Congressional Black Caucus Health Braintrust, chaired by Congressman Louis Stokes, of Ohio. The celebration of National Black Nurses Day on Capitol Hill and in our local communities includes invitations to the press and to elected officials, and a public forum. The members of the Congressional Black Caucus and the representatives to Congress join us at the press conference and public forum on Capitol Hill on the Thursday before National Black Nurses Day. Our association president, Congressman Louis Stokes, other members of Congress, federal officials, the presidents of other black health professional organizations, and our community partners discuss proposed legislation and issues that affect African American and other communities. Members and participants have the opportunity to dialog with members of Congress at the forum. In the afternoon, we visit with Congressional representatives to discuss the impact of legislation on our communities.

It was this strategy, of holding press conferences and public forums, that we utilized throughout the country during the health care reform debates. Each chapter was sent briefing materials on the issues. Chapter presidents and national board members spoke at press conferences and appeared on local cable networks and public access stations. Members told their stories of individuals and families burdened by poverty and hopelessness and the lack of health care. In conjunction with our community partners, we held 52 town hall meetings in urban and rural communities across the United States in 1993 and 1994. More than 23,000 individuals attended these forums. Members of the legislatures in the states listened to the citizens and the health care providers. These town hall meetings served as a catalyst for collaborative community action. We believe that the data from community members about the potential effects of changes in health-care delivery were critical to continuing our efforts to influence health and social policies.

National Black Nurses Foundation Health Authority Model

The National Black Nurses Association and the National Black Nurses Foundation worked together to develop a model of care delivery that supports the needs of underserved Americans. A grant application was submitted to the W. K. Kellogg Foundation and subsequently awarded to the National Black Nurses Foundation. We utilized the collaborative model, with other black health professional organizations, to convene a group that met for 3 days and developed a consensus document. The model, referred to as the National Black Nurses Foundation Health Authority Model, combines the involvement of both public and private sectors at two levels, finance and service delivery. The National Black Nurses Foundation model, financed by both public and private funds, has the potential to resolve key barriers to accessing health services, such as the lack of insurance for working poor and the lack of enabling services (transportation, child care, and social services). This model

supports the inclusion of all willing health providers and advocates for culturally competent health care services, outreach, and health education activities. The role of the consumer in defining and evaluating his or her own community's health is emphasized in the governance and service delivery aspects of the model. Emergent roles for nurses and social workers are proposed in the areas of case management, advanced practice, and health services research (National Black Nurses Foundation, 1995).

A copy of this model was distributed to the members of the 104th Congress and to the speakers of the state legislatures. The model was presented at national meetings of our collaborative members, such as the National Association of Black Social Workers and the National Medical Association. We again utilized our local chapter leadership and local coalitions to disseminate the information. Chapters had copies of the National Black Nurses Foundation model and were encouraged to use it as a discussion tool as they began their annual legislative activities in their states. Members were encouraged to volunteer for advisory committees and to have their names submitted for appointments to state committees working on health care issues. A number of our chapter members have been successful in getting appointed to local and state committees.

Summit II on Reforming Health Care Workforce Regulations

The release in December 1995 of the Pew Report *Reforming Health Care Workforce Regulations: Policy Considerations for the 21st Century* (Finocchio et al., 1995) was another opportunity for the National Black Nurses Association to get involved in influencing policies in our state. This report looks at the regulatory system's role in protecting the public's health. The report proposes reforms of the country's regulatory system. Policy options are presented through recommendations in 10 issue areas. These issue areas are standardizing regulatory terms, standardizing entry-into-practice requirements, removing barriers to the full use of competent health professionals, redesigning board struc-ture and function, informing the public, collect-ing data on the health professions, ensuring practitioner competence, evaluating regulatory effectiveness, and understanding the organiza-tional context of health professions regulation.

In September 1996 the University of Califor-nia at San Francisco Center for the Health Pro-fessions, State Initiatives, solicited requests for proposals for organizations to hold debates/dis-cussions or to develop a plan to respond to the Pew document. The National Black Nurses Foundation, with support from the National Black Nurses Association, submitted a pro-posal and was awarded a small grant to bring together our coalition members: African Ameri-can nurses, doctors, dentists, lawyers, pharma-cists, and state elected officials. This summit, held in February 1997, produced a consensus document that has been circulated to all gover-nors, members of the 105th Congress; members of the National Black Caucus of State Elected Officials; members of the Black Congress on Health, Law, and Economics (National Black Nurses Association, National Medical Associa-tion, National Dental Association, National Bar Association, National Pharmacists, Association of Black Professional Firefighters, National Podi-atric Association, National Optometric Associa-tion); and our community partners.

The group discussed each of the policy op-tions for the 10 issue areas. Some of the major points on which consensus was reached in-cluded support for the entry into practice for nursing at the baccalaureate level, opposition to institutional licensure, and opposition to the proliferation of unlicensed health care workers. An important part of the consensus document is a plan recommended for use by the members of the National Black Nurses Association and other professionals in their respective states. This ac-tion plan builds on the coalition model that we have used in the past. Association chapters are being asked to facilitate meetings with their members and the members of other African American health professional groups to discuss the Pew report. The consensus statement is to be used as a discussion piece that would facili-tate the work needed in each state before and when state legislative bodies begin to consider reforming health care workforce regulations.

Conclusion

The National Black Nurses Association and the National Black Nurses Foundation believe that we can work together with our chapter members, other health professionals, and our community partners to develop consensus state-ments and appropriate responses to recom-mended policy changes and pending legislation. We believe that we have developed the skills and the partnerships to hold our elected officials accountable for their actions or lack of action. The continued staggering morbidity and mortal-ity rates in African-American communities require us to work within and outside of our current organizational frameworks to change policies at our state and national levels.

References

Finocchio, L.J., McMahon, T., Gragnola, C.M., & Task-force on Health Care Workforce Regulation. (1995). *Reforming health care workforce regulations: Policy considerations for the 21st century.* San Francisco: Pew Health Professions Commission.

National Black Nurses Foundation. (1995). *National Black Nurses Foundation Health Authority Model: A health delivery system for underserved ethnic popula-tions.* Washington, DC: Author.

Chapter *33*

POLITICAL ACTION COMMITTEES

BARBARA THOMAN CURTIS AND BARBARA LUMPKIN

May 5, 1993, was a beautiful day in the nation's capital, and for the nursing profession it was a banner day. What a thrill it was for the 300 registered nurses from all areas of the country to watch Virginia Trotter Betts, RN, MSN, JD, President of the American Nurses Association (ANA), the Health and Human Services Secretary Donna Shalala, and President Bill Clinton walk through the doors of the Oval Office of the White House into the Rose Garden to proclaim National Nurses Day. The ceremony, which included extensive remarks by President Betts, Secretary Shalala, and President Clinton, was for many of the politically active nurses present a summit on the political mountain that nurses have been climbing since 1974, when they first formed a political action committee (PAC) within the ANA (then called the Nurses' Coalition for Action in Politics). Those present at the ceremony represented the thousands of members who had been energized by the ANA endorsement in 1991 of Bill Clinton and Al Gore for president and vice president.

At the same time those nurses were listening to President Clinton, other nurses were meeting in the Executive Office Building with First Lady Hillary Rodham Clinton to help formulate what would emerge as the Health Security Act. The ANA endorsement of the Clinton-Gore ticket, spearheaded by the ANA-PAC, surely had invigorated nurses and their participation in the 1992 elections. The President and Mrs. Clinton were demonstrating their appreciation through both of these events.

This chapter discusses the role of PACs in influencing policy, the guidelines for forming and operating PACs, and the processes for candidate endorsement and support. For additional information on PACs and current discussions of campaign finance reform, see Chapter 21: Contemporary Issues in Government.

WHY HAVE PACs?

The formation of PACs is one means by which groups gain access to elected officials. The primary task of a PAC is to endorse and support candidates for elective office who support the legislative agenda and beliefs of the group making the endorsement. PACs enable voters to be involved in the democratic process. By giving cash and campaign support, voters participate in the electoral process. The result is heightened interest in who is running for office and their stand on issues. The ultimate and most important demonstration of support is to vote and encourage others to do the same. For nurses, this can be their first political experience.

PACs can be created at any level of government: local, state, or federal. The election laws under which they operate are determined by the governmental level of the candidates being supported. For instance, the ANA-PAC operates under federal election laws, which allow ANA-PAC to endorse only candidates for federal office: members of Congress and the President and Vice President. State nurses associations, if they have a state PAC, can endorse only candidates for such state races as gubernatorial and legislative. Local nursing organizations can form local PACs, which would operate under local laws to endorse candidates for such local races as mayor, city council (if that is the form of local government), and even county judge or coroner races.

Money received and dispensed through PACs is tightly controlled by election laws. In 1996, federal PACs numbered approximately 4,520 (up from 2,551 in 1980 and 113 in 1972), with approximately 600 related to associations. AMA-PAC, the PAC of the American Medical Association, is one of the oldest health-professional PACs. It was formed in the early 1960s. In the 1995–1996 election cycle, AMAPAC contributed more than $2.3 million to Congressional campaigns and ranked third among the 25 largest PACs. ANA-PAC ranked eighth among health PACs. During the 1992–1994 election cycle, ANA-PAC ranked third.

Groups with PACs reflect a wide spectrum of interests: labor, business, environment, trade associations, women, independents (primarily conservative groups), and education. Because so many elections are decided by just a few votes, active interest groups can rightfully claim that their support made the difference in races for Congress and state legislatures. Clearly the large PACs represent large numbers of contributors. Candidates know it, they respect it, and they respond to it.

PACs exist to solicit and distribute funds to candidates running for public office. The election laws that enable PACs to exist require strict reporting and disclosure documents. The law explicitly requires that organizations, like the ANA establish, administer, and solicit contributions to "a separate, segregated fund to be utilized for political purposes by a corporation or labor organization." The monies cannot be placed in an organization's operating account.

PACs work to influence the outcome of elections. They research and watch the political races closely to see who will advance their organization's legislative agenda. Information is gathered and is passed on to the board of trustees to make the decision as to who should be endorsed and, if so, what should be the amount of a contribution. In Congressional races a maximum of $5,000 per election (primary, special, or general) may be contributed. Elections are

costly. In 1996 the average U.S. Senate race cost $4.3 million, with some races costing in excess of $20 million. In 1996, incumbent House members spent at least $750,000 each for reelection campaigns, and several challengers spent more than $1 million. ANA-PAC enables nurses to pool resources and maximize the benefits. A large contribution from ANA-PAC in the name of nursing gives nurses more political clout than smaller, individual campaign contributions. In federal elections a contribution to a candidate in Massachusetts will benefit nurses all over the country. For the 1996 election cycle, ANA-PAC raised more than $1,004,000.

ANA-PAC

The Nurses' Coalition for Action in Politics was established in 1974 as the political action arm of the ANA. In 1985 the ANA House of Delegates voted to change the name to ANA-PAC to reflect the connection to the ANA. ANA-PAC endorses and contributes to federal candidates who are friends of nursing and who, it is hoped, will listen to nursing's perspectives on health and social policy issues. ANA-PAC is a vital strategy to create power and influence for nursing.

All money donated to ANA-PAC comes from voluntary contributions by state nurses association (SNA) members. Federal law prohibits solicitation of funds from people other than SNA members, nor can money collected from association membership dues be used to support candidates. Contributions from families and friends of members can be accepted but not solicited.

There are 11 members of the ANA-PAC Board of Trustees, six elected from sitting members of the ANA Board of Directors and five chosen by the ANA-PAC board. The board is bipartisan. It considers for endorsement every seat in the House of Representatives (435) and the Senate (100). Endorsements are made every 2 years, when all seats in the House are decided and at least 33 in the Senate.

Within the ANA, the Department of Political and Grassroots Programs works with ANA-PAC to ensure that nurses are a political force. This department helps nurses learn and then use effective political skills. Staff members work with the SNAs to help nurses become more effective campaigners and lobbyists.

N-STAT AND CDC/SC NETWORKS

An organization's lobbying staff in Washington, D.C., cannot be effective without broad-based grassroots support from members. One of the most effective and respected grassroots efforts is ANA's Congressional District Coordinator/Senate Coordinator (CDC/SC) and Nurses Strategic Action Team (N-STAT) networks. Their goal is to organize nurses to help elect ANA-PAC–endorsed candidates and to inform members of Congress about policy issues of concern to nursing. CDC/SCs monitor the political scene and, through the SNAs and the ANA Department of Political and Grassroots Programs, provide ANA-PAC with information and recommendations to be used in the endorsement process.

N-STAT is a more expansive network developed to increase participation of SNAs and enable nurses' voices to be heard on Capitol Hill. More than 40,000 nurses in 1996 composed the N-STAT Rapid Response Team. When nurses join N-STAT, they receive *Action Alert* and *Legislative Update,* detailing specific legislative issues to enable them to be adequately informed. N-STAT communicates nursing's message to members of Congress. CDC/SC designees play a leadership role in soliciting individual N-STAT Rapid Response Team members; planning district meetings; setting up telephone trees; promoting nursing's issues to the local press; and coordinating election activities.

CDC/SCs are ANA's link to local politics and to the member of Congress from the district. The CDC/SC, or designated N-STAT participant, serves as a resource person for position statements on health-related issues. For example, one legislator called on the CDC for information about the plight of homeless and chronic mentally ill persons. Another consulted a nurse about the incidence of domestic violence and asked

her opinion about what legislation should be initiated.

When ANA-PAC considers endorsing Congressional candidates, an ANA designee (usually the CDC/SC) interviews the candidates; assesses their viability; and makes a recommendation to the ANA-PAC. After ANA-PAC endorses a candidate, the CDC/SC may work on the candidate's campaign and recruit other nurses to help in electing an endorsed candidate. Involvement in the grassroots network has been a training ground for some nurses to run for office (see Chapter 25 vignette: One Nurse's Journey to Becoming a Policymaker).

THE ENDORSEMENT PROCESS

The process of interviewing candidates and making endorsements is a basic activity of all PACs. Generally, representatives from the parent organization and the governing body of the PAC determine endorsement policies.

Issues to be considered when making endorsements should include how winnable the race is, the ability of the candidate to mount an effective campaign, the amount of money the candidate is able to raise, and the candidate's willingness to accept PAC contributions.

The ANA-PAC's endorsement policy mandates that board members review a confidential report on each candidate, using a variety of measures. These include input from the CDC/SC and from the SNA, the candidate's voting record, and his or her position on specific issues. After this review, the board votes on whether to endorse and contribute money and, if so, how much money. ANA-PAC (as with most PACs) has a limited amount of money to dispense, so it is important that the money go to the races where it will count the most. For candidates who receive a donation, the amount of money varies according to established criteria, but it cannot exceed the amount set by law.

Special attention is paid to certain kinds of candidates. For example, because 93% of professional nurses are women, ANA-PAC carefully reviews all women candidates. Women traditionally have had more difficulty raising money than men, so the impact of a monetary contribution to women is greater. ANA-PAC may invest in a well-qualified woman even if her chance of winning is considered a long shot. In such cases the PAC contribution may make a difference.

The ANA-PAC has established the following priorities for endorsement:

- Those races where an endorsement can make the difference for the candidate. For instance, a candidate with a difficult race, who has shown consistent support for the legislative agenda of the parent organization, would be a top priority.
- Incumbents who face little or no serious opposition.
- Those incumbents with a positive voting record (as defined by the legislative agenda of the parent organization).
- Candidates who support nursing or are responsive to nursing input and who are challenging known adversaries of nursing.
- Candidates supportive of the organization's legislative agenda who are running for an open seat (no incumbents running).
- An *incumbent* who holds a leadership position or has the potential to do so (e.g., a member of a key committee or a committee chair).
- A *challenger* who holds a leadership position in a political party or has the potential to do so, is supportive of key nursing issues, or has a background in health care issues.

Endorsement can take several forms:

- *Major endorsement* signifies significant financial assistance and commitment to work on the campaign.
- *General endorsement* may provide minimal financial contributions but some "in-kind" support, such as PAC mailings to constituents of the endorsee, organizational help in mobilizing constituents, or help with campaign activities.
- *Name-only endorsement* for candidates who either do not need funding or have a lower priority for support.

- *Independent expenditures* are the costs to advocate for the election or defeat of a candidate that are incurred without the coordination, consultation, cooperation of a candidate, or candidate's committee.

One of the most significant steps in the endorsement procedure is delivering a written endorsement or a check to the candidate. Timing of this activity is crucial and is coordinated by the campaign staff to provide the best visibility for both the candidate and the nursing PAC. There may be occasions when an early endorsement could be critical, such as in a race for an open seat. Participation of the nursing community in endorsements is crucial. After a decision for endorsement is made, the ANA notifies nurses in the district. The purpose is to encourage nurses to become involved in the campaign.

The Interview

The interview is an important component of the endorsement process, but it has an additional purpose: to increase the candidate's knowledge about nurses and their expertise in policy and politics.

The interview team typically consists of two to five persons. They decide in advance who will be the leader, or chair, for the meeting. The leader introduces each member of the team at the beginning of the interview, and the members ask the candidate prepared questions. Time limits need to be scheduled in advance, including time after the interview to review and record comments. If possible, candidates for the same race should be interviewed on the same day by the same team of interviewers.

After introductions, the candidate may deliver a brief opening statement. The interview is an opportunity to learn the candidate's position on issues of concern to nursing. It is critical not to comment on the candidate's answers (this should be reserved for the postinterview session), although it is important to follow up on vague or incomplete answers to questions.

At the close of the interview, the team should tell the candidate when to expect a decision.

Follow up with a letter of thanks. A decision of endorsement should be made both in writing and by calling the campaign.

An important consideration related to the endorsement includes gaining media exposure. Consider the type of media for the announcement, the timing and location for the announcement, and the individuals who should present the check. It is preferable to allow the candidate some control over these activities. For example, the candidate's public relations staff may develop a media event to publicize the nursing PAC's endorsement, involving nurse volunteers who plan to work in the candidate's campaign. Both for nursing and the candidate, it is usually best to get as much media coverage as possible.

Presidential Endorsement

The ANA has participated in presidential politics since 1984. The ANA House of Delegates voted to "promote the selection of a qualified woman who supports the ANA National Nursing Agenda as a vice presidential nominee in the 1984 presidential election." Thus, in September 1984, the ANA Board of Directors voted to endorse the Walter Mondale–Geraldine Ferraro ticket for the offices of President and Vice President of the United States. This was the first time that the association had endorsed a candidate in a Presidential race.

That year, the ANA also voted to develop a procedure for the endorsement of a Presidential candidate in the 1988 Presidential election. It was recognized that the process for endorsing a candidate for the highest office in the land needed to be a carefully designed one. The following procedure has been developed for Presidential endorsements: (1) analysis of political climate, (2) analysis of voting records, (3) sending candidates a questionnaire, (4) publication of voting records and questionnaire results, (5) polling of SNAs, (6) interviewing of candidates, (7) adoption of ANA-PAC position, and (8) ANA-PAC oversight of campaign activities.

Analysis of Political Climate. The national political climate is analyzed, considering the cost/benefit ratio to the nursing profession of a Presidential endorsement.

Analysis of Voting Records. The voting records of all identified (announced and unannounced) Presidential candidates are analyzed in relation to the ANA National Nursing Agenda for Health Policy (legislative agenda) and legislative and regulatory priorities. The ANA-PAC Board of Trustees reviews and approves the analysis.

Sending of Candidate Questionnaire. The ANA-PAC board structures a questionnaire based on ANA's legislative agenda and priorities. The questionnaire is sent to all potential candidates.

Publication of Voting Records and Questionnaire Results. A summation of voting records and questionnaire responses is published in *The American Nurse.* A clip-out coupon is provided as approved by the ANA-PAC board for SNA members to indicate a preference of candidates. The coupon is remitted to the SNA.

Polling of State Nurses Associations. ANA-PAC polls the SNAs to determine the outcome of the preferred candidate balloting.

Interviewing of Candidates. The ANA-PAC chairperson and the ANA president interview the preferred candidates of both parties, on the basis of SNA polling. The interviews include the candidate's response to ANA's legislative agenda and priorities, examination of the campaign's finances and organization, listing of the groups supporting the candidate, and assessment of the candidate's ability to win his or her party nomination. The ANA president and the ANA-PAC chairperson report back to the ANA-PAC board.

Adoption of ANA-PAC Position. The ANA-PAC board considers the data compiled from policy positions, voting records, questionnaire responses, SNA polling, and candidate interviews. The ANA-PAC board adopts one of the following positions:

- No endorsement or support of any candidate
- Support of one or more candidates in the primaries, with consideration of endorsement after the primaries but before the party conventions
- Support of one or more candidates in the primaries, with consideration of endorsement after the party conventions
- No support of any candidates during the primaries but consideration of endorsement after the party conventions
- Support and endorsement of one candidate during the primaries and party conventions

ANA-PAC Oversight of Campaign Activities. ANA-PAC participates in campaign activities consistent with the availability of funds and level of endorsement.

Although ANA's Presidential endorsements have been controversial, the advantages of making them include the opportunity to influence the Presidential election and the endorsed candidate's party, increased access to the Administration should the endorsed candidate be victorious, and increased influence with endorsed members of the candidate's party in Congress.

The ANA has taken risks through its endorsement in the previous four Presidential elections. Having endorsed the winning team in 1992 and 1996, ANA can measure increased opportunities for nurses' involvement at high levels of decision making.

FUND-RAISING STRATEGIES

Raising money is a key function of all PACs. People are always trying to come up with new ways to raise money, and in a tight economy, many groups compete for the same dollar. Creative ways to raise funds, however, are really variations of the same themes: direct mail, special events, and personal solicitation.

ANA-PAC fund-raising activities have run the gamut from gala affairs—a luau in Honolulu and

a rodeo in Houston—to a celebrity auction in Washington, D.C. One of the easiest and quickest activities is to plan a "challenge" at large gatherings. Nurses are reminded that it costs money to demonstrate strength. Individual nurses take their turn to announce their contribution to the PAC and to challenge their colleagues to match it. In a little more than 15 minutes, ANA-PAC has been able to raise $28,000 in contributions from approximately 700 nurses at an ANA House of Delegates meeting. The PAC of an SNA held a similar challenge during its annual meeting and raised more than $4,000.

Telephone solicitation has also been an effective means of fund raising for ANA-PAC. Although many people express negative feelings about telemarketing, it has proved to be effective for ANA-PAC. A key component is to have a concise and familiar message so that one's interest in the message is stimulated when the call is answered. Association members who quickly realize that the message is about their profession are more likely to listen carefully to the entire message. It was through telemarketing that ANA-PAC first raised more than a million dollars for the 1994 election cycle. The one negative aspect is that this method of fund raising is one of the most expensive.

Since 1989, when the ANA Leadership Circle was established, it has become obvious that the most effective fund-raising effort for a high level of contribution to the PAC is straightforward solicitation. Nurses are realizing that politics is not a spectator sport. Creativity in fund raising will always have its place, but the best approach will always be a straightforward request for funds. Many dollars are needed from SNA members if nursing is to maintain and increase its effectiveness, promoting awareness and action on consumer concerns and promoting and safeguarding nursing.

Many SNAs have dues check-off procedures where a small portion of dues money goes to the PAC. Members have the option to refuse the contribution to the PAC. Such a dues check-off provides SNA PACs with consistent funds to make contributions to candidates. In some states, SNA PACs are among the best funded health care PACs in the state.

The primary mechanisms for fund raising are described below. In addition, the box below provides some additional tips for fund raising.

FUND-RAISING TIPS

- Determine the amount you want to raise, and state it publicly.
- The most effective method of fund raising is one-to-one, direct, personal contact with a potential donor. (It is much harder for people to say no face to face.)
- People expect to be asked to give money, and most people don't give unless you ask. Don't be shy. If you believe in your cause and your organization, then you should be asking for support and contributions of money.
- Always ask individual donors for more than you expect them to contribute (people will never give more than what you ask them to give).
- When doing a fund-raising event, expenses should not exceed one third of the price of the ticket; otherwise, you will not make enough money to justify the effort required.
- People like raffles and 50/50 drawings, which produce many small individual contributions. They can be included in any fund-raising event. You will take in more incidental money from those in attendance. These can also be done at meetings and other types of gatherings.
- Keep asking. You can vary the techniques of fund raising (mail solicitation, phone calls, personal contact), but be sure to ask repeatedly.
- Be sure to keep records of those who contribute. Never give your list of donors away; lists are power. (If some other group asks for money, the persons on your list may give to them and not to you next time.)
- Be sure to thank people in person if possible. Send a thank-you note immediately. If the fundraiser is for a candidate, the campaign should send a thank-you note from the candidate.

Direct Mail

If a direct mail campaign is planned far enough in advance, it can be a smooth and efficient way to raise money for candidates or a PAC. Using a known list, such as the organization's membership, enables the cost of solicitation to be calculated fairly accurately. When a direct mail campaign is planned, it is important to provide sufficient time for the following: obtaining labels, writing the solicitation letter and preparing other materials to be included; printing the letter, literature, envelopes, and return envelopes; and sorting the envelopes for bulk mailing. Direct mail companies perform all these tasks, but their services can be expensive. Volunteers should be recruited, particularly for the time-consuming tasks of stuffing envelopes and sorting zip codes.

It is wise to include suggested donations on the pledge card. The PAC should be bold but should also take into account a particular state's economy and an average nurse's weekly salary.

It is also important to devise a record-keeping system before the mailing is done. As responses are received, the name and address of each donor should be recorded so that each respondent can be contacted again the following year. Most laws require this information on all contributions.

Special Events

Special events are fun and can provide visibility and supplemental funds for the PAC. Long-term planning is essential to ensure a smoothly run event. Events may be built around a special appearance by a person who will attract a crowd, a benefit performance where an amount is added to the cost of the ticket for the donation, or a group activity (auctions, house tours, garage sales, walks, marathons). It must be remembered that money can be *solicited* only from association members, not the public at large.

Many N-STAT leaders (CDC/SCs) host receptions in private homes. This enables the nurse to entertain elected officials and politically active nurses in a relaxed atmosphere. Such events can raise up to $5,000 with relatively little effort.

Personal Solicitation

The most effective way to raise money is to ask for it. It costs little and has a high return. The most important factor in personal solicitation is a group of trained volunteers who believe in what they are doing. Many people will say that they will do anything except ask for money. The key is to make sure solicitors have a full understanding of what they are doing and why. A training session is essential.

Personal solicitation can be done in several different ways. The organization's membership list can be broken down into local calling areas, and solicitors can spend a specific number of hours on the telephone. It is always important that volunteers know in advance what is expected of them and how many hours their task will take. Personal solicitation is often used to follow up on a direct mail campaign. If that is the case, make sure that the names of nurses who have donated by mail are removed from the telephone list.

Another follow-up to direct mail is solicitation of nurses at a specific location. Care should be taken that solicitation is done methodically rather than randomly. A special approach may be taken with nurses in a position to give more than an average contribution. Once such nurses have been identified, the solicitor should visit that nurse at home or over lunch or dinner. The solicitor should describe the PAC's program, how the money is spent, and the results to date. A specific amount, determined in advance, should be requested.

FUTURE OF PACs AND CAMPAIGN FINANCE REFORM

Much of the debate today regarding campaign finance reform centers on "soft money" contributions to *political parties.* Though some PACs do contribute to political parties, many con-

tributors are wealthy individuals or corporate interests. Many see these contributions, often in significant amounts, as a direct attempt to buy influence for special interests. Finding a means to accomplish real reform without violating our constitutional Bill of Rights is a significant challenge for reformers. There is consensus among elected officials and the public that campaigns are much too expensive; however, limiting costs will be difficult now that most campaigns are waged through electronic media. Another idea that surfaces is limiting the time frame for campaigns, but such limits could face court challenges.

PACs were designed to provide members of organizations and professions with a mechanism for pooling their individual contributions so that the interests of the organization or profession could be enhanced by a significant contribution to a candidate or issue. PACs have been enormously successful in this area. PACs encourage the participation of small donors and make campaign money accountable to the public. Eliminating PACs will prohibit the working people of our country from playing a vital role in our political process. PACs are a vehicle for leveling the playing field between nurses and wealthy citizens and businesses. Nursing, especially, has coordinated political activities with legislative initiatives vital to consumers and the profession. Through participation in PACs, nurses have collectively gained visibility and respect at the state and national levels. Thus the ANA and the ANA-PAC oppose placing restrictions that would eliminate PACs.

Nevertheless, many individuals, and groups such as Common Cause, have joined the movement to ban PACs in the name of campaign finance reform and ethics. Because the majority of PAC funds go to incumbents, PAC critics stress that incumbents have an unfair advantage over challengers for elected office. It is ironic that PACs are now identified as the problem, when they were the result of election and ethics reforms in 1974 after Watergate. Watergate, it must be remembered, was the result of fundraising activities designed to solicit huge contributions from the wealthy elite and to launder corporate gifts of significant proportions.

ANA-PAC is working with a group of association PACs to monitor current proposals to limit or ban PACs. Though reform will no doubt occur, some proposals may even enhance the influence of ANA-PAC. One such proposal, which has considerable support, would limit the percentage of campaign contributions that could come from a PAC. For example, if only 25% of a candidate's funds can come from PACs, most candidates will seek organizations and professions with which they want to be publicly identified. Because nurses are respected by the public, many candidates seek an association with nursing. For his 1992 Senate race, Senator Bob Graham, of Florida, decided to solicit early support from only three PACs: the ANA-PAC, the Sierra Club PAC, and the teachers' PACs.

Are PACs merely a vehicle for "special interests"? Is ANA-PAC? Yes, the interest of America's nurses are special: securing safe, quality, and affordable health care for everyone; ensuring that communities have the resources to care for their own populations; ensuring that our public health systems stay strong enough to promote healthy lives; and ensuring that our highways and workplaces are safe. Involvement in ANA-PAC is one way that nurses are speaking with one strong voice about the critical health care concerns facing our nation. That collective voice must not be silenced.

Even if PACs are eliminated, ANA must continue to set aside dedicated funds for political activity and education of the 40,000 members of N-STAT across the country. This is a formidable army of campaign strategists and workers that can wield great influence in promoting the profession's legislative agenda. By soliciting just 10 friends to contribute $10 each to candidates, N-STAT members could collectively contribute nearly $4 million as well as thousands of hours of campaign work and strategy. Investing in the education and training of a network of nurse political activists will ensure that the profession will have a role in shaping America's health care system as we enter the twenty-first century.

CONCLUSION

Through ANA-PAC endorsements and the increased activity of the PACs of SNAs, nursing's political clout is gaining status and power. Nurses are demonstrating their willingness to accept both political responsibility and accountability for making quality health care accessible for all Americans. They are seeking and winning appointed and elected positions at all levels of government.

The nursing profession's political influence is growing through its use of PACs at the state and national levels. We must continue to exercise this process and prepare to utilize different strategies if and when PACs are significantly restricted or eliminated.

UNIT V CASE STUDY
Nursing Organizations in Action

INTRODUCTION

DEBRA M. CAMPBELL

Nursing organizations meet a variety of needs for their members. One of the most substantial is that of advocacy for our profession and our patients. The saying that *there is strength in numbers* holds true in policy development. By working collectively to use the political power that comes with 25,000 oncology nurses, 770 nurse massage therapists, or 520 colleges of nursing, the chances for success in policy change or development are greatly enhanced.

Once again the editors of this book invited national nursing organizations to share their experiences in initiating or changing a policy that affects nursing or the public's health. This chapter contains 15 vignettes, each highlighting how nurses have used political strategies to influence the regulatory and/or legislative processes.

Policy development begins with the organization's own internal process of defining its priorities, key issues, and positions. Some organizations are actually groups or coalitions of nursing organizations such as the National Alliance of Nurse Practitioners. They depend on a governing body of representative members to establish priorities. Many organizations rely on their board of directors or their legislative committees to define key policy issues. The Society of Pediatric Nurses, a young organization, has spent its first 5 years increasing its membership, educating members on the critical policy issues, and developing a grassroots network. This organization is just beginning to have an impact on local issues and is working to be more active on the state and federal levels. However, it takes time to establish sufficient

credibility and political presence to change policy.

Many of the vignettes detail policy changes on the federal level. These nursing organizations worked with the Health Care Financing Administration, the Occupational Health and Safety Administration, the Food and Drug Administration, and the U.S. Congress. On the state level, nursing organizations worked with the state boards of nursing, state legislatures, and state departments of health and human services. To be effective, nursing organizations must have a political and legislative presence on the federal, state, and in many cases the local and institutional levels where nursing practice takes place.

It can take a long time, sometimes decades, to achieve a desired policy outcome. Nurses, through organized efforts, have been working since the 1970s to achieve prescriptive authority in the states. With varying degrees of independence from physicians, all but one state legislature has approved nursing's efforts. Yet some policies can be enacted quickly if the need is well defined and there is public and legislative support.

Engaging in policy development can be an emotionally charged experience. These efforts are often the result of many volunteer hours of planning, strategizing, and lobbying. They may involve hundreds or thousands of nurses writing letters, signing petitions, or meeting with their legislators. Policy changes may also be initiated by a small group of dedicated nursing leaders. Regardless, the endeavor can be exhausting. Nurses cannot afford to lose perspective and give up on their efforts. Even though the process can become a battle of "us versus them," nurse activists must realize, as seasoned political strategists do, that the next legislative session or regulatory review period brings new faces and new opportunities to the policy table.

The following vignettes cite examples of nurses' policy successes. Each organization used similar tools to achieve these successes. Nurses must use political skills to establish connections with key decision makers, and they must also become adept at lobbying and educating these decision makers and constituencies. Nurses need insight into the legislative and regulatory processes on the state and federal levels. That is why a synopsis of the Nurse in Washington Internship (NIWI) concludes this chapter. NIWI is an intensive 4-day educational program that provides a firsthand experience with the political and legislative processes. The program, held in Washington, DC, highlights grassroots political skills, coalition building, and lobbying on Capitol Hill.

Nursing organizations work for their nurse members, but individual nurses must be willing to work through their organizations to change policy. With persistence and the right tools, success can be yours.

American Assembly for Men in Nursing

DAVID O. SPROUSE

The American Assembly for Men in Nursing (AAMN) was founded in 1974 to provide a forum for nurses, male and female, to discuss and refine the professional, educational, and conceptual aspects of nursing practice. The objectives of AAMN are to encourage men to become nurses, to join together with other nurses in strengthening and in humanizing health care, to support men in nursing, and to educate society about the benefits of having men in nursing. In addition, AAMN has become an advocate for continued research, education, and dissemination of information about men's health issues at the local and national levels. As AAMN continues to evolve, the need for grassroots networking and for communicating the needs of men in nursing has become a central, galvanizing issue.

Men in nursing and male nursing students have assembled for AAMN's annual conferences for the past 22 years. During these conferences, the subject of discrimination against men in the profession inevitably arises. Many who attend the conferences have related personal experiences and also their firsthand knowledge of discrimination against other men in nursing. Generally, the male nurse or student responds either passively or actively, either by accepting the discrimination, by changing jobs or schools to avoid confrontation, or by pursuing legal action. However, few actually seek legal action.

One of the most publicized cases involved a male licensed practical nurse (LPN) who was fired from his position as a labor and delivery (L&D) nurse because of gender. He sued the hospital and won his case in court. Yet, in another case, when a male registered nurse sued a hospital for gender discrimination after he was fired from L&D because of gender, the court ruled in favor of the hospital. Another male LPN, who worked at a long-term care facility and was denied a promotion because he was male, sued and won his case.

Though L&D nursing is an integral part of every nursing school's curriculum, even today many male nursing students are denied the opportunity and experience of the birthing process. What's more, most men in nursing and male nursing students report having experienced assignment to a heavier case load; consistent requests for help with moving, turning, and ambulating patients and restraining unruly patients; and/or assignment to the "difficult patients."

Discrimination against men in nursing and against male nursing students, particularly in the area of L&D nursing, is not supported by the Association of Women's Health, Obstetric, and Neonatal Nurses (AWHONN). AWHONN issued a position statement in 1995 that states in part that "gender is not a qualification requirement to practice as a nurse and gender discrimination in employment is unlawful." Furthermore, AWHONN believes that nurses, regardless of gender, should be employed in women's health, obstetric, and neonatal nursing on the basis of their ability to provide such care to the clients.

As a further support of the argument against discrimination, the recent Virginia Military Institute (VMI) discrimination case heard before the U.S. Supreme Court used a nursing discrimination case to support the ruling against VMI. In the VMI case, Justice Ruth Bader Ginsburg referred in part to *Mississippi University for Women v. Hogan* (1982). Mr. Hogan was denied admission to the university's nursing program because he is male. He sued, and the case went to the Supreme Court. The Hogan decision held that admissions could not be based on "archaic and stereotypic notions" of "proper" roles for men and women. Incidentally, the Hogan case's author for the majority was Justice Sandra Day O'Conner, the first woman to serve in the Supreme Court. Justice Ginsburg stated that discrimination cases must apply a " 'skeptical scrutiny' under which the state must demonstrate an 'exceedingly persuasive justification' for any official action that treats men and women differently."

In 1997 the Illinois General Assembly attempted to pass an amendment to House Bill 0089 that would have allowed the requirement of female supervision for male staff providing care to female patients in long-term care facilities. Essentially, this bill would have discriminated against men in nursing and would have encouraged employers not to hire a man because he would require supervision and, in effect, increase staffing costs.

When an Illinois member of AAMN alerted the national office of AAMN about the bill, a telephone, mail, fax, and E-mail campaign was coordinated between AAMN officers, members, and other nursing organizations. The campaign targeted key members of the Illinois Assembly, providing them with AAMN's position on the bill, a copy of AWHONN's position statement, and a copy of the VMI court case decision. AAMN encouraged them to amend or defeat the bill's discriminatory provisions. After several weeks of grassroots action, the office of the Majority Floor Leader of the Illinois General Assembly informed AAMN that the bill had been defeated, never having come out of committee because of a lack of support to bring it to the floor.

To heighten awareness of discrimination issues, AAMN has developed, and continues to expand, a grassroots network that will act to scrutinize policymaking bodies, from the institutional to the national level. Male nurses have made important contributions to nursing education, research, knowledge, and leadership. Clearly, discrimination against men or any other minority in nursing should not be allowed to continue. Comprising 5% of the total nursing population of 2.2 million, men in nursing need to support the national organization that represents them and to become involved in grassroots networking to monitor fair and impartial practices in the nursing world.

AMERICAN ASSOCIATION OF COLLEGES OF NURSING

ANNE M. RHOME

MEDICARE FUNDING OF GRADUATE NURSING EDUCATION (GNE)

For the past 12 years, the American Association of Colleges of Nursing (AACN), representing baccalaureate and graduate nursing education institutions throughout the country, has worked toward the redirection of Medicare funds now focused on entry-level nursing education to the clinical training of graduate nurses. Advanced practice nurses (APNs) (nurse practitioners, clinical nurse specialists, nurse anesthetists, and nurse midwives) represent categories of providers not in existence when Medicare educational payment policy was designed; the educational costs of these new providers are, with the exception of nurse anesthetists, not covered by Medicare.

AACN's position is that this innovation would provide an ongoing revenue source, not subject to the uncertainties of the annual appropriations process, to expand the production of APNs, a vital resource for meeting future Medicare and other population needs.

When Medicare legislation was enacted in 1965, it was with the intent that Medicare support clinical training of physicians, nurses, and other health personnel. Thus Medicare payments were made to hospitals to reimburse a portion of the costs of nurse education to promote quality inpatient care for Medicare beneficiaries. Since the inception of Medicare, nursing education has shifted almost entirely to community colleges, senior colleges, and universities. Yet Medicare reimbursement for nursing education programs is limited by the "provider-operated rule," which directs most of the funding to diploma programs that produce entry-level nurses who are trained in hospital-oriented care, not primary care or ambulatory care, where many needs of the future Medicare patients lie.

In fiscal year 1996 the Health Care Financing Administration, the federal agency responsible for managing the Medicare and Medicaid programs, estimated that it provided $220 million to hospitals in support of nursing education costs. At the same time, Medicare estimates that it spent approximately $7 billion on physician residency training. It is AACN's belief that the $220 million, four times the amount of money provided by the Nurse Education Act, an appropriated fund for nursing programmatic support, would be much better spent by directing these monies to the clinical education of the APN, who can provide the care most needed by the Medicare beneficiary and others.

Through the years, AACN has urged Congress and the Administration to consider chang-

ing hospital Medicare reimbursement policy to reflect current needs of the Medicare population. Three major AACN initiatives have culminated in moving the Medicare reimbursement policy issue forward. The first initiative, as a direct result of AACN's effective lobbying efforts, brought about the passage in 1988 of the Tax Technical Corrections Bill, with an amendment sponsored by Senators Lloyd Bentsen, of Texas, and John Chafee, of Rhode Island, that would create five demonstration projects for 5 years to allow Medicare "pass-through" reimbursement for graduate nurse training. (*Pass-through* refers to Medicare reimbursement that is not a part of the prospective payment to hospitals but, rather, is "passed through" to hospitals for incurring training costs.) This initiative allowed reimbursement from the Medicare program to a provider (i.e., a hospital) for reasonable costs incurred while providing graduate clinical training for nurses enrolled in an approved master's or doctoral program in an educational institution. These "reasonable costs" included stipends, salaries of supervisors, and classroom space. This authority provided for five graduate training projects between hospitals and schools of nursing. Each hospital-supported activity was eligible to receive up to $200,000 per year for a period of 5 years (1989 to 1994).

The five demonstration projects selected were Fairfax Hospital and George Mason University; Hermann Hospital and the University of Texas Health Sciences Center; Vanderbilt University Hospital and Vanderbilt University; Grady Memorial Hospital and Georgia State University; and Presbyterian-University Hospital and the University of Pittsburgh. Graduate nurse clinical education occurred in inpatient settings. The report of the results of the demonstration projects, due to Congress in July 1995, is not available because a final accounting of costs has not yet been completed. However, preliminary results indicate that the hospitals experienced a lower turnover rate in nursing staff, recruitment benefited, costs of orientation were lowered, and patient education efforts were successful. AACN plans to use the demonstration projects as models of Medicare funding for clinical graduate nurse education (GNE) for future lobbying.

The second initiative occurred when President Clinton sponsored the Health Security Act of 1993. As a result of AACN's work, along with a coalition of 10 national nursing organizations, President Clinton agreed to include a GNE account of $200 million for the training of APNs. Funding would have been directed to the academic program and would have been determined by the number of students and the cost of educating students. Academic programs would have been able to use monies to pay tuition and fees, student stipends, the cost of faculty supervision at the provider site, and program expenses. The program also would have been able to pay any type of clinical site, including community-based sites, that incurs costs for the support of GNE programs (e.g., preceptor time). Because of other factors, the Health Security Act was not passed by Congress, but members of both houses supported the GNE account.

The third initiative began in late 1996, when the House Ways and Means Committee and its subcommittees on health and oversight requested that the Institute of Medicine (IOM) recommend a method of distributing monies from a graduate medical education (GME) trust fund to teaching hospitals and for the selection of entities to receive education payments. The committee also asked IOM to look at other considerations, such as to what extent payments are being made for graduate training in other health professions. Consequently, IOM asked AACN and other organizations to submit data, studies, and policy statements that might be relevant to the allocation of GME funds. AACN staff and member deans of schools of nursing contributed information to IOM, supporting the redirection of current monies for clinical APN education. The report, made available in April 1997, recommended support of

APN clinical education through a GME trust fund and will suggest that monies be directed to the entity incurring the costs of clinical education.

At the same time that IOM worked on its report to the House Ways and Means Committee, AACN lobbied members of that committee and the Senate Finance Committee regarding redirection of funds. Most members are showing an interest in working with the nursing community as they debate Medicare reform during the 105th Congress. In addition, AACN has reconvened the coalition of 11 nursing organizations, known as the GNE coalition, which collaborated on the Health Security Act in 1993. The GNE coalition is in the process of establishing a consensus on the GNE issue, so that nursing may lobby collectively for a GNE fund.

Although the outcome of AACN's years of effort on GNE remains uncertain, major policymakers, from the President to the IOM and Congress, now seem ready to acknowledge the validity of the concept of GNE. The lesson is that doing one's homework, developing a sound concept that is timely and logical, and building a diverse coalition to move the issue can bring a concept into consideration and possibly implementation. AACN is committed to moving the issue forward, resulting in a better prepared nursing work force that improves health care and accessibility.

AMERICAN ASSOCIATION OF OCCUPATIONAL HEALTH NURSES

JERRY WILLIAMSON AND KAE LIVSEY

Occupational health nurses are key to successful workplace health and safety programs. The largest group of health care providers at the work site, and often the only health care provider at the workplace, occupational and environmental health nurses develop and manage programs to promote and protect the health and safety of workers and the environment. The occupational health nurse's "field" experience, coupled with business expertise, brings practical perspective and cost-effective solutions for the prevention of workplace illness and injury. Despite having an important role in interpreting regulations and implementing compliance activities in their work settings, occupational health nurses did not actively participate in developing these regulations until the early 1980s.

In 1982 the Occupational Health and Safety Administration (OSHA) issued a highly controversial standard that highlighted this lack of input into federal policymaking. The Hazard Communication Standard, requiring employers to inform and educate workers about the hazardous substances to which they are exposed in the workplace, specifically excluded occupational health nurses in the definition of "health professional." This deliberate action alerted occupational health nurses and their professional association, the American Association of Occupational Health Nurses, Inc. (AAOHN), to the critical need for their involvement in establishing policy at the national level. In an effort to increase understanding of the roles and contributions of occupational health nurses, AAOHN set three specific goals:

- Change the Hazard Communication Standard to include occupational health nurses in the definition of health professional.
- Secure the appointment of an occupational health nurse to the National Advisory Committee on Occupational Safety and Health (NACOSH), which advises, consults with, and makes recommendations to OSHA on matters relating to the administration of the Occupational Safety and Health Act.
- Secure the appointment of one or more occupational health nurses to the management staff at OSHA.

In 1983, AAOHN launched a highly visible communications campaign targeting three key audiences: nurse members and the legislative and executive branches of the federal govern-

ment. Members were informed and educated through AAOHN's monthly newsletter, and they participated in a successful letter-writing campaign to Congress. AAOHN sent news releases to nursing and other trade press outlets and mailed newsletters to Congressional offices. Personal meetings were held with OSHA officials, White House staff, and members of Congress who served on OSHA oversight and appropriations committees. AAOHN also hosted visits of high-level OSHA officials to actual work sites of nurse members.

As a result of these efforts, two occupational health nurses were appointed to the NACOSH: one in December 1984, who served a 2-year appointment, and another in November 1985, who served two consecutive 2-year terms. Unfortunately, because of political factors, the committee met very little and contributed little to policymaking during this time. OSHA proposed revisions to the Hazard Communication Standard, which included occupational health nurses as health professionals in December 1985. The third goal, which took more time to achieve, continued to evolve.

AAOHN lobbying efforts directed at members of the House and Senate Appropriations Committee resulted in the inclusion of specific language in their reports for fiscal years 1985, 1986, and 1987, acknowledging the contributions of occupational health nurses to occupational health and safety. The reports also encouraged OSHA to appoint an occupational health nurse to the NACOSH and to hire an occupational health nurse for its staff. OSHA continued to ignore the committee's display of support for hiring an occupational health nurse, so language *directing* OSHA to hire an occupational health nurse in a policymaking position first appeared in the Senate Appropriations Subcommittee Report for fiscal year 1989, released in June 1988. By August, the first occupational health nurse was hired at OSHA as a health scientist within the Office of Occupational Medicine. However, this organizational structure limited opportunities for nursing input on policy decisions, and the position was reassigned to the director of the Directorate of Technical Support. In addition, the OSHA nurse intern program was established to provide additional opportunities for nursing input to agency activities.

To ensure continued visibility, AAOHN submitted testimony to the House Appropriations Subcommittee on Labor, Health and Human Services and Education in 1989 and testified before the corresponding Senate subcommittee in 1990 and 1992 to request adequate funding for education and training for occupational safety and health professionals.

The next logical step was to establish a separate office of occupational health nursing. Occupational health nursing had no official standing in the agency, and its existence continued to be threatened. Again, one prospect was placement under the Office of Occupational Medicine. AAOHN continued to lobby Congressional offices to promote an independent office viewed as equal to all the other occupational health professionals. In 1993, AAOHN requested, and the Senate Appropriations Subcommittee report included, language to support the creation of a separate office of occupational health nursing. OSHA announced establishment of the office in April 1993.

During this 13-year time frame, AAOHN also built alliances to further its goals. The American Nurses Association (ANA), as an advocate for the workplace health and safety of nurses and other health care personnel, identified the need for a nursing presence at OSHA as a common goal. The organizations worked together and met with top OSHA officials and members of Congress to build support. AAOHN also created partnerships within OSHA to convince others within the agency of the need for nursing input into policy decisions.

By 1996 the Office of Occupational Health Nursing was well established. However, Congressional efforts to dismantle OSHA and cut the agency's budget once again threatened the office, which had never been fully staffed. The nurse intern program also lacked the full support of the agency. Though medical resident interns were guaranteed funding, the nurse intern program was unable to secure a commitment of funding. AAOHN and ANA mounted a grassroots campaign requesting members to contact the White House and OSHA. OSHA received more than 600 letters of support for the office and for the nurse internships.

AAOHN also met with the then assistant secretary of OSHA, Joe Dear, to discuss staffing of the Office of Occupational Health Nursing, continued funding for the intern program, and, once again, securing the appointment of an occupational health nurse on the NACOSH. As a result, the office received funding for three full-time staff members and a commitment to fund six nurse internships. In addition, an occupational health nurse, who is a member of AAOHN and an owner of a small business, was appointed to a management slot on the NACOSH.

The next challenge is to extend the nursing presence in OSHA by increasing the number of occupational health nurses employed in the agency's regional offices, where they can provide consultation, training, and compliance assistance to employers in all parts of the country. With surprisingly adequate funding for fiscal year 1997, OSHA planned to fill more than 100 compliance positions throughout the regions. AAOHN requested that its constituent associations meet with their OSHA area directors to educate them about the role of occupational health nurses. Federal OSHA officials also agreed to encourage the regional directors to consider occupational health nurses when filling these compliance positions.

Occupational health nursing now has a presence at OSHA. The Office of Occupational Health Nursing has been lauded for its work as one of the most productive offices at the agency. At a recent AAOHN leadership conference,

Assistant Secretary Joe Dear acknowledged the important role that occupational health nurses play in OSHA's ability to meet its mission and protect our nation's workers. As the players change in the agencies and in the Congress, new alliances will have to be built to maintain this presence. The battle is long, hard, and never ending. These goals could not have been achieved without the dedication of many occupational health nurses and the work of both the AAOHN and ANA.

AMERICAN COLLEGE OF NURSE-MIDWIVES

KAREN S. FENNELL

Section 4073 of the Omnibus Budget Reconciliation Act (OBRA) of 1987 provided for the coverage of nurse-midwives' services under the Medicare program. Payments for covered services were made on the basis of a fee schedule established by the secretary of the Health Care Financing Administration (HCFA). The effective date for coverage under the amendment was July 1, 1988. The law provided the HCFA secretary with little guidance as to how the fee schedule should be established, except to stipulate that payment for nurse-midwife services cannot be greater than 65% of the applicable prevailing charge for the same service when performed by a physician. The law further specifies that payments must be made on an assignment-only basis.

The 1987 amendment defines covered nurse-midwife services to mean those "which the nurse-midwife is legally authorized to perform under state law (or the regulatory mechanism provided by state law) as would otherwise be covered if furnished by a physician or as incident to a physician service." The statute also defines a nurse-midwife as a "Registered Nurse who has successfully completed a program of study and clinical experience meeting guidelines prescribed by the Secretary, or has been certified by an organization recognized by the Secretary, and performs services in the area

of management of the care of mothers and babies throughout the maternity cycle."

Federal Medicare policy regarding payment for practitioner services is extremely important because of the precedents that are established for other public programs and private payers. Interpretation of the federal law by the HCFA was problematic for the American College of Nurse-Midwives (ACNM) because it defined covered midwife services as only those provided in the maternity cycle. It excluded gynecological and newborn services, a significant portion of the care that nurse-midwives provide. Before the law was implemented, the ACNM sent a letter to the HCFA administrator about this issue. The letter stated:

> Thus, we believe that Congress intended to cover all services that certified nurse-midwives are permitted to perform under state law, providing such services would be otherwise paid for by Medicare when furnished by a physician. . . .
>
> We strongly believe that failure to provide coverage of a service when provided by a certified nurse-midwife, who is legally permitted to provide such a service, could, in our judgement, deny Medicare beneficiaries the freedom to choose among alternative health care providers and prevent the Government from taking full advantage of the cost savings that can accrue when nurse-midwives rather than physicians provide Medicare covered services.

In July 1988 the department officially responsible for policy development relating to implementations of Section 4073 rejected the position expressed by the ACNM about the scope-of-coverage issue. An argument was made that the law limited coverage of services provided only during the "maternity cycle" and that a similar scope-of-service limitation is spelled out in the Medicaid regulations regarding such services. The department never issued regulations, although policy guidance was issued to Medicare carriers containing instructions to limit scope of coverage to the maternity cycle.

The ACNM had no choice but to seek legislative relief to change the department's views about the coverage of services. In 1988 the ACNM Board of Directors established this issue as the number one priority. It took 5 years of lobbying and grassroots action for the ACNM to obtain passage of this legislation. A metropolitan Washington, D.C., group of certified nurse-midwives was organized to assist in lobbying Congress and to serve as contacts to the ACNM state legislative liaisons.

In 1989, ACNM attempted to get a technical amendment that would have clarified the original intent of the OBRA 1987 language. Though successful in the Senate Finance Committee, the House Ways and Means Committee voted against such a provision in conference committee. Then, in 1992, Congressman Bill Richardson, of New Mexico, who served on the House Energy and Commerce Committee, introduced HR 5825 to expand covered services under the Medicare and Medicaid programs. However, many members of Congress and their staff viewed certified nurse-midwives as providing only maternity services. In an effort to educate Congress and the public, a new brochure was developed about other certified nurse-midwife services.

The next hurdle was accurately describing services that certified nurse-midwives perform outside the maternity cycle. Frequently, ACNM staff and certified nurse-midwives talked about providing gynecological services, family planning, and services to newborn infants. Discussing family planning services led congressional staff to conclude erroneously that certified nurse-midwives were providing abortion services. ACNM then changed their literature and lobbying efforts to focus on the less controversial parts of their practice such as cancer screening. A majority of members of Congress approved and supported certified nurse-midwives in seeking payment for these services.

Though the ACNM believed the battle had been won, the Congressional Budget Office (CBO) cost estimate for a 5-year period was more than $13 million. The ACNM knew that this was not accurate but had no data to dispute it. In 1993 the ACNM gave the staff of the Senate Finance Committee background data and an estimate to challenge the CBO figures. Senators Rockefeller, of West Virginia, and Grassley, of Iowa, were able to reduce the estimates to less than $8 million for 5 years.

In OBRA 1993, certified nurse-midwives finally won the battle over covered services. The ACNM is now working on increasing the level of payment from 65% to 97%. This has been difficult to achieve because of budget cuts to the Medicare program. However, ACNM does believe that with perseverance this goal can be achieved.

AMERICAN NEPHROLOGY NURSES ASSOCIATION
KATHLEEN T. SMITH

The American Nephrology Nurses Association (ANNA), originally founded in 1969 as the American Association of Nephrology Nurses and Technicians, is the professional organization representing nearly 10,000 registered nurses who are involved in the care of patients with renal disease. As such, it is the largest group of nephrology professionals in the nation. The primary work environment for the majority of ANNA members is outpatient hemodialysis units, although many work in acute care settings such as dialysis or transplant units.

ANNA's involvement in health policy issues dates back to the early 1980s, 6 years after the creation of the federal end-stage renal disease (ESRD) program. The ESRD program is the only program that entitles all eligible persons with a specific diagnosis (in this case, permanent kidney failure) to Medicare. This heavy dependence on Medicare reimbursement led

ANNA and other groups in the renal community to become involved in federal government affairs, particularly those activities related to Medicare policy. In addition, ANNA began its grassroots development in the early 1990s by focusing on its state chapters and educating its nurse members. This foundation positioned the association to respond to state-level issues that were brought to the ANNA board's attention by its grassroots members.

Throughout 1996, most of this activity centered around the issue of unlicensed assistive personnel (UAP) because of the attempt by state legislatures and regulatory agencies to regulate their practice. Because nephrology nurses have always shared their practice setting with technicians, ANNA felt compelled to communicate that experience with policymakers. ANNA members served on task forces dealing specifically with UAP in the dialysis setting in a number of states, including New Mexico, Connecticut, and Ohio. ANNA had two primary concerns in responding to the various state activities: protect the practice of the registered nurse and, more specifically, protect nurses practicing in the dialysis setting.

ANNA found that it was necessary to educate policymakers about the need to regulate or limit the practice of UAP. For example, some states attempted to regulate UAP directly through legislation that would require licensure, granting independent scopes of practice to dialysis technicians. ANNA's response was that such action would essentially remove these allied health care workers from the purview of nursing. In addition, granting licensure would make it difficult for nurses in states with clearly defined delegation rules, such as Ohio, to delegate tasks to this new category of practitioner. Other states used regulatory boards, like the boards of nursing, to limit the practice of UAP through indirect means. This usually took the form of clarifying and codifying in regulation the delegation authority of the registered nurse. In presenting testimony to a panel of legislators

in Pennsylvania, an ANNA member successfully pointed out that the state's proposed limits on delegation would have been too restrictive in the dialysis environment.

In an effort to clarify its stance on UAP, ANNA developed a position statement entitled "The Role of Unlicensed Assistive Personnel in Dialysis Therapy" in 1996. It states that UAP must function under each state's nurse practice act (and therefore be regulated by the board of nursing) and under the direct supervision of a registered nurse. It opposes the licensure of UAP. ANNA agreed with a 1993 American Nurses Association report that included a recommendation to "support an approach utilizing the least restrictive form of regulation for unlicensed assistive personnel." As an alternative to licensure, ANNA recommended that states regulate dialysis technicians as they do nursing assistants in nursing homes. This nursing home regulation, mandated by the Omnibus Budget Reconciliation Act of 1987, requires states to keep a registry of nursing assistants who have completed the required training and competency assessments. Ohio and Oregon, for example, have accepted this alternative and are no longer considering separate licensure for dialysis technicians. ANNA's position statement has been essential in the association's educational efforts as it responds to various state proposals.

ANNA communicated and coordinated with the state nurses association and the board of nursing in each state before initiating any grassroots action. This was done to gain insight into any related activities previously undertaken in the state, to present a consistent response from the nursing community on these issues, and to educate the groups about the specific nature of the dialysis practice setting. Further collaboration was accomplished when ANNA joined with the National Association of Nephrology Technicians and Technologists in issuing a position statement on the use of unlicensed personnel in dialysis.

ANNA's involvement in government affairs and policymaking through the years, as well as its development of grassroots support at the state level, positioned ANNA to respond to the issue of UAP. Further, because the scope of nursing practice is determined at the state, not the federal, level, the association anticipates continued activity in the remaining states. ANNA has learned how important it is for nurses to work together and with their allied health partners, to define and protect their nursing practice, and to communicate this to policymakers at all levels of government.

ASSOCIATION OF CHILD AND ADOLESCENT PSYCHIATRIC NURSES

ELIZABETH BONHAM AND LINDA M. FINKE

The Association of Child and Adolescent Psychiatric Nurses (ACAPN), at 26 years, is the oldest of the four psychiatric nursing specialty organizations. The primary purpose of ACAPN is to provide advocacy for the mental health of infants, children, adolescents, and their families. This is accomplished through public policy, legislation, clinical practice, education, and public awareness. More than 12 million youth in America have treatable but undiagnosed mental disorders. These disorders primarily include conduct disorders, depression, and hyperactivity–attention deficit disorders, as well as chronic mental health problems such as autism. Many of these children are sent to the juvenile court system or have behavior problems in schools that are not prepared to assist them. In addition, children's mental health issues are buried when public discussions center on insurance portability, access to mental health care, and reimbursement of providers for treating mental illnesses on the same level as physical illnesses.

To address these challenges, ACAPN has created two committees within its organizational structure: the Research/Education Committee and the Advocacy/Practice Committee. Mem-

bers of the Advocacy/Practice Committee developed an "advocacy packet," which is available from ACAPN's national office. The packet serves as a road map for nurse members to use in their grassroots lobbying efforts on the local, state, or federal level. It includes tips for verbal and written communications with legislators, suggestions for legislative networking, a sample letter to a member of Congress, and ACAPN position papers. The position papers address a range of issues that are important to the practice of child and adolescent psychiatric nurses, such as "seclusion and restraints" and "registered nurse staffing patterns." Frequently the ACAPN receives information from other nursing organizations, advocacy groups, or mental health associations that is developed into an "action alert," which gives instructions to members regarding a course of action. For example, when the Institute of Medicine sought testimony on nurse staffing adequacy in inpatient psychiatric units, an action alert was sent to members, requesting that they write or call their member of Congress and call or send fax messages to colleagues about the ACAPN's position.

ACAPN has worked to increase federal funding for the education and training of child and adolescent psychiatric nurses. In cooperation with the Society for Education and Research in Psychiatric Nursing (SERPN), ACAPN secured a $25,000 grant from the National Institute of Mental Health (NIMH) to host a national meeting on education and research for psychiatric nurses. The meeting was held in 1990, with participants including child and adolescent psychiatric nurse educators, parents of children with mental disorders, and psychiatric nurses who provide patient care.

Participants developed nursing education recommendations for child and adolescent mental health content for undergraduate and graduate nursing programs, including specific content and clinical learning experiences. The need for graduate education in child and adolescent psychiatric nursing at the master's and doctoral levels was emphasized, and sample curricula were developed. The recommendations included service guidelines for staffing psychiatric units and the promotion of standards of care for treatment. The research recommendations requested national funding for research in child and adolescent psychiatric nursing and the promotion of interdisciplinary research.

As a result of the 1991 conference and continued lobbying by ACAPN and other psychiatric nursing organizations, a steering committee was formed by the NIMH to increase nursing research in the field. Previously, funding was targeted only for psychiatrists, psychologists, and social workers. Through ACAPN's efforts, psychiatric nurses were added to the list of core mental health researchers.

In addition, in 1993, a program was implemented by the NIMH called the New Researcher Mentor Partnership. After an initial training workshop, the program took doctorally prepared nurse researchers and paired them with NIMH research staff. Approximately 50 nurse researchers attended the workshop in Washington, D.C., and 10 were chosen to receive funding to conduct research in child or adolescent mental health.

ACAPN's mission has historically been to provide advocacy for a population that is vulnerable, voiceless, and voteless. Even though national trends reflect increasing support for and understanding of the causes and treatment of mental illnesses, there is much work to be done. Through public policy, education, and research, ACAPN will continue its efforts to advance the issues of children with mental health disorders.

ASSOCIATION OF OPERATING ROOM NURSES
CANDACE L. ROMIG

The Association of Operating Room Nurses, Inc., (AORN), became a leader in 1996 on the issue of electrosurgical smoke evacuation.

AORN convened meetings in 1996 and 1997 of public and private stake holders to discuss the issue of and needed actions on surgical smoke. AORN participated in a coalition formed to influence government actions in 1996. In addition, AORN has continued to educate its members on the dangers of surgical smoke.

Since the mid-1980s, researchers and health professionals have focused on surgical smoke produced by lasers, because DNA from the human papillomavirus had been found in surgical smoke after wart removal procedures. Of course, concern spread through the medical community that operating room personnel could become infected with the human papillomavirus and maybe even hepatitis viruses or the human immunodeficiency virus. Adding to the concern about surgical smoke was increasing anecdotal reports of registered nurses and other operating room personnel experiencing more respiratory infections, eye soreness, shortness of breath, and even spontaneous abortions.

Surgical smoke, whether created by lasers or electrosurgical units (ESUs), is the result of tissue heated to 100° C, at which point cell membranes burst and produce a vapor containing cellular particles. Different surgical procedures and equipment produce different dispersions of aerosolized tissue. The three primary components of surgical smoke are (1) particulate matter, including carbonized tissue, blood, and viruses and bacteria that have the potential of being infectious, (2) steam released by the disintegration of tissue, and (3) toxic substances, chemicals, and gases that potentially may be hazardous or even carcinogenic. Operating room personnel often are first aware of surgical smoke through its extremely unpleasant odor.

Many personnel, who spend hours in the operating room inhaling surgical smoke for long periods, consider the protection of masks and respirators to be unsatisfactory. They have come to depend on surgical smoke evacuation equipment as the most reliable means of protection from smoke plume.

AORN and the AORN Foundation sponsored a roundtable discussion on surgical smoke in Denver, in January 1996. Many stake holders were invited to attend, including researchers, perioperative nurses, government regulatory officials, and industry representatives. Discussion focused on surgical smoke research and concerns about the quality of air in operating rooms and other facilities. The 1-day meeting resulted in a consensus that (1) smoke from ESUs should be treated the same as smoke from lasers, (2) government agencies (e.g., the Occupational Safety and Health Administration [OSHA]) should apply the same regulations to smoke from ESUs as are applied to laser smoke, and (3) further investigations should be conducted on the hazards of surgical smoke.

Eugene Moss, of the National Institute of Occupational Safety and Health (NIOSH), and Kenneth Ross, of ECRI, a nonprofit agency that evaluates medical equipment, called for more well-designed scientific studies of electrosurgical smoke and the effects on operating room personnel and surgical patients. At the time, these officials believed that there were too many unknown factors to support a federal mandate. Dr. Ralph Yodaiken, of OSHA, promised to review the guidelines governing the use of lasers in light of the possible hazards of ESUs. However, Dr. Yodaiken also wanted more scientific evidence of actual hazards pertaining to ESU smoke.

Shortly after the January 1996 meeting, the Coalition for the Protection of Operating Room Personnel was formed to lobby the federal government and to educate individuals interested in improving the health and safety standards in surgical arenas. Almost entirely funded by the private sector, the coalition pursued political rather than scientific solutions to the problem. The activities of the coalition included meeting with federal officials and contracting with a lobbyist to help direct activities. AORN and the American Nurses Asso-

ciation joined the coalition in the fall of 1996. These nursing organizations were supportive of coalition activities and have continued to urge local support through official mailings and action alerts.

The Coalition for the Protection of Operating Room Personnel has experienced modest success. It spearheaded a letter to OSHA through Congressman Carlos Romero-Barcelo, of Puerto Rico, asking that electrosurgical smoke be included in the revision of the OSHA laser guidelines. Amendments to the guidelines governing laser smoke have been drafted to include ESUs. As of March 1998, OSHA had not officially released these guidelines. NIOSH and the Centers for Disease Control and Prevention did release a hazard bulletin to their facilities network with warnings about the dangers of surgical smoke and advice on using smoke evacuation systems in conjunction with room suction systems to alleviate the potential problems.

The February 1997 meeting was held to discuss collaborative efforts regarding smoke-related safety issues in the operating room and to review new research. In addition to perioperative nurses, researchers, industry representatives, and government regulators, participation was broadened to include representatives from the American Society of Anesthesiologists, the Association of Surgical Technologists, the Joint Commission on Accreditation of Health Care Organizations, and the American College of Surgeons. The physicians' point of view was an important addition to the debate, especially because they initially did not support using the smoke evacuators in surgical settings, noting that they are noisy and impair vision. Their voice was important in urging additional research. Moreover, they were receptive to nurses' concerns about health problems arising from exposure to surgical smoke for long periods.

At the meeting's end, Dr. Yodaiken directed the participants to determine whether surgical smoke caused significant work absences or a significant number of injuries, whether equipment was available to alleviate the problem, and what would be the economic impact of potential government regulation. As a result of the strong message that government representatives gave to manufacturers and researchers, formal discussion about the design and implementation of more scientific research, as a preliminary step to achieving national smoke evacuation standards from OSHA, has begun.

AORN has taken the lead in identifying this health and safety issue affecting operating room nurses and has moved to define the debate. AORN will continue to work with its members, the Coalition for the Protection of Operating Room Personnel, and other health care provider groups to ensure that OSHA releases the guidelines on electrosurgical and laser smoke and to guarantee that patients and employees are protected from the hazardous effects of electrosurgical smoke in the operating room.

NATIONAL ALLIANCE OF NURSE PRACTITIONERS

JUDITH S. DEMPSTER

The National Alliance of Nurse Practitioners (NANP) was formed in 1985 as an alliance of organizations to foster communication among professional nurse practitioner groups. Collectively the NANP member organizations represent more than 25,000 nurse practitioners of all specialties. The 1997 organizational members are the American Academy of Nurse Practitioners, American Association of Occupational Health Nurses, American College Health Association, National Association of Pediatric Nurse Associates and Practitioners, and National Conference of Gerontological Nurse Practitioners. The Nurse Practitioner Associates for Continuing Education is a sustaining member.

NANP's purpose is to promote the health of the nation through primary care by promoting the visibility, viability, and unity of nurse practitioners. NANP is committed to achieving cost-effectiveness in health care, improving the organization and delivery of health care ser-

vices, and supporting the education of health professionals. The uniqueness of NANP is that a governing body of representatives from each member organization operates on a consensus model to facilitate NANP activities. These representatives form a critical link to their organizations and are a means to inform and mobilize a broad base of nurse practitioners from the national level through the grassroots level for needed policy and legislative action.

A major activity of the NANP is in the area of government relations. Strategies to shape health policy are based on the organization's annual legislative platform and are carried out through cooperative lobbying and grassroots activities of the constituent member organizations. NANP also coordinates its efforts with other appropriate nursing and health care organizations. Since its inception, NANP has united to work on issues such as providing health care for vulnerable populations, providing funding for nurse practitioner education, identifying nurse practitioners as essential primary care providers in all health care delivery settings, inserting nondiscriminatory language to support nurse practitioner practice in legislation, and ensuring reimbursement for nurse practitioner services.

Expanded reimbursement of nurse practitioners through Medicare is an example of NANP's successful legislative and health policy activities. In the mid-1980s, NANP supported the first federal legislation (Senate Bill 101) that addressed direct reimbursement for nurse practitioner services. This bill called for direct Medicare reimbursement for services provided by nurse practitioners in long-term care facilities. This legislation was signed into law, and subsequently, reimbursement for nurse practitioner services provided in rural areas was achieved.

With data supporting the quality and cost-effectiveness of nurse practitioner care and the recent legislative victories, NANP focused on identifying legislators who would introduce Medicare reimbursement legislation for nurse practitioners regardless of geographic location, practice site, or specialty. NANP worked diligently with legislative staff and members of Congress to draft specific legislative language, acquire cosponsors for each bill, facilitate the movement of legislation, and mount an effective grassroots campaign with individual members of the constituent organizations to support the proposed legislation.

In many instances, achieving a legislative goal is a slow and tedious process. Such has been the case with direct Medicare reimbursement for nurse practitioners. Through the years, the constituent members of NANP did not lose hope. They looked at each piece of legislation as a viable step toward the goal. Member organizations kept the momentum and maintained visibility by continuing to lobby legislators while members of Congress continued to introduce and reintroduce legislation that would allow for direct reimbursement for nurse practitioner services. Finally, in August 1997, President Clinton signed into law the Balanced Budget Act of 1997, which included comprehensive reimbursement for nurse practitioner services by Medicare.

NANP's legislative and health policy efforts are ongoing. New priorities, which include interstate authority of nurse practitioners and utilization of telemedicine or telehealth technology by nurse practitioners, are being addressed. Because health policy and legislative efforts will be needed to advance the role of the nurse practitioner and to enhance health care delivery, NANP is positioned to foster and support efforts of member organizations to provide a united front.

NATIONAL ASSOCIATION OF NURSE MASSAGE THERAPISTS

BONNIE MACKEY

The National Association of Nurse Massage Therapists (NANMT) is a nursing organization whose 700 members retain a specialized body of knowledge and skill that encompass a diverse, analytical, and intuitive nursing and bodywork educational background. Nurse massage therapists hold registered nurse (RN) licensure and have completed at least 500 additional hours of postgraduate education and training in soft tissue mobilization/myotherapy, bodywork, and other therapies found integrated into a holistic nursing framework in various practice settings such as private practice, hospital, or other clinic-based settings. Though the NANMT promotes the practice, education, research, and political interests of its members, for the past 10 years, the organization has had to work for recognition and acceptance of the practice of nurse massage therapy within the nursing community.

In 1993 the "Standards of Practice for the Nurse Massage Therapist" were written and approved by the NANMT, and a 500-hour core curriculum was approved in 1994. In addition, joining the National Federation for Specialty Nursing Organizations, whose mission is to promote specialty nursing practice and contribute to the health of the nation, was paramount to the recognition of nurse massage therapy. These efforts helped to achieve legitimacy for the practice of nurse massage therapy on a national level. However, it was on the state level that the special pursuit, occupation, service, and health care delivery of the nurse massage therapist remained constrained.

Recognition of the nurse massage therapist's education and practice by the state boards of nursing is beneficial to both the health care consumer and the nurse massage therapist. By recognizing nurse massage therapy as a component of contemporary nursing practice, the state boards of nursing ensure consumer protection for safe and appropriate practice. Further, it ensures that the nurse massage therapist operates within the legal realm of the state nurse practice act.

The NANMT approached the state boards of nursing, requesting that therapeutic massage, soft tissue mobilization, and other bodywork therapies be acknowledged as nursing interventions. General information about nurse massage therapy education and practice was sent to each state board. A letter of intent, requesting that the nursing agency formally recognize these therapies as nursing modalities on the basis of the completion of well-defined postgraduate education and training, was attached. Thirteen states issued a written statement of recognition for support of nurse massage therapy education and practice, some did not respond, and others clearly denied that these therapies were nursing interventions.

In the State of Florida, where massage therapy has been regulated for more than 50 years, the Florida State Board of Nursing (FSBN) ruled that nurse massage therapy should be under the jurisdiction of the Florida State Board of Massage. In 1995, this issue was challenged and the FSBN determined that the inquiring nurse massage therapist, having been certified by the National Certification Board for Therapeutic Massage and Bodywork, was within the practice laws that govern the RN. In this case the nurse massage therapist could legally practice in Florida, but RNs without this national certification were not regulated by either the state boards of nursing or the massage board. Further, the FSBN did not recognize that RNs are exempted from the licensing and other requirements of the State Massage Registration Law.

Individual and collective efforts continue to strengthen the credibility of and support for the practice of nurse massage therapy in Florida. One approach was to adopt a broader view and recognize nurse massage therapy as a component of holistic nursing. Holistic nurses in Florida petitioned to form the Florida Nurses Association's Council for Holistic Nurses, and in May 1997 it was approved. The council's goal was to unify and to create a voice for issues related to holistic nursing practice, education, and legislation in Florida. In addition, a state meeting was held in which Florida members of the American Holistic Nurses Association and the NANMT networked with council members to define common projects and goals.

During the past several years, the NANMT has garnered support from the state boards of nursing in 13 states for the practice of nurse massage therapy. However, in the remaining 37 states the organization must focus the efforts of its energetic and dedicated membership on using either the regulatory or the legislative process to achieve further recognition. With trends continuing to show the beneficial effects of massage therapy in health promotion and disease prevention, the NANMT is well positioned to move into this next phase of grassroots action.

NATIONAL ASSOCIATION OF ORTHOPAEDIC NURSES

NANCY E. MOONEY

The National Association of Orthopaedic Nurses (NAON) is the professional organization representing over 8,000 registered nurses whose practice area includes the care of patients with arthritic conditions, bone diseases, traumatic injury, and associated musculoskeletal diseases. The foundation for NAON's public policy efforts is the desire to encourage the enactment of legislation and regulation that promotes the musculoskeletal health of the general public and advances the nursing profession. NAON has always worked with related organizations to achieve common goals. In 1993 NAON began a productive relationship with the National Osteoporosis Foundation (NOF).

NOF has long had, as one of its goals, the standardization of Medicare's inconsistent coverage of bone mass measurement testing by establishing a uniform coverage policy for all local Medicare insurance carriers. Beginning in 1995, NAON members participated with NOF in the Osteoporosis Action Campaign. The campaign included an annual effort to collect signatures on a petition to Congress urging reimbursement for bone density testing, a national osteoporosis prevention education program, and expanded medical research. Thousands of signatures were gathered each year at NAON's annual meeting. Though legislation was introduced in the House and the Senate during the 104th Congress, the legislation was not enacted.

In 1996, NOF held a National Public Policy Forum as a first step in the development of a grassroots response network at the local level. NAON was a sponsoring organization for the forum and solicited grassroots volunteers for NOF from its membership. In addition, NAON served on the advisory committee for the 1997 forum.

NOF and NAON were successful in having the Bone Mass Measurement Standardization Act introduced once again in the 105th Congress. A NAON member who was also an NOF key contact from Montana was cited during the 1997 National Public Policy Forum as having been influential in getting Senator Max Baucus, a member of the influential Finance Committee, to support the legislation. During the May 1997 NAON annual meeting, more than 150 postcards were sent from attendees to their congressional representatives in support of the Bone Mass Measurement Standardization Act. This mailing was timely because Congress was just beginning its budget deliberations. This legislation was ultimately included in the budget reconciliation bill passed by Congress in the summer of 1997.

NAON is particularly proud of its work with the NOF in passing the Medicare Bone Mass Measurement Standardization Act. In addition, this relationship led to NAON's involvement with Strong Women, Inside and Out. This group is a coalition of more than 100 national organizations, representing consumers and health care professionals working at the state and federal levels to combat osteoporosis through education and advocacy. Though nurses have many opportunities to be advocates for their patients at the bedside or in the institution, these efforts have afforded many NAON members the opportunity to learn what it means to be a health advocate for a larger population. Through these collaborative efforts, NAON has been an active participant in improving life for the 25 million Americans affected by osteoporosis.

NATIONAL ASSOCIATION OF STATE SCHOOL NURSE CONSULTANTS

PHYLLIS J. LEWIS, MARY ELLEN HATFIELD, AND JUDITH A. MAIRE

The mission of the National Association of State School Nurse Consultants (NASSNC) is to provide a national forum for state-level nurse consultants to share information and develop an expert consensus on issues affecting the practice of school nursing as they relate to the overall health and educability of the nation's school-age children and youth. The NASSNC fosters the contribution of individual members through a network of information sharing and provides a standard approach to issues affecting the health and well-being of students.

By establishing guidelines or position papers, school nurse consultants have been able to influence policy and therefore school health. An example of an effective NASSNC position statement is "Medicaid Reimbursement for School Nursing Services." It was written in 1993 to assist states in the process of developing plans to reimburse school nursing services.

In 1992, individual state plans were rapidly being developed to obtain reimbursement for categories of rehabilitative services defined as "any medical or remedial services recommended by a physician or other licensed practitioner of the healing arts for any maximum reduction of physical or mental disability and restoration of any individual of his/her best function level" (Section 4719 of the U.S. Omnibus Budget Reconciliation Act of 1990). Similarly individual school districts across the country were developing their own plans to recover some of their costs incurred in serving students with disabilities. These state and individual school district plans maximized state dollars and brought federal dollars to help serve those Medicaid-eligible children who were recipients of health services in the schools.

The need to clarify the school nurses' role and ensure reimbursement for school health nursing services quickly emerged and provided the catalyst for the development of a position by the NASSNC. The following position statement was written:

> The National Association of State School Nurse Consultants (NASSNC) believes that school nursing services should be provided to all students and that Medicaid funds should be incorporated as a funding source for school nursing services provided to eligible children. The list of nursing services and procedures in this document, therefore, should be reimbursable by Medicaid to school districts. These services are outlined in categories of 1) case finding, 2) nursing care procedures, 3) care coordination, 4) patient/student counseling/instruction, and 5) emergency care. We adhere to this philosophy, and promote incorporation of these services as Medicaid-reimbursable services provided by qualified professional school nurses.

At this time, only a small number of services that school nurses provided, if any, were being considered for reimbursement by national and state policymakers. After the position statement was developed, reviewed, and approved by members, the NASSNC concurred that reimbursement for a broad scope of nursing services or any other reimbursement plan for school nursing services should be a part of all state plans for Medicaid.

The use of this position statement has been widespread. Delaware was one of the first states to have a state-wide plan around school nurs-ing services, with multiple categories and reimbursement including health education provided by school nurses. Some states were slowly expanding the initial reimbursement for minimal services to include additional categories. In South Carolina the state plan was based on this position statement and its five categories of services. However, implementation was delayed because of evolving state plans for medical care. In Connecticut, nursing services were first included in the school-based health services Medicaid reimbursement program for eligible special education students in 1996, partly because of the NASSNC position statement.

The Medicaid reimbursement position statement was used to amend a policy in the State of Washington Department of Social and Health Services (DSHS), defining the school nursing activities that the DSHS should reimburse. The rationale contained in the statement and the listing/description of school nursing services were clear and compelling enough for the DSHS to expand the list of reimbursable services for special education students. The statement also helped expand administrative matching funds to services for Medicaid-eligible students in regular education. Though the position statement was not the only factor involved, it contributed significantly to the understanding and promotion of school nursing services as reimbursable services in school settings.

The NASSNC is a small organization with approximately 40 nurse members employed in state departments of education and health. With access to E-mail and telephones, state nurse consultants effectively share their solutions to school-based health issues across state borders. Currently Minnesota and Florida are developing state plans seeking Medicaid reimbursement for school nurse services and are using the NASSNC position statement as a resource. In addition, school nurse consultants are pursuing data collection to support the effectiveness of their efforts to increase health care services and improve the health of the student population.

ONCOLOGY NURSING SOCIETY

PAMELA J. HAYLOCK AND
KATHERINE McDERMOTT BLACKBURN

The Oncology Nursing Society (ONS), with more than 25,000 registered nurses and other health care professional members, is the largest cancer-related specialty organization in the world. Members have historically been intimately connected to the patient-care aspects of cancer treatment. The 1986 implementation of diagnosis-related groups (DRGs), with subsequent reimbursement restrictions by third-party payers for cytotoxic agents, was a catalyst for members' political activation to ensure that people with cancer have access to optimal chemotherapy protocols.

In 1991 the Government Accounting Office indicated that one of every eight people with cancer had not been offered the most effective known therapy. The U.S. Food and Drug Administration (FDA) package insert, or its "label," is used by private and government-sponsored third-party payers to determine the reimbursement potential of prescribed drugs. There are reimbursement differences from payer to payer, from state to state, and even within a single payer's region in one state. The FDA approval process, in which a drug's efficacy in one disease entity is demonstrated, includes approval of a package insert that describes appropriate indications for use of the drug in question. The FDA approval process is lengthy and expensive, and pharmaceutical companies are unlikely to put an agent through a second approval process to demonstrate its worth for a second or third indication. Once the FDA approves a drug, it is available for prescription on the basis of a physician's discretion.

The "off label" use of anticancer drugs is common and standard practice: at least 60% of drugs used in the treatment of cancer are used in ways other than that indicated on the FDA label. However, variable interpretation of reimbursement policies based on the FDA label is one of many barriers preventing people with cancer from receiving optimal therapy. Rather than assume financial risks, physicians may select less effective, though reimbursable, cancer treatment protocols. Hospital or clinic formularies disallow selection of "off label" protocols. In addition, managed care's emphasis on the integration of health care financing and cost containment with the delivery of care makes the reimbursement potential of various treatment options even more contentious.

The Medicare Cancer Coverage Improvement Act, drafted in 1992 by Representative Sander Levin, of Michigan, and enacted in 1994, mandates that Medicare and Medicaid alter reimbursement strategies for cancer chemotherapy. Provisions of this legislation mandate payers' reimbursement for drugs if the drug use in question has FDA approval; is supported by one or more citations in at least one of three major compendia *(The American Hospital Formulary Service Drug Information; The AMA Drug Evaluations; the U.S. Pharmacopoeia Drug Information);* or is supported by clinical evidence reported in peer-reviewed medical literature. As the legislation made its way through the legislative process, ONS members rallied in support. The ONS government relations committee identified "off-label use of anticancer drugs" as a priority issue and, in turn, generated a concise, one-page fact sheet describing the values of off-label usage. Members used the ONS fact sheet, "Reimbursement for Clinical Trials and Off-Label Drugs," to articulate consistently the ONS position in grassroots lobbying efforts that included letters, telephone calls, telegrams, and visits to key legislators.

Because the Employee Retirement Income Security Act (ERISA) exempts self-insured companies from federal legislation, persons not insured by Medicare or Medicaid—some 60% of the population—are unaffected by the Cancer Coverage Improvement Act of 1994. State-based uniform coverage of anticancer-drug legislation must be enacted to amend insurance laws to mandate more complete coverage for cancer patients not covered by Medicare and Medicaid. An effective, coordinated effort involved passage of California's uniform coverage bill, AB 1985. California's population has nearly 10% of the nation's new cancer cases each year, making California a key focus in efforts to promote appropriate cancer treatment. Through collaboration of the ONS and the Association of Community Cancer Centers, California ONS members worked to support passage. The fact sheet prepared in response to federal legislation remains an effective tool to help members articulate salient facts. After the bill was introduced to the California Assembly in 1992, an ONS "action alert" system was activated. Action alert notices from the ONS government relations staff went to each of California's 2,500 ONS members. The action alert described the issue, invited the member's participation in the ONS response, reiterated the ONS position, and provided a copy of the fact sheet and a sample letter that was to be personalized and sent to state legislators and the governor. Copies of members' letters were sent to the ONS national office to track the response. At least 100 letters were sent to the governor as the legislation awaited his signature. The bill was enacted in January 1993. ONS members used similar strategies to support uniform-coverage legislation in other states, including Illinois, Hawaii, Massachusetts, and Indiana. By early 1997, 20 states had uniform coverage legislation in place, with comparable initiatives pending in at least seven additional states.

Current political philosophy advocates minimal federal governmental intrusion. It is rea-

sonable to expect that health care reform measures will most likely be addressed in state and private-sector policymaking arenas. While maintaining vigilance over and responding to federal initiatives, the ONS is developing and implementing strategies that help the ONS and its members to advance its mission, the promotion of excellence in oncology nursing and quality cancer care, through grassroots and state-level advocacy efforts.

SOCIETY OF GASTROENTEROLOGY NURSES AND ASSOCIATES

VIRGINIA A. WALTER

During the 1980s, gastrointestinal (GI) endoscopy was developed as a primary diagnostic and therapeutic tool for the treatment of GI diseases. Manufacturers, nurses, infection control practitioners, and physicians each developed their own protocol for the maintenance of GI endoscopes. These protocols were different and at times conflicting in their requirements. In 1990 the Society of Gastroenterology Nurses and Associates (SGNA) formed a task group as part of its product utilization committee to create a unified standard of practice based on science and broadly endorsed by all these groups. The task group included members from product manufacturers, the U.S. Food and Drug Administration (FDA), the Centers for Disease Control and Prevention (CDC), the Association of Practitioners in Infection Control, and the users of GI endoscopes.

As a result of the findings of this task group, the FDA requested the American Society for Testing and Materials (ASTM) to lead a consensus group to develop standards for cleaning and disinfection of GI endoscopes. In 1994 the "Standard for Cleaning and Disinfection of Flexible Fiberoptic and Video Endoscopes Used in the Hollow Viscera" was completed and published. SGNA was an active participant in developing this consensus standard.

Concurrently the FDA assumed responsibility for regulating liquid chemical germicides (LCGs). LCGs are used for high-level disinfection of GI endoscopes, high-level disinfection being the standard for reprocessing these instruments. Data and scientific evidence were published at this time to indicate that some LCGs label claims could not be verified. As a result, the FDA requested that the manufacturers of LCGs submit to the "510K process" to validate the claims of their products. The 510K process is the review process used by the FDA to substantiate the manufacturer's claims for a product before it can be sold in the U.S. marketplace. As a result of this review process, the FDA called for the removal of several LCGs from the market, and manufacturers of others were required to modify their claims.

The LCG glutaraldehyde is the LCG most commonly used to reprocess GI endoscopes. After the FDA review of this product, the FDA required that the 2% alkaline glutaraldehydes have a claim of 45 minutes' immersion time to achieve high-level disinfection. This claim was based on a worse-case-scenario testing, which is standard testing protocol for the FDA. The then-current standard immersion time for achieving high-level disinfection was 20 minutes, but the new label claim would greatly increase the turnaround time for these expensive instruments used in GI endoscopy. Additionally, and most important, the FDA's testing did not replicate the standard procedure used for reprocessing GI endoscopes.

The standard protocol for reprocessing GI endoscopes required that the endoscopes be washed meticulously before immersion in an LCG. The worse-case-scenario testing by the FDA eliminated the washing process completely. Published research, however, indicates that meticulous washing of endoscopes can remove up to 99% of the bioburden.

This government-required change in practice doubled the reprocessing time for GI instruments, thereby severely affecting the ability of gastroenterology professionals to perform GI endoscopy procedures in a timely and cost-effective manner. This was of great concern to the GI community in light of the average cost of instruments—$15,000, with some specialized instruments costing in excess of $65,000. Doubling the reprocessing time would mean that GI facilities would need to increase the number of available instruments greatly in order to perform the same number of procedures on a daily basis.

The American Society for Gastrointestinal Endoscopy (ASGE) initiated the formation of an ad hoc committee to assess and interpret available research related to reprocessing of medical instruments and to recommend infection control standards for GI endoscopy settings. Members of the ad hoc committee included representatives from the leading GI professional associations, such as the SNGA and the American Gastroenterology Association, the Association of Practitioners in Infection Control and Epidemiology, and representatives from the CDC and the FDA. All members of the committee were committed to analyzing all relative published data and reviewing current practice. The goals were to reach a consensus on a safe and cost-effective standard of practice and to make recommendations to the respective association memberships.

In 1995 the ad hoc committee published a position statement stating the need for meticulous cleaning of endoscopes before immersion in a 2% glutaraldehyde solution for 20 minutes to achieve high-level disinfection. This endorsement of the decreased soak time requires strict adherence to the defined washing protocol and the appropriate testing of LCGs before immersion. The committee further endorsed a need to have a specific education and quality assurance plan in each GI endoscopy setting. The final work of the committee was to develop a user-friendly document that would encompass all the infection control issues in the GI endoscopy setting and that would serve as a guide for reprocessing and infection control in any GI endoscopy setting.

The SGNA led the task of developing this document, which would serve as the consensus standard of practice. It was agreed that to effect change and implement standardization in the endoscopy community, the standard must be broadly endorsed by scientists, manufacturers of instruments and LCGs, infection control practitioners, physicians, and nurses.

The SGNA proceeded to develop the infection control document, which was reviewed by the ASTM committee on endoscopes and endorsed by the SGNA Board of Directors in December 1996 and the ASGE Board of Governors in February 1997. The standard was published in the March-April 1997 issue of *Gastroenterology Nursing*. The foundation of standardizing safe, efficient, and cost-effective infection control practice in GI endoscopy settings has been achieved through the collaboration of diverse professionals in nursing, medicine, infection control, manufacturing, and government.

Further, the professional medical and nursing organizations have requested the FDA to revise the testing procedure related to GI endoscopes. It was recommended that testing replicate the standard of practice related to endoscope reprocessing, which requires a meticulous washing process before immersion in an LCG. In the fall of 1996, the FDA responded that this recommendation was being taken under advisement.

SOCIETY OF PEDIATRIC NURSES

SUZANNE FEETHAM, BARBARA VELSOR-FRIEDRICH, AND SALLIE PORTER

The improvement of health outcomes for children and their families is a compelling concern in a health and social policy environment of constricting and restricted resources. National policy, or, more significantly, the lack of a comprehensive health policy related to the unmet needs of our nation's children, was a major force behind the development of the Society of Pediatric Nurses (SPN) in 1990. Also, at that time, there were policy changes at the national level of the American Nurses Association, resulting in changes in its organizational structure. It became clear to nursing leaders in pediatrics that, without a specialty organization, pediatric nurses were going to be without adequate direction or voice.

Most important to the organizers was their concern for improving the care and health outcomes for children and their families. They recognized the overwhelming unmet social and health needs of children and families, including the increased acuity of hospitalized children with rapidly decreasing lengths of stays; the increasing numbers of children with chronic illness and disabilities and the diminution of services to these children; and the renewed focus on the preventive and primary care needs of children, especially those in poverty. Because of these needs, SPN was established with a broad-based structure resulting in attention to general health and prevention issues not addressed by other nursing organizations.

Significant effort has been directed to organizing and educating nurse members to address policy issues affecting the health of children at the institutional, state, and national levels. The policy goals of SPN range from disseminating information on policy issues, to informing members of strategies to affect policy, and to positioning its members to provide policy leadership. SPN also increases its potential to influence policy through its partnerships with other organizations and disciplines such as the American Academy of Pediatrics, the National Association of Children's Hospitals and Related Institutions, the Child Health Council, and the Nursing Organizations Liaison Forum.

As a young organization, SPN has a need to inform members about their important role in influencing public policy. This activity is central to building an infrastructure to affect the health of children. Steps include the preparation of a document, "Public Policy for the Pediatric Nurse," explaining roles for nurses as individuals and as part of a group and the establishment of the Policy Action Network (PAN) to provide a rapid response to policy issues. The PAN includes top-down and members-up alert systems for identifying and responding to child health issues.

Because SPN is a small organization of 2,200 members, some delineation of priorities is required to improve opportunities for influence and to balance relevancy and SPN resources. One of the first questions that the policy committee addressed was the prioritization of the various child health issues. During a 5-year period, the society is focusing on increasing the rate of immunizations, preventing firearm injuries, and preventing unintentional injuries. Policy statements and action plans were developed for each issue and disseminated to members and other organizations. SPN addressed the issue of injury prevention by working collaboratively with other groups committed to the cause, specifically by participating in a regional injury prevention organization. Chicagoland Safe Kids, a local coalition of the National Safe Kids Campaign, is an organization that supported the introduction of bicycle helmet legislation in Illinois. Although the legislation did not pass, policymakers and consumers were educated about this issue. In addition, SPN continues its networking relationships with the National Safe Kids Campaign, as well as with other organizations concerned with child injury prevention.

Although responding quickly to issues is critical, it is also important for SPN to provide leadership to other organizations and disciplines, to policymakers, and to other stake holders. With the current educational efforts directed to nurse members and the establishment of the three priority issues, SPN is creating an infrastructure suitable for policy leadership. With time and growing resources,

SPN hopes to be a force for initiating or improving children's health policy at all levels of government and, in doing so, to improve the health of children and families.

NATIONAL FEDERATION FOR SPECIALTY NURSING ORGANIZATIONS: NURSE IN WASHINGTON INTERNSHIP

KATHLEEN T. SMITH

The Nurse in Washington Internship (NIWI) began in 1985, and since that time more than 1,200 nurses have enjoyed the NIWI experience. The internship was developed by and continues to be sponsored by the National Federation for Specialty Nursing Organizations (NFSNO), a national coalition of 37 individual specialty nursing associations, representing approximately 400,000 registered nurses. NFSNO developed the concept of NIWI as a way of educating the leaders of its member organizations about health care policy issues that affect the practice of nursing. The federation contracts with the Legislative Services Division of *Nursing Economic$*, in Washington, D.C., to conduct the program.

The purpose of the NIWI is to prepare nurse citizens to become more involved in the legislative process. NIWI impresses on nurses the value of their clinical knowledge and experience to the makers of health policy. NIWI interns are educated in ways to influence the policymaking process at the state and federal levels both as individual constituents and as members of specialty nursing organizations.

The NIWI provides a unique blend of didactic education and practical experience. The interns are supplied with a rich array of current literature that provides a background for the intensive seminar. Before arriving in Washington, the interns are encouraged to schedule appointments with their two Senators and their member of the House of Representatives. Interns are encouraged to bring position statements from their organizations on issues of concern to them; these statements form the basis of discussion when the interns visit their legislators.

Other highlights of the NIWI include presentations by nationally recognized speakers working in all branches of government at both the state and federal levels, as well as by speakers from various advocacy groups. Many of the invited faculty members are nurses, and some are even NIWI graduates. Role models and mentors abound during the internship experience. The Nurses in Washington Roundtable Dinner is an annual NIWI event that offers the nurse interns an opportunity to network with policymakers, NIWI alumni, and nursing leaders from the greater Washington metropolitan area. In addition, the White House briefing is always a popular and significant part of NIWI.

Nurses who attend NIWI do not need to be knowledgeable about government issues or processes. Although most interns attend as representatives of their specialty nursing organization, there is no requirement for attendance other than the desire to learn and to put the knowledge into practice on returning home.

In addition to the formal education offered at NIWI, interns continually remark about the diverse education, experiences, and issues shared among their peers. The opportunity to network with fellow interns and speakers has been highly valued by the participants. The NIWI experience bonds these nurses much like their clinical experiences have done during their careers. NIWI graduates continue to network long after their week in Washington.

A number of nursing specialty organizations provide scholarships to enable more of their members to become interns. In addition, since 1995 the authors of *Policy and Politics for Nurses* and the publisher, W. B. Saunders Company, have offered a $1,500 scholarship on behalf of all the book's contributors through NFSNO as a demonstration of their commitment to the education of nurses in health policy.

Further information about NIWI can be obtained from the NFSNO national office at 609-256-2333. See Appendix A for additional information on political and policy internships.

Unit *VI*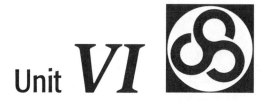

POLICY AND POLITICS IN THE COMMUNITY

Unit VI

describes policy and politics in communities, from local to international. It embraces the adage "Think globally, act locally." It begins with a discussion of some of the issues confronting communities and challenges the values that underlie some of the continuing conditions and struggles of many of the people in this nation and the world. The vignette following this chapter describes one nurse's work as an advocate for safe urban policies for bicycling in her community.

Chapter 35 provides a framework and strategies for working with communities as partners and is filled with examples of nurses implementing these strategies with care and vision. It is followed by a vignette that describes how a public health nurse worked with a community on environmental concerns, within a framework of environmental justice.

Foundations support innovations in promoting the health of communities that often lead to changes in public and private policies. Chapter 36 describes how foundations work, their impact on health care, and how to work with them.

Global perspectives are becoming increasingly important to local communities and nations. International issues and perspectives on health and health care are discussed in Chapter 37. It includes a discussion of the role of the oldest international health organization—the International Council of Nurses—in influencing nursing and health worldwide. Two vignettes provide stories of policy and politics with this international perspective. The first describes one nurse's experience with the politics of Guatemala regarding one of the most important health-promoting skills that people need—literacy. The second vignette is a personal account of a nurse with origins in Armenia who later emigrated to the United States and became involved in influencing policies and politics worldwide. She describes her experience as a delegate to the United Nations' Fourth World Conference on Women.

Unit VI concludes with a case study describing the politics of developing birthing centers. It demonstrates the importance of community support and perseverance.

Two End Case Studies synthesize the concepts discussed in this book. The first is based on two nurses' experiences in starting a nurse-managed health center for uninsured persons in a community in Pittsburgh. The second describes the interweaving of policy and politics around the issue of HIV/AIDS and includes the role of nurses in shaping the debate and responding to this disease.

Chapter *34*

CONTEMPORARY ISSUES IN THE COMMUNITY

JANET GOTTSCHALK AND SUSAN SCOVILLE BAKER

This chapter presents an overview of the challenges and opportunities for nursing in the global community. The authors offer a broad perspective of some worldwide concerns and challenges and offer examples of how nurses and others have addressed these challenges. Although a global community development perspective is offered, the context is also firmly couched in terms of the political and economic history and traditions of the United States. Any meaningful, effective interaction within the global community requires first an understanding and acceptance of one's own cultural and historical context.

Tremendous socioeconomic and political changes have taken place in the United States and the world during the past several decades. These changes not only have affected the lives of millions of Americans but also have altered our place in, and the perceptions of, the global community. This chapter will address some of those substantive societal changes along with their associated socioeconomic health problems.

THE CHANGING AMERICAN LANDSCAPE

Less than 50 years ago, one could walk into almost any community or neighborhood in the United States and expect to find clear examples of the basic American values that helped build a nation respected throughout the world. The combination of individual choice and hard work plus the "magic" of a free market system was believed to be all that was needed to make the "American dream" a reality. Americans, recalling their own immigrant heritage, proudly repeated the well-known phrase on the Statue of Liberty: "Give us your tired, your poor . . ." and, because the future seemed filled with endless possibilities, welcomed others to become a part of the great "melting pot" that was America.

Although persons lived generally in communities, it was the individual, in true American fashion, who was free to define his or her personal and political goals. Individual rights, guaranteeing the freedom and space to pursue personal goals, were passionately protected. The United States was, after all, the "Land of Opportunity," and "equal opportunity" was a constitutional right of every American citizen and newcomer to our shores.

Although there were often major problems caused by the rapid growth of the nation, activists and social reformers always seemed to rise in large enough numbers to stir America's social conscience to the plight of those less fortunate and enact the necessary legislation to ease their burdens.

In the early years after World War II, the United States was the model of freedom and democracy for newly emerging nations. Praised for its unselfish generosity and humanitarian efforts, the United States was a nation with the technical expertise and "know-how" not only to assist in the rebuilding of Germany and Japan but also to lead the way in global industrial and economic development.

Russia's *Sputnik* may have spurred the United States on, but the long-established U.S. public school system was solid and strong enough to support intensive educational and scientific efforts that led to a successful first landing on the moon. Was there anything the United States could not achieve? Was there any area in which the United States was not "Number One"?

In recent years, however, problems too serious to be ignored have begun to tarnish the image of American society. Distinctions and, at times, violent conflicts between different groups are beginning to make some people question many of the most deeply held beliefs in the United States.

If everyone is free to pursue his or her individual goals, what is to happen to those persons who—by reason of race, class, gender, sexual orientation, illness, or other circumstance—stumbled along the way to achieving the American dream? Does society, as a whole, have a responsibility to and for those persons? If there is agreement that a responsibility does exist for such people, should it be our national, state, or local governments that initiate and fund the needed social programs?

In a society where basketball players sign multi-million-dollar contracts at the beginning of their professional careers and citizens across the country vote to build new sports arenas instead of schools, we still seem helpless to deal positively with the numbers of homeless persons sleeping on the streets and in alleyways. During the 1996 presidential campaign, candidates vied with each other to declare their commitment to "American values," and yet little or no national agreement exists as to exactly what these values are. Many of our public school systems are crumbling and in danger of being placed under the protection of the courts. Even our nation's capital, unable to meet its fiscal and social responsibilities with the resources available to it, has been, like a number of our cities, in danger of bankruptcy. Our Social Security system is financially threatened, and many senior citizens fear that their future Medicare and/or Medicaid benefits will be inadequate for their needs. In

fact, our generations-long national belief in people's right to "entitlements" or "guarantees" of assistance by our government is now doubted by so many that President Clinton during his second inaugural address emphasized that we live in a land of equal opportunity and not of "guarantees." How dulled has our social conscience become?

As some become rich and a privileged few become super rich, a widening income gap is dividing our country, with the middle class racing to stay in place and the poor being left far behind. Children, as so often happens, are among those who suffer the most from this increasing poverty. What a scandal it is that, in the richest country in the world, children's hunger is not only widespread but increasing. According to the Bread for the World Institute, "Child poverty is more widespread in the United States than any other industrial country," with more than 1 of 5 children, or 21.5%, in the United States classified as poor. This translates into approximately 13.6 million American children who are hungry or at risk of being hungry each day. With the exception of Africa—a continent convulsed with wars, tribal conflicts, and famine—there is no other area in the world where child hunger has increased so dramatically in the past 25 years. ("U.S. Child Poverty . . .," 1996). Given such an obvious lack of commitment to the well-being of our children, it should come as no surprise that our elected representatives have not yet found it important to ratify the "Convention on the Rights of the Child," developed in 1990 by the nations of the world at a Children's Summit convened by UNICEF.

Many other Americans fare little better. While many of our wealthier Americans, living in gated enclaves, attempt to protect themselves and their homes from the deterioration, crime, and violence of our crumbling cities, some economists point out that our current economic cycle is one of "jobless growth." While our politicians proudly tell us that "welfare as we know it is dead," others, perhaps more able to see the "welfare problem" in its broader dimensions, alert us to the grim reality that the disappearance of work in our ghettoes and inner cities is reaching catastrophic proportions. They further warn that there will be serious consequences for all Americans if we do not include the complex issues of job creation, skill development, housing, safety, and child care in our efforts to end welfare "as we know it" (Wilson, 1996).

TROUBLING QUESTIONS

In these times of abundance for some, is a nation that was originally committed to "justice for all" responsible to change its policies and programs that perpetuate and create unjust and unequal situations and structures?

If the United States, as a nation, is proud of its "melting pot" heritage, why has it become so difficult to accept immigrants and eventual citizens who seek better lives for themselves and their children through hard work and through the contribution of their talents and cultures? The majority of those currently seeking immigration to the United States are not fleeing military violence but deep, often subhuman, misery and poverty, caused in their countries by inefficient and corrupt national elites, an economic globalization of trade that appears to benefit only the richer nations and corporations, population and urbanization pressures that overwhelm national capacities and resources, and structural adjustment programs that privatize social services and further impoverish poor persons.

At the same time that we open our borders to "free trade" and plan for the building of new bridges, interstate highways, and canals to facilitate the easy movement of commodities between nations, why do we limit the access of the people of those same nations to our country? While painfully aware of the deepening poverty and social disintegration in much of our own country, are we so skeptical of our ability to resolve our problems that we are afraid to share our opportunities with people fleeing an often subhuman existence?

Why must we build fences across much of our 2000-mile border with Mexico—fences high enough to stop people but not drugs? Is our fear of the "newcomer" child—Hispanic or otherwise—so great that we need to legislate against bilingual education, militarize our southern border with immigration officers, and deny welfare benefits to those who, having entered our country legally, are considered future citizens?

Another troubling question is why, 500 years after the "discovery" of North America by Columbus, descendants of the original Native Americans and those African Americans brought in chains to U.S. shores have not generally achieved even middle-class status.

CHANGING U.S. ROLE IN THE GLOBAL COMMUNITY

These economic and ideologic dilemmas, along with an increasing cynicism of government at all levels, have deepened the confusion many have regarding the role of the United States in the world. Coupled with a growing awareness of possible corruption at the highest levels of U.S. government and business, this confusion and, at times, isolation from what is happening in the world today may actually be leading the people of the United States deeper into societal contradictions.

Since World War II the world has witnessed an economic "contest" between those nations committed to the principles of free trade and unlimited access to markets and those committed to more socialistic or government-controlled economies. However, the fall of the Berlin Wall and the breakup of the Soviet Union have led to so many ongoing social and political changes in Europe that the United States has been left as the world's one undisputed superpower—economically and militarily. Unfortunately, though, the tax dollars spent on maintaining our military superiority leave fewer tax dollars to rebuild our deteriorating cities, highways, and educational systems and to provide health/medical care for all our citizens, especially the approximately 41 million with no or inadequate health insurance. Drugs, crime, violence of all kinds, unemployment, underemployment, homelessness, and numerous forms of environmental pollution are now common, often intractable, problems in American cities and towns. Even worse, our social scientists and economists note an increasing gap between the rich and the poor in American society, with the consequent development of what some observers call a permanent underclass.

While the basic infrastructure in much of the United States continues to deteriorate, multinational economic interests are merging with or buying up U.S. corporations and real estate. At the same time, powerful economic blocks of nations developing in Europe and Asia are attempting to displace the United States from its once universally accepted role as leader of the global economy. Currently, though, American dominance seems assured because the American growth model appears well suited to produce information technologies considered essential for continued economic growth in a single, high-speed global marketplace (Friedman, 1997). Such a process of globalization of the world's economies, or the absorption of all countries into one economic entity, has, in fact, become the defining feature of the last days of the twentieth century—a reality that anyone involved in social or political action must consider.

ARE WE READY FOR THE TWENTY-FIRST CENTURY?

Caught up in what some consider an irreversible process, we are told we must prepare ourselves for the challenges of the twenty-first century—challenges based on competition in an increasingly integrated world. While the "winners" in this competition acquire more and more riches and power, the "losers" are those countries and peoples across the world and in the United States who are prematurely used up by work and want. Increasingly excluded from the universal marketplace, the "losers" are the hapless victims of "global downsizing" (Seabrook, 1996).

Communism may have died in the Western world as a consequence of the breakup of the Soviet Union, but many are asking: What checks now exist internationally on the excesses of unchecked capitalism? What has become of our earlier vision of building a world where all peoples and nations can thrive in peace, harmony, and health? In this era of economic and cultural globalization, in which some transnational corporations are richer than most nations, how can these same nations control their own destinies? When nations, weakened or strengthened by these global economic factors, unite in an international organization such as the United Nations, what power can such an organization have as a peace broker or peacemaker if it has no financial resources? During the Cold War, we were eager to "help" those nations in danger of becoming too friendly to Russia. Now that the Cold War is over and the geopolitical importance of many of these poorer nations is less, do we continue to believe in contributing to the human development of *all* peoples, wherever they may be on our increasingly fragile planet?

As individuals and, some might say, as a people, many Americans continue to be confused as to our place in today's world. Given the dizzying rate of change the world is experiencing and the complexity of issues in a globalized society, the world of tomorrow will present us with even more challenging and perplexing questions.

UNHEALTHY RESPONSES TO CHANGE

Some, faced with the enormity and pace of global change, feel powerless to change the course of events and are tempted to retreat into isolation and the safety of the known. Others, feeling equally powerless, find strength and support in adherence to increasingly conservative, isolationist, and individualistic beliefs and organizations. Concern for their own personal security, as well as that of the public at large, has led some American citizens to participate in the development of militias, secessionist groups, and other antigovernment groups; to support capital punishment and the building of more prisons instead of the funding of crime prevention programs; to organize in favor of the National Rifle Association and against the Brady bill; and even to feel justified in committing terrorist acts directed against government institutions, private agencies, and others with whom they disagree.

Attacks on affirmative action policies are common throughout the country, and racism, much to our national shame, continues unabated, exacerbated, perhaps, by the increasing inequality between the rich and the poor in our country. Racism now also includes the fear of immigrants who have achieved economic success by adhering to the American virtues of hard work and perseverance. Classism, once thought antithetical to the American dream, can be seen in our often judgmental views of the "poor," the "welfare cheats," the economic "deadbeats" of our society. And, of course, sexism, as manifested in discrimination and abuse of all kinds, is omnipresent in American society. Unfortunately, the continued or increasing presence of these "isms" in our society may be directly related to a highly individualistic orientation fostered by an emphasis on economic growth for a few, with the hope that the many will someday benefit.

SHIFTS IN HEALTH CARE POLICY

These dramatic changes in both American society and the world have had a substantial impact on the nation's overall health status and its various health care systems. In addition to the external influences discussed above, paradigm shifts in the structure and financing of health care itself are currently transforming the delivery of U.S. health services with major consequences for the professional practice and education of all health professionals.

On the positive side, there is a major shift from institutional inpatient care to community-based outpatient care. The focus of such care, especially at the institutional level, is population based, with emphasis on disease prevention and illness management that is as efficient, effective, and economical as possible.

Unfortunately, competition for control of the health care "market" is destroying smaller health care facilities, limiting people's access to their traditional health care institutions and providers, and endangering the quality of American health care. Through a concentration on market share, buyouts, and mergers, highly integrated for-profit systems are transforming the appearance of American health care institutions, leaving them with little or no accountability to the communities in which they are located.

In a country that has seen decades of discussion and acrimony regarding the appropriate development of national health policy and adequate insurance coverage for all its citizens, market forces have stepped in and are radically changing American health care. Concurrent with this massive privatization has come decreased funding for public health and an apparent decrease in public responsibility for the nation's health. Given the probabilities of decreased levels of future funding for Medicare at the national level and decreased funding for Medicaid and other "safety net" programs at the state and national levels, the growing economic inequality between the races and classes of our country, plus the very real threat to quality health care that exists in our currently privatizing health care systems, we should expect to see major changes in our national and local health indices.

Many in our most vulnerable populations today carry enormous and, at times, overwhelming burdens: teenaged mothers with young children, persons with chronically physically and mentally ill relatives, caregivers of elderly or physically challenged persons, and partners of the "socially outcast," such as persons with human immunodeficiency virus infection or with acquired immunodeficiency syndrome, homeless persons struggling with a mental disorder or substance abuse, and unemployed workers or those without adequate wages to support themselves and their families. Unfortunately, it does not appear to be good politics these days to express too much concern for our poorest and most vulnerable citizens or, worse yet, to express concern for those who have legally entered our country but are not yet U.S. citizens.

HOPEFUL SIGNS IN COMMUNITIES

Although we should not minimize the disturbing trends so evident in many parts of the United States today, we should not join the ranks of the cynical and pessimistic who see little hope for positive change in our country. On the contrary, we should carefully identify the many strengths of communities throughout the world so that, together with others, we might build a more just and equal society.

When the term *globalization* is used, it usually refers to the integration or absorption of all countries into one entity in *economic* terms. There is, however, another form of globalization increasingly present in the world today, one that holds promise for the well-being of our planet. It is a heightened awareness of the fact that, wherever we are in the world, most of us struggle with many of the same difficulties, watch the same sunrises and sunsets, and share the same dreams for ourselves and our families.

This global awareness, in its turn, is stimulating the growth of so many "people's organizations" throughout the world that some social commentators are saying the increasing influence of these organizations should be considered one of this decade's major features. As a category, these groups, known as "Civil Society Organizations," are becoming major players in our world, and their influence is being noted at all levels of government. These groups include the citizens marching in the streets of the former Yugoslavia, the mothers silently standing in the plazas of Latin America to demand information about their missing children, the women of Liberia who said to their leaders, "Enough of war," and the thousands who represented the concerns of organized groups in their own countries at the United Nations conferences on the environment, population, human rights, poverty, housing, and women.

Not content to leave the resolution of the world's pressing problems to diplomats, people throughout the world are insisting their voices be heard in local town councils, state legislatures, national parliaments, and the United Nations. Their interests and perspectives range from the need to provide small loans for struggling minority groups to banning land mines and chemical weapons. With orientations that range from the far right to the far left, these people are attempting to transform the future according to their beliefs and desires. Women, veiled according to strict Muslim custom, and yet operating camcorders, mingle with Western-clad activists lobbying for children's rights, better housing, cancellation of nations' debts, preservation of the ozone layer, and an end to economic growth at the expense of people's lives and well-being.

Many, firmly convinced of their own abilities and those of the people they represent, are seeking alternatives to "business as usual." Such emphasis on the seeking of alternatives is especially evident in the health field. In the villages, small cities, and urban megalopolises of our world, health activists, preparing for the Fourth World Conference of Women, insisted on the need for more holistic and alternative technologies and for more health care across women's life span, not just during their childbearing years. Moreover, as was clearly evident in Beijing when 50,000 persons gathered for the Fourth World Conference on Women, attention to gender issues is no longer a goal only of Western women's groups. Calling for an increased emphasis on their human rights, women are organizing throughout the world to rectify the unjust situations found in their homes, workplaces, and the halls of power, whether in government or in industry.

It is not just women's groups, however, who are seeking alternatives to so much that is unjust in our societies. Locally, regionally, nationally, and internationally, neighborhood organizations, faith communities, self-help groups, labor unions, and professional associations, to name a few, are today organizing themselves with renewed commitment to attaining their goals. Aware that a few voices can easily be muted and ignored, they are linking together in partnership and solidarity across national boundaries, ethnic divides, and religious distinctions.

NURSES AS CATALYSTS IN COMMUNITIES

With so much ferment in our world today, it is an extraordinarily exciting time to be alive. Possibilities abound for nurses, in both their personal and professional lives, to unite with others in the building of a more just, more peaceful, more healthy society. In communities everywhere, nurses are transforming these possibilities into realities. A group of nurses in a small city in Brazil launched a project in the city parks to teach people that they could improve their health through life-style change rather than being dependent on professionals and clinics and prescriptions. In southern Mexico, the faculty of a university school of nursing were joined by thousands in the university community to launch an effective demonstration for the professionalization of nursing education. In towns on both sides of the border between the United States and Mexico, nurses and lay community health workers from both nations are joining together in binational campaigns to address public health issues. Nursing students are joining students of other health care professions in community initiatives. And a new university on the Atlantic coast of Nicaragua has identified nursing as one of the natural resources of the region.

Nurses are always on the front lines in times of crisis. Historically, crises have also offered the greatest opportunities for the advancement of nursing as a profession. In partnership with other nurses and with local, national, and international communities, the closing years of the twentieth century offer exciting challenges and opportunities for nursing.

REFERENCES

Friedman, T. L. (1997, February 9). Dear Dr. Greenspan. *The New York Times* [Foreign Affairs].

Seabrook, J. (1996, August). Internationalism versus globalism. *Around Africa*, 3–4.

U.S. child poverty rate highest in industrial world. (1996, October 21). *Monday Developments*, 4(20), 1, 11.

Wilson, W. J. (1996, August 18). When work disappears. *The New York Times Magazine*, 26–31, 40, 48, 52–54.

VIGNETTE
Bicycling, Public Policy, and Health: The Nurse as Community Activist
Irene Van Slyke

I have bicycled for as long as I can remember. I grew up in Indonesia and in the Netherlands, where you rode a bicycle to school and after shopping threw your groceries in a bicycle basket to take them home. Bicycle parking in most Asian countries is like parking a car in the United States. You either lock the bicycle and leave it in the street or park it with a bicycle attendant for a fee.

I never thought much about bicycles as a mode of transportation. Bicycling was a necessity. Much later, as a nurse, I appreciated bicycling not only as transportation but also as a vehicle of public health. But back then I wondered when I would be rich enough to get a car. The solution: you immigrate to the United States, make a lot of money, and buy a car, of course.

I immigrated to the United States in 1964 and, within 6 months of working as a nurse, was able to buy a $50 car. Soon thereafter I did what every American dreams of: drove on a four-lane highway; went to drive-in-movies, drive-in restaurants, and drive-by mailboxes; and lived in a house with a garage on a street without sidewalks. Who would want to walk or bicycle if you can sit in a car? But the dream comes at a price, I realized much later. The unbridled highway-building effort and the proliferation of cars gobbled up open space, destroyed communities, produced air pollution, and encouraged the unhealthy habit of spending much time sitting in a car.

Activists have a lot in common with people who try to convert others to their religion. What makes someone become a community activist is usually a personal experience with an issue, as well as a dream of how to make a better world and a healthier society. What protects activists from burning out is the belief that one person can make a change for the better. An effective activist is someone who is willing to fight for incremental changes that make up crucial pieces of the solution. An activist is also someone willing to speak up about not only what is wrong but what is right.

Activists spend a lot of time discussing a new and better way, examining what people do now versus how it can be done. Because people are comfortable with what they are used to doing, activists need to have all the arguments ready to help people see a better way. This means gathering facts and presenting them in new and creative ways to achieve a solution to a problem. Offering a solution gives people hope that they can do little things that are good not only for themselves but also for their neighborhood and the country.

The path from being a nurse to becoming an activist, helping individuals while also working for the greater good, is one that many nurses follow. This is how I got involved.

For many people in the United States, bicycling is a recreational activity. I had a bike, but I rode it on weekend trips outside New York City. One bicycle rider I knew invited me on a bike ride to "discover your own backyard—Brook-

lyn." It was wonderful to ride through neighborhoods, hop off my bike when I saw something interesting, and visit sites I had never known existed, all within easy riding distance. I enjoyed it so much that he invited me to a meeting of Transportation Alternatives, a local bicycling advocacy group in New York City.

Only about 10 people attended the meeting, but that is where I first heard about people committed to other modes of transportation: bicycling, walking, roller blading, and riding subways, ferries, and trains. They discussed the many impediments in their way, from car drivers and police officers unaware of a bicyclist's right to the road, to federal policies that favor car driving. One thing that stuck in my mind was that car ownership in Europe is comparable to car ownership in the United States, but in many European countries 40% of short trips are made by bicycle or by walking. In the United States, only 11% of short trips are made by bicycle, even though 40% of all trips in the United States are less than 2 miles in length. People in Europe chose to leave their cars at home. I was hooked. Here was a whole new way of looking at things, a new way of doing things, a whole new world!

As a nurse, I was well aware of how the lack of physical activity adversely affects public health. What I had not known is that physical activity has been engineered out of American life, as one activist put it. We must actively put it back in our lives.

Although in Africa and Asia bicycles are a major means of transportation because of a lack of money, in Europe the high number of people walking and bicycling is due to conscious policy decisions by the countries' leaders to incorporate alternatives into transportation networks. At train stations, by and large, you do not find parking garages; you will find a bus depot with connections to surrounding communities. In the Netherlands, railway stations provide bicycle parking in front of the station, but parking garages are a short walk away or might not be there at all. This kind of system provides a "seamless" multimodal transportation network for people without cars. When entering a residential area, you might find a narrowing of the road, traffic circles, or bumps to slow down car traffic. These engineering features tell car drivers that they are entering a residential area and to respect the road as an extension of front yards, where children, senior citizens, and other pedestrians share space with cars.

In the United States, on the other hand, people value convenience, and they think that cars bring convenience. To maximize convenience, policies have favored car drivers over pedestrians; for example, obstructing traffic is a crime. Gas taxes fueled highway construction, and new highways enticed more car drivers to use them. Highway building creates traffic, not transportation. The distinction is that transportation carries people where they want or need to go; traffic, on the other hand, is a mindless moving about which creates bottlenecks at rush hours and popular destinations without addressing people's needs.

To begin to address traffic and transportation problems, Congress passed the 1991 Intermodal Surface Transportation Efficiency Act (ISTEA, pronounced "ice tea"), which for the first time shifted policy away from building more highways that would accommodate more cars. The Act declared the U.S. highway system complete and gave states more flexibility in spending transportation dollars, required public participation in the decision-making process, and provided funds for transportation projects that improve air quality, health, and safety.

The passage of ISTEA has made public dollars and local and statewide bicycling and pedestrian coordinators available to local activists. However, progress has been slow. Coordinators have worked on encouraging local advocates, and advocates often must make their local officials aware of the flexibility in funding and must show public support for "traffic calming," or a slowing down of car traffic, and for pedestrian and bicycle projects. Moreover, although ISTEA suggests planning for an inclusive transportation policy, there are no mandates to follow; instead, money is available for innova-

tion. This approach necessitates considerable local advocacy.

Advocacy can take many forms, but with transportation advocacy I like to follow the advice of a traffic engineer: First look at policy, and then find money to implement policy. Next, determine the necessary engineering changes in the road. Last, enforce the rules.

These steps seem simple to follow, but they are not. For example, when my neighborhood civic group advocated the enforcement of rules against bicycle riding on the sidewalk, my first reaction was that the bicyclists' behavior was a manifestation of unsafe road conditions. I pointed out that complaints came from pedestrians. We looked at car and pedestrian accident data and asked Project for Public Spaces, an advocacy group for pedestrians, to help us interpret the data and to suggest solutions.

Not surprisingly, we found that the city's policy had been to favor car traffic over pedestrians and bicyclists. New York City's transportation department, in an effort to speed up traffic, had increased green time for cars, which resulted in speeding. This drove the bicyclists onto the sidewalk. Furthermore, restrictive parking policies and excessive speeding were hurting businesses and causing a high number of accidents. The debate about bicyclists on the road shifted. The research led us to ask, What is the city doing to make the road safe for pedestrians and bicyclists, and how can traffic become transportation friendly and thereby more business friendly?

Before specific solutions are found, it is helpful to agree on some general principles. For example, in New York City

- The road should be designed for the legal traffic limit of 30 miles an hour.
- Traffic and parking rules should incorporate the needs of car drivers, pedestrians, bicyclists, and skaters, as well as handicapped persons riding in wheelchairs.

General principles will help the group focus and will provide a standard to evaluate proposed solutions.

In defining the problem and locating solutions, government can be your best friend and your worst enemy at the same time. The policy and money might be in place, but the engineering steps can be the hardest to accomplish. The temptation for advocates is to think that changes can be accomplished quickly once the other side "sees the light." Nothing is further from the truth. Entrenched bureaucracies will tell you that the road was meant for traffic and that traffic has to move. The solution will come in small steps and through the political process.

Once the problem has been defined and the policy you want to change pinpointed, it is smart to suggest a pilot program, even if you have chosen a specific solution. Let's say that you want traffic lights retimed so that cars move at less than 30 miles an hour. Avoid arguing with a traffic engineer about how it can be done while he tells your group why it cannot be done. In this kind of situation, advocacy means locating the political will to effect change. Approach your local politician who oversees the department of transportation. Present the problem and the solution and try to get him or her on your side. Ask a politician what political hurdles must be scaled, whether a pilot project is possible, and whether money can be found in the budget; then do what is asked. For example, if a politician is not convinced about public support of your solution, ask whether a petition or a meeting with concerned citizens can be convincing. Politicians are naturally cautious and do not like to take a stand unless they can defend their decision if a backlash occurs.

Significant public support for change is always necessary. In building public support, start from the bottom and work your way up. Locate key community leaders or endorsements from small groups, and then approach larger groups for support. Never underestimate the power of "word of mouth." I always ask people to talk to everyone they know. If you have a relevant message and outreach is done well, the news will spread quickly even without media coverage. For a small project, neighborhood support is enough; for bigger projects, you might need to form a coalition of groups that support your principles. In either case, in advocacy you can combine building public support with building political support.

You can demonstrate how your solution works and how a politician can look good while working with your group. Bicyclists have a motto: Same road, same rights, same rules. It means that all vehicles on the road must know that they need to share the road—that no one has a monopoly. What better way to illustrate this than to have politicians participate in Bike-to-Work Week by riding in traffic and following the rules of the road?

When you are planning an event, think big, include everybody, and try to institutionalize the event. For example, I participated in the first Bike-to-Work Week in May 1990 in New York City. Transportation Alternatives, of which I was a board member, raised funds for a free breakfast for anyone who showed up with a bike at 8 AM at five locations in each borough of New York City. All were strategic locations on roads where cyclists and bike messengers regularly ride. We were assured of a crowd. We spent many hours discussing how we would convince everyone else that bicycle commuting is not only fun but feasible. Volunteers searched out parking garages where bikes could be parked safely and asked health clubs whether they could offer free showers and a locker for Bike-to-Work Week.

We decided, above all else, to be upbeat. We would publish a brochure stating everything positive about bicycle commuting. One thing we all agreed on was how good a person feels with regular exercise. The brochure said: "Bike commuters save money on fares, tolls, and gas while keeping fit. They save time, avoid subway crowds, and arrive at work energized. Employers of bike commuters are rewarded with increased employee punctuality, reduced transportation costs, lower absenteeism, and increased productivity and mental well-being."

Volunteers produced a 30-second public service announcement to send to television stations, featuring bicycle commuters from all five boroughs—men and women, young and not so young, and African Americans, Asians, and white persons. I drew up several story ideas for the newspapers: interviews with bicycle commuters; a list of bicycle-friendly businesses, from restaurants and theaters to art galleries; and interviews with bicyclists as commuters, bike messengers, and recreational travelers. Further, we offered the media the opportunity, at our free breakfasts, to see a variety of bikes, from uprights to recumbents, and from folding bikes to tandems.

We wrote letters to all politicians and to the department of transportation, announcing the first Bike-to-Work Week and inviting them to attend the breakfast or to ride to work. This was followed by a mailing of the brochure and telephone calls. We made a special effort to get the mayor and borough presidents to attend. Although we were not totally successful in getting politicians to ride, some did so while others sent representatives. In this way, we found city workers who were bicycle commuters and made new contacts for advocates working on the inside of city government to effect changes. New York being New York, we found someone who manufactured bicycles that could be used for small moving jobs or for short-distance deliveries. He agreed to show off his vehicles as well.

To our great surprise the blasé New York media loved the story. The media coverage greatly helped our cause even if it did not convince many people to ride and use their bikes as a mode of transportation. Bike-to-Work Week has now been largely taken over by the department of transportation as a yearly event, as it should be.

Advocates strive to institutionalize policies and events making them part of the new rules people live by. Yet, institutionalizing punitive measures often work against the desired goal. There is an endless debate between bicycling advocates and public health officials who advocate mandatory helmet laws. At many meetings and conferences where bicycling advocates meet, discussions regarding mandatory helmet laws are actively discouraged because the two camps are set in their positions without being willing to concede points to the other side.

As health professionals we would not want to encourage someone to start a potentially dangerous activity without requiring safety precautions. Therefore public health professionals tend to focus on institutionalizing changes by pushing for laws requiring car safety belts and mandatory helmet laws. These laws stipulate that everyone should wear a helmet while riding a bike or buckle up in a car, and those who do not comply can be fined. Bicycle advocates, on the other hand, know how difficult it is to convince people to become bicycle commuters. They tend to favor education first. In 1996, Transportation Alternatives vigorously opposed a New York City mandatory helmet law and won. When news of a proposed law to mandate helmets for bicyclists appeared on an Internet mailing list moderated by Transportation Alternatives, bicyclists mobilized to send E-mail messages to legislators, organized to testify at a hearing regarding the measure, wrote letters, and made telephone calls. As a result, the proposed law was withdrawn.

Nurses know, as do other health professionals who focus on prevention, that telling people what they ought to do does not mean they will follow the advice. The patient needs to have motivation, encouragement, and information that is helpful. So it is with advocacy. In my experience, what works is to offer people something fun to do and an activity that makes them feel good. For example, inviting people on a short ride (such as the one I went on, which advertised discovering your own backyard) is a good idea. Before the ride we offer a quick safety check: do the brakes work, and is the saddle at the right height? We talk about following traffic rules, riding single file, and how to fit a helmet properly. We stress that reliance on a helmet for safety is not enough. Then, after taking a short ride to a point of interest, we talk about our experience of riding on local streets. What does not work is to demonstrate graphically the dangers of bicycling without a helmet. One helmet advocacy group suggests standing on a crate, dropping a watermelon on the ground, and, with the red mush splattered on the floor, pointing out what your brains will look like when you fall from a bicycle without a helmet.

I also found that appealing to people to bicycle for health or to save money is only mildly motivating. People invariably tell you that they decided to bicycle regularly because they enjoyed themselves. And what helps people continue is to help them learn how they can enjoy themselves more by discovering new pleasures.

An event to announce a new map with bicycle routes of neighborhood sites and an appeal for input to add to the map is a good way to get people out of their cars and on the road. These kinds of activities build community support for walking and bicycling and for some of the engineering changes that bicycling and walking advocates would like to see, such as bicycle paths, wider sidewalks, and traffic calming.

There are several national advocacy organizations for biking. The Bicycle Federation of America (BFA) is a policy-oriented group that has the following motto: "Working to create bicycle-friendly and walkable communities through planning, research and program development, professional development, and technical assistance and advocacy." The Pedestrian Federation of America, an offshoot of the BFA, gives similar support to pedestrian advocacy groups.

The League of American Bicyclists (LAB), a national organization of more than 30,000 bicycle advocates, has adopted a new motto: "Healthy communities and the freedom to ride." LAB provides assistance to groups that would like to organize a bike day, week, or month. The group organizes a national Police on Bikes Conference to promote neighborhood safety and publishes a bimonthly magazine *Bicycle USA*. LAB also campaigns to certify "bicycle-friendly communities." To qualify, a town's officials must send LAB documentation that they have taken specific measures to promote bicycling and bicycle commuting, such as observing National Bicycle Month, having a bicycle coordinator on staff and a citizens' bicycle advisory committee, and spending at least $1 per capita per year on bicycle facilities and events. Bicycle-friendly cities include Seattle, Washington; Portland, Oregon; Davis, California; and Tucson, Arizona. LAB would like to see at least 400 bicycle-friendly communities throughout the United States.

Sources of Information about Bicycling

League of American Bicyclists (LAB), 1612 K Street N.W., Suite 401, Washington, DC 20006. E-mail: BikeLeague@aol.com; World Wide Web http://www.bikeleague.org

The Bicycle Federation of America, 1506 21st St., NW, Suite 200, Washington, DC 20036; phone: 202-463-6622; E-mail: bikefed@aol.com

Surface Transportation Policy Project (STPP), 1100 17th St., NW, 10th floor, Washington, DC 20036; phone: 202-466-2636; E-mail: stpp@transact.org; World Wide Web: http://www.transact.org

Chapter *35*

WORKING WITH THE COMMUNITY FOR CHANGE

Mary Ann Christopher, Judith L. Miller, and Theresa L. Beck

School-based comprehensive family service institutes, establishment of a neighborhood school-based health center, a smokeless stove project in Nepal, an environmental cleanup project in urban neighborhoods, community-conducted health fairs, revitalization of an urban school—such have been the community collaborations facilitated by registered nurses (Courtney, Ballard, Fauver, Gariota, & Holland, 1996; Flick, Reese, Rogers, Fletcher, & Sonn, 1994; Klevens, Morina & Cashman, 1992; May, Mendelson, & Ferketich, 1995). In the current climate there are several imperatives that make the ability of nurses to collaborate with communities a particularly relevant and marketable skill. Shrinking revenues for acute care hospitalization, third-party payers concerned with meeting the needs of populations, and reduced reimbursement for services are the variables driving the health care industry to redefine itself (Purdy, Adhikari, Robinson, & Cox, 1994).

This increased emphasis on community is validated in the strategic plans set forth by managed care organizations, the public health sector, and Healthy People 2000. Increasingly, managed care organizations will be expected to address the needs of disenfranchised persons. Meeting the needs of vulnerable subpopulations will require aggressive community outreach efforts and grassroots coalition building. As states seek to redefine the role of the public health sector, increased emphasis will be placed on promoting population-based and community-based initia-

tives. The public health sector will focus more on the monitoring function and less on the delivery of direct personal care services.

As the imperative to work with communities becomes more solidly the foundation of effective health care reform, public health agencies will increasingly attempt to facilitate partnerships linking community health services with coordinating public policy that focuses on effective community collaboration. An emphasis on increased population-based and community-based prevention of disease, injury, disability, and premature death will force a realignment of the role and responsibility of the public health sector. The only way that total system costs will be controlled is to focus significantly on the prevention of illness conditions, which will improve the collective state of health (Primomo, 1995).

Further, an examination of Healthy People 2000 reveals that the ability to implement those objectives is tied to effective community collaboration at the local level. In fact, the report that launched the initiative stated, "Recent research and demonstration projects addressing chronic diseases indicate the preventive approaches that hold the greatest promise are community based, community wide and focus on both individual behavior and societal influences" (Healthy People 2000, in Delgado, 1995). The report went on to say that "prevention programs for minorities are most effective if developed for and with the community."

A FRAMEWORK FOR WORKING WITH COMMUNITIES

What framework should nurses use to build on their strong tradition of community-based leadership? The ability to work effectively with communities is tied to the mastery of three basic concepts: (1) the differentiation between community and population, (2) a broad conceptualization of health, and (3) a methodology that fosters participation.

Community and Population

Understanding the differential concepts of community and population is critical to effective community collaboration. *Population* refers to a collective of individuals with common properties, whereas *community* exists when individuals share a locale and engage in patterns of social interaction, share a common identity and participate in interdependent activities, and work toward shared goals and collective activities. It is this concept of community grounded in locality development that has been the hallmark of effective community collaboration. This model has its emphasis on problem solving by a cross section of community members in a geographical area (Kang, 1995). The failure of Medicaid managed care to have an impact on the immunization rates of children is due in part to managed care organizations' focus on population rather than community. In other words, within a given geographical area, a managed care organization would focus on the needs of its beneficiaries only. Uninsured or underinsured children within that community would not have the benefit of outreach.

At the Visiting Nurse Association of Central New Jersey (VNACJ), an effort to establish a neighborhood advisory council linked to every regional office for the visiting nurses required modification based on the population-versus-community concept. Because of the diversity of socioeconomic, ethnic, and cultural needs of the populations served from individual regional offices, it was evident, through a reduction in participation rates in the councils, that people identify with neighborhood-specific issues. As a result, a strategy has been developed to establish several neighborhood advisory councils in a community, rather than just one council.

Yet another example of this phenomenon was experienced by a neighborhood primary care program based in Massachusetts. Funded by the W. K. Kellogg Foundation, this staff sought to engage community members in the identification of local needs. Implementation of an environmental cleanup project provided evidence that community members responded more appropriately to a street-specific focus rather than a community-wide initiative. As a result, this group has modified its approach to look at smaller advisory groups that are much more geographically confined because of the varying needs in an area (Klevens et al., 1992). Even though this approach is labor intensive, it is the only strategy deemed to be effective.

Conceptualization of Health

Another critical skill in working with communities successfully is to conceptualize and define health broadly. Nurses who are the most effective with community collaboration are those who have a comfort level with program designs that define roles in nontraditional ways. A broad conceptualization of health is based on a definition that encompasses physical, emotional, social and spiritual dimensions of well-being. The importance of the ecological relationship between individuals and their social and physical environments often results in programs' being focused on social and living conditions in the community rather than on the delivery of health care (Flick et al., 1994).

An example of this focus on social and living conditions in the community is an activity that VNACJ engaged in 10 years ago under funding from the Robert Wood Johnson Foundation. Titled the "Supportive Services Program for Older Adults," this project centered around a needs assessment conducted on elderly persons in our service area. Whereas staff identified programs such as geriatric case management, medical adult day care, and respite care as the critical products to be offered through the program, seniors themselves overwhelmingly identified chore and home repair services as their critical need. As a result, the program Your Senior Connection took on a home-repair focus rather than a traditional professional-health-care focus. The outcome of this initiative was that in maintaining the physical structures of seniors' homes, their overall health status was affected positively through reduced falls, less frequent relocation, and lower reported emotional stress.

Another example involved the VNACJ's Mobile Outreach Clinic Program, whereby nurses deliver on-site health assessment and case management to more than 2,000 deinstitutionalized mentally ill residents living in single-room occupancies and boarding homes. When communities identified that the needs of the community were better met by relocating selected numbers of deinstitutionalized mentally ill persons to other counties, the nurses' role changed from a traditional health focus. A nurse actually accompanied the residents on a van throughout the state, easing the anxiety that accompanied their relocation and assisting them in the selection process of a new home. The nurses' presence fostered the residents' ability to make an informed choice. In addition, it demonstrated to communities at large and to policymakers that anticipatory planning must accompany any major policy shift.

A third example goes back to the neighborhood health center funded by the Kellogg Foundation in Boston, where staff of the neighborhood health center engaged members of the community to identify needs. While staff identified issues of substance abuse and acquired immunodeficiency syndrome (AIDS), community members were more concerned with the problem of environmental trash. Thus was born the TLC ["Trash, Lots, and Cars"] project. The health center staff participated in the project by actually working side by side with residents to pick up trash and by mobilizing community leaders to address the need (Klevens et al.,

1992). Through staff participation in the environmental cleanup, the health center emerged as a focal point in the community and the staff members demonstrated their commitment to be an integral part of the community.

Yet another project was the "rural elderly project" in Alabama, funded initially to maintain the independence of elderly persons. The project developed an intergenerational focus in response to community demand. Outcomes of the project included the development of volunteer coalitions to address the activities-of-daily-living needs of elderly persons, to create after-school and summer tutoring programs for children, to develop a referral system to link communities to provider agencies, and to establish a school-based community health center. These outcomes have facilitated the attainment of the project's initial goal, which was to develop a rural health and human services delivery system that was family centered, coordinated, and accessible (Farley, 1995).

Participation Methods

Finally, the third competency that has implications for effective community collaboration is the development of the collective mind-set. The two dimensions of that changed mind-set are the focus on aggregate needs and participative intervention. It is often in ministering to individuals that nurses have the ability to mobilize and facilitate community involvement that contributes to the health of the aggregate (Drevdahl, 1995). The goal of building community collaboration is achieved because barriers are reduced, trust is increased, and common goals are shared.

VNACJ has spent the last several years developing a Neighborhood Nursing philosophy of care, which is built on exactly this premise (Reinhard et al., 1996). As an example, one nurse found that, in her caseload, significant numbers of elderly persons were malnourished, which resulted in frequent hospital readmissions. This observation, based on her care of individual patients, led her to work with the community to develop through local churches an extensive program of home delivered meals for patients who did not meet the eligibility requirements of the federal entitlement program for senior services. Staff working with individuals in communities have the opportunity and responsibility to act on trends that are individually manifested but geographically significant. For example, a community health nurse, after having witnessed the social isolation and depression of seniors living in the only unlocked housing facility in a high crime area, petitioned the town council and the county to secure the building.

The second dimension of the collective mindset is a true belief in the power of partnerships and participation. Participatory approaches are most effective because they increase interpersonal relationships and feelings of personal and political confidence. As an example, neighborhood nurses at VNACJ participate in town parades and city celebration days, often on weekends and holidays. These activities further validate for the community that the organization is a partner and that the nurse is engaged in the fabric of community.

Partnership is defined as the negotiated sharing of power between health professionals and community members (Courtney et al., 1996). The basic condition of partnership is trust, whereby members become confident that other participants will uphold formal and informal agreements. The mutuality in contributions to the partnership means that the professional does not take on all the responsibility, the accountability, or the authority. Partners share a mutual role in determining goals and actions, with the ultimate goal being to enhance the capacity of communities to act more effectively on their own behalf (Kang, 1995).

Issues that must be resolved for community collaboration to work are power and control, protection of turf, competition among partners, and challenges of sustainability (Gauthier & Metteson, 1995). A critical action step is to identify what each partner wants from the relationship. Participation and collaboration are a transformative process in which the community

ceases to view itself as a victim and learns ways to identify and solve problems. Such a process considers cultural relevance not as a barrier but as a matrix through which problems are solved. The feelings of community members are changed from helplessness to efficaciousness (May et al., 1995).

This movement away from victimization was evidenced recently during strategic planning in a blighted urban municipality. Community members insisted on the inclusion of strengths—not just on the traditional problem list and negative statistics. Programs flowing from these assessments must build on strengths rather than be focused solely on need.

It is critical that nurses involved in effective community collaboration guard against the trap of falling into the rhetoric of empowerment. This rhetoric just reinforces the power of the professional and strengthens the view that the professional knows best. According to McKnight (1995), the rhetoric of empowerment has caused competent communities to be invaded, captured, and weakened by mottoes that speak of collaboration and empowerment but actually reinforce feelings of powerlessness (Courtney et al., 1996). Needs of organizations are met, rather than the needs of communities.

An example of the power of collaborative mutuality was demonstrated in a project conducted by community health nurses in a local Hispanic community. As part of an annual festival, a committee of community leaders and health care professionals developed a health fair based on their assessment of need. Although satisfaction rates were positive, overall participation was low. In the second year a committee of peer outreach workers, nurses, and community members determined, through an extensive focus group process, the thrust that the fair should take. More community members actually participated in presenting the fair, with the result that participation increased by 400% (May et al., 1995).

Yet another example of transforming the professional role into a partnership role occurred in an Hispanic urban center when school officials approached nurse practitioners to conduct a school-based health fair. Aware that an overall objective in the community was to increase parental involvement in the school, the nurse practitioners formed a planning committee of parents, invited parents to administer health surveys at the fair, and guided the health club students to run the first-aid booth. The results of this project were so positive that the health fair was replicated in other elementary schools (Courtney et al., 1996).

This mutuality among partners/patients was highlighted when VNACJ and five other service providers were approached by a regional funder to identify a community project. Sensitive to the community's spoken concern that funded activities should be "of the people," the service providers engaged the community in the development of a community leadership program. Applications were distributed throughout the city of Asbury Park, New Jersey, inviting residents to be leaders with an idea to benefit the community. Enthusiasm abounded and many applied, with 10 leaders being selected. After a weekend retreat the leaders met weekly for 12 weeks to learn the history and resources of the city, community development, and leadership skills. The provider agencies, who serve as repositories of the funding, provide a project site and mentorship for the leaders. Among the community projects that the leaders have launched are the following: senior-citizen women working with young, school-aged girls in a program called "Be Yourself, Support Yourself"; a creative cultural arts program for elementary-school children; a "fun to fitness" group of girls aged 5 to 14 years to learn about their bodies and minds; a Haitian program for children aged 14 to 18 years to encourage them in the development of greater cultural understanding and to teach them how to interact within the community; an entrepreneurial training course for older youth, aged 18 to 21 years, to teach them how to set up their own vendor business; a read-aloud group for children aged 6 to 12 years; a performance art program; and an environmental program entitled "We Sea," in which children aged 7 to 12 years are exposed to hands-on activities along the beach. The outcomes of this project were threefold: resolution of community need, development of community pride and well-being, and development of future community leaders.

COMMUNITY ORGANIZING

Participation and collaboration of this kind are supported, not by a traditional medical or health planning model, but by a community organizing approach. In the medical model, community participation is minimal and the health professional maintains control. Community participation is greater in the health planning model; however, the intent is to maximize the resources of the professionally defined program, not those of the community itself. In contrast, in the community organizing approach, the community is mobilized through community participation and control, and the professional is the resource and catalyst for change; the program and direction come from the community itself (Flick et al., 1994).

An example of the community organizing approach is a community health center launched in a medically underserved area by VNACJ. The center is a freestanding organization with a board of trustees derived from local community-based organizations and the community itself, and the role of the nurse practitioners in the center has taken on a form much different from that in other community health centers in a similar geographical locale. For instance, one of the nurse practitioners spends time weekly at the boys' club, the girls' club, and a middle school to provide education on relevant topics such as health and sexuality. In yet another example, the executive director, a nurse practitioner, provides outreach to senior citizens on the issues of substance abuse, medication compliance, and social isolation. This center has truly taken the form of the community it serves because of a board structure that provides the community a forum for input and control.

Another method of ensuring that program and direction come from the community itself is to hire from the community in which an organization operates. This is the basic reason for the success of the peer-worker programs that have been so effective with maternal child health issues and AIDS outreach (Behrman, 1993; Zimmerman, 1993).

Community organizing and participation require three phases of development: locality development, social planning, and social action. In the locality development phase, the outcome is the cultivation of community capacity to provide self-help, with the professional assuming the role of coordinator and enabler. Social planning involves data collection, with the professional assuming the role of fact gatherer and facilitator. During the social action component, there is a shift in the relationship in an attempt to address social injustices and to create institutional change, with the health care professional assuming the role of activist. Community collaboration thus becomes a self-perpetuating process in which residents initiate future activity after the organization's formal role has been completed (Drevdahl, 1995).

Throughout this process, several action steps must be initiated. It is critical that an exploration of environmental conditions that contribute to illness or interfere with wellness be undertaken. Coalitions must be formed to engage the community in the process. Critical dialog must be facilitated with community members, and conditions that interfere with full participation must be changed. Finally, because of the interrelationships among local issues and national and international trends, the global environment must be evaluated relative to the grassroots problem that has been identified. Critical discussions focusing on methods available to change larger sociopolitical structures must be conducted (Drevdahl, 1995).

For instance, the economic situation in a locality, state, or nation has a significant impact on how people live and feel. An example of the relationship among issues is the Welfare to Work initiative occurring nationally. In New Jersey the process for rolling out the Welfare to Work initiative is overseen on a local level by work-

force investment boards comprising welfare beneficiaries and the private and public sectors. A critical issue now being raised is how this initiative will be sustained in the face of large corporate and similar employer downsizing in the area. These are the kinds of discussions in which nurses must meaningfully participate.

VISIONARY LEADERSHIP

Visionary leadership is imperative in effective community collaboration. The visionary leader is one who remains simultaneously tenacious and decisive, as well as caring and flexible. Gardner (1990) summed it up: "They say the purposes of the group are best served when the leader helps the followers to develop their own initiative. It strengthens them in the use of their judgement and involves them to grow and become better contributors."

A recent example at VNACJ involved a collaborative venture with a local Hispanic church. Church leaders and a local physician had identified the need for an on-site primary care center to be situated in a trailer in the church's parking lot. Inquiries by VNACJ about the possibility of collaboration resulted in the organization's management being sought for a consultation role. Initially the VNACJ manager assumed the role of directing the group, designing a nurse practitioner–physician collaborative model, and preparing proposals to foundations. What quickly became apparent was that the physician and the church leaders felt threatened by what they perceived to be a control issue by the manager.

In a meeting between church leaders and the VNACJ administration, the administration asked a simple question: "What would you like us to do?" That simple question, aimed at returning the locus of control to church leaders, resulted in VNACJ's role being defined by the group. VNACJ will continue as a participant, providing on-site nursing, immunization services, and community-based outreach.

A great deal of the success of the leader involves her attention to the external environment (Farley, 1995). Four basic dimensions have been identified as contributing to visionary leadership: management of attention, of meaning, of trust, and of self (Bennis, 1991).

Management of attention is defined as the ability to focus on the vision even in times of uncertainty and chaos. The critical vision that must underlie any community partnership is the fact that professional-citizen mutuality can be sustained even during the transition process. In fact, professional-citizen mutuality must be maintained not only to sustain partnership but to achieve the ultimate vision. VNACJ, in response to community need, developed and began to implement plans for a nurse-managed, community-based primary care center in a high-risk, isolated urban municipality. Stresses within the community were such that political uncertainty existed: controversy among agencies, residents, and city government was the norm. Fourteen city and school elections and reelections had taken place in less than 4 years. In response to the challenge, VNACJ leadership met frequently with both elected officials and city management. However, the players and the agenda often changed from meeting to meeting. Management focused on repeating the same message of our vision and mission. In addition, management joined with residents and colleagues at meetings to state the vision and mission. Foremost in those statements were family and community needs as the core reason for the proposal. The vision prevailed, and the center was awarded a certificate of occupancy by the city and a designation as a Federally Qualified Health Center by the federal government. Keeping mission and community partnership foremost, VNACJ then invited the local health department and the area hospital into partnership—a significant gesture because both had been opponents during the competitive process.

Management of meaning has to do with the ability to communicate. Continuous communication is critical so that professional and citizen participants understand and have input into the direction of the program. For more than 10 years a VNACJ manager had served on the boards and committees of three counties, as well as at the state level. Recognized as an expert in the management of services for persons and families with AIDS or human immunodeficiency virus (HIV), she achieved success in creating partnerships among fiercely competitive organizations as a direct result of her communication style. Through discussion, negotiation, caring, and understanding, she exhibited active listening, which creates a constant feedback loop for participants. She also extended her communication outreach to the grassroots-county and state-level constituencies. As a result of her management of meaning, this regional HIV/AIDS consortium is recognized as a model in the state.

Management of trust is facilitated by ensuring that all stake holders have a place at the table. Community collaboration is enabled by having the same players involved in the community through time (Farley, 1995). On December 11, 1992, the importance of management of trust to the promotion of positive community health outcomes was elucidated as a northeaster ravaged the coast of central New Jersey. VNACJ staff were mobilized to action. Outreach to the American Red Cross, area police departments, and emergency management services resulted in the VNACJ nurses' staffing multiple shelters throughout the area. Because of the decade-long relationships in the communities, staff were able to mobilize local merchants and pharmacists to donate and deliver infant formula, clothing, pharmaceuticals, food, and water to the facilities. Many of these efforts necessitated that these persons be transported by means of police department vehicles from their homes to their places of business. On an infrastructure level, VNACJ brought stakeholders together after the disaster to plan procedures for the future. Issues that were addressed included the temporary placement of frail elderly persons in county long-term care facilities, the emergency release of medications and supplies from area hospitals, and a formalized relationship with VNACJ and the American Red Cross.

Management of self revolves around the leader's understanding of and sensitivity to her own strengths and weaknesses. If the nurse leader is particularly adept at managing and responding to the global environment but is less adept at managing operational details, she must pair her own abilities with the abilities of the group. The leader must always be sensitive to enhancing the visibility and accomplishments of the entire group. This technique has been validated by George (1983): "Successful organizers are those willing to enjoy the reflective glows of others' successes, those that find satisfaction not only in their production but in the production of others."

A program launched by a VNACJ pediatric nurse practitioner (PNP) provides intensive home visiting to vulnerable new patients. Although the PNP brought extensive clinical, managerial, and public health experience to the program, she was not a layperson living within a low-income, blighted urban area. She recruited community members, training them to provide ongoing support and anticipatory guidance. At state and county meetings, the PNP described the success of the program in terms of the peer worker and family accomplishments.

NURSING'S ROLE IN THE COMMUNITY

Working with communities provides the most fertile opportunity for the nursing profession in the next millennium. According to the results of the Pew Health Professions Commission (1996), key competencies that health care professionals will need by the year 2000 include the following: expertise in healthy life styles, preventive and primary care, improved communication skills, and enhanced community health and partnership abilities involving complex negotiations.

The sentiments of the Pew Commission are echoed by former World Health Organization chief nursing scientist Maglacas, who suggests that the process of enabling people to increase control over their health represents the mediating strategy between people and their environment. She goes on to emphasize the critical importance of political advocacy in the role of the nurse in the year 2000 (McMurray, 1991).

Cognizant of the changing expectations of the competencies of registered nurses, Northeastern University College of Nursing, in collaboration with Boston University School of Medicine (Gauthier & Metteson, 1995), established four community health centers with the city department of health and hospitals to revamp nursing education. A center for community health, education, research, and science was created, enabling students participating in this project to spend half of their total clinical time in one neighborhood.

Increasingly it is being urged that the concepts of poverty, caring, and activism be included as building blocks of nursing curricula, with home visits and health strategies the teaching tools employed to reinforce these core competencies (Erickson, 1996). VNACJ, with funding from the W. K. Kellogg Foundation, has developed a competency-based practice model based on the novice-to-expert continuum. Among the skills required for the expert community health nurse are networking, critical thinking, community development, assessment (of individual, family, and community), care planning, leadership, caseload management, clinical and intervention skills, teaching, case finding, and screening.

The role of mentorship will become increasingly critical as society expects nurses to master the art not only of processing information but also of establishing networks and fostering interdisciplinary collaboration (McMurray, 1991). At the foundation of effective community collaboration must be clinical competence. This credibility is essential for nurses as the community turns to them as a resource (McMurray, 1991).

Because of the changing imperatives in the health care delivery system, nurses are uniquely positioned to build on their strong tradition of community-based partnerships. Three concepts that require mastery in this role are a keen understanding of the differentiation between community and population, a broad conceptualization of health, and the development of a collective mind-set. Nurses must seek and understand aggregate data and the community organizing approach. A sensitivity to the larger sociopolitical environment is critical.

Strategies that are essential to succeeding in this role include drawing partners from the grassroots community itself, addressing the needs *of* the community (not *for* the community), facilitating community members' ability to be advocates for themselves, and maintaining relationships with stakeholders through time. As a society, we must be committed to maintaining the well-being of communities—the infrastructure of our culture.

REFERENCES

Behrman, R. E. (1993). *The future of children.* Los Altos, CA: Center for the Future of Children, The David and Lucille Packard Foundation.

Bennis, W. (1991, Winter). Learning some basic truism about leadership. *Phi Kappa Phi Journal, 13.*

Christopher, M. A., & Beck, T. L. (1997). Managed care: Its impact on visiting nurse associations. *Home Health Care Management & Practice, 9*(2), 45–50.

Christopher, M. A., Reinhard, S., McConnell, K., & Mason, D. (1993, January). The community as partner. *Caring,* 44–49.

Cochran, A. (1995, Spring). Empowering patients and nurses through community education. *The Journal of Nurse Empowerment,* 85–86.

Courtney, R., Ballard, E., Fauver, S., Gariota, M., & Holland, L. (1996, June). The partnership model: Working with individuals, families, and communities toward a new vision of health. *Public Health Nursing, 13*(3), 177–186.

DelGado, J. L. (1995, March/April). Meeting the health promotion needs of Hispanic communities. *American Journal of Health Promotion,* 300–311.

Drevdahl, D. (1995, December). Coming to voice: The power of emancipatory community interventions. *Advances in Nursing Science, 18*(2), 13–24.

Erickson, G. P. (1996, June). To pauperize or empower: Public health nursing at the turn of the 20th and 21st centuries. *Public Health Nursing, 13*(3), 163–169.

Farley, S. S. (1995, June). Leadership for developing citizen-professional partnerships: Perspectives on community. *Nursing & Health Care, 16*(4), 226–228.

Flick, L. H., Reese, C. G., Rogers, G., Fletcher, P., & Sonn, J. (1994, Fall). Building community for health: Lessons from a seven-year-old neighborhood/university partnership. *Health Education Quarterly, 21*(3), 369–380.

Gardner, J. W. (1990). *On leadership.* New York: Macmillan.

Gauthier, M. A., & Metteson, P. (1995, November). The role of empowerment in neighborhood-based nursing education. *Journal of Nursing Education, 34*(8), 390–395.

George, I. R. (1983). *Beyond promises: A guide for rural volunteer program development.* Montgomery, AL: Alabama Office of Voluntary Citizen Participation, State of Alabama Commission on Aging.

Glick, D. F., Hale, P. J., Kulbok, P. A., & Shettig, J. (1996, July/August). Community development theory: Planning a community nursing center. *Journal of Nursing Administration, 26,* 44–50.

Jenkins, M. L., & Sullivan-Marx, E. M. (1994, September). Nurse practitioners and community health nurses. *Community Health Nursing and Home Health Nursing, 29*(3), 459–471.

Kang, R. (1995). Building community capacity for health promotion: A challenge for public health nurses. *Public Health Nursing, 21*(5), 312–318.

Klevens, R., Morina, & Cashman, S. (1992). Special contribution: Transforming a neighborhood health center into a community-oriented primary care practice. *American Journal of Preventive Medicine, 8*(1), 62–65.

May, K. M., Mendelson, C., & Ferketich, S. (1995, February). Community empowerment in rural health care. *Public Health Nursing, 12*(1), 25–30.

McKnight, J. (1995). *The careless society: Community and its counterfeits.* New York: Basic Books.

McMurray, A. (1991). Advocacy for community self-empowerment. *International Nurse, 38*(1), 19–21.

Partners in the community. (1995, April). *Critical Care Nurse/Critical Visions,* 16–18.

Pew Health Professions Commission, Third Report. (1994). *Critical challenges: Revitalizing the health professions for the twenty-first century.* Philadelphia: Pew Foundation.

Primomo, J. (1995, April). Ensuring public health nursing in managed care: Partnerships for healthy communities. *Public Health Nursing, 12*(2), 69–71.

Purdy, A. F., Adhikari, G., Robinson, S., & Cox, P.

(1994, Fall). Participating health development in rural Nepal: Clarifying the process of community empowerment. *Health Education Quarterly, 2*(3), 329–343.

Redman, B. K. (1993, May/June). How to bring primary care back to patients. *Journal of American Health Policy,* 42–45.

Reinhard, S., Christopher, M. A., Mason, D. J., McConnell, K., Toughill, E., & Rusca, P. (1996). Promoting healthy communities through neighborhood nursing. *Nursing Outlook, 44*(5), 223–228.

Russell, K. (1994). Community care management and the emergence of new partnerships for health. *Public Health Nursing, 11*(2), 140–141.

Skelton, R. (1994). Nursing and empowerment:

Concepts and strategies. *Journal of Advanced Nursing, 19,* 415–423.

Suppiah, C. (1994, February). Community mothers: Working in partnership with community mothers. *Health Visitor, 67*(2), 51–53.

Whelan, E. M. (1995, March-April). The health corner: A community-based nursing model to maximize access to primary care. *Public Health Reports,* 184–188.

Zerwekh, J. V. (1992, February). Public health nursing legacy, historical practical wisdom. *Nursing & Health Care, 13*(2), 84–91.

Zimmerman, M. (1993, April). Opening doors for healthier families: How to start a resource mothers program. *Implementation Guidelines,* 9–13.

VIGNETTE

Environmental Health Policy: Environmental Justice

Lillian H. Mood

In late December 1995 the South Carolina Department of Health and Environmental Control (DHEC) received an application from SERR, Inc., for a permit to construct and operate a landfill. The landfill is proposed to receive debris, including asbestos, from construction and demolition projects. By the time the application was received, two important steps had already been taken. First, the applicant had bought a tract of land just outside the city limits of the county seat in a small rural county and adjacent to a neighborhood known as the Helena community. Second, the applicant had applied to the county council and had received a *letter of consistency,* stating that this project was consistent with the county's solid waste management plan, a prerequisite in state statute for DHEC consideration of the permit application.

Other actions had also been taken. A group of citizens from the nearby neighborhood, the Involved Citizens of Helena, had appeared before the county council, asking the council not to approve the project and asking the applicant to

choose adifferent site for his business. The council's response was to send a second letter to DHEC, expressing "unanimous opposition to the location." The applicant's response, as reported in the local newspaper, was that he "would not come into a community where he was not wanted."

The citizens left the council meeting feeling relieved, thinking they had averted what they saw as a damaging addition to their neighborhood, only to learn afterward that the application had been submitted and the county administrator had informed DHEC that the second letter did not rescind the required letter of consistency. I had been alerted to the brewing situation by one of our field staff who sent me the news account of the council meeting, but my active involvement began with a call from the permitting staff in our state office, asking for help with a citizen request for a "public hearing" on the permit application.

My job is entitled "director of risk communication and community liaison." I work in the

Deputy Area of Environmental Quality Control (EQC) in the state agency charged with responsibility for public health and environmental protection, which includes responsibilities delegated by the U.S. Environmental Protection Agency (EPA). After 22 years in public health nursing, in home health services, and on the commissioner's staff, I transferred to EQC because, in the deputy commissioner's words, the environmental programs "needed a nurse." He was speaking of an increased requirement and demand for public participation in regulatory decision making. Through the years his staff of engineers and other environmental scientists had experienced the recurring nightmare of public meetings where they were battered by anger, accusations, and criticism. "Is it safe, or not?" "Why are you taking so long?" "Just make them stop polluting!" "I don't trust you government people." The messages were, You are not doing enough, you are not acting quickly enough, you are not letting people know enough, and we don't trust you!

Why a nurse? My position is not discipline specific, but my background means that I am comfortable in communities and with citizens in settings where many of our environmental experts feel least comfortable. Calls to my office may come from citizens, from our field and/or state program staff, from legislators, or from agency management. I am a safe place and a safe person to call and ask for information or help or to report a problem. Callers may identify themselves or not, though I always ask if there is a way that I can get back in touch with them. Part of the job is responding to specific concerns. A call may involve a complaint, an inquiry, or the need to get information out to the public on a permit, a spill, or a cleanup plan.

When a call relates to a specific site or situation, I put great importance on *being there*, and so it was with the call about the Helena landfill. After getting a little background information from my co-worker, I asked who had requested the public hearing and was given the name and telephone number of a retired schoolteacher and administrator. I called Mr. R and asked whether I could visit him to hear and understand his concerns.

I went to Mr. R's home, armed with the knowledge that our staff was willing to have a meeting even before we reached a point in the process where the law calls for a "public hearing." The date, place, and format were up to me to coordinate. As I sat at Mr. R's dining room table and looked at and listened to the evidence of the citizens' effort, I was impressed with the energy, insight, and commitment of this community to preserve the character of a place they were trying to maintain and improve. I got an even more vivid picture as we drove through the neighborhood and around the site. The Helena community traces its history to the mid-1800s; it was once a township. It has always been a predominantly African American community (99%+), and many residents have a low income. A number of community members who have achieved greater prosperity have chosen to build homes and remain in the community. They are proud of the three churches in the neighborhood and of the plans to build a new middle school nearby. The sense of place, of belonging, and of community spirit is strong. Also strong is the belief that we can accomplish much if we work together, within the community and with institutions such as elected bodies and state agencies. Quiet dignity and persistence were strengths evident on my first contact and were consistent throughout my work with my citizen colleagues in Helena.

We did hold a public meeting on an evening convenient for the residents and in their preferred meeting place (the county courthouse). Those attending included more than 100 citizens, our staff, the applicant, the county administrator, members of the county council, the state senator, a candidate for the state house of representatives (formerly an attorney for DHEC), and the local news media. Citizen attendance was boosted by Mr. R's assistance in distributing flyers that were prepared by our media relations staff. I served as the moderator for the lively and sometimes heated exchange of issues and information.

When the evening ended, we had a clear map of the issues, which fell into three major policy areas: land use, technical requirements of environmental law and regulations that are designed to protect the public health, and environmental justice.

Land use policy is primarily and predominantly a responsibility of local government. Restrictions on use of land and planning for orderly growth are the products of local ordinances, both city and county. The county council determines where the boundaries lie between commercial, industrial, and residential areas in an unincorporated area. In this county, and in a number of others in South Carolina, councils have been silent on this policy issue. There are no land use ordinances to guide development, restrict how an individual may use his property, or protect his neighbors from an undesirable use.

Environmental law and regulations are administered by a combination of state and federal jurisdictions. The waste management laws are state statutes, and DHEC is delegated the authority by the EPA to enforce the applicable federal requirements. Issues such as protection of wetlands and groundwater, management of stormwater runoff, and protection of air quality are addressed in this policy arena. Permits issued by DHEC to landfill owners and operators specify requirements for construction and operation to protect public safety and environmental quality. DHEC field staff monitor compliance with the requirements of the permits and for any evidence of environmental damage. Enforcement action for violations can be civil action, through the process defined by the State Administrative Procedures Act, or criminal, if the permit holder "willfully and knowingly" violates the law. Every permit requirement and every enforcement action must withstand the scrutiny and challenge of legal appeals by the applicant or any person or group with legal standing to appeal. The appeals go through staff review, to DHEC's citizen board, which is appointed by the governor and approved by the state senate to govern the agency, and on to the court(s) with jurisdiction.

Environmental justice is a concept that invokes the protection of the federal Civil Rights Act to ensure that low-income and minority communities do not bear a disproportionate burden of environmental pollution or degradation. In 1994 President Clinton added substantial weight to this principle in Executive Order 12898 by requiring every federal agency to make "environmental justice part of its mission by identifying and addressing, as appropriate, disproportionately high and adverse human health or environmental effects of its programs, policies, and activities on minority populations and low-income populations." There is not yet a body of case law clarifying what conditions and what criteria are sufficient to support a decision based on ensuring environmental justice.

Two unexpected possible solutions also emerged from that early public meeting. A county councilman said that DHEC should have communicated directly with the council rather than the administrator on the apparent contradiction in the letters we received. We said we would revisit that issue with the council. Citizens began to hope that the council would rescind the letter of consistency, which would stop the DHEC permitting process but would likely lead to the applicant's filing suit against the council. The second possible solution came as an offer by another councilman to meet with the applicant to discuss a possible "land swap" for a more suitable site. Again, hopes rose that an amicable solution could be found. Although, in this case, neither of these solutions has reached fruition, I am convinced, and continue to advocate, that convening parties with disparate agendas and facilitating civil discussions can lead to win-win outcomes unavailable if we employ only adversarial methods to resolve issues.

An expected question from the citizens in the public meeting was directed to us as regulators: "Do you have or would you want a landfill in your neighborhood?" We responded that we would not want to share our neighborhoods with a landfill. This acknowledgment of common ground on the undesirability of landfills in residential areas was important because it not only affirmed the reasonableness of the citizens' objective but also has kept the focus on what we have the legal authority to do, not on what we might *want* to do. It has also freed me to state openly and candidly, in my conversations with citizens and elected officials and in staff policy discussions, that my agenda is to find a legally defensible way to "do the right thing."

At the time of this writing, this story has not reached its conclusion. We did confirm with the county council members their decision that the proposed landfill is consistent with their plan for waste management. We recognize that they see benefits in avoiding litigation, in gaining the 50¢-per-ton revenue for the county from the landfill's operation, and in attracting additional industrial development by having the infrastructure for industrial waste disposal.

The environmental justice questions are being pursued in several ways. Our staff prepared maps, using Geographic Information Systems (GIS) technology, to examine patterns of landfill locations and the demographics of the population. We did not find a pattern of siting in minority communities. One of our senior managers and I took the maps to Mr. R and a minister from the citizen group and went over what we had done, so that they would have this information before the hearing. The issue of whether census block data are specific enough to make judgments about nearest-neighbor populations was raised in the hearing, and the citizens' attorney signaled an intent to make environmental justice an issue. The citizens, however, have put their initial focus on unfair treatment, treatment that discriminates on the basis of race, on the county council's actions. They have filed a complaint with the U.S. Justice Department, citing Title VI of the Civil Rights Act.

Our staff completed its review of the technical issues and issued public notice of a draft permit, with a prescribed comment period and a public hearing. Again with the assistance of Mr. R, flyers were distributed and a notice was published in the newspaper. This time there were about 200 citizens who spoke "on the record," citing the reasons for their opposition to the landfill. My role was to work with the citizens to get the speakers in the order they wished, to welcome people, to honor one citizen's request that he begin by offering a prayer, and then to explain how the procedure for a formal hearing would be different from our earlier meeting. Then I listened. A hearing officer and a court reporter took responsibility for managing the hearing. I felt admiration for the thoroughness with which the citizens got every point that I could think of into the formal proceedings. It was also gratifying to see the support they had assembled: the leader of a statewide environmental advocacy organization, a competent and articulate attorney to serve as their legal counsel, and the newly elected state representative, who has become their effective advocate. In addition, we have responded to inquiries on their behalf from a U.S. Senator and from legal counsel in the governor's office.

The staff's work after the hearing was to consider each of the issues raised, prepare a written response, and reach a final decision on whether the permit should be issued. In that process, two new laws affected the application: one was a more restrictive limit on the area of wetlands that could be affected, and the second was a provision that the landfill area (the "footprint") could not be within 1000 feet of the nearest residence. The combined effect of these two factors resulted in a decrease by nearly one third in the area available for landfill use. Despite these limitations, the applicant revised his plans accordingly and continued his pursuit of a permit.

When the staff completed their review and their response to all the issues noted at the hearing, the permit engineer, two senior management staff, and I met with representatives of the Involved Citizens group to go over the changes in the application and the staff conclusion that all the permit requirements had been satisfied. In addition to four members of the citizens' group, we were joined by the state representative and one of the white owners of the adjacent land. The representative requested that we delay a decision until we obtain a court opinion on the status of a regulation cited at the hearing. The adjacent-land owner asked that we allow him additional time to negotiate a different site with the applicant, and the Helena citizens expressed their despair that any public concerns would affect the outcome.

When we displayed two maps showing the effect of the two new laws on the landfill area, the landowner said: "Wait a minute! My father just put a mobile home on the shore of the pond at the corner of the property. I know it is within 1000 feet of the landfill!" On inspection, and after verification that the mobile home met the definition of a "residence" (a well, a waste disposal system permit, and a county seal), the applicant was notified that the permit could not be issued because the plans as presented violated the 1000-foot buffer. Within hours the applicant submitted a revised application that met the requirement and further decreased the area of the footprint by 20%.

The staff called me on vacation to tell me that the permit had been issued, and when I returned, I learned that the citizens had filed an appeal.

Any of several outcomes can be envisioned at this point in the process:

1. *The applicant could withdraw his application or find a different site.* The owner of the adjacent land has met with the applicant to propose alternative locations. The applicant's attorney (also a former DHEC attorney) told me that he would advise his client to take that option if a reasonable alternative is available. Another suggestion has been that the citizens offer to help defray the applicant's environmental investigation costs for a new site with resources they would otherwise invest in litigation. At present, the applicant seems unwilling to consider an alternative site.

2. *The county council could decide to rescind its letter of consistency.* Although there was renewed energy among some of the citizens at the hearing to approach the council once again, I admit that I think there is a low probability of such an outcome.

3. *The administrative law judge hearing the appeal could find that the regulation cited by the citizens' attorney and their representative is grounds for denial of the permit.* The regulation cited has not previously been applied in similar applications. The DHEC legal staff is examining the implications of its application in this case. The finding and recommendation of the administrative law judge would have to be upheld by the DHEC governing board. If the citizen position is supported by the board, the applicant is almost certain to appeal to the courts. The citizens have stated that they will continue their appeal if their position is not supported by the board.

The appeals process will mean investment of time and resources by all parties in an ultimate win-lose outcome. If the permit is finally granted, we can expect that our field staff will invest considerable effort and time in monitoring the landfill's operation and in responding to complaints. The citizens have assured us that they will continue to oppose the landfill, "even after it is permitted." In their words, they "do not intend to be good neighbors." They will never welcome an entity that "kills people's dreams. When you kill dreams, you kill people. What child can hope and aspire to achieving when his daily view is a 'dump'?"

In reviewing my own and my professional colleagues' participation in this project, I hear five recurring themes of public expectations, and I use them as my personal quality indicators. Repeatedly, in many different ways, citizens tell me they expect us to:

1. Listen
2. Take them seriously
3. Treat them with respect
4. Give them straight information
5. Do what we say we will do

My assessment is that we have been true to these standards with the Helena community.

When agency regulatory decisions are in litigation, communications are more formal and less open. I have indicated in a letter to the citizens that I am still available to them, but I know it is not likely that they will look to me for any assistance. The legal documents in an appeal will state "DHEC vs. the Involved Citizens of Helena." If they are successful in their appeal, it will seem that they won in spite of the actions of the agency charged with protecting them, not with our help and support.

I will continue to articulate the citizens' perspective in policy discussions, and I will be an advocate for aggressively using whatever tools we have to prevent the problems this facility may bring. I will be working with staff who feel the stress of the legal limits of their regulatory authority to address community priorities in a political climate that is sensitive to "government interference" in individual property rights and where great value is placed on economic development. Part of my job will be to explain the process as it unfolds and to interpret the reasoning behind the decisions to a variety of people. Perhaps most important, I will continue to search for ways to ensure that a broad definition of healthy communities is supported in public policy.

Chapter 36

POLICY, POLITICS, AND FOUNDATIONS

SHIRLEY GIROUARD AND PAULINE M. SEITZ

Public policies emerge from a complex set of interactions. Often not recognized is the important influence of philanthropy on the development and implementation of policy. The Robert Wood Johnson Foundation's work promoting school-based health clinics illustrates the potential significance of foundation activities on local, state, and federal policy. School-based clinics, adopted by communities across the country, have demonstrated their value and the value of the advanced practice nurses who provide care in these clinics. The result has been that local school districts have raised money through taxes and other levies to support the clinics, state legislatures have reexamined the laws and regulations governing the practice of nurses in school-based clinics, and federal agencies have funded school-based clinic services.

Foundations in the United States have played and continue to play a major role in influencing the health care system. Thus nurses and nursing are directly and indirectly affected by the decisions that foundations make about what and who they choose to fund. As the organization, delivery, and financing of the health care system undergo rapid change, funding for innovative ideas, research, and education is changing as well. Devolution and other changes in financing also influence the current funding climate. Philanthropy, influenced by policy and political action, needs stake holders—such as nurses—to be involved in a variety of ways to maximize their influence on philanthropic decisions about what and whom to fund.

Foundations are private, not-for-profit organizations that provide support for the work of other not-for-profit organizations such as nursing schools, hospitals, health care organizations, and research centers. Foundations generally support activities and innovative ideas not usually addressed by government or other traditional funding sources. As Dr. Leighton Cluff, former president of the Robert Wood Johnson Foundation, states: "Only by having a group of institutions that are free to try quite different routes from those required of government can we be assured that we are protected from the hazards of an increasingly centralized decision making process" (Cluff, 1996, p. 32).

Although the proportion of funds available through philanthropic organizations remains relatively small in comparison to total health care spending—less than 1%—the role of foundation funding has taken on greater importance in recent years. With the downsizing of government that began in 1994, there is increasing pressure to find new sources of support for projects traditionally funded by public dollars. Decreased funding for clinical research is being reported and is expected to increase with the growth of managed care. This relates to the decline in revenues, which many believe will threaten the ability of health care organizations to meet their research and teaching missions. Public funds, particularly those of the federal government, answer more immediate needs of the nation, such as those associated with Medicare and Medicaid. In addition, a large portion of public money is targeted for biomedical research, as opposed to fostering programmatic innovations or health services research—both more likely to be done by nurses and to have a greater and more immediate impact on nursing practice and education.

Contributing to the current climate are growing pressures on health care organizations to reduce spending. Thus, fewer dollars are available at the organizational level for innovations and research. As Dr. Cluff (1996) states, this situation:

> makes it difficult for certain kinds of new untested ideas to gain the support needed for an adequate trial or implementation. This also makes it difficult to provide opportunities for individualized, locally-tailored initiatives in health care to emerge. . . . In contrast to public agencies, health-oriented foundations can put their resources into programs that have the long-term objective of improving health care in the future.

Nurses have increased their influence on philanthropy in recent years as foundation officers, as leaders of major foundation initiatives, and as grant recipients. Given the changing climate in health care and the competition for funding, these efforts are increasingly important. The benefits that result from seeking and obtaining grants and working with and within foundations accrue at three levels. Society benefits when the knowledge and expertise of the nursing profession are applied to solving the challenges facing the health care system. The profession of nursing will benefit from the status and recognition associated with obtaining grants and being affiliated with prestigious grant-making organizations. Individual nurses who successfully compete for grants will obtain support for their research or program and gain recognition associated with outside funding.

This chapter will provide an overview of foundations and general information and additional resources that may be of use to readers interested in grant-making activities and philanthropic support. In addition, the ways that foundations have an impact on nursing education and practice will be used as examples of major philanthropic efforts that influence the nursing profession and the health care system. The chapter will identify some of the ways in which nurses and the profession are engaged in influencing the work of foundations. In conclusion, the chapter will provide suggestions for enhancing the profession's and the individual nurse's roles in philanthropy.

FOUNDATIONS IN THE UNITED STATES

Foundation Giving

There are presently 38,807 grant-making foundations in the United States (Renz, Qureshi, & Mandler, 1996). The total number of foundations grew by 3.3% from 1993 to 1994, and $11.3 billion was given in grants—an increase of 1.6% from 1993 to 1994. Private support, of which foundation grants are a small portion, represents less than 20% of the revenue of voluntary organizations. As reported by The Foundation Center (Renz et al., 1996), there have been a number of significant recent trends that are important to nurses and nursing:

- Support for education and human services has increased.
- Support for health care has declined sharply, from 18.2% of all grant dollars to 15.2%, the lowest ever reported.
- Funding for children and youth has increased.
- Funding for minorities has declined.

Types of Foundations

The term *foundation* can be confusing, especially since organizations of providers and others have begun using the term in their titles. Foundations and other types of charitable organizations differ operationally and legally. In addition, there are differences in the types of private foundations that influence their development and philanthropic giving. The Foundation Center (Renz et al., 1996) defines private foundations as organizations that are nongovernmental and not for profit. These organizations derive their funds, dispersed primarily through grants, from endowments. Grants are generally made to nonprofit organizations for activities that serve the public good, such as education, social programs, and health care.

There are four basic types of foundations in the United States, each with its own unique characteristics (Renz et al., 1996):

1. *Independent foundations* are the most numerous. They are independent grant-making organizations that aid charitable activities. The funds to support (endow) these foundations generally come from an individual or family. Funding decisions may be made by the donor, a board, or others acting for the foundation. Approximately 70% of these foundations limit their grant making to a local area. The Robert Wood Johnson Foundation and the Ford Foundation are examples of large, independent foundations with a national focus.
2. *Company-sponsored foundations,* also called corporate foundations, are established by a business for philanthropic purposes. Although funded by the business, they are separate legal entities. Funds come from the for-profit activities of the organization. Funding decisions are generally made by corporation officials but may also be made by other representatives on the foundation board. Examples include the Baxter Foundation, Inc., and the Merck Company Foundation.
3. *Community foundations* are publicly sponsored, deriving their financial support from a number of donors. They generally make grants in a specific community or region, with decisions made by representatives from the community. The New York Community Foundation and the San Francisco Foundation are examples.
4. *Operating foundations* are established for a specific purpose, such as conducting research with funds from a single source and public donations. They use their own resources to conduct research or provide services, with decisions made by an independent board. Few grants are made outside the foundation. Examples include the David C. Cook Foun-

dation, the Rockwell Foundation, and the Howard Hughes Foundation.

Foundation Priorities

Private foundations play a major role in the development of health policy and health care programs by providing support for ideas and activities not generally within the domain of government or other organizations. Foundations maximize their influence by:

- Contributing to the health policy debate through identifying, evaluating, and analyzing health and related issues
- Developing, testing, evaluating, and disseminating new ideas and models
- Facilitating, coordinating, and convening leaders in the field to stimulate change

These approaches are made operational by funding activities such as research, demonstration and evaluation projects, conferences, publications, and the education and training of health professionals. Foundations provide general, capital, and program support; provide funds for student aid, research, technical assistance; and support program evaluation. Decisions regarding funding priorities relate to the nature of the foundation and the influence of its board or other decision makers. In larger foundations, staff members play a major role in the decision about funding priorities and the awarding of grants.

In recent years, funding for health represents only 15.2% of grant dollars, a significant decline from the 25% for health in the 1980s (Renz et al., 1996). The Foundation Center reported the following distribution of these grant dollars in 1994:

- 35% to hospitals and medical care
- 20% to medical research
- 12% to mental health
- 9% to specific diseases
- 7% to public health
- 7% to reproductive health care
- 4% to policy and management

- 4% to general and other rehabilitative services
- 2% to health care financing

The following major foundations include health in their funding priorities:

- The W. K. Kellogg Foundation, with assets of $6,034,576,655 (1995). Funding priorities include projects designed to improve human well-being through adult continuing education, problem-focused community-based health services, a wholesome food supply, and broadening of the leadership capacity of individuals.
- The Robert Wood Johnson Foundation, with $5,257,995,582 (1995) in assets. Established as a national philanthropy in 1972 and today the largest U.S. foundation devoted to health care, the Robert Wood Johnson Foundation concentrates its grant making in three areas: to ensure that all Americans have access to basic health care at reasonable cost; to improve the way services are organized for and provided to people with chronic health conditions; and to promote health and reduce the personal, social, and economic harm caused by substance abuse—tobacco, alcohol, and illicit drugs.
- The Pew Charitable Trusts, with assets of $3,778,481,571 (1995). In the spring of 1997, officials announced that they were evaluating their national health and human services program to determine how best to respond to the significant changes taking place in the health care and social services environments. During this planning process they will not be making new awards for national activities in the areas of care of elderly persons, care of infants and children and their families, and community development.
- The John D. and Catherine T. MacArthur Foundation, with $3,297,625,923 (1995) in assets. Six major initiatives include the health program for research in mental health and the psychological and behavioral aspects of health and rehabilitation.

- The Rockefeller Foundation, with assets of $2,523,653,744 (1995). Activities are concentrated on science-based international development in agriculture, health, and population sciences; arts and humanities; and equal opportunity.
- The Andrew W. Mellon Foundation, with $2,485,168,000 (1995) in assets. In health funding, the emphasis is on medical and public health education and research and on population control.

THE IMPACT OF FOUNDATIONS ON HEALTH CARE

History

Historically, philanthropy has contributed importantly to the health status of both the United States and the world through research on the control or cure of disease. The attack on the massive epidemics that wracked the world only a few generations ago was led by the Rockefeller Foundation. The Rockefeller Sanitary Commission and the International Health Board significantly reduced the scourges of hookworm, malaria, and yellow fever. The Rockefeller Institute of Medical Research remains a world-class center for research into the basic phenomena of living systems and how they are expressed in disease.

The swift expansion of government funding for medical research since World War II, particularly through the National Institutes of Health, has made the role of foundations in this area much less prominent. However, they have maintained a leadership position in a few fields in which the government has elected not to play a role. For example, the government has not led the way in the fields of reproductive biology and contraceptive technology.

Efforts to strengthen education for the health professions have probably been the most sustained endeavor of the work of foundation philanthropy in the health arena. In 1910, under a project funded by the Carnegie Foundation for the Advancement of Teaching, Abraham Flexner completed a landmark report, *Medical Education in the United States and Canada,* which challenged medicine to develop as a science-based profession, firmly rooted in the university. During the ensuing years, the General Education Board, a Rockefeller philanthropy, invested more than $100 million to help this concept take hold as a national standard.

By the 1950s, however, it was apparent that the phenomenal growth in the scientific-technological content of medical practice was driving medical schools and the medical profession toward a complex and fragmented system of sophisticated specialty care. General and primary care were vanishing as domains of teaching and practice, and communities across the country were having difficulty in obtaining generalist physicians.

The response of foundations was rapid and important. The Robert Wood Johnson Foundation and the Kaiser Family Foundation, among others, initiated major grant programs to prepare generalist physicians in such key practice fields as internal medicine, family medicine, and pediatrics. Simultaneously, programs were initiated to ensure that the primary care needs of underserved minority communities were met. Support was given to medical schools (such as Meharry Medical College) that trained the greatest number of minority physicians, as well as to mainstream schools. The Macy Foundation, the Commonwealth Fund, and the Robert Wood Johnson Foundation were among the foundations that supported these efforts.

Foundations and Nursing Education

The role of foundations in nursing education has been less robust than in medicine; nevertheless, it continues to be an important factor in nursing's struggle to establish itself as a learned profession. The Rockefeller Foundation helped advance the concept of nursing as a university-based discipline through its support for the Committee for the Study of Nursing. The committee's report, prepared by Josephine Goldmark and issued in 1923, recommended the establishment of university schools to prepare nurse leaders. A few such schools were founded, for example, the Yale School of Nursing, but relatively little progress was made. After World War II the Russell Sage Foundation commissioned another study of nursing. Headed by Lucille Brown, this study also recommended that the preparation of nurses be based in institutions of higher education. This has been achieved less by the university than by the rise of the community college, a movement that was fostered particularly by the W. K. Kellogg Foundation.

Preparation of nurses at the graduate and advanced graduate levels has been a principal interest of several foundations. The aim has been to prepare scholar-clinicians in the field who can bring leadership to nursing research, teaching, and practice. The Robert Wood Johnson Clinical Nurse Scholars Program (now completed) was a significant effort in postdoctoral education, and its Nurse Faculty Fellowships Program (also completed) was a master's-level initiative to equip a cadre of faculty for leadership roles in preparing clinical nurse specialists in primary care. Graduates of this program helped to establish nurse practitioner education within the mainstream of the nation's graduate programs in nursing.

Professional education in public health nursing was started under foundation auspices. The first school of public health was founded in 1913 at Johns Hopkins University with funding from the Rockefeller Foundation. In the ensuing years, Rockefeller provided major funding for 22 additional university schools in 17 countries. Recently, the W. K. Kellogg Foundation established a program featuring collaborative training among schools of public health, local health departments, and community health services.

Foundations and Health Care Services

Many foundations, in addition to their pioneering work in research and their long-term interest in the education of health professionals, have contributed to the nation's systems and arrangements for providing health services. For example, the prototype of the American community hospital was developed by the Commonwealth Fund through long-term support for more than a dozen model hospitals across the country. The features of these institutions, including open staffs and community boards, were adopted in the federal Hill-Burton legislation in 1948.

The Commonwealth Fund and the Kaiser Family Foundation took an early interest in prepaid group practice. The fund's support for the Harvard Community Health Plan helped this institution emerge as a standard setter for the burgeoning growth of health maintenance organizations. The Robert Wood Johnson Foundation has participated with scores of local and regional foundations in testing and implementing improved care systems to address a number of needs, such as regional emergency medical response systems and school-based primary care clinics.

Recent Trends and Issues

More recent grant-making interests and trends in philanthropy have included increased attention to our national capacity in health services research, the reformulation of medical education, and attention to vulnerable groups—elderly persons, mothers and infants, persons with chronic mental illness, homeless persons, and families. Foundations also are beginning to work on many of the behavioral problems that have enormous negative health consequences for society, among them human immunodeficiency virus infection and acquired immunodeficiency syndrome, the use of addictive substances, child abuse, and family dysfunction and violence.

Changes in the organization, delivery, and financing of health care, particularly the move to managed care, have prompted a number of foundations to fund projects to assess the access, quality, organization, and delivery of health care services. The Robert Wood Johnson Foundation's project to track health system changes and the Kaiser Family Foundation's Medicaid project are examples of major initiatives in this area. One of the major changes that may result in both an increase in philanthropic dollars and changes in the focus of health care funding relates to the sale of not-for-profit health care facilities to for-profit entities. These conversions, described as a transaction shifting all or most of the assets of a not-for-profit health care organization to for-profit purposes (Claxton, Feder, Shactmon, & Altman, 1997), raise a number of political and policy issues of concern to nurses. For example: How will the money from the sale be used? Who will determine how the money is used? Nurses will need to be aware of and involved in the process, including influencing state and federal laws and regulations that establish the legal environment for health care organizations and regulate the conversion of hospitals.

If appropriate interventions do not take place, the charitable assets of health care organizations may be lost to the community. As a condition of the sale, many states are requiring that a foundation be established to offset the loss of the charitable contribution to the community and to convert profits for community benefit. According to Stephen Isaacs (author of *Health Care Conversion Foundations,* a report funded by the Robert Wood Johnson Foundation for dissemination through Grantmakers in Health), there were 79 conversion foundations as of July 1997. Ten of these conversions were formed in 1994, nineteen in 1995, and seventeen in 1996. These new foundations had combined assets in excess of $9.3 billion dollars at the end of 1996. If these new foundations give out 5% of their assets annually, as private foundations are required to do by law, their donations will bring $465 million per year into American philanthropy (S. Isaacs, personal communication, 1997).

California, where large conversions have taken place, illustrates how legislative action can influence the direction of conversion. Vigilant consumer advocacy for a legislative mandate that required Blue Cross of California to distribute the full value of its assets to a charitable trust resulted in the availability, from conversions, of almost $4 billion dollars for health care philanthropy in California. This has not been the case in states such as Georgia, where legislation enabled Blue Cross/Blue Shield to convert to for-profit status with no obligation to use its assets for the public benefit (Tein, 1997). Alert health professionals and consumers can "follow the money" when transformations of nonprofit assets to for-profit statuses are proposed and be ready to press for public hearings to ensure that the public has a voice in the disbursement of the assets and appointment of board members for the new foundation.

NURSING AND PHILANTHROPY

The mission statements of national philanthropies are often stated in fairly global terms to allow the organization flexibility in translating its philosophic goals into specific program funding activities. For example, the role of the Robert Wood Johnson Foundation is to "improve the health and health care of all Americans." The mission of the Pew Charitable Trusts is to seek the "empowerment of the individual—the right and ability of the individual to achieve or express his or her full potential." The W. K. Kellogg Foundation is concerned with the application of knowledge to solve the problems of people. The Helene Fuld Trust awards grants "to promote the health, education and welfare of enrolled student nurses who are being taught to care for the sick and injured at the bedside."

The Pew Charitable Trusts

The health professions, and consequently the nursing profession, are a consistent focus area of philanthropies interested in American health care. In 1990 the Pew Charitable Trusts created the Pew Health Professions Commission, which, through a series of reports, has recommended changes in the health professions' education and work force policy. The recommendations for the nursing profession in the 1996 report entitled *Critical Challenges: Revitalizing the Health Professions for the Twenty-first Century* include the following:

- Recognition of the value of the multiple entry points to professional practice

- Consolidation of professional nomenclature so that there is a single title for each level of nursing preparation and service
- Distinction between the practice responsibilities of the different levels of nursing by focusing associate preparation on the entry-level hospital setting and nursing home practice, baccalaureate preparation on hospital-based case management and community-based practice, and master's preparation for specialty practice in hospital and primary care, with strengthening of existing career ladder programs to make movement through these levels as easy as possible
- Reduction in the size and number of nursing education programs (1,470 basic nursing programs as of 1990) by 10% to 20%, with the closings coming in the associate-degree and diploma programs and attention paid to the geographic distribution of programs in making these decisions
- Encouragement of the expansion of the number of master's-level nurse practitioner training programs by increasing federal support for students
- Development of new models of integration between education and the highly managed and integrated systems of care that can provide nurses with appropriate training and clinical practice opportunities
- Recovery of the clinical management role of nursing and recognition of the role as an increasingly important strength of training and practice at all levels

The Robert Wood Johnson Foundation

The Robert Wood Johnson Foundation (RWJF) has supported a large portfolio of grant initiatives in the health professions. During the previous 25 years, close to 25% of the $2.1 billion the foundation has awarded has been targeted for expansion or improvement of the health-care work force. These program investments in medicine, nursing, and dentistry are reviewed in an essay in *Health Affairs,* entitled "Grants to Shape the Health Care

Workforce" (Isaacs, Sandy, & Schroeder, 1996). Isaacs et al. note that RWJF played a vital role in establishing the credibility and acceptance of nurse practitioners in the mid-1970s through grants to six nursing schools to establish master's-level primary care nurse practitioner training.

A 1995 initiative, "Partnerships for Training: Regional Educational Systems for Nurse Practitioners, Certified Nurse-Midwives, and Physician Assistants," continues the foundation's support of advanced practice nurses. The program recognizes the difficulties encountered by rural and inner-city communities in recruiting and retaining nurse practitioners and nurse midwives. It encourages regional partnerships between educators and employers of nurse midwives, nurse practitioners, and physician assistants to develop and implement strategies for addressing the access, financing, academic, and policy barriers that deter qualified students from entering the professions. The program, authorized at a level of $14 million for a 3-year period, supported planning projects at 12 sites and will fund implementation grants in eight regions encompassing 13 states.

Colleagues In Caring: The Regional Workforce Initiative, a 1996 initiative of the Robert Wood Johnson Foundation, is designed to help nursing schools, hospitals, and other nursing service institutions to initiate concerted work force development systems. The initiative recognizes that nurses need to be prepared to practice in a wide variety of settings and to assume multiple roles. It also acknowledges the importance of an ongoing assessment of a labor market's need for nurses, the capacity of nurses to meet these needs, and the area's educational infrastructure to produce the numbers and types of nursing professionals needed. The program supports the development of formal consortia among nursing schools that (1) enable individual nurses to pursue a continuum of education throughout their careers, from licensure in practical nursing through the doctorate, (2) prepare registered nurses to meet all the regional nursing care needs (acute, long-term, chronic, primary care, and public health), and (3) develop a regional

cadre of registered nurses for leadership roles as clinicians, educators, and service managers. Twenty consortia are supported through the initiative, which has a total authorization of $6 million. RWJF's Ladders in Nursing Careers program (1993–1997) replicated a career advancement program for health care employees that was initially developed by the Greater New York Hospital Association.

The Kellogg Foundation

Project 3000 by 2000: Health Professions Initiative is a joint endeavor of the W. K. Kellogg Foundation, the Robert Wood Johnson Foundation, and the Association of American Medical Colleges (AAMC). The goal of the initiative is to increase minority participation in the health professions. The strategy is enhancement of the academic preparation of minority students and nurturing of their interest in health careers throughout the 12-year pipeline of high school, college, and medical school. Initially developed for education in medicine by the AAMC in 1991, the program has been expanded to ensure that students learn about other opportunities in the health professions. The program challenges medical, nursing, and other health professions' schools to join together and partner with local school systems and colleges.

The Commonwealth Foundation

Fellowship and scholarship programs play an important role in preparing individual nurses to act as change agents in their professional environment and in larger health systems. Recognizing the need for a cadre of nurses who are comfortable and conversant in management and finance, the Commonwealth Foundation supported the development of dual masters' degrees in nursing and business administration at 26 nursing schools. Scholarship support for nurses obtaining a master's degree in business administration was also provided by the Commonwealth Foundation.

Collaborative Efforts

Qualified nurses are eligible for Health Policy Fellowships, offered through a competitive application process by the Pew Charitable Trusts and the Robert Wood Johnson Foundation. Both programs are administered through the Institute of Medicine. Corporate philanthropy also supports fellowship programs. One of the largest is the Johnson & Johnson Company's program for nurse executives, which is conducted at Leonard Davis Institute of the University of Pennsylvania's Wharton School. During the 4-week fellowship program, nurse executives attend workshops in economics, finance, organizational change, and management. Nurses who have made outstanding contributions in their local communities can also apply to the Robert Wood Johnson Foundation's Community Health Leadership Program, which provides recognition for the contribution that community leaders make in achieving the foundation's goals.

MAXIMIZING NURSING'S ROLE IN PHILANTHROPY

Opportunities to Influence Foundations

Nurses can also influence foundations by serving as foundation staff, on advisory committees, and as consultants and participants in foundation-funded projects. Such positions can influence who and what the foundations fund. Most foundations use outside experts to review proposals, provide technical assistance, develop programs, and sit on advisory committees. By getting to know foundation staff and exposing them to nurses' potential to serve the needs of the foundation, nurses can make themselves available for such influential roles.

Employment with a foundation provides an excellent opportunity to learn about grant making and contribute to health care through grant-making activities. Nurses have as much to contribute to philanthropy as any other health care provider. Many nurses have the knowledge and skills needed to become successful staff members at foundations that focus on health or related areas. Nurses interested in such roles should contact individual foundations regarding the possibility of future positions.

Nurses and nursing often play an important role in the programmatic activities of foundations interested in health care. This involvement includes grants to nurses and covers a wide range of programming in education, practice, research, and policy. Some examples of nurses currently working in leadership positions at American Foundations include Rebecca Reimel, president of the Pew Charitable Trusts; Rheba DeTornyay, trustee of the Robert Wood Johnson Foundation; Gloria R. Smith, vice president for programs, the W. K. Kellogg Foundation; and Susan Sherman, president of the Independence Foundation.

The Grant Process

Foundations may actively solicit proposals through a request for proposals or other competitive programs. In addition, individuals or organizations may be asked to submit proposals, and unsolicited proposals may be encouraged. Because the focus and funding strategies of foundations vary, nurses interested in seeking foundation support should obtain additional information from the foundation itself. Research should be done to identify which foundation has funding priorities related to the project to be funded. Grant seekers should consider the content area the foundation is interested in, the geographical area the foundation funds, and whether or not the foundation supports the type of funds being sought (startup funds, research, capital). A number of excellent foundation and funding directories and lists of recent grants are available (see "Sources of Information About Foundations," at the end of the chapter). Information can also be obtained on the Internet. For example, the Foundation Center (http://fdncenter.org) maintains a web site that includes a variety of information about foundations and grant making.

Numerous articles and books describe how to

write a grant proposal. In general, the content of a proposal includes the following descriptions:

- The problem that the proposed project will address
- The goals and objectives of the project
- The research method or intervention
- The qualifications of the applicant and the institution
- How the project will be assessed or evaluated
- Dissemination plans
- The budget and plans for sustaining the project (if appropriate) beyond the period of grant support

When approaching a foundation for grant support, keep the following in mind:

- Foundation staffs are not likely to speak the same language as nurses. (Write so that laypeople can understand.)
- Assume that the reviewer knows little about nursing education or practice. (Explain the potential impact of the nursing intervention.)
- Many health problems require multidisciplinary responses. (Involve others in your intervention.)
- The generalizability of research findings and programs will be enhanced by sample size. (Collaborate with nurse colleagues.)
- Be sure your proposal is consistent and comprehensive. (Relate the problem to the intervention, to the budget, and so on.)

The Politics of Philanthropy

Nurses can use foundation resources and influence foundations in a variety of ways. The key to working with foundations is to understand their mission, goals, and strategies. The interests of the individual nurse or organization must fit those of the foundation being approached for funding. The politics of grant seeking is not unlike a political campaign:

- Have a good project (candidate).
- Have a project that fits the foundation's mission (a platform that appeals to the majority of voters).

- Know the foundation and make contacts with individuals employed there (know your constituents and get out to meet them).

A "good project" is one that fits with the purpose, mission, and direction of the foundation and is of importance and interest to the prospective nurse grantee. Directories, indexes, and other documents available in public and university libraries can be used to identify possible sources (see "Sources of Information About Foundations," at the end of the chapter). Details regarding past, present, and future areas of funding are usually contained in the annual reports of foundations. Personal contact with people who know the world of philanthropy and with foundation staff can be used to identify appropriate funders. Moreover, one must be willing to modify a proposed project so that it reflects the mission or guidelines of a particular foundation.

When evaluating a grant proposal, the foundation officials will need to decide whether the project matches their agenda and whether it addresses a significant need in an innovative way. In addition, they will need to know the applicant's capacity to conduct the project and his or her credibility as a grant recipient. Some foundations support organizations with a record of grant success. If you are new to the use of grants, partnering with experienced grant recipients will be helpful.

The nursing profession's ability to obtain grants and to influence the direction of foundations is similar to the ability to influence the policy process and its outcomes. Consistent effort, knowledge of the context of grant making, and active engagement in all aspects of foundation work are essential for influence. Nurses can apply their growing sophistication in political action to the world of philanthropy. Applying the nursing process—assessment, planning, intervention, and evaluation—to grant making can provide individual rewards and accrue the social, professional, and individual benefits necessary to move the profession and its contributions forward.

CONCLUSION

The role of nurses in influencing health policy and health care will be enhanced if nurses became more involved in the work of philanthropy. The resources and influence of private foundations can be more widely used by nurses. Opportunities to be foundation grantees, consultants, and staff exist at the national, state, and local levels. Nurses should take advantage of these opportunities so that nursing's unique contributions are included in future health policy decisions.

As the health care system continues to change, the role of philanthropy is increasingly important to assess the implications of change on the nation's health and on the nursing profession. Philanthropy provides a unique opportunity for nurses to influence health policy and related decisions. Using our growing political and policy knowledge and skills, we can contribute to the future directions of health care through philanthropy.

REFERENCES

Brown, E. L. (1948). *The Brown report: Nursing for the future.* New York: Russell Sage Foundation.

Claxton, G., Feder, J., Shactmon, D., & Altman, S. (1997). Public policy issues in nonprofit conversions: An overview. *Health Affairs, 15*(2), 9–28.

Cluff, L. (1996, 4th Quarter). Health, health care and philanthropy. *Reflections,* 32.

Flexner, A. (1910). *Medical education in the United States and Canada,* (Bulletin No. 4). New York: Carnegie Foundation for Advancement of Teaching.

Girouard, S., Keenan, T., & Seitz, P. (1993). Policy, politics and foundations. In D. Mason, S. Talbott, & J. Leavitt (Eds.), *Policy and politics for nurses* (2nd ed.). Philadelphia: W. B. Saunders.

Goldmark, J. (1923). *Goldmark report: Nursing and nursing education in the United States.* New York: Macmillan.

Isaacs, S., Sandy, L., & Schroeder, S. (1996). Grants to shape the health care work force: The Robert Wood Johnson Foundation experience. *Health Affairs, 15*(2), 279–295.

O'Neil, E. H., & Hare, D. M. (Eds.). (1990). *Perspective on the health professions.* Durham, NC: Pew Health Professions Program, Duke University.

Pew Health Professions Commission Third Report. (1996). *Critical challenges: Revitalizing the health professions for the twenty-first century.* Philadelphia: Pew Foundation.

Renz, L., Qureshi, S., & Mandler, C. (1996). *Foundation giving.* New York: The Foundation Center.

Tein, C. (1997, July–August). Asset storm. *Foundation News and Commentary,* 32.

SOURCES OF INFORMATION ABOUT FOUNDATIONS

Organizations

Council on Foundations
1828 L St., NW
Washington, DC 20036-5168
(202) 466-6512

The Foundation Center
79 Fifth Ave.
New York, NY 10003-3050
(212) 620-4230

Grantmakers in Health
1100 Connecticut Avenue, NW
12th Floor
Washington, DC 20036
(202) 452-8331

Periodicals

The Chronical of Philanthropy
1255 23rd St., NW
Washington, DC 20037

Foundation News and Commentary
(Council on Foundations)
1828 L St., NW
Washington, DC 20036-5168

Foundation Giving Watch
835 Penobscot Building
Detroit, MI 48226

Internet Resources

Association for Healthcare Philanthropy: go-ahp.org

Foundation Center: fdncenter.org

Philanthropy Journal Online: philanthropy-journal.org

Other References

The foundation directory (2 parts, annual). New York: Foundation Center.

Nauffts, M. (Ed.). (1994). *Foundation fundamentals.* New York: Foundation Center.

Freeman, D. (1991). *Handbook of private foundations.* New York: Foundation Center.

Chapter 37

NURSING, HEALTH, AND HEALTH CARE IN THE INTERNATIONAL COMMUNITY

JANE WEAVER

As Nobel Laureate Joshua Lederberg stated, "The microbe that felled one child in a distant continent yesterday can reach yours today and seed a global pandemic tomorrow" (Centers for Disease Control and Prevention [CDC], 1994, p. 2). Thus a local view is dangerous and naive. Now, more than ever, all communities need to remain abreast of seemingly distant poverty, instability, violence, and disease. The decay of one country is, in a way, infectious in itself.

Today social reality is "globalization"; nurses and nursing cannot help but become more involved with other cultures and international health issues. Although the capacity for improving international health has never been greater, tremendous problems remain. For instance, life expectancy is actually declining in some areas, and not just in countries ravaged by acquired immunodeficiency syndrome (AIDS). In terms of meeting basic human needs, 25% of the world's people still lack safe water,[1] access to basic sanitation has actually fallen to 34%, and ever greater numbers are without clean air to breathe (United Nations Children's Fund, 1997). In terms of human behaviors influencing health outcomes, major concerns are harmful life-style choices, domestic violence, 115 million antipersonnel land mines, and ethnic conflicts where children are soldiers, millions are displaced from their homes by fear, and destruction of agriculture, transport, education, and health infrastructures occurs.

The victory of democracies in the Cold War has not translated into less conflict. Rather, pent-up nationalistic and religious conflicts held in check by superpower confrontation are erupting repeatedly in almost every corner of the world (Gagnon, 1994–1995). Further, research has shown that people making the transition to a democratic form of government are particularly likely to become involved in war (Mansfield & Snyder, 1995).

With the demise of the Cold War and its threat of nuclear annihilation, many countries are revising their concepts of national security (Goduc, 1992). Global health problems, failing development, the environment, drugs, and crime are recognized as transnational threats (Albright, 1994; Institute of Medicine, 1997). Government officials further include population growth, family breakdown, and the proliferation of nuclear, biological, and chemical weapons outside the military as security issues for all nations (Clinton, 1994).

International health is increasingly being politicized with the realization that global conditions matter on Main Street. Had such a far-reaching approach to human welfare been in place previously, the emergence of infection with human immunodeficiency virus and of AIDS may have been detected as early as the mid-1960s, when it was known to African doctors as *slims disease*, giving the scientific community a 10- to 20-year head start in combating the virus. Apart from humanitarian concerns, such enlightened self-interest could now be saving thousands of lives and annual economic costs of $30 billion or more in the United States alone (National Council for International Health [NCIH], 1997).

Ultimately, globalization will mean that domestic and foreign health problems become inseparable. Therefore gaining an understanding of international health concerns is essential to nursing and all citizens for the twenty-first century.

AN OVERVIEW OF GLOBAL HEALTH ISSUES*

The key theme for the next century will be the growing imbalance between population and resources. World population has doubled since 1957, and every year the planet gains another 81 million inhabitants, taking only 11 years to add another billion. The largest generation in history will soon enter their childbearing years; by the year 2000, the World Bank estimates, one seventh of the world will be teenagers (Rockefeller Foundation, 1997).

Economics of Health

Historically, international health models depended on two variables, categorizing populations in terms of their economic development and age distribution. First, countries without significant industrialization and urbanization, and hence with low rates of productivity and income, usually lacked the ability to provide the infrastructure to fight disease, such as sanitation, food safety, secure shelter, education of health care providers, transport of medical supplies, and hospitals for their populations. Countries that had developed such capacities were generally far healthier. Second, disproportion between the very young population and the productive working-age population, which had to feed and care for children, also explained poor health. For example, in Great Britain the under-five mortality rate is 7 deaths per 1000 births, whereas Kenya's rate is 90 per 1000 births. This

variance could be conceptualized simply as a function of the two countries' developmental stage, birth rate, and percentage of children.

More recently, such variance has been attributed to developing countries' curtailing social services to meet lenders' (e.g., the World Bank's) goals and demands for the structural adjustment needed for sustainable development. Often, these lending policies have led to such an immediate decline in human welfare that millions in the developing world, frequently children, now live in the streets, foraging for survival (World Federation for Mental Health [WFMH], 1996). Likewise, disinvestment by industrialized governments in local infrastructure during the past 15 years has left large numbers of people living in squalor, highly vulnerable to disease and violence (United Nations Children's Fund, 1997).

Today, we know that neither the transition from an agrarian to a prosperous industrial system, nor the age balance in a population, ensures health for all. The infant mortality rate is still twice as high among U.S. black persons as among U.S. white persons (Bodenheimer & Grumach, 1995), and 24% of children less than the age of 6 years in the United States live in poverty (United Nations Children's Fund, 1997). In Sweden, Belgium, Greece, France, Italy, and Finland, at least 22% of the population aged 24 years or younger are unemployed, whereas in Spain 43% of the younger population have no job (United Nations Children's Fund, 1997). Economically and socially depressed cities are ripe for disease, with potentially devastating effects for national productivity and stability, plus psychological consequences for a whole generation of adults who have little independence.

Political and Geographical Stability

Although economic sufficiency and stability are essential, they are not an assurance of well-being. Maintaining health requires governmental and political security. Unfortunately, political violence and civil war have eroded other safe-

---

*Julia Davis, Washington, DC, assisted with the research and writing of this discussion.

guards. In countries like Bosnia and Rwanda, staggering numbers of the able, working-aged citizenry have been killed in war, in labor camps, or in massacres. Political instability is rarely contained by geographical borders. Ethnic cleansing has resulted in mass migration away from violence and genocide, leaving behind people who have neither the materials to endure nor the tools to rebuild. Lacking any promise of political stability, countries can obtain little relief support or attract economic investment. After initial outpourings of assistance when human tragedies like those in Somalia appear in the headlines and on television, donor fatigue and indifference set in.

Infectious Disease

Most people in the world die prematurely of opportunistic, infectious diseases. Many could be spared with clean water, basic sanitation systems, minimum levels of nutrition, basic vaccinations, and prophylaxis against a few vectors. Tuberculosis (TB), once thought on the verge of eradication, now kills 52,000 each week. The reemergence of TB in the developed world is related to a combination of many factors, but the movement of people, more than 2 million each day crossing national borders (Institute of Medicine, 1997), is key. Similarly, the sex workers of Burma and Thailand have crossed borders, spreading comorbid TB and HIV and proving that neither country's efforts to isolate the population of the other is an effective public health strategy (Over & Piot, 1993).

The epicenter of the AIDS epidemic is still on the horizon, threatening to wipe out a significant part of the working-aged population in Sub-Saharan Africa and Asia. Nevertheless, the trend of growing numbers of AIDS fatalities clearly emerged in 1996, when AIDS accounted for more deaths globally than malaria and for one fourth of all deaths ever attributed to HIV disease (MacGinnis, 1996).

Globally, women and children are the most at risk. Research continues to confirm significant vertical transmission through breast-feeding,

meaning that HIV-infected women[2] can risk their child's life either by breast-feeding or, if they cannot afford substitutes, by not breast-feeding. Even where powdered formula is free, many HIV-infected women have no way to properly reconstitute it (either no water, no means to render the water safe, or physical incapacity). "In about 30 developing countries, HIV/AIDS is threatening and even reversing" decades of health progress against neonatal mortality, malnutrition, and deaths prevented by immunizations (United Nations Children's Fund, 1997).

Chronic Diseases and Mental Illness

The next most frequent worldwide causes of death are diseases of the circulatory system (heart disease and stroke), cancer, and diabetes. Often referred to as life-style illnesses or chronic diseases, these are increasingly common and burdensome in the aging populations of Japan, Europe, and North America and in developing countries that have taken up Western nutrition and smoking habits. Each year, cancer's impact on world mortality rates grows; by 2000, annual cancer deaths will total 7.2 million, with two thirds in the developing world (World Resources, 1997).

Mental illness is also a growing cause of global morbidity and death. In 1990, unipolar major depression was ranked fourth among causes of global illness; it is projected to rank second by 2020 (Murray & Lopez, 1996). Once understood as a risk for populations of industrialized nations alone, neuropsychiatric disorders may affect one fourth of the earth's population (WFMH, 1997 [Fact Sheet]). This calculation is staggering when one considers that 75% of these cases are in the developing world, with little access to diagnosis or treatment (WFMH, 1996). Children and adolescents are particularly vulnerable because poor living conditions and violence take their emotional toll at younger ages and with more frequency than ever before (WFMH, 1997). A recent study of depression in adolescent immigrants from Bosnia suggests that 25% of survivors have posttraumatic stress disorder, and 17% have clinical depression (Weine et al., 1995). In countries that report youth suicide, it is repeatedly one of the top three causes of death (WFMH, 1997).

The Changing International Health Agenda

While the insidious cycle of poverty, resource depletion, low wages, unemployment, and civil unrest continues and increasingly affects the United States, one hopeful change is more attention to the critical connections among population, women's and children's health, and economic development. Most countries now recognize that for every year of schooling, not only does a woman's own health status improve, but that of her entire family improves. Further, low-cost methods, including breast-feeding, immunizations, oral rehydration, and better child spacing, have proved particularly effective for promoting the health of families. Nurses could be essential in expanding such care through a commitment to (1) universal provision of desired family planning,[3] (2) reduction of sexual exploitation and abuse, and (3) more advocacy for equity in education and employment opportunities.

AVENUES FOR INTERNATIONAL COLLABORATION

The International Council of Nurses

Fortunately, nursing as a profession has recognized the value of international collaboration since at least 1899, when the International Council of Nurses (ICN) was formed in London. In fact, ICN is the oldest and largest professional health organization in the world. Nurses may visit ICN in Geneva, Switzerland, or experience it by attending its global meetings every 4 years (quadrennials) or by subscribing to its magazine, *International Nursing Review*. ICN now represents nurses in more than 120 countries; most recently, nursing associations from Namibia, South Africa, Angola, Slovenia, Yugoslavia, and Slovakia joined.

Every 2 years ICN holds a Congress of National Representatives (CNR). Members[4] send in topics for discussion and proposals to be placed on the agenda. The CNR may pass, reject, or modify the proposed resolutions, but, once adopted by majority vote, they become official positions of the international nursing community.[5] At the 1995 CNR in Harare, Zimbabwe, ICN adopted a resolution condemning female genital mutilation (FGM); U.S. nurses then shared the resolution with legislators. Subsequently, Congress passed a law making FGM a criminal offense[6]; some states made it a state crime as well.

In 1995 a Harvard study showing the tremendous toll of mental illness, almost 9% of the total global disease burden, had just been released (Harvard School of Medicine Department of Social Medicine, 1995). In the same year, CNR adopted a timely position statement on the importance of educating and utilizing nurses in national mental health programs. Such resolutions help nurses lobby for improved training and utilization in their own countries. Resolutions on shift work and temporary employees are helpful in negotiations on working conditions because uniform demands on employers by the profession internationally (e.g., for basic equipment like respiratory masks, gloves, needle-disposal safety devices, or hepatitis immunizations) can effect change far more rapidly than less global efforts. ICN's 1983 "Statement on the Nurse's Role in Safeguarding Human Rights" contributes to customary international law (Hoffman, 1995).

ICN's greatest accomplishment, though, has probably been in enhancing the professionalism and prestige of nursing globally. This has been achieved through publication of a code of ethics and upgrading of educational standards for nursing. As recently as 1993, nurses' training could start at age 13 years in some countries. Many countries now require completion of secondary school and attainment of age 17 years to enter nurses' training, whereas ICN's standard is that "[p]rogrammes of nursing education should generally parallel those for other professions as

PROMOTING A GLOBAL NURSING PERSPECTIVE

1. Increase teaching of cross-cultural awareness and competencies in basic nursing programs, basing teaching on international nursing research. Then incorporate more multicultural content, as well as refugee and immigrant health issues, in nursing licensure and certification examinations, as well as in practice.

2. Familiarize all nursing students and nurses with the ten or so basic international instruments for health advocacy and international humanitarian law (see box entitled "Basic International Health Policy Documents for Nurses"). Require inclusion for program accreditation, and incorporate knowledge of these international advocacy tools into licensure and certification examinations, as well as into practice.

3. Work toward international consensus in the nursing academic community on evaluating credits and policies for transferability of nursing course credits. Increase international collaboration in graduate nursing research and teaching nurses a second language.

4. Ensure that graduates of basic nurses training are competent in primary health care and community leadership roles. Increase community-based student placements, mandating multicultural experiences and participation in policy-influencing activities. Promote a population-based epidemiological system approach for nursing practice and research (American Academy of Nursing, 1997).

5. Formulate a construct of international health that encompasses nursing's core concepts and values,* and then integrate it into nursing schools, activities of nursing associations and organizations, and all multinational health enterprises. This construct should consider the relationship between immigration and health, and between core fair labor standards and health. Increase collaboration between nursing organizations in addressing issues relative to migration, immigration, humanitarian aid, the environment, and global resource depletion.

6. Increase the numbers and geographic representation of nurses in global professional or health care regulatory activities, such as the ICN regulatory project; the International Regulatory Conferences, held in London (1995) and Vancouver (1997); and conferences/projects of the Center for Quality Assurance in International Education (Washington, D.C.).

7. Support nurses who are not yet organized to build professional nursing associations and become ICN members. Although nurses can certainly collaborate internationally without being members of a state or national nurses association, there is no substitute for ICN, which can deliver a unified message from almost 5 million nurses.

8. Integrate advocacy for international health, and enforcement of human rights law, into nurses' political action activities at both state and national levels. Enter foreign policy debates to influence aid spending; support policies that promote families, the care and integration of immigrants, and respect for refugees' cultural histories and migration experience.

9. Support public health, including policies that protect the environment, promote ecological balance, educate the public about benefits of global health thinking, and prevent emerging microbial diseases and drug resistance (American Academy of Nursing, 1997).

10. Increase numbers of nurses who are aware of, apply for, and are awarded international project funding, such as WHO short-term travel and Rockefeller Foundation and Fulbright fellowships.

11. Mobilize consumers to convince communities worldwide that nursing services provide added value and cost-effectiveness. This must be accomplished both locally and globally. A key component is the power hierarchy's acceptance of universal nursing classification systems and quality indicators allowing nursing participation in consumer, multidisciplinary, and intersectoral venues, where identified, quantified, and measurable variables can be compared and where the efficacy of professional nursing with individuals, families, and communities can be documented globally.

Box continued on following page

PROMOTING A GLOBAL NURSING PERSPECTIVE *(Continued)*

12. Ensure nursing involvement in international health research. Increase the number of visiting foreign nursing scientists in national programs such as the National Institutes of Health (Fogarty International Center, 1997; Institute of Medicine, 1997). Disseminate nurses' scientific findings outside the nursing community, through vehicles like literacy classes, the World Wide Web, or HealthNet (operated by Satellife).†

13. Increase the number of nurses in United Nations staff positions, particularly filling WHO nursing vacancies, either by pressuring WHO or by finding private granters/funders to support nursing positions' becoming and remaining occupied and adequately staffed and resourced. Increase nursing's role in health surveillance, ecology and disease prevention, and the design of human habitats.

14. Ensure nursing representation on health infor-

matics and information systems committees and task forces, including international telehealth regulatory negotiations. Nurses must participate in the development of electronic and computerized patient records and of health-status tracking systems, especially in regard to standardization and confidentiality, because nursing will comprise the largest profession working with such data globally.

15. Increase nursing representation on trade advisory committees for all government agencies involved in drafting and negotiating trade in services agreements, including any labor and environmental clauses or side agreements.

16. Increase health advocacy in the international economic and political arenas, including applying for United Nations grants, supporting regional development bank and World Bank health projects, and holding nations accountable for international health commitments.

---

*ICN has identified as universal nursing concepts the following: acceptability, altruism, appropriateness, caring, effectiveness, efficiency, equity, health goals, humanity, and respect for persons (ICN, 1996b).

†SatelLife is a Boston-based nonprofit operating HealthNet, a computer network providing vital health information, in cooperation with medical publishers, to health care workers in at least 28 countries in Africa, Asia, and Latin America. As an Internet gateway, SatelLife provides health care workers in the developing world with an inexpensive "on ramp" to the information superhighway. (See http://www.healthnet.org [C. Woolery, personal communication, May 7, 1997]).

to setting, level, academic credentials, control and general standards" (CNR, 1985, quoted in ICN, 1996a, p. 12). "Throughout history very few fields have achieved professional status outside of traditional academic structures and there is no reason to assume that nursing is so powerful or so profound to be any different" (Stevens, 1985, quoted in ICN, 1996a, p. 12). Considering that, in most countries, nurses and midwives constitute more than 50% of the entire professional work force (Nurses Foundation of Japan, 1993), global acceptance of nursing as a profession would foster tremendous opportunities to exercise power and influence global health—provided the profession was organized, strategically focused, and politically astute.

ICN also assists nurses to demonstrate the value of nursing services and implement research-based practice. One way it does this is

through annual distribution of International Nurses Day kits. These kits highlight a different global health concern each year, informing the issue, presenting nursing lessons learned from around the world, and summarizing the latest relevant nursing theories, research, and projects. As nurses celebrate May 12 (Florence Nightingale's birthday) each year, the kits are extremely effective in generating self-esteem and public recognition of the profession as a political force concerned about mobilization for public health.

In the policy arena, ICN has been tireless in improving nurses' leadership and managerial skills. The joint ICN–W. K. Kellogg Foundation Leadership for Change project is currently grooming nurses for more public policymaking roles by teaching negotiating techniques, management principles, and other self-actualization skills to Central and South American nurses, with the expectation to duplicate the program in Africa.

ICN's current major project is to develop a universal nursing language, the International Classification of Nursing Practice (ICNP) (ICN, 1997a). This system will facilitate obtaining globally the data needed to identify the domains of nursing, to identify and quantify nursing interventions, and to measure the health outcomes of nursing care. ICNP has already been translated into 12 languages, and European nurses are beginning to test the system.

World Health Organization

Formed shortly after World War II as a specialized agency of the United Nations (UN) and headquartered in Geneva, the World Health Organization (WHO) actually has six more countries (191) belonging to it than are members of the UN. The role of WHO is to set technical and ethical standards and to propose guidelines and codes of good practice in all areas of health (Nakajima, 1996). WHO has traditionally been headed by a physician director general, the largest percentage of its professional staff are physicians, and, until 1992, no systematic data on nursing were collected (WHO, 1995).

Dr. Miriam Hirshfeld, a nurse from Israel, served as chief scientist for nursing, coordinating 40 worldwide nursing positions, mostly in the six WHO regions, as well as a global advisory group on nursing and a network of 31 WHO collaborating centers for nursing and midwifery.[7] Unfortunately, the failure of some countries, like the United States, to pay their full UN and WHO dues assessments, has allowed excuses of budgetary constraints to result in the

---

BASIC INTERNATIONAL HEALTH POLICY DOCUMENTS FOR NURSES

1. Universal Declaration of Human Rights (1948), particularly Article 25.
2. United Nations Covenant on Civil and Political Rights (adopted 1966, entered into force 1976; ratified by the United States in 1992; 999 United Nations Treaty Series [UNTS] 171, 1966).
3. United Nations Covenant on Economic, Social, and Cultural Rights; particularly Article 12, Right to Health (adopted 1966, entered into force 1976; United States has not ratified; 999 UNTS 3, 1966).

   Together, the preceding comprise the International Bill of Rights (Buergenthal & Shelton, 1995).
4. Geneva Conventions (1864, 1949) and Two Protocols (1967, 1977); United States has ratified the Conventions, not Protocols (American Academy of Nursing, 1997, p. 24; 75 UNTS 287; 1125 UNTS 53; 19 UNTS 6223).
5. Convention Relating to the Status of Refugees (1951); plus United Nations High Commissioner on Refugees guidelines on health matters (American Academy of Nursing, 1997, pp. 20–21; 189 UNTS 137).
6. International Convention on the Elimination of All Forms of Racial Discrimination (adopted 1965, entered into force 1969; United States ratified in 1994; 660 UNTS 195).
7. Declaration of Alma-Ata (1978).
8. Convention on the Elimination of All Forms of Discrimination Against Women (adopted 1979, entered into force 1981; U.S. President has signed, but Senate has never given advice and consent; 34 United Nations General Assembly Official Record [No. 46] at 193).
9. Declaration on the Rights of the Child (UN, 1959) and The Convention on the Rights of the Child (adopted and entered into force 1989; U.S. President signed, but Senate has never given advice and consent) See www.unicef.org/crc for text of convention.
10. ICN Code of Ethics (1953, last reviewed 1989) and Position Statements.
11. WHO International Code of Marketing of Breastmilk Substitutes (1981).
12. United Nations world conference documents, such as Nairobi's Forward Looking Strategies, Cairo Plan of Action, Copenhagen Declaration, and Beijing Platform of Action.

elimination of six nursing posts, and many of the remaining 40 posts have been left unfilled (WHO, 1996b). In 1997, U.S. default on its WHO treaty obligation was $145 million (Institute of Medicine, 1997).

Every May, WHO holds a World Health Assembly (WHA), where resolutions important to nursing are debated. More nurses should lobby to have nurses on their country's official delegation. Traditionally, ICN has sponsored a nurses' meeting so that nurses can solidify positions on certain issues and influence their countries' votes. That strategy proved successful in 1996, when nurses garnered unanimous renewed commitment to strengthen nursing and midwifery (WHA, 1996, Resolution 49.1).

A particularly important WHO policy statement that **all nurses should be familiar with** is the *Declaration of Alma-Ata,* adopted in 1978 and named after the city in Kazakhstan where its formulation took place. This declaration prioritizes accessible community-based primary health care services for all and equity in the distribution of health resources and health care manpower. Most of the proposed minimum package of health services can be delivered by nurses and midwives (World Bank, 1993), because it is generally accepted that government expenditures for high-technology interventions are often inappropriate.

ICN strongly supports the principles and values heralded at Alma-Ata. Nursing's health orientation and primary care message, once the core of nursing, seemed orphaned in many countries. Nursing had become too closely associated with urban hospitals, where nurses fulfilled technically complex roles in managing modern equipment and were not prepared to deliver primary care or assume leadership roles apart from formal institutional settings. A majority of many countries' nurses provided only curative services to a small percentage of the urban population (ICN, 1996a). Between 1979 and 1985, WHO and the ICN worked together to delineate a range of competencies that nurses needed across eight essential elements of primary health care services. More than 253 nurses from 75 countries were involved in leadership training for primary health care. In Europe, more than 50 countries formulated new nursing curriculums to broaden the base of nursing education and focus on primary care. Thus closer alliances with international colleagues could provide U.S. nurses with direction in assuming the accountability and the rewards of providing a larger share of health care, as midwives and health visitors in England, nurse practitioners in Korea, and community nurses in Africa have already done.

National strategies to reach Alma-Ata's "Health for All" goals created campaigns such as "Healthy People 2000" in the United States. Where implemented, these campaigns had a major impact on nursing practice. However, most countries, including the United States, will fall short, not only because of monetary constraints, but because health care delivery and educational systems based on medical models have had difficulty in refocusing on universally accessible basic health services. Further, social conditions are proving to be stronger determinants of health than are health services.

National Council for International Health

The National Council for International Health[8] (NCIH) is a United States–based coalition of government agencies, businesses, nongovernmental organizations and private volunteer offices, professional associations, and universities to improve international health. NCIH publishes *Healthlink,* a quarterly international health newsletter; *AIDSLink,* a bimonthly newsletter on the HIV pandemic; and *Career Network,* a monthly international health jobs listing in both paper and electronic form. By participating in NCIH's activities, especially its annual conference, nurses achieve visibility and voice in multidisciplinary and multisector international health problem-solving forums.

Other Avenues for International Nursing

Opportunities to influence health policy also occur during major international conferences such as the social, children's, and environmental summits, and especially the four women's conferences.[9] To maximize this political venue, it is critical that nurses be on their countries' official delegations, as Linda Tarr Whelan, RN, and American Nurses Association President Virginia Trotter Betts, JD, MSN, RN, were for the United States in Beijing. Nurses thus directly drafted international documents such as the Beijing Platform of Action and negotiated their health content and adoption. Subsequently, nurses have been participating in implementation efforts (President's Interagency Council on Women, 1995) and in holding governments accountable for their commitments (U.S. Department of State, 1995).

Another avenue for international nursing collaboration is Sigma Theta Tau (STT), a 76-year-old international nursing honor society with chapters at baccalaureate-level nursing schools around the world. STT is particularly known for its international nursing research conferences, and increasingly STT chapters are inducting nurses from overseas as a prelude to conducting collaborative international nursing projects (STT, 1997).

Finally, clinical specialty groups have established international organizations. For example, the International Federation of Nurse Anesthetists is made up of national association members from 22 countries (McAuliffe & Henry, 1996). Other nursing specialties may recognize more than one chapter per country. The International Association of Forensic Nurses directly admits individual nurses, regardless of national or local chapter membership. Emergency nurses and midwives now administer identical certification examinations in several countries. Nurses should consider that choices regarding organizational structure, accreditation, and certification criteria represent a policy perspective on international health itself. Basically there are four paradigms: the national framework, the legalis-

tic, the capitalistic, and the global or humanistic approach (American Academy of Nursing, 1997, p. 8; Godue, 1992). Current forces challenge the first.

INTERNATIONAL WORK FORCE ISSUES AND POLICIES

Increasing global migration has both personal and professional ramifications for nurses. First, there are challenges from more patients and clients from different cultures, including the need to recognize and take precautions against new, reemerging, and drug-resistant infectious diseases like hanta virus disease, TB, malaria, cholera, and *Salmonella* and *Escherichia coli* food poisoning (CDC, 1994; Sokolove, 1994; Zuber et al., 1996). Almost all of the 17 outbreaks of measles in the United States in early 1996 (Marwick, 1996) are believed to have originated from foreign exposure.

Second, there are competitive threats and opportunities because of the importation of nurses during personnel shortages, or exportation of health care personnel to achieve a favorable impact on a country's trade balance. Recruiting for nurses is going on at any given time for at least six countries—currently, Malta, the United Kingdom, Oman, Australia, Saudi Arabia, and the United States. After the turn of the century, it will be the rule, rather than the exception, for U.S. nursing students and registered nurses to live overseas at some point in their nursing career. For those who do not work overseas, it will be the norm to have co-workers from abroad.[10]

Impact of Migration on Nurses as Caregivers

Between 1981 and 1990, a total of 7,338,000 immigrants came to the United States, the most in any decade since 1901 to 1910 (Immigration and Naturalization Service, 1997). In Boston alone, as many as 27,000 Russian refugees were resettled in one year. A recent conversation with a public health nurse from New Zealand, working in Arlington County, Virginia, revealed that only one person in her entire caseload was born in the United States; the remainder came from 15 different countries.

When translators are difficult to come by, nurses caring for non-English-speaking clients, whether as school nurses, public health clinic nurses, emergency department nurses, or nursing home or hospice nurses, may become extremely anxious when they cannot take histories, complete assessments, or involve patients in planning as they have been trained to do. The feeling of cross-cultural inadequacy can be stressful and can so significantly interfere with the delivery of individualized care as to compromise its quality. To further add to the complexities of delivering competent cross-cultural care, nursing research has shown that caregivers must not only understand specific cultural differences but also assess and plan interventions based on which stage of transition or acculturation that immigrants or refugees are experiencing (American Academy of Nursing, 1997). To achieve better nursing, most, if not all, of the visiting public health nurses in Arlington, Virginia, are bilingual.

Impact of Migration on Nurses as Employees or as Entrepreneurs

A nurse in Russia earns about $20 a month, but many of the nurses haven't been paid in a year! Experienced nurses in Latin America may earn about one fifth of the salary of teachers (ICN, 1996a). In Africa, nurses face 80-hour workweeks, brutal civil strife, and huge civil service salary cuts and job loss during structural adjustment. Uganda lost 40% of its nurses in 1986. Between 1991 and 1995, 7% of Zimbabwe's nurses left (ICN, 1996b). In developed countries, nurses have been converted to part-time status as hospitals downsize. Under the North American Free Trade Agreement (NAFTA), more nurses are crossing borders to work than are workers in any other profession. Hospital cafeterias in London are like a miniature United Nations, with large numbers of

Australian, Indian, eastern European, German, Finnish, and Irish nurses and nursing students[11] (J. Humphries [Royal College of Nursing, United Kingdom], personal communication, April 15, 1997). Demand for nursing services, combined with good salaries in some economies of the Middle East and the Pacific Rim, attract nurses from both developing and developed countries. In one Saudi city alone, there are 2,000 U.S. nurses and 1,000 Canadian; another 1,000 Australian nurses are scattered throughout Saudi Arabia (Drees, 1997). In short, nurses are on the move.

Clinical experience alone has been sufficient qualification, but soon the need for linguistic, cultural, and primary or managed care competencies will drive the competitiveness of the global nurse marketplace. Already advertisements for U.S. nursing jobs increasingly specify Spanish language skills; a $2,000 annual bonus seems standard. Educational preparation also influences competitiveness as the trend to move nurses training into the college setting expands globally. Increasingly, a 3- or 4-year university degree is the required or predominant basic training level to become a nurse (in Australia, Chile, Canada, Iceland, New Zealand, North Dakota, Spain, and the Philippines). Canada, the United Kingdom, and the entire Federation of Southeast Asian Nurses Associations have identified 3-year university training or the baccalaureate degree as a requirement for entry by the year 2000 (ICN, 1996a).

Nurse Migration and Trade Agreements

In 1994 a new treaty, the General Agreement on Trade in Services, was signed, and a standing body—the World Trade Organization—was created with powers to monitor, implement, and enforce trade agreements, including the settling of disputes. These multilateral, indeed global, agreements govern the movement of capital and labor, as well as goods, and they will have a significant impact on nurses and the nursing profession in the twenty-first century. Although ICN recognizes the right of individual nurses to migrate, it also acknowledges related problems, such as "brain drain" and exploitation (ICN, 1996b). The latter was recently well documented when Filipino nurses in Chicago won their lawsuit accusing U.S. employers of paying them $4 an hour less than the prevailing wage rate for registered nurses, and a huge visa-fraud, RN-smuggling operation was exposed in 38 states (American Nurses Association, 1998).

One political issue for nurses is whether trade agreements should include requirements for mandatory enforcement of fair labor standards. Core fair labor standards are (1) prohibition of the use of forced, or compulsory, labor, (2) the right of association and to organize, (3) the right to bargain collectively over work conditions, (4) the right to equal remuneration without discrimination on the basis of sex, race, or religion, and (5) a minimum age for the employment of children (Prah, 1996). Another key International Labor Organization (ILO) standard is the right to acceptable conditions of work with respect to minimum wages, hours, and occupational safety and health (ILO, 1997). Inclusion of such guarantees by signatories of trade agreements is a contentious issue internationally, even within countries. As a compromise, NAFTA has side agreements on labor and environmental protections, but this practice has been strongly criticized as ineffective.

Already there are efforts to expand NAFTA to include Chile and some Caribbean countries, to develop a Free Trade Area of the Americas by 2005, and to develop the Transatlantic Free Trade Area (TAFTA) by 2020. Whether nursing will be on the list(s) of occupations that will qualify for special visa privileges under these trade agreements is still to be determined. Another political issue is whether nurses entering the United States, especially those who attended U.S. nursing schools, will continue to have the same prescreening requirements for nursing licensure that are presently in place. Voluntarily, Caribbean nurses have instituted reciprocity of licensure. First, a standardized basic nursing curriculum was introduced in 1989, followed by standardized entry-to-practice examinations in 1993. Reportedly, no barriers to migration of registered nurses among 13 Caribbean countries remain—a unique educational and regulatory achievement for nursing.

CONCLUSION

For most nurses today, the urgent and increasing need to provide culturally appropriate primary care within pluralistic communities means that there is much to gain from international collaboration. First, mutual health problems may be more readily or more effectively solved when nursing's collective, multicultural knowledge base is used. Second, the profession can be greatly strengthened and its impact on global politics/policies enhanced by better training and development of consistent and unified advocacy strategies. Nurses constitute more than 50% of the world's health care work force (WHO, 1994) but have yet to mobilize those numbers politically for a universal cause. Finally, as part of the human family in this global village, closer family ties can offer every nurse love, support, and understanding during both professional development and one's personal lifetime journey.

NOTES

1. Nurses should not assume that "developed" countries will never experience problems with access to safe drinking water. In 1993, waterborne cryptosporidiosis in Milwaukee caused prolonged diarrheal illness in approximately 403,000 persons, with 4,400 requiring hospitalization (CDC, 1994); ultimately 100 immunocompromised victims died. Much of the urban infrastructure on the U.S. East Coast is in decline; in the national capital, the water supply was so contaminated that the District of Columbia Health Department had to issue warnings in 1996 not to drink the tap water. Some U.S. cities cannot support the construction of additional toilets or showers.

2. Actually, every new mother must face this choice, unless she is sure that she and her sexual partner are, and will remain, uninfected with HIV for the duration of breast-feeding, or that she can, and will remain able to, provide safe substitutes for breast milk.

3. I believe that a global commitment by the nursing profession to ensure that every woman who wants family planning or protection from immediate transmission of sexually transmitted diseases (STDs) will have them is crucial to the world's health. My belief is based on the following information, mostly from the 1997 Rockefeller Report:

The personal and social costs of STDs, especially HIV infection, far outweigh costs of prevention.

Every year, 7 million infants die because their mothers either were not physiologically ready for pregnancy or lacked obstetrical care.

Every single day, 1,600 women die—almost 600,000 every year—of pregnancy-related causes. The leading cause of maternal death, postpartum hemorrhage, is most common among poor women who have undergone many closely spaced births. For every woman who dies in childbirth, approximately 30 more suffer serious maternity-related injuries, infections, and disabilities.

More than one of every four births is unplanned; one in four children is unwanted. Of the 50 million women who abort pregnancies each year, 75,000 die while attempting it where abortion is illegal and unsafe. All totaled, between 100 and 200 million women who would like to space or limit childbearing are not using modern contraceptives (Institute of Medicine, 1997). Making family planning services available to all who need them is the first step in the Cairo Program of Action, endorsed by 180 countries in 1994.

In a global economy that rests on information and technology, those (families, communities, and nations) who cannot invest in their children's education will fall behind. Population growth today only raises the hurdles to reach economic self sufficiency and prosperity. Where governments have committed to national family planning programs with free or subsidized contraceptive choices, as in Thailand, slowed population growth has allowed economic growth and greater human development choices.

Because it is unlikely that the industrializing or industrialized world will voluntarily reduce its resource consumption soon, further population growth has the potential to engender more poverty, more hunger, a more degraded environment, and violent competition for resources. Poverty is the single major determinant of individual, family, and community health, and already one fifth of humanity lives in poverty (Rockefeller Foundation, 1997; Siantz, 1997).

4. ICN members are national nurses associations, one per country. Individual nurses can participate in ICN only by being members of the national association that is the ICN member for their country. In the United States, this means joining the state nurses association, which is a constituent of the American Nurses Association, a founding member of ICN.

5. A notebook containing all 50-plus ICN position statements can be purchased for approximately $20 by writing ICN at the following address: 3 place Jean-Marteau, CH 1201 Geneva, Switzerland. Most ICN publications are available in ICN's three official languages, English, French, and Spanish; still, many member nursing associations, as in Japan, Denmark, and Brazil, must translate ICN materials into their own language before distributing them.

6. Assembly Bill No. 2125 (California, 1995); Immigration Reform and Immigrant Responsibility Act of 1996 (United States, 1996).

7. The strategic plan of the WHO global nursing network has the following goals: (1) to develop collaborative projects in primary health care and identify resources to support implementation; (2) to strengthen the effectiveness of the network's program of work, processes, and financial resources; (3) to develop a message and a plan for external communication with media and the political arena; (4) to strengthen communication methods to increase knowledge of each other; (5) to establish planning cycles and methods; and (6) to develop paradigms of action and decision making (Global Network of WHO Collaborating Centres for Nursing/Midwifery Development [1995]: *Strategic Plan of the Global Network.* Seoul, Korea: Global Secretariat, Yonsei University).

8. National Council for International Health, Suite 600, 1701 Connecticut Ave., NW, Washington, DC 20006; phone, 202-833-5900.

9. Conference on Environment and Development (Rio de Janeiro, 1992); United Nations Conference on Human Rights (Vienna, 1993); International Conference on Population and Development (Cairo, 1994); World Summit on Social Development (Copenhagen, 1995); United Na-

tions Conference on Human Settlements—Habitat II (Istanbul, 1996); First World's Conference for Women (Mexico City, 1975); Second World Conference for Women (Copenhagen, 1980); Third World Conference for Women (Nairobi, 1985 [parallel nongovernmental-organization forum convened by a nurse, Dame Nita Barrow, of Barbados]); and Fourth World Conference for Women (Beijing, 1995).

10. The Commission on Graduates of Foreign Nursing Schools, established to prescreen foreign-educated nurses desiring to work in the United States, opened the International Commission of Healthcare Professions to be a screening agent for other health professionals (Commission on Graduates of Foreign Nursing Schools, 1997).

11. The European Community facilitates mutual recognition and ready transfer of academic credits, increasing the movement of nursing students between member countries. The European Community has mandated unrestricted movement of professionals, including nurses, for almost 25 years. Laws there require mutual recognition of nursing licenses unless the absence of language competence would preclude functioning with the national patient population; that language barrier is believed responsible for far less movement than is permitted and was expected.

REFERENCES

Affara, F., & Styles, M. (1992). *Nursing regulation guidebook: From principle to power.* Geneva: International Council of Nurses.

Albright, M. (1994, November 7). Principle, power, and purpose in the new era. *U.S. Department of State Dispatch, 5*(45), 744–747.

American Academy of Nursing (Ed.). (1997). *Global migration: The health care implications of immigration and population movements.* Washington, DC: Author.

American Nurses Association. (1998, January 15). *American and foreign nurses abused by massive visa fraud.* Washington, DC: Author.

Basch, P. (1990). *Textbook of international health.* New York: Oxford University Press.

Bodenheimer, T. S., & Grumach, K. (1995). Access to health care. In *Understanding health policy.* Norwalk, CT: Appleton & Lange.

Buergenthal, T, & Shelton, D. (1995). *Protecting human rights in the Americas: Cases and materials* (4th ed. revised). Arlington, VA: NP Engel Publisher.

Carnegie, M. E. (1996). *The path we tread: blacks in nursing worldwide, 1854–1984* (3rd ed.). New York: National League for Nursing Press.

Centers for Disease Control and Prevention. (1994). *Addressing emerging infectious disease threats. A prevention strategy for the U.S.* Atlanta, GA: U.S. Department of Health and Human Services.

Characteristics of foreign-born Hispanic patients with tuberculosis in eight U.S. counties bordering Mexico, 1995. (1996, November 29). *Morbidity and Mortality Weekly Report, 45*(47), 1032–1036.

Clinton, W. (1994, September 26). Building a secure future. *U.S. Department of State Dispatch, 5*(39), 633–636.

Commission on Graduates of Foreign Nursing Schools. (1997, Winter). *International Evaluator, 1*–3.

Drees, C. (1997, August 14). Money and adventure lure Western nurses to Saudi. *Reuters Feature,* at http://www.infoseek.com; printed version available from author.

Fogarty International Center. (1997). *Directory of international grants and fellowships in the health sciences.* (NIH Publication No. 97-3027.) Washington, DC: National Institutes of Health.

Gagnon, W. (1994–1995). Ethnic nationalism and international conflict: The case of Serbia. *International Security, 19*(3), 130–166.

Godue, C. (1992). *International health and schools of public health in the U.S.* Unpublished manuscript.

Harvard University School of Medicine Department of Social Medicine. (1995). *World mental health: Problems and priorities in low-income countries.* Boston: Harvard University.

Hoffman, M. (1995). International humanitarian law and the nursing profession: The current framework and challenges ahead. In American Academy of Nursing (Ed.), *Global migration: The health care implications of immigration and population movements.* Washington, DC: Author.

Holleran, C. (1993). Nursing and the international community. In D. Mason, S. Talbot, & J. Leavitt (Eds.), *Policy and politics for nurses* (2nd ed., pp. 636–645). Philadelphia: W. B. Saunders.

Immigration and Naturalization Service. (1997). *Immigration fact sheet.* Available at WWW URL http://www.ins.usdoj.gov/stats/300.html.

Institute of Medicine, National Academy of Sciences. (1997). *America's vital interest in global health:*

Protecting our people, enhancing our economy, and advancing our international interests. Washington, DC: National Academy Press.

International Council of Nurses. (1996a). *Nursing education: Vol. I. Current and future trends.* Geneva: Author.

International Council of Nurses. (1996b). *The value of nursing in a changing world.* Geneva: Author.

International Council of Nurses. (1997a). *International Classification of Nursing Practice, Alpha Version.* Geneva: Author.

International Council of Nurses. (1997b, May). *WHO's predicted increase in chronic diseases accents need for caring and prevention.* Press Release, No. 9. Geneva: Author.

International Labor Organization. (1997, June). Globalization and labour: New universal ground rules needed. *World of Work, 20,* 12–14.

MacInnis, R. (1996, November–December). UN AIDS director urges: "Keep AIDS on the agenda." *AIDS-Link, 42,* 1.

Mansfield, E., & Snyder, J. (1995). Democratization and the danger of war. *International Security, 20*(1), 5–38.

Marwick, C. (1996, September 11). National effort to immunize adolescents begins. *Journal of the American Medical Association, 276,* 766.

McAuliffe, M., & Henry, B. (1996). Countries where anesthesia is administered by nurses. *Journal of the American Associations of Nurse Anesthetists 64*(5), 469–479.

Murray, C., & Lopez, A. (Eds.). (1996). *The global burden of disease.* Geneva: World Health Organization.

Nakajima, H. (1996, September–October). Health, ethics, and human rights. *World Health, 5,* 3.

National Council for International Health. (1997). Testimony at U.S. Senate Subcommittee Hearing hosted by Senator Leahy, May 15, 1997.

Nurses Foundation of Japan. (1993). *Nursing in the world.* Tokyo: Author.

Over, M., & Piot, P. (1993). HIV infection and sexually transmitted diseases. In D. T. Jamison, W. H. Mosley, A. R. Measham, & J. L. Bobadilla (Eds.), *Disease control priorities in developing countries.* Oxford: Oxford University Press.

Prah, P. (1996, April 3). Western hemisphere labor leaders seek labor protection "guarantees." *BNA News, 64,* A-2.

The President's Interagency Council on Women. (1995). *Follow-up on U.S. commitments made at the UN Fourth World Conference on Women, Beijing, September 4–15, 1995.* Washington, DC: The White House.

The Rockefeller Foundation. (1997). *High stakes: The United States, global population and our common future.* New York: Author.

Siantz, M. (1997). A global profile of the immigrant/migrant child. In American Academy of Nursing (Ed.), *Global migration: The health care implications of immigration and population movements.* Washington, DC: Author.

Sigma Theta Tau. (1997, 2nd Quarter). *Reflections,* 5–23.

Sokolove, R., Mackey, D., Wiles, J., & Lewis, R. J. (1994). Exposure of emergency department personnel to tuberculosis: PPD testing during an epidemic in the community. *Annals of Emergency Medicine, 24*(3), 418–421.

Stevens, B. (1985). Does the 1985 nursing education proposal make economic sense? *Nursing Outlook, 3*(1), 124–127.

Truong, D. H., Hademark, L. L., Mickman, J. K., Mosher, L. B., Dietrich, S. E., & Lowry, P. W. (1997, March 5). Tuberculosis among Tibetan immigrants from India and Nepal in Minnesota, 1992–1995. *Journal of the American Medical Association, 227,* 735–738.

United Nations Children's Fund. (1997). *The progress of nations.* New York: United Nations.

U.S. Department of State. (1995). *United States commitments announced at the Fourth World Conference on Women, Beijing, China.* Washington, DC: Author.

Weine, S., Becker, D. F., McGlashen, T. H., Vojvoda, D., Hartman, S., & Robbins, J. P. (1995). Adolescent survivors of "ethnic cleansing": Observations on the first year in America. *Journal of the American Academy of Adolescent Psychiatry, 34*(9), 1153–1159.

World Bank. (1993). *World development report 1993: Investment in health.* Washington, DC: Author.

World Federation for Mental Health. (1996). World Mental Health Day 1996: Women and mental health kit. (Available from the World Federation of Mental Health, 1021 Prince St., Alexandria, VA 22314.)

World Federation for Mental Health. (1997). World Mental Health Day 1997: Children and mental health kit, fact sheet and global burden of mental and emotional disorder table. (Available from the

World Federation of Mental Health, 1021 Prince St., Alexandria, VA 22314.)

World Health Assembly. (1996). *Strengthening nursing and midwifery* (WHA 49.1). Geneva: Author.

World Health Organization. (1994). *Nursing within the World Health Organization* (HRH/NUR/94.1). Geneva: Author.

World Health Organization. (1996a, 21 February). *Implementation of resolutions report by the Director General, II, WHA 45.5 and WHA 48.81,* pp. 4–9 (A49/4). Geneva: Author (Director General).

World Health Organization. (1996b, 21 February). *Nursing posts in WHO in 1996, by region and grade* (A49/4). Geneva: Author.

World Health Organization. (1997). *Report on the tuberculosis epidemic.* Geneva: Author.

World Resources: 1996–97. (1997). *A guide to the global environment.* Available at http://www.wri.org/wri/wr-96-97/hd_txt4.html.

Zuber, P. L., Knowles, L. S., Binkin, N. J., Tipple, M. A., & Davidson, P. T. (1996, December). Tuberculosis among foreign-born persons in Los Angeles County, 1992–1994. *Tuberculosis Lung Disease 77*(6), 424–530.

VIGNETTE
The Power of Literacy
Jody Glittenberg

Nurses around the world daily confront injustice and inequality, as such conditions undermine the human spirit and damage the health of all. We have found ways to bring such sociopolitical issues into awareness through programs of community and public health; we have fought for the rights of humankind by taking these concerns to the seats of power for political action. Sometimes we plant seeds for health without ever seeing the harvest of the work; yet, at other times, we are privileged to see such efforts come to fruition. My story is of such a planting and of such a harvesting, I hope that the message gives hope to many who have worked ceaselessly but with little to show for their toil. My vignette describes my experience in 1975 in the highlands of Patzun, Guatemala, a village of Cakchiquel Mayan Indians, with a short sequel in 1997 in the same area. It begins with the announcement of the Nobel Peace Award to Rigoberta Menchu.

Her face, her words, the traditional red dress with bright blue embroidery—yes, she is *patzunera,* a woman from Patzun, Guatemala. She, Rigoberta Menchu, the 1992 Nobel Peace Prize awardee, wrote *I, Rigoberta,* with such passion, chastising people in power, anywhere and everywhere around the globe, about inhumane treatment of all indigenous people. Yes, I believe that Rigoberta must have been one of the children assembled every Wednesday in 1975 on the earthen floor, home of Hortensia Caj, the president of the Mother's Club of Patzun. Looking at the cover of her moving book reminded me of the story entitled "Thumbprints on Newsprint," which I tell in the book I wrote (1994), *To the Mountain and Back.*

Thumbprints on Newsprint

Edith, the British midwife who worked with the Behrhorst Program, held an "under-five" clinic every Wednesday in Patzun, to assess the health of children five years old and under and to educate mothers about proper feeding and child rearing. [p. 128]

The clinic was held in the courtyard of one of the Cakchiquel Mayan mothers, Hortensia, who was president of the Women's Club (my etic term for the social group of women in town, Patzun) and a mother of three children, all under the age of five. Her family was wealthier than most in the town; their compound home was large, with a spacious courtyard that was often filled with bundles of corn from the harvests. Hortensia was friendly, smiling, and open to new ideas. During the harvest season she worked hard in the fields, beside her husband, Ernesto. Her home was spotless, her dress impeccable. Hortensia was a role model for women in Patzun, the town known to be a place of Indian power and a threat to the national government. It was natural with such a large home that the Women's Club meetings be held there. The Club was organized by women interested in learning together about such topics as health care and ways of improving their own education. The Club had two goals: health care for the children and literacy for themselves. [pp. 129–130]

Although Cakchiquel was the spoken language the women wanted to learn Spanish. This wish was the same as expressed by Rigoberta Menchu in her book (1992): "They've always said, 'poor Indians they can't speak,' so many speak for them. That's why I decided to learn Spanish." [p. 157]

My role was to assist Hortensia, in setting up the storage shed in the courtyard into a measuring and weighing room. Each mother brought her children under the age of five— some had as many as three—into the shed; the inside was clean and dry. The scales were simple; there was little expense in the equipment. The only expense to the mother was fifteen cents for a month's supply of vitamins, if the mother chose to buy them. No medications were given at this clinic; the goal was to teach mothers how to improve the daily care of their children by giving them nutritious food. Immunizations for childhood diseases such as diphtheria, measles, smallpox, whooping cough, and polio were given at the public health clinic.

Outside the weighing and measuring shed were two chairs and a table, where Edith would talk privately to each mother about her children's health. Edith would then listen with a stethoscope to the heart and lung sounds, and also examine the mouth, throat, and ears of each child. The child's height and weight were recorded on a card kept by the mother. If Edith found a child was not growing at an expected rate, she would advise the mother about seeking medical care. The clinic was a means of screening children for potentially serious problems, such as malnutrition, intestinal worms, and infection. The mothers and children considered Edith a friend; she would talk with everyone, and they would laugh with her.

The under-five clinic lasted for about an hour, after which the mothers would form a circle on the earthen floor inside Hortensia's house. The children would play outside, safe in the courtyard. Rather than sitting and gossiping, the women were all learning to read. Yes, what an exciting experience! In Patzun 95 percent of women over the age of twenty were illiterate. Younger children were attending local schools and learning to read and write, but older women had been kept away from such opportunities; Hortensia was one of those women. The members of the Women's Club were determined to be able to read and write, as was evident by their faithful attendance. Week after week, they arrived carrying their well-worn reading booklets.

It was clear that for the women of Patzun becoming literate was tied with improving the lives of their children. They also expressed a desire to become more independent when business deals were conducted in Spanish, which often included written agreements. These women were expert weavers and sold their products to the many tourists who stopped in the town's plaza. The *patzuneras* knew that if they were literate in Spanish they could carry on negotiations with powerful businessmen and also tourists.

Edith and I used comic books in teaching the women to read. The simple language plus the appealing pictures made concepts easier to grasp. Writing was a little harder, but each week we could see progress. Women were starting to sign their names. The openness they showed in confronting their illiteracy was exciting. They would laugh about mistakes and tease one another.

Hortensia would greet us each Wednesday morning around nine. Her round, rosy cheeks and wide-open smile were a welcoming sight.

One day, however, she wasn't there—but on our arrival, we saw six Jeeps parked outside the compound.

Edith cried, "Oh, oh! There's trouble!"

As we opened the big gate into the compound, Hortensia was not there; instead, combat soldiers armed with machine guns lined the compound wall. There were about twenty soldiers and the leader, a giant man about six and a half feet tall, stood aiming a machine gun right at Edith.

Edith, in her usual, nonchalant manner, said a customary greeting, "Good morning. How are you today?"

The leader, a stern-looking man, stepped forward and said, "We have come to arrest you for practicing medicine without a license."

Hortensia and the other women were now pressing against the wall, having come out of the house, but they were huddled away from the soldiers, looking very frightened. The children peeked out from behind their mothers' skirts, which they were hugging tightly, obviously frightened as well.

"That's silly," replied the brave midwife. "What do you mean 'practicing medicine'? I'm a midwife, and I'm here only to weigh and measure the children and to teach the mothers how to prevent malnutrition. You know the president's wife has nutritional programs all over the Republic. Why do you think I am practicing medicine?"

The tall man, the chief public health officer of the department, replied sternly, "Let me see what you do and how you do it!"

As on all other Wednesdays, Edith and I went about our work, setting up the scales, the measuring tapes, and the table and chairs. We placed the vitamins on the table. The chief said triumphantly, "I see that you do have bottles of pills."

"Those are only vitamins," Edith explained emphatically. We went about our business.

"And who are you?" the public health officer asked, pointing at me.

"I'm an anthropologist from the United States." I answered with a tremble in my voice (a safe answer). "And I help to weigh and measure the children in the shed."

"Hmph!" he snorted.

Several children and their mothers timidly went through the usual routine of talking with Edith and getting weighed and measured.

After about fifteen minutes, the chief officer came forward and said, "We are closing you down, because you do not have proper sanitary conditions here."

Edith chuckled, "You know that the water in the fountain is from the city and the seat of the latrine has a stamp on it that reads, 'Inspected by the Public Health Department.' If these aren't sanitary, then what is?" The officer looked frustrated. Finally he said, "Well, you don't have proper lighting in the shed for weighing and measuring the children. Come in and I'll show you." We followed him into the shed. The officer closed the shutters and slammed the door shut. Edith, the tall officer, and I stood in pitch darkness for several minutes. I had to stifle a giggle, as we stood shoulder to shoulder in the darkness.

"I guess you're right." replied Edith with resignation. I didn't say a word.

With triumph the tall health officer and the twenty machine-gun-toting soldiers silently left the compound. Edith explained to the women that we could not meet anymore until this matter was cleared by the officials. "I hope that you continue to learn to read and write on your own and together. We'll return as soon as the matter is cleared up." Several women had tears in their eyes, but none spoke. "We must leave right away," said Edith, "because the soldiers will soon return to see if we have gone, as they have ordered us to. I don't want to be arrested. I'd suggest that everyone just go home—quietly." [pp. 132–133]

Edith and I returned and told the story to Doc Behrhorst, Lutheran medical missionary who had developed the World Health Organization model primary health care program. "I'm disappointed," said Doc, "but I guess we could have predicted that he would try to corner us somehow, so he used the Women's Club to do it. What a coward. We'll stay quiet for a while and see what the Indians themselves do." [p. 133]

Several weeks later, Edith came to my house, very excited: "Look what Hortensia and the women did!" She pulled out of her car a huge roll of white newsprint paper and began to unroll it on my living-room floor. Thumbprint after thumbprint marched down the side of the paper and now and then a "beginning" signature. One hundred, 300, 500, no, 800!! Eight hundred thumbprints marked the women's protest to the cancellation of literacy classes. Eight hundred illiterate women had expressed their power—their right to learn to read and write. They protested with their thumbprints, for they knew what the power of learning could bring to them, their families—their children. Others too—such as the public health officer— knew that literacy would empower women, and thus cowardly chose to keep the women powerless, at least for as long as possible. When I left Guatemala in 1975, the under-five clinic was still prohibited from reopening, and no one was helping the women to overcome their illiteracy. [p. 133]

Twenty-two Years Later

In March 1997, twenty-two years after the closing of the Mother's Club, as I stood in the National Assembly of Congress in Guatemala City, I saw an Indian congresswoman dressed in her native dress; she spoke clearly, in Spanish, to those assembled about a law that needed their support. She obviously was literate and very powerful. The Peace Accord, ending a 35-year civil war, was signed December 29, 1996, and both sides were burying all weapons. I knew that those who had tried to hold back the power of the word, such as the army officer in 1975, were powerless when faced with a just and righteous cause—peace. But it took Rigoberta and thousands like her who refused to succomb to illiteracy to overcome the injustice of power-hungry people in whatever part of the globe they are found.

I believe it is the covenant that we, as nurses, have made to the *people* to help foster and empower them to seek justice as part of health care. I still believe, as I wrote in 1986:

> Our role as advocates for the powerless, the underprivileged, the disenfranchised has been a part of our history of nursing, . . . our heri-

tage. . . . We cannot be content with mere flaming words and undirected passion. Now we must use our emerging role as leaders . . . to take our responsible causes to the seats of power and lawmaking with clear thinking and articulate arguments. We cannot be narrow in our vision but rather deal with the vast potential in all humans. It is with this philosophy of advocacy that we, as nurses, assist people in determining and participating in their care, identifying their own needs, and using their own resources. For health is found when people are empowered to participate in their own health decisions, whether it is to have a pap smear or to replace weapons with plows. It is found when infants have loving faces for bonding, or when children have knowledge about their own bodies, or when women have equal rights and are assured of sensitive health care, or when young people grow up without the fear of war, or people of all ages and skills find meaningful work, and when those illiterate find new worlds of wonder and power through learning to read and write, or when old people are no longer lonely and devalued, or when the mentally ill are protected from their own abuse.

Nurses are a strong force in assuring that social justice exists, is retained, and is felt worldwide. Our voices, our intellect, our commitment must assure that globally a new sense of balance prevails. We must refuse to go backwards by defining health in relation to the limits of the hospital wall or the narrow definition of an illness. We must see our role as key health promoters worldwide. Our leadership is vital; our time is now. [Glittenberg, 1986, p. 1]

References

Glittenberg, J. (1986). A decade of transformation. *Nursing Praxis* [New Zealand], *3*(3), 2.

Glittenberg, J. (1994). *To the mountain and back.* Prospect Heights, IL: Waveland Press.

Menchu, R. (1992). *I, Rigoberta: An Indian woman in Guatemala* (Edited and with an introduction by Elisabeth Burgos-Debray. Translated by Ann Wright). London: Verso. (Originally published in 1983 as *Me llamo Rigoberta Menchu y asi me nacio la concienca.* Barcelona: Arco Vergara).

VIGNETTE

The Fourth World Conference on Women: The Road to Beijing and Beyond

Anie Kalayjian

As the United Nations (UN) representative for the World Federation for Mental Health (WFMH), I had the privilege to be a delegate to the Fourth World Conference on Women (FWCW), held in Beijing, China, as well as to the Non-Governmental Organization (NGO) Forum on Women, which took place some 60 kilometers away in Huairou, China.

My interest and involvement in international issues has been long-standing, but my involvement with the UN started only in 1990. At that time I was a visiting professor at Pace University's Leinhard School of Nursing and a member of the WFMH. While reading the WFMH Quarterly Report, I came across a report by Dr. Kay Greene, who was then a member of the UN NGO Committee on Aging and the main representative for WFMH. I wrote to her, expressing interest in her work and sharing with her my research on the survivors of the Ottoman Turkish Genocide of the Armenians, as well as the Mental Health Outreach Program for Armenia, which I founded after the 1988 earthquake and the Azeri-Armenian conflict. In less than a week I had a call from Dr. Greene. We met, and, on the basis of my interests, expertise, and research, I was immediately recruited as a UN representative; a year later, I was elected as the secretary/treasurer of the UN NGO Committee for Human Rights.

Since the 1985 adoption of the Nairobi Forward-Looking Strategies (FLS) for the Advancement of Women to the Year 2000 at the Third World Conference on Women, I have been interested in the document and have followed its progress very closely. This plan of action laid out a framework that can be used by national governments to design concrete programs and policies in all spheres of women's involvement to bring the Nairobi goals within reach by the beginning of the twenty-first century. In the ensuing years, there have been major political, economic, social, and cultural changes that have had both positive and negative effects on women.

At the Beijing conference there were three major negotiating groups: the European Union, the United States, and G-77, a group of developing nations and China. Major disparities between the G-77 and the West lay in the areas of reproductive health and resources commitment. Much agreement was reached in the area of physical health, but not as much in mental health. Although one could see and hear the slogan "Health is a human right and not a commodity," people meant physical health—the right to reproduce, breast-feed, and be free from diseases like HIV disease and breast cancer. The conference did not address the emotional and psychosocial components intertwined with physical health. The Beijing Declaration and Platform for Action included a critical statement about women's reproductive rights: "The explicit recognition and reaffirmation of the right of all women to control all aspects of their health, in particular their own fertility, is basic to their empowerment." But, in contrast to previous conferences, there was no inordinate emphasis on reproductive and mothering roles, as though these were the sole contributions of women in society. Instead, this conference built on themes explored at the Third Women's Conference in Nairobi—Equality, Development, and Peace.

The mission of the FWCW related closely to my own beliefs on promoting human rights for all people, especially women: achieving equal status for women; creating processes enabling women to participate fully and actively in decision making within the family and community, at national, regional, and international levels; and empowering women and men to work together as equal partners.

The aforementioned goals of the Plan of Action had a special meaning for me. I am an Armenian-American whose family was driven from its home twice: first when Ottoman Turks slaughtered more than 1.5 million Armenians in 1915 for religious, territorial, and other reasons, and later by the Syrian government because of its subtle oppression of and discrimination against women. My father was among the 20% of Armenians who survived. Surviving the forced marches through the Arabian deserts, he settled in Syria. My mother was the child of a survivor who had also settled in Syria, where I was born. Being an eyewitness to the Syrian-Israeli conflict as a child, I felt the traumatic impact of wars and conflicts. Far too often we had to hide in subbasements as Israeli planes flew so low that some of our windows shattered. Growing up in Syria, I also tasted the bitterness of gender discrimination. Oppression was everywhere, especially for women and girls. In accordance with the cherished double standard of that time, my brother was allowed to go out and play when the area was safe from the enemy, but I was forbidden to do the same. Why? Simply because I was a girl. Most of my female classmates were forced to get married after completing the eighth grade. I was fortunate to have a brother who, as a U.S. citizen, sponsored our emigration from Syria.

My Middle Eastern sisters were not as fortunate, nor were those in Asia. In Asia, where baby boys have always been preferred, baby girls are killed in any of the following ancient ways: feeding them poisonous oleander berries, smothering them in their afterbirth, not feeding them, aborting them, or just neglecting them.

I became internationally involved to make a difference in issues concerning women globally. As an official delegate to the WFMH at the UN's FWCW, I witnessed more than 40,000 women from around the world, coming together to pursue an agenda for equality, peace, and harmony. I was able to take part in the UN plenaries and caucuses. An important task of the caucuses was to examine and recommend revisions to the language of the Platform for Action because this was the document to be used to set worldwide priorities for addressing women's issues. This process began a year before the FWCW. Documents were received before the caucuses, they were reviewed, and controversies regarding issues of equality, health, and development were bracketed. When the conference began, the platform contained more than 438 sentences, or parts of sentences in brackets, indicating areas of disagreement—many of which were on health issues. By the end of the conference, almost all brackets were gone. This process was long and complicated but fruitful. During the caucuses, the indigenous people, as well as government officials, were educated about these issues. Then the plenaries took place. The goal of the plenaries was to revise the documents, to work on the language, and to include mental health issues, instead of focusing only on reproductive health, which had been the focus of the UN Third World Conference on Women.

In Beijing, I observed with excitement and astonishment as 40,000 women representing more than 180 countries came together. I was excited by the experience of the solidarity, unity, and power of women. As an active member of the UN NGO Working Group on Women, Human Rights, and Mental Health, I was instrumental in organizing two panel discussions addressing issues specific to women. The panels were extremely well received, and the quality of participation was high. Global networking groups were established to address issues concerning women and mental health. Some 2 years after the Beijing conference, the women in these networking groups have remained in touch with one another, collaborating and participating in other international conferences and meetings around the world.

In Beijing, I met nurses from Egypt, the United States, and Armenia. But I am sure there were many nurses with whom I interacted without realizing that they were nurses; it seemed as though professions were secondary. We went beyond what we did, or what degrees we held, or which schools we had attended. We were a group of women, gathered to address the human rights of all men, women, and children, and seeking peace, love, and harmony.

In the global village of the twenty-first century, nurses can act collectively and globally to ensure that information not nuclear weapons, assertiveness not aggression, and sharing not domination are used for empowerment and for linking people into a holistic and humane unit worldwide.

UNIT VI CASE STUDY
The Community and Childbearing Centers
*Ruth Watson Lubic and Lisa Summers**

The Childbearing Center (CbC) in New York City is a health care innovation that changed policy in maternity care delivery worldwide. The CbC is a freestanding birth center, a home-like facility where family-centered care is *de rigueur* and the care team includes the families being served (Lubic & Ernst, 1978).

The services provided, which grew out of caring and concern for families, brought about social change in at least two ways. First, alternatives to the conventional system for healthy childbearing families were provided—alternatives that give birth back to women. Second, the services supported the leadership role of certified nurse-midwives (CNMs) in designing new forms of care and thus caused a shift in control and power among medicine, nursing, midwifery, and families. Even the CbC's most vociferous opponents agreed that nurse-midwives, through competitive demonstration, sharply escalated the humanizing of in-hospital maternity services (Lazarus et al., 1981).

This case study, in describing the development of the birth center concept, emphasizes the community context and strategies. Woven into the birth center story, however, are examples of how nurse-midwives have worked effectively in other spheres of political action. Two organizations, the Maternity Center Association (MCA) and the National Association of Childbearing Centers (NACC), have, under the leadership of nurse-midwives, played a dramatic role in this health care innovation. These organizations and the leaders of the birth center movement have been highly effective in working with government leaders to shape health care policy. Finally, though the early leaders of the birth center movement were motivated by their desire to offer an alternative to childbearing families rather than to serve professional needs, the story of the birth center is also the story of the creation of a new workplace for nurse-midwives. Creating and controlling the workplace has facilitated autonomous practice and the ability to provide a model of care that nurse-midwives see as ideal for healthy childbearing families.

The founders of the birth center movement have, from the beginning, worked to influence policy. After first demonstrating the viability of the birth center, this has been done in six major ways:

1. Establishing a networking organization to provide support to fledgling birth centers
2. Evaluating centers through a prospective multisite study and other research
3. Facilitating replication through workshops on how to establish freestanding birth centers
4. Providing accreditation based on standards developed by a multidisciplinary group
5. Assisting states to develop rules and regulations for licensure
6. Ensuring reimbursement by informing third-party payers about cost-effectiveness and safety aspects

---

*The opinions in this article are those of the author and except where directly quoted should not be interpreted to represent the opinion of the American College of Nurse-Midwives or any member of its Board of Directors.

DEMONSTRATION PROJECT

Demonstration is the key to change. Ideas are important, but you must breathe life into them through demonstration if you expect to gain attention and to effect change.

Though the cost-effectiveness of birth center care is receiving a good deal of attention today, the birth center concept did not grow out of the needs of society for relief from the high costs of health (usually spelled "medical") care. Nor did it grow from the needs of professionals to secure their futures, though it has provided a comfortable workplace for nurse-midwives. The birth center grew from the needs of childbearing families.

In the 1960s and early 1970s, many families complained about the conventional in-hospital, illness-oriented maternity care, and some began to turn to do-it-yourself home births. Two or three decades earlier, home birth had been an everyday event, although a waning one. By the late 1960s, however, a decade after the MCA had closed its home birth service because of lack of demand, home birth was regarded by most health professionals as extreme, an exhibitionist tactic of a lunatic fringe. Rather than address families' concerns about the inappropriate medical view of pregnancy and birth as a pathologic event—a disease to be controlled by more and more application of technology—medical leaders told birth center proponents over and over, "Educate them; they are ignorant!"

The birth center as an innovation (it is not an invention) grew out of the failure of the public to convince most physician leaders of the need for an option, but it grew, as well, out of nurse-midwifery's success in understanding the complaints of families and acting on them. This nurse-midwives did; the rest is history—brief, but history nonetheless.

In anthropological terms, nurse-midwives were and are involved in effecting planned change. The board of directors of the MCA considered a return to a home birth service (which had been operated between 1931 and 1959), as well as a freestanding maternity hospital. After lengthy discussions with the families they sought to serve and careful consideration of safety, the birth center was designed. In brief, the CbC was designed to give birth back to women in a setting best described as a maxihome, not a minihospital.

The CbC provides comprehensive maternity care to families anticipating a normal pregnancy and birth in an out-of-hospital setting. For demonstration, it was set up in MCA's 92nd Street home in Manhattan and included the following features to offset the complaints and concerns heard from childbearing families:

- An orientation for full discussion of the service—its benefits and its risks
- Early enrollment—not later than the 22nd week of pregnancy—to allow sufficient time for prenatal education
- Provision of history and general consent forms to be examined at home before the first visit
- Screening at the first visit and all succeeding visits
- Prenatal care, including education for birth and parenthood
- Preparation of siblings
- Care provided by nurse-midwives, with obstetrical and pediatric consultation and hospital backup constantly available
- Families' access to their own records, including charting of self-collected weights and urine test results
- Social service support if necessary
- Appropriate use of diagnostic technology
- Fees one third to one half the charges for in-hospital care
- Labor and birth monitored and attended by a nurse-midwife in a private birth room, with family members of choice present [The mother defines family as she wishes—consanguineous and/or fictive.]

- No routine use of intravenous fluids, shaving, enema, or episiotomy
- Birth in position of choice
- Newborn examination on site
- Return home in up to 12 hours
- Home visit by a public health nurse within 24 hours
- Postpartum visits at between 7 and 10 days and at fifth or sixth week

When the CbC was opened in 1975, after 2½ years of preparation, MCA was uncertain whom it would attract or whether it would be successful. Change, especially because it portends redistribution of power, generates opposition. That opposition, MCA learned, can take many forms and be fiercely applied. A political anthropological analysis of the barriers and conflict relating to the establishment of the center demonstrated that powerful groups do everything they can to retain their control and that they feel justified in so doing (Lubic, 1979). A number of lessons can be learned from an analysis of the conflict surrounding the CbC:

1. In planning any change in the health care delivery system, expect obstruction from the groups in control.
2. Obstruction to change will be brought to bear at all levels: legal, moral, ethical, professional, and financial.
3. The means employed to obstruct—even dishonest activities—will be seen to justify ends.
4. Bureaucracies are particularly susceptible to manipulation by powerful groups.
5. Groups in control will attempt to assert authority whether or not there is evidence for their assertions.
6. Formal intention, even of the Congress, will be subverted if it interferes with the seats of power. (Medicaid reimbursement, to which the CbC was entitled as an Article 28–established diagnostic and treatment center, was withheld for 2½ years.)
7. Financial backing is necessary for successful innovation.
8. Regulation of professional groups must be developed, just as for business or other self-serving groups; that is, backup services for innovations must be legislated. (They were legislated in 1988 by the New York State Department of Health, and MCA in 1990 had to bring the regulations to bear.)
9. Professional groups are susceptible to the excitement of new technologies and must be constrained against their premature and inappropriate use.
10. A focus on health and humanitarian services oriented to people is accorded low priority by groups in power.
11. Professionals who have achieved their career goals are less dependent on the approbation of their fellows and thus are more inclined to support innovation.
12. Innovative services that promise safety, satisfaction, and economy through altering patterns of care are resisted out of all relationship to their actual size and potential for provision of care (Lubic, 1979).

The CbC was a target of activities designed to prevent reimbursement, interfere with grant proposals, discredit it with the people it planned to serve, raise questions regarding competence, sully personal and professional reputations, discourage the cooperation of those needed for consultation, and prevent the studies necessary to demonstrate safety. Even when the demonstration is a success, these same problems are experienced to varying degrees by those who replicate it.

EVALUATION

Early on, evaluation of MCA's childbearing center was effectively stopped by those opposing it. First, they interfered at the funding level; that is, those in power used their authority and actually advised foundations against supporting the demonstration and its evaluation. (Nevertheless, the John A. Hartford and W. K. Kellogg foundations, 8 years later, did fund a national prospective study.) Second, obstetrical leaders refused to provide access to the populations necessary for comparative study or randomized, controlled trial, even when this would have relieved overtaxed in-hospital services.

Without a possibility for randomized, controlled trials and matched-pair, or cohort, studies, midwives turned to the only recourse left: descriptive data collection (Bennetts & Lubic, 1982; DeJong, Shy, & Carr, 1981; Faison, Pisani, Douglas, Cranch, & Lubic, 1979). Even when these studies were prospective and in large numbers, detractors criticized them as inadequate, untrustworthy, and scientifically naive.

In the mid-1980s, however, the NACC embarked on a prospective multisite study of birth center outcomes. Eighty-four centers participated, and an analysis of outcomes of almost 12,000 women entering labor in freestanding birth centers was published late in 1989 as a "special report" in the prestigious *New England Journal of Medicine* (NEJM) (Rooks et al., 1989). The report was accompanied by a detracting guest editorial written by distinguished obstetricians (Lieberman & Ryan, 1989).

In the February 1990 issue of the *American Journal of Nursing,* Editor-in-Chief Mary B. Mallison published an editorial regarding the study. The editorial, entitled "Gate Crashers," has an important lesson for those interested in policy and politics for nurses:

> The guest editorial accompanying the NEJM article should be required reading for all students of real politic. It questions the significance of a study in only half of the nation's birth centers. Imagine questioning a study of 12,000 consecutive patients with one common diagnosis in "only half" of the nation's hospitals! The editorial also expresses fears about the safety of transfers from freestanding birth centers to hospitals, raising the specters "rare

but critical complications." Yet, the outcomes in this study were outstanding! . . .

> The NEJM editorial also fears that no ideal study that compares birth center to hospital outcomes will ever be possible. The unspoken conclusion is left hanging in the air: Tell the public the data are inadequate and always will be. . . . So we have here a near-perfect example, right in front of our noses, of what sociologist Paul Starr calls the triumph of accommodation of organized medicine to unpalatable truths. [Mallison, 1990, p. 7]

Political behavior is related to competition for scarce resources. When research results might reveal weaknesses in the conventional system, the research may well be prevented, delayed, altered, or otherwise manipulated. When practice-oriented research (which is an accurate descriptor of the CbC, MCA's laboratory for ideal nurse-midwifery practice) threatens to alter patterns of care or shift control, it will be opposed. When that research concerns an innovation designed and promulgated by members of groups other than those in power, it will be even more vigorously opposed. Opposition is almost always cloaked in protestations of clinical or quality-of-care concerns. So it was in the guest editorial on the national study of birth centers (Lieberman & Ryan, 1989).

REPLICATION: THE STORY OF NACC

The leaders of the birth center movement realized that a successful demonstration project was just the beginning; they would have to facilitate the concept's growth and development by teaching others to establish birth centers, emphasizing that the service must be carefully designed and scrupulously monitored for quality and adherence to its philosophy and goals. This was especially important as hospitals and physicians picked up the model and replicated it.

A great deal of education is required to interpret the midwifery practice on which birth centers are based and its difference from what is known as low-risk obstetrics. This education is provided in the form of several workshops each year. That statement, quickly and easily made, does not properly reveal the 6 years of arduous and complex organizational effort required to establish, first, the Cooperative Birth Center Network in 1981 (under a grant from the John A. Hartford Foundation) and then, in 1983, the NACC. The NACC also works to provide the data that are essential to convincing policymakers and purchasers of care. Annual surveys are conducted and made available to policymakers such as the Health Insurance Association of America, which in 1989 published the first report on maternity care costs demonstrating the cost-effectiveness of free-standing birth centers (Minor, 1989).

It has now been more than two decades since the CbC opened. Across the country, more than 145 birth centers are known to NACC, with an additional 100 in the development process. Internationally, MCA and NACC have consulted in Australia, New Zealand, England, Scotland, Holland, Belgium, Sweden, Germany, and Italy. NACC workshops have included attendees from Mexico and Peru, and many visitors from both developed and developing countries have visited birth centers to see for themselves. MCA, in keeping with its mission to demonstrate innovative forms of care and, if successful, to spin them off to another organization, has recently transferred the site and ownership of the CbC to a New York City hospital while retaining it as a freestanding model. Actually, two hospitals contended for the CbC. One would have moved it in-hospital; the other was chosen.

In addition to MCA and NACC, other organizations have played an important role. Professional associations holding their own standards for practice may be influential and may need proof of the safety of new models. In the CbCs experience, support came first from nursing and later from nurse-midwifery. It has not yet come from organized medicine. The American Public Health Association, however, which is a multidisciplinary organization, provided an effective forum for those active in the birth center movement, publishing guidelines for licensing centers (American Public Health Association, 1983).

ACCREDITATION AND LICENSURE

Concerned about ensuring quality care and faced with uneven state and local regulations and the lack of any appropriate program for accreditation for birth center facilities, NACC spawned an accrediting body, the Commission for the Accreditation of Freestanding Birth Centers (now the Commission for the Accreditation of Birth Centers), in 1985. The commission, originally supported by a coalition of funding agencies, was structured to provide representation of leaders from professional groups (including obstetricians, pediatricians, CNMs, and nurses), childbirth educators, and consumers. It adopted NACC's national Standards for Freestanding Birth Centers as the basis for the process of accreditation. The commission offers workshops to assist birth centers in preparing for accreditation and provides training for site visitors. Accreditation is a voluntary process that provides evidence of quality to families, to other health care providers, and to third-party payers.

Licensure, on the other hand, is a regulatory process that varies widely from state to state. Some states have no regulations that provide for the licensure of birth centers; others recognize the NACC standards. Regulations for licensure tend to focus on the physical facility and do not generally provide the assurance of quality inherent in the accreditation process. For these reasons, insurers may require accreditation. NACC has also been active in the area of birth center licensure, offering its expertise to individuals at the state level who seek to formulate regulations.

FINANCING AND REIMBURSEMENT

When nurses are seeking to effect planned change, funders are an important group to reach. This includes both foundations and governmental agencies that award program monies in response to proposals and reimbursement agencies that insure individuals for health care through either public programs (Medicaid, Medicare) or private programs (Blue Cross, commercial insurance companies, health maintenance organizations). Either type will require data regarding both safety and cost and may be called on for support of evaluation. An early study done by Luc Cannoodt, under the auspices of New York Blue Cross/Blue Shield, was important. It demonstrated the cost of birth in the CbC to be 37% of that of in-hospital normal childbirth (Lubic, 1983).

The direct effect on foundations of political activity against the CbC remains, although it is diminished. Twenty years of experience and good outcome data have, to a great extent, put foundations at ease. Another significant development is the greater frequency with which foundations turn to nurses or nurse-midwives, in addition to obstetricians and pediatricians, when they seek advice on matters relating to maternal and child health. The W. K. Kellogg Foundation, which began providing major assistance to MCA in 1986, was an early leader in its direct attention to the importance of nursing in designing maternal and child health projects.

Critical to the survival and growth of birth centers is third-party reimbursement for birth center care. Because of NACC's diligent work, the Civilian Health and Medical Program of the Uniformed Services (CHAMPUS) published rules and began reimbursing accredited free-standing birth centers in 1988. Other insurers base their reimbursement on evidence of accreditation as well.

NACC also works to provide the data that are essential to convincing policymakers and purchasers of care. Annual surveys are conducted and made available to policymakers such as the Health Insurance Association of America, which in 1989 published the first report on maternity care costs demonstrating the cost-effectiveness of freestanding birth centers (Minor, 1989).

In the past 5 years, the cost-effectiveness of birth center care has received increasing attention. A recent analysis suggested that, on average, hospitals are 38% more expensive and less appropriate models of care for a low-risk birth (Stone & Walker, 1995). The willingness of third-party payers to reimburse for birth center care, and in some cases to provide incentives for enrollees to use birth centers, has been responsible in large part for the growth of birth centers.

This development has been, however, a double-edged sword. It requires more than a financial incentive to set up a birth center. Hospitals, in their zeal to capture their share of the maternity market, have set up "birth centers" that may or may not be consistent with the model demonstrated by MCA. Birth centers are being linked with ambulatory surgical services and have, in some cases, provided little more than a new setting for birth. The *successful* mainstreaming of the birth center concept is of great concern. As signified by a name change (dropping "Freestanding"), the Commission on the Accreditation of Birth Centers is planning to make its accrediting services available to all birth centers in order to provide the public with a means to measure quality and to identify those birth centers providing care consistent with the midwifery model.

RESPONDING TO THE NEEDS OF LOW-INCOME FAMILIES: LESSONS IN EMPOWERMENT

Although families did come to the CbC from all five boroughs of New York City and its safety, satisfaction, and economy were proven, comparatively few low-income families were attracted to it. Therefore, in 1978, MCA began to plan for a center to be placed in a low-income neighborhood. It was 10 years before the opening of the Childbearing Center of Morris Heights in 1988. Once again, the naysayers were busy: "You can't put a birth center in a low-income neighborhood; the women are all at high risk." In many respects, the opposition to this plan was even stronger than opposition to the original CbC. It was easy to see that low-income families have been stereotyped in a way that intensifies their disempowerment.

MCA nevertheless set out to find a health care organization in a low-income neighborhood that would collaborate in establishing a CbC with the intent that MCA would transfer the service to its partner if it proved successful. The Morris Heights Health Center, on Burnside Avenue in the South Bronx, a federally funded community health center that was moving to a larger building across the street from its original address, was agreeable to being part of the venture. Grants from foundations and the New York State Health Department provided the seed money necessary for startup. Backup, the *sine qua non* of birth center establishment, was secured from Bronx-Lebanon Hospital, and in 1988 the Childbearing Center of Morris Heights (CBCMH) opened. Today it is a genuine community resource operated by the Morris Heights Health Center.

The story of the CBCMH teaches an important lesson about grassroots organizing. Outsiders who attempt to intervene in a community may not be welcome there; community involvement has been crucial to the success of the CBCMH. First, a task force of women from the area who had given birth in the 92nd Street CbC was set up to advise on the program and decoration of the CBCMH from the time that planning was begun. Then, as community women began to give birth in the center, they joined the task force and eventually changed its name to the Community Action Committee. During MCA's tenure of ownership, this committee was a vital part of the center, its collective wisdom listened to carefully by staff. Employing neighborhood women as nurse-midwife as-

sistants and support staff was also important to success.

It is clear that there are many low-income families who are both capable of passing the physical screening and interested in participating in all aspects of the program. The values of these families are not different from those of the middle class, especially as to wanting healthy children and positive birth experiences. It is also clear, however, that outreach is important in low-income areas in order to educate families about any new service, particularly one that deviates so remarkably from conventional care. Grandmothers-to-be play an important role with their expectant daughters and should be invited to participate in center activities.

A newborn infant represents hope to most families, and birth is seen as a spiritual and religious event, as well as a physical, emotional, and social one. A personalized, caring service empowers women and families. Staff, in turn, are empowered.

The role of this last concept, empowerment, is now, more than 20 years after the CbC's establishment, being recognized by the medical profession. John Wennberg, a physician interested in outcomes and patient choice in treatment, stated at a 1991 symposium, "Health Care in the 90's: Economics, Ethics and Quality":

> The mark that American medicine will leave on world medicine in this decade is that for the first time the patient is an active agent in medical decision-making. The whole social pattern of our country is moving in that direction. We are a restless group of people who want to participate in our own futures. As a result, a very fundamental revolution is going on.

In North Texas one can find an example of a birth center that was created by nurses and nurse-midwives who vowed to continue providing care to medically indigent women when the only public hospital in the area closed. This innovative, nurse-managed clinic began with CNMs and nurses volunteering their time in a prenatal clinic and has expanded to provide a variety of services, including a family birth center (Capan, Beard, & Mashburn, 1993).

Culturally sensitive primary care has been provided by CNMs in south Texas for almost 30 years at Su Clinica Familiar, one of the most comprehensive community and migrant health centers in the United States. The one-stop shopping, which includes case management, social services, pharmacy, laboratory, and radiography, also includes a birth center (Burk, Wieser, & Keegan, 1995).

Plans are currently under way in the nation's capital to establish a birth center and well child care, linked with community-based organizations providing a drop-in center, day care, and early childhood education facilities.

MAINSTREAMING THE BIRTH CENTER CONCEPT

Ernst (1996) noted that "redecorating and refurbishing the acute care setting is a step in the right direction but does not bring about the fundamental change needed. The real change must be in the attitude of the care providers." Garite, Snell, Walker, and Darrow (1995, p. 414), in their discussion of a university-affiliated freestanding birth center, comment that, "although many community hospitals have redesigned or set aside areas within the hospital that they often call birthing centers, these should not be confused with freestanding birthing centers because they are not likely to provide similar cost savings, reductions in technology use or reduced cesarean rates." Fullerton and Severino (1992), using the same research method as that used for the National Birth Center Study, reported on a comparison group of more than 2,000 low-risk women admitted to hospital care during the same period and concluded that "hospital care did not offer any advantage for women at low risk and was associated with increased intervention."

Some birth centers are both hospital sponsored and NACC accredited; hospital sponsorship does not preclude "true" birth center care. An analysis of birth center data from the National Survey of Women's Health Centers, however, uncovered significant differences between hospital-sponsored and nonhospital centers (Khoury, Summers, & Weisman, in press).

The BirthPlace, in San Diego, California, is an example of a successfully mainstreamed birth center. Though it struggles to maintain personalized, family-centered care in the face of large numbers of clients and low reimbursement, the BirthPlace has successfully integrated four systems of care: (1) a private practice of CNMs and obstetricians, (2) the public community clinic system, (3) the tertiary university hospital, and (4) a freestanding birth center (Dickinson, Jackson, & Swartz, 1994).

IMPLICATIONS FOR THE PROFESSION OF MIDWIFERY

The birth center movement has had a profound effect on the profession of midwifery. In particular, it has created a new work place for midwives and has spawned new midwifery educational programs. It has provided an enhanced opportunity to shape workplace policies, work environment, and workplace culture.

THE BIRTH CENTER AS WORKPLACE

Just as families have found the hospital an unsatisfying place to give birth, nurse-midwives have sometimes found the hospital a difficult place to practice midwifery. Even in hospitals with birthing rooms and programs that cater to healthy low-risk women, the nurse-midwife's practice may be curtailed by physicians, who have the power to define risk and to set policies regarding standard intervention in the birth process. On the other hand, the home, traditionally the site for midwife-attended births, has its own set of challenges for nurse-midwives. Because of travel time and the highly individualized nature of preparation for home birth, home-birth midwives must keep their practices fairly small, are always concerned about two clients going into labor at the same time, and may struggle to support themselves economically.

Katz Rothman, from her perspective as a medical sociologist, has described the development of the birth center as a compromise between home and hospital, suggesting that the birth center may provide the ideal work setting for nurse-midwives. Birth centers provide many of the advantages that hospitals offer practitioners: shared responsibility, close collegial relationships with other nurse-midwives, and long-term collective negotiations for physician consultation services. In addition, birth centers provide a pleasant environment for births and, perhaps most importantly, professional autonomy (Rothman, 1983).

NEW MODELS OF MIDWIFERY EDUCATION

The birth center concept caught on at a time when the demand for a short supply of nurse midwives was high and when most educational programs did not prepare student midwives for out-of-hospital practice. Recognizing a responsibility for ensuring the delivery of a service for which the public appetite had been whetted, MCA was part of a consortium, including the Frontier Nursing Service, the Frances Payne Bolton School of Nursing at Case Western Reserve University, and NACC, to stimulate innovations in nurse-midwifery education and to test the Community-based Nurse-Midwifery Educational Program (CNEP). The model was developed during a period of several years and was piloted beginning in 1989, having received accreditation from the Division of Accreditation of the American College of Nurse-Midwives (ACNM). By 1992, the first class had graduated and successfully passed the certification examination administered by the ACNM Certification Council, Inc. (ACC).

The CNEP offers nurses with a bachelor of science in nursing degree the opportunity for self-paced instruction within their own communities. Units of instruction are divided into educational sequences and modules, which students complete at their own rate. Students gain clinical experience first in birth centers or other nurse-midwifery services for instruction in normal childbirth and then in conventional hospital settings, both within reach of the students' community. The program is usually completed in 20 to 34 months, and graduates meet educational requirements for certification by the ACC. Students may also elect a master of science degree in nursing on completion of specified courses offered through the Frances Payne Bolton School of Nursing, Case Western Reserve University. This program, while realizing substantial cost savings for students and the educational system, has enrolled a relatively large number of students. By 1997, the program had graduated 503 nurse-midwives. In 1996, 29% of the CNMs certified by the ACNM Certification Council were graduates of the Frontier School of Midwifery and Family Nursing and the CNEP (Tatum, K., personal communication, 1997). Distance learning is becoming increasingly popular; since CNEP's inception, other distance-learning programs have been established to educate nurse-midwives (Treistman, Watson, & Fullerton, 1996).

THE USE OF POWER

Nurses must not only enter the world of health politicians but must do so in a politic fashion. There is an important difference between the words *politic* and *politician*. A *politic* person is wise, prudent, sagacious in devising and pursuing measures, and diplomatic. The word *politician,* as distinct from *statesman,* is frequently used in a derogatory sense and with the implication that the person is seeking personal or partisan gain. As we move into the arena of shaping health policy and dealing with the inevitable competition and conflict that will result from our presence and activism, the synonyms for *politic* are those which we nurses should emulate: *prudent, wise, sagacious, provident, diplomatic, judicious, wary, well devised* and *discreet.*

The articulation of the art of nurse-midwifery within the world of health care policy was not a simple matter. Education is the vehicle by which the art is ensured continuity, and service delivery is the living demonstration of the art at work. The farther that nurse-midwives move from settings in which they are caring for childbearing families, the more difficult it is for others to grasp the art. Because we are the vessels of our art, interpretation is achieved through our presence and demeanor.

Mary Breckinridge, the founder of the Frontier Nursing Service, and Hazel Corbin, former general director of MCA, are two outstanding examples of politic women in the history of nurse-midwifery who were responsible for shaping health care policy. Their accomplishments are with us today primarily because of their diplomacy, their recognition of the role of consumers in getting the job done, and their sensitivity to the needs of childbearing families. They have provided the tools we need to carry the work forward. To do so, there must be access to the halls and committee rooms where the powerful sit.

In 1995, such access was greatly facilitated when the Assistant Secretary of Health, Philip Lee, named Ruth Lubic as an expert consultant in the Office of Public Health and Science. From her office in the Humphrey Building, she is, as Dr. Lee wrote in the announcement of her appointment, available to speak about the establishment and operation of childbearing centers and the important aspects of empowerment for families and communities involved in the development and use of these services.

In nursing's search for a place on political agendas, its role models are essentially self-interest groups. But the art of nursing is other-centered, not self-centered. Nursing must learn from the example of the self-interested, without succumbing to its lure, that a taste of power (even a minor political skirmish won) can whet the appetite. Because another art, that of negotiation, is denigrated in favor of confrontation and adversarial postures, consumers on the sidelines quickly discern the similarity between professionals, as both individuals and groups, in any jockeying for a favored position. They worry that the result will be the same: exploitation of the public.

What goals do we have in mind in seeking political muscle? The art of nurse-midwifery would say "the improvement of quality and access for all childbearing families and the lowering of cost in the health care delivery system." But there are midwives who, in their eagerness to gain control over their practice settings, destroy that very setting through impulsive and impatient behavior, perhaps showing irritation with physician or nursing colleagues because of their failure to accept the concept of a team relationship. As difficult as it may be to remain even tempered, diplomacy and discretion are essential.

Nurses must be patient—as patient as were Hazel Corbin and the MCA board of directors during those 40 years between the establishment of the first school of nurse-midwifery and the recognition of the profession by organized obstetrics in 1971. Prudence, wisdom, determination, and persistence, even in the face of adversity, are essential attributes of the politic nurse-midwife. How fortunate it is that the art of nurse-midwifery has taught us these qualities as we attend laboring women, assisting them in giving birth. Nurse-midwives are not by nature impulsive, impatient, reckless, or irritable; the art of being "with woman" does not permit such qualities. Wisdom, discretion, and diplomacy, qualities that equip one to shape health care policy, are required. To succeed, we have had only to use the tools of our art.

We must also understand how political debates are framed and take care in how we choose to expend political capital. The recent debate over drive-by deliveries and the ensuing legislation mandating payment for a 2-day hospital stay after normal childbirth is a sad example of legislation by anecdote and an enormous missed opportunity (Kun & Muir, 1997; Lubic, 1997). The issue is not the length of the hospital stay, but, as we like to frame it, (1) how childbirth has become a medical and surgical procedure that requires hospitalization and (2) how we prepare mothers and their families for the role of parenting, beginning early in the prenatal period and continuing through the postpartum period. Birth center families expect and welcome early discharge because they have been well prepared for it. Insurers have covered the necessary education and counseling when the cost of providing these services was included in a comprehensive fee for the entire maternity package. Legislators and insurers may have ensured women 2 days in the hospital but cannot be left believing that they have given childbearing families what they need.

We close, as does Mallison in the final paragraph of her editorial on the national study of women entering labor in freestanding birth centers:

> The stunning outcomes of this study of primary care by nurse-midwives deserve to be shouted, not whispered, not smothered in honeyed "yes-buts" and "if-onlys." Much of the shouting will be up to nurses. For nurse-midwives are the nursing profession's wedge into the system of gatekeeping that has, so far, been almost entirely physician-controlled. This study of a whole different system of care can crash some gates. Use it. [Mallison, 1990, p. 7]

References

American Public Health Association. (1983). Guidelines for licensing and regulating birth centers: Policy statement adopted by the Governing Council of the American Public Health Association. *American Journal of Public Health, 73*(3), 16–18.

Bennetts, A. B., & Lubic, R. W. (1982). The free-standing birth centre. *Lancet, 1,* 378–380.

Burk, M. E., Wieser, P. C., & Keegan, L. (1995). Cultural beliefs and health behaviors of pregnant Mexican-American women: Implications for primary care. *Advances in Nursing Science, 17*(4), 37–52.

Capan, P., Beard, M., & Mashburn, M. (1993). Nurse-managed clinics provide access and improved health care. *Nurse-Practitioner, 18*(5), 50–55.

DeJong, R. N., Shy, K., & Carr, K. C. (1981). An out-of-hospital birth center using university referral. *Obstetrics and Gynecology, 58*(6), 703–707.

Dickinson, C. P., Jackson, D. J., & Swartz, W. H. (1994). Making the alternative the mainstream: Maintaining a family-centered focus in a large freestanding birth center for low-income women. *Journal of Nurse-Midwifery, 39*(2), 112–118.

Ernst, E. K. M. (1996). Midwifery, birth centers, and health care reform. *Journal of Obstetric, Gynecologic, and Neonatal Nursing, 25,* 433–439.

Faison, J. B., Pisani, B. J., Douglas, R. G., Cranch, G. S., & Lubic, R. W. (1979). The childbearing center: An alternative birth setting. *Obstetrics and Gynecology, 54*(4), 527–532.

Fullerton, J. T., & Severino, R. (1992). In-hospital care for low-risk childbirth: Comparison with results from the National Birth Center Study. *Journal of Nurse-Midwifery, 37*(5), 331–340.

Garite, T. J., Snell, B. J., Walker, D. L., & Darrow, V. C. (1995). Development and experience of a university-based, freestanding birthing center. *Obstetrics and Gynecology, 86*(3), 411–416.

Jeffords, J. M. (1997). A senator's perspective. *Public Health Reports, 112,* 289.

Khoury, A. J., Summers, L., & Weisman, C. S. (1998). Characteristics of current hospital sponsored and non-hospital birth centers. *Maternal and Child Health Journal, 1*(2) 89–99.

Kun, K. E., Muir, E. (1997). Drive-by deliveries. *Public Health Reports, 112,* 277–283.

Lazarus, W., Levine, E. S., Lewin, L. S., & Lewis and Associates. (1981). *The Childbearing Center case study* (Vol. 2). Washington, DC: The Federal Trade Commission.

Lieberman, E., & Ryan, K. J. (1989). Birth-day choices. *New England Journal of Medicine, 321*(26), 1824–1825.

Lubic, R. W. (1979). *Barriers and conflict in maternity care innovation.* Unpublished doctoral dissertation, Columbia University, New York.

Lubic, R. W. (1983). Childbirthing centers: Delivering

more for less. *American Journal of Nursing, 83*(7), 1053–1056.

Lubic, R. W. (1997). A missed opportunity. *Public Health Reports, 112,* 284–287.

Lubic, R. W., & Ernst, E. K. M. (1978). The childbearing center: An alternative to conventional care. *Nursing Outlook, 26*(12), 754–760.

Mallison, M. B. (1990). Gate crashers [Editorial]. *American Journal of Nursing, 90*(2), 7.

Minor, A. F. (1989). *The cost of maternity care and childbirth in the United States.* Washington, DC: Health Insurance Association of America.

Rooks, J. P., Weatherby, N. L., Ernst, E. K. M., Stapleton, S., Rosen, D., & Rosenfield, A. (1989). Outcomes of care in birth centers: The national birth center study. *New England Journal of Medicine, 321,* 1804–1811.

Rothman, B. K. (1983). Anatomy of a compromise: Nurse-midwifery and the rise of the birth center. *Journal of Nurse-Midwifery, 28*(4), 3–7.

Stone, P. W., & Walker, P. H. (1995). Cost-effectiveness analysis: Birth center vs. hospital care. *Nursing Economics, 13*(5), 299–308.

Triestman, J., Watson, D., & Fullerton, J. (1996). Computer-mediated distributed learning: An innovative program design in midwifery education. *Journal of Nurse-Midwifery, 41*(5), 389–392.

END CASE STUDY

The Rainbow Kitchen: Developing a Neighborhood Health Center

Theresa Chalich and Joyce Penrose White

Homestead, Pennsylvania, like many other towns strung along the Monongahela River, was hard hit when the steel industry, its industrial base, was shut down in the 1980s. As a result of economic decline, these towns experienced significant reductions in the health care available to their citizens. Homestead, however, has benefited from a coalition of nurses, physicians, and community residents who have worked to improve access to health care. In this case study, we describe the development of a storefront clinic, its transformation into the Rainbow Health Center, and the new assaults threatening its mission of providing health care to all who need it.

FIRST EFFORTS: 1982

The summer of 1982, like most summers in the towns in the Monongahela Valley, which is carved into the hills of western Pennsylvania by the Monongahela River, was hot and muggy. The small group of worried steel workers, facing the worst slump in steel making they had ever encountered, left meetings in airless union halls and walked past the Homestead Works. Homestead, just across the Monongahela River ("Mon" River) from Pittsburgh, had depended on the manufacture of steel for more than 100 years. Only in the past two decades had work in the mills finally paid good wages and provided benefits, including health insurance for workers and their families. The town was accustomed to the boom-or-bust cycles that typified dependence on a single industry, and few realized that this time was different. The early 1980s saw changes in the global economy, the beginning of multinational corporations, and a failure to develop industrial infrastructures to respond to these changes, which ultimately resulted in the permanent collapse of Homestead's steel industry (Hall, 1997).

The mills that had lit up the night skies with their plumes of steam for almost 100 years were eerie in the darkness; the faint glow of the night watchman's flashlight moved from building to deserted building. Theresa watched, too, listening to the worried voices telling each other that things would turn around soon. She knew that some families had already lost their health benefits, and that mothers were concerned about where to take sick children for care. The seeds of what was to become the Mon Valley Unemployed Committee's first health care effort were sown during those long, hot summer evenings.

THE COMMUNITY RESPONDS: 1984

Months and then years passed, and the open hearths and blast furnaces remained cold and untended. The growing insecurity united many forces in the Mon Valley, and by 1984 Theresa and a group of unemployed workers had set up a storefront office in Homestead and organized a soup kitchen on a corner of Homestead's main street, Eighth Avenue. Anticipating that the kitchen would be a vehicle to work on grassroots solutions to the economic crisis, the organizers named it the Rainbow Kitchen. The name symbolized their hopes that it would, like Jesse Jackson's Rainbow Coalition, unite the diverse constituents of the area in setting a legislative and political agenda. For now, its staff served hot meals, handed out bags of groceries, and negotiated with banks threatening to foreclose on mortgages. Working the night shift in the neuropsychiatric unit of the local Veterans Affairs Hospital, Theresa spent her days in the kitchen.

Since 1982 Theresa had worked as a health care advocate for the unemployed after she and a group of workers founded the Mon Valley Unemployed Committee's first health care committee. Her determination to be an advocate grew as she saw children going unimmunized, parents slumping into depression and chemical dependence, and chronic illnesses left untreated. The committee arranged for those whose insurance benefits had run out to be cared for free of charge by a cadre of Mon Valley's doctors. Theresa learned which hospitals had not fulfilled their Hill-Burton* obligation to provide free and reduced cost care. When she found that doctors were exhausting their sample supplies and patients were unable to afford to have their prescriptions filled, she and nurse volunteer Marilyn Sullivan began the Rx Council of Western PA, a nonprofit agency that continues to provide emergency prescription assistance through pharmacy vouchers or contributions by pharmaceutical manufacturers.

The networking involved in these early advocacy efforts provided Theresa with a growing list of concerned health care professionals, institutions, and social service agencies. In addition, it made her aware of the economics of providing care to people in need.

An early activity of the Mon Valley Unemployed Committee was the formation of a women's group to address the needs of both unemployed women steel workers (the last hired in what had been an exclusively male work force, women were now among the first laid off) and wives of steel workers. With their feminist

---

*The Hill-Burton Act of 1946 provided federal monies for the construction of hospitals and health centers. Facilities built with these funds are required to provide some free or reduced-cost care to those in need.

backgrounds, Theresa and counselor Jan Carlino decided to sponsor a series of sessions designed as feminist, consciousness-raising groups, reminiscent of the 1970s. But, contrary to their plans, the group of women expressed concerns over losing medical insurance and the impact of this loss on their families. The women did not want to talk about themselves. Theresa quickly learned that the community's needs were not always well served by one's personal agenda.

In 1984, Theresa wrote an organizing guide, *People's Health Care: Problems and Solutions,* to be used in developing advocacy programs for others who were working with uninsured persons. Studying for a master's degree in public health at the University of Pittsburgh, she continued her interest in Homestead; her master's thesis was a door-to-door health needs assessment of 542 households. The findings were both expected and sobering. Fourteen percent of the respondents no longer had any health insurance. Forty-one percent had experienced delays in getting medical care, dental appointments, and prescribed medications.

TRYING A POLITICAL SOLUTION: 1990

Theresa, in a move consistent with the political activism of the Rainbow Kitchen, ran for the state legislature in 1990. Concerned that her referral and advocacy work were not adequately meeting the ever-expanding needs of workers and families who had suddenly joined the ranks of the medically indigent, she sought a seat in the state house of representatives, where her goal was to work on a statewide effort for universal health care legislation.

Theresa's campaign slogan was "Nurses Save Lives." Her campaign platform called for comprehensive women's health care that included reproductive choice, not popular in her conservative, blue-collar, and strongly Roman Catholic district. She lost her electoral bid and returned to implementing a local approach to what she continued to believe was a state and national problem.

THE RAINBOW CLINIC: 1990

Disappointed by Theresa's defeat but determined that the recommendations of her survey be implemented, a group of nurses decided to take the health care needs into their own hands. A jeweler whose store had been next to the Rainbow Kitchen had gone out of business, victim of the crumbling economy. The store, built in the 1930s, was a long, narrow space that could be converted into a clinic where health education, screenings, and basic physical examinations could be provided. The ambitious goal was to promote healthy life styles and to detect illness in its early stages. This clinic would serve as a base for Theresa's referral and advocacy work.

Theresa obtained a $5,000 grant for refurbishing the interior walls and floor and installing bathroom facilities. Even so, the clinic's physical atmosphere was grim when the clinic opened on May 5, 1990. It began with a 100% volunteer staff and was open only on Saturdays. Gradually the days of operation came to include some afternoon and evening hours as doctors in specialties from pulmonology to infection control volunteered to provide free primary care on a walk-in basis. Clinic hours further expanded when residents from a local hospital's family practice program provided volunteer evening hours and the chair of medicine at the University of Pittsburgh agreed to pay for the volunteer physicians' professional liability insurance. A local foundation paid Theresa's first year's salary as clinic director. Theresa would be the only paid staff person until 1994.

On opening day the equipment consisted of one desk, a stethoscope, and a sphygmomanometer. Additional donations were a hemoglobin screening machine, an ancient but operating 12-lead electrocardiograph, a spirometer, a glucometer, weight and height scales, and Snellen charts. Needed pharmaceuticals were donated by health care professionals and institutions or purchased with monies obtained through fund raising.

The early 1990s found Theresa and the volunteers struggling to provide a semblance of primary care in a storefront building without the convenience of a laboratory, modern diagnostic equipment, or even examination rooms. Patients came in large numbers for physical examinations that they needed for employment, prison work release, and school. Health screening and education programs increased. A mobile mammography van, parked outside the clinic twice a year, provided free mammograms. Many visits were for the treatment of chronic illnesses, such as diabetes and hypertension, but patients' lack of health insurance made needed diagnostic testing and follow-up care difficult. Theresa continued to use her network of hospital and social services, but the task of providing comprehensive care was daunting.

As Theresa cast about for long-term strategies for the clinic's survival, wrote grant proposals, and struggled to provide services to an ever-increasing number of patients, she continued her political involvement, organizing activities for senior citizens in Pittsburgh who were working on the passage of a Pennsylvania legislative initiative to prevent doctors from overcharging on Medicare payments. Success was achieved with the passage of the Medicare Overcharge Measure in 1991.

HOPES FOR HEALTH CARE REFORM: 1992

The increased volume of uninsured patients seen in the clinic reflected the nation's growing number of uninsured persons. In the early 1990s, the national figure was 35 million. The 1992 Presidential and Congressional races were associated with calls for health care reform. The media told of people denied access to health care because they had neither insurance nor money. Pittsburgh television stations and newspapers called the clinic, looking for local hard-luck stories. Many, including Theresa, had reason to hope that our country would at last develop a national health care program. Politicians seemed to be speaking the activists' language, and the 1992 Presidential primary race brought Democratic candidate Jerry Brown to the clinic. He presented his campaign program and was in turn presented with a copy of Dr. Jack Geiger's thesis (1992) on primary care.

Theresa was secretary of the local chapter of Health Care for All, a group that promoted a single-payer comprehensive national health care program based on the Canadian model. A cold, clear Saturday in October 1992 found three Canadian health professionals speaking to small groups in Homestead and other Pittsburgh working-class communities about their system.

William Coyne, a U.S. Congressman whose district encompasses Homestead, is a supporter of a single-payer system, and Theresa continues to meet with him both to lobby for a national health insurance program and to describe nursing's agenda for health care reform. Unfortunately, the health care reform winds blew out as quickly as they had blown in. The Clinton Administrations's health care reform proposal quickly became controversial and subsequently died.

BEGINNING NURSE PRACTITIONER COLLABORATION

In the fall of 1990, Joyce Penrose White responded to an advertisement for a nurse practitioner to volunteer in helping to establish a women's health program at the Rainbow Clinic. After Joyce proposed her plans for a women's care program, she and Theresa set about arranging physician consultation. The law regulating the practice of nurse practitioners in Pennsylvania requires that nurse practitioners have physician supervision.

The initial proposal for physician oversight was directed to the women's hospital associated with the University of Pittsburgh Medical Center. Joyce and Theresa were told that no mechanism existed for partnering with a community-based clinic and its nursing care model. A second attempt to work with the University of Pittsburgh involved a proposal to the School of Nursing dean to transform the clinic into a community nursing center. The 1980s had seen a number of schools of nursing develop such centers, often used as sites for faculty practice and clinical experiences for students. Concerned about assuming financial responsibility for a clinic that depended on fundraisers to raise rent money and that served a patient community without health insurance, the dean rejected Joyce's plan.

Joyce and Theresa finally ended up in the office of Dr. Joseph Russo, director of obstetrics and gynecology at the Hospital of Western Pennsylvania. With a long history of advocating the integration of advanced practice nurses into primary care and a deep commitment to underserved women and teenagers, Dr. Russo agreed to provide telephone consultation and to accept referrals of patients whose problems were outside the nurse practitioner's scope of practice.

Protocols were established for the delivery of care that included a full spectrum of women's primary care services, including pelvic and breast examinations, pap smears, testing and counseling for sexually transmitted diseases (STDs), birth control services, and prenatal and menopausal care. The clinic evaluated eligibility for the women, infants, and children (WIC) program; provided tetanus, influenza, and pneumonia immunizations; and offered free pregnancy testing and condoms. The women's health care program startup hours were one-half day a week.

RAINBOW BRIDGE PROJECT: 1993

The collaborative work by Joyce, Joe Russo, and Theresa led to the submission of a grant proposal in 1992 to expand the women's health care program. The proposal incorporated their beliefs that women's health care should include both reproductive and nonreproductive care, that obstetrics/gynecology residents should learn to care for women in community-based settings, and that women should be actively engaged in caring for themselves and their neighbors.

In 1993 the Rainbow Clinic was awarded a 3-year $357,000 grant from the Western Pennsylvania Hospital Foundation for the Rainbow Bridge Project to accomplish the following:

- Expand women's health care services
- Promote a caregiving model in which the physician is a member of a community-based care team
- Identify high-risk groups and develop a strategy to achieve optimal use of a comprehensive women's health care program
- Improve the clinic's on-site laboratory and facilities
- Develop and implement a community outreach worker program

In the implementation of the grant, a number of changes took place. Joyce Barrow, a family nurse practitioner, was hired at 16 hours a week to augment "the other Joyce's" volunteer hours. Residents in obstetrics/gynecology provided consultation to the nurse practitioners and became involved in health education programs both in the clinic and in the community. Renovations were completed by the end of 1993. Three examination rooms with doors replaced the screened-off examining space through which everyone had walked to reach the bathroom. A laboratory that met the level I criteria of the Clinical Laboratories Improvement Act was set up on site. The center added a private intake room, a bathroom accessible to the physically challenged, and an education/counseling room. A corner of the waiting room was set aside for children. It was stocked with books, games, and toys and displays children's artwork on the wall. The name of the Rainbow Clinic was changed to the Rainbow Health

Center at the completion of the renovations, which identifies it as a community health center that promotes positive, healthy life styles.

Fifteen area women were recruited and trained to be community outreach workers. Theresa had observed that these women were already actively working on issues of health care access at the clinic and were interested in working as advocates for those in need. Theresa organized the workers into "block watch programs," where they became health care advocates for a block of their residential neighbors. Their work was to address barriers to care and to increase use of services at the clinic and at other health care institutions. Together with Theresa and volunteer nurses, they worked with teenagers and women in a variety of settings: the local high school, senior citizens' centers, the housing project, and child and parenting centers.

COMMUNITY HEALTH CENTER REACHES OUT TO COMMUNITY: 1996

The Rainbow Bridge Project enhanced the clinic's reputation as accessible and user friendly. By 1994, patient use of all services—women's health, walk-in medical care, podiatry, and dermatology—was steadily increasing, and the center was able to increase the family planning services provided by becoming a subcontract agency of the federally funded Title XX Family Health Council. Joann Brooks, an outreach worker, was hired as the office manager and receptionist.

One of the activities that brought the clinic into the community was a health care utilization survey (Chalich, 1989) done in 1994 and 1995 by the Rainbow Bridge outreach workers and volunteer registered nurse staff. The purpose of the survey was to assess the health care needs and practices of the residents in the health center's catchment area. The age-appropriate health practices design was developed by using the "Healthy People 2000" objectives as a template. The findings of 224 households, released in March 1996, indicated a need to increase preventive services such as lead screenings, immunizations for both the young and elderly, pap smears, colorectal screenings, and dental care (Chalich & Gula, 1996). The community indicated an increased need for safety and police protection and for drug and alcohol services. The center has used the findings to increase its promotion of cancer screenings on site and to organize immunization clinics in the local housing project. The results indicated that some area residents were unaware of the center's services, which suggested a need to better publicize the health center's work.

In 1996, several of the clinic's nurses and women from the community with Pittsburgh's Community Literacy Center wrote a handbook entitled *Getting to Know You: A Dialogue for Community Health,* to be used for improving communication and for addressing the barriers between health care providers and female consumers (Higgins & Chalich, 1996). Theresa's conviction that teenagers' and women's knowledge of their bodies either improves or impedes health care led her to organize this literacy project. The project was originally conceived as the clinic's own version of *Our Bodies, Our Selves* to address "health care illiteracy" issues. Joining forces with the Community Literacy Center resulted in a booklet in which women wrote their own poignant stories of painful experiences when seeking health care, of discrimination aimed against women of color or mothers on welfare, and of being victims of family incest and domestic violence. The handbook includes a section on communication strategies that describes ways in which the scenario of a particular story could have played out better for both patient and health care worker and provides examples of cultural differences, common myths about women's health issues, and dialogs on cancer, pregnancy, STDs, abuse, depression, and chemical addictions. The handbook is currently being used in nursing classes in several of Pittsburgh's universities.

NEW CHALLENGES

By 1995, managed care began to play a bigger role in the region's health economics. Concern about its impact on the quality of care given to new mothers and their babies prompted the Pennsylvania legislature to conduct statewide hearings on early after-delivery discharges from the hospital that were being mandated by health maintenance organizations (HMOs). Theresa, because of her grassroots involvement, was asked to present testimony at the Pittsburgh hearing. The Pennsylvania General Assembly went on to pass a law forbidding HMOs to require early discharge when the physician considered it to be against the patient's best interests.

Despite this progressive piece of legislation, Pennsylvania in 1996 chose to reduce state spending by withdrawing medical assistance from the 200,000 recipients often referred to as the "working poor." These were people who did not qualify for cash assistance because they were employed but whose incomes were so low that they were eligible for medical assistance. Theresa actively organized against the proposed cut, testifying that this action was a way of punishing people for working. She noted that the center was already caring for hundreds of people who were employed, some at two jobs, but who were without health care benefits and were earning too little to purchase insurance privately.

Currently Pennsylvania has mandated the enrollment of all medical assistance recipients into managed care plans by the year 2000, with enrollment in the Pittsburgh region to be completed by 1998. Confusion and uncertainty have resulted. In 1996 Theresa joined the Working Group on Health in the Monongahela Valley, urging that neighborhood forums be conducted to orient the residents to HMO operations so that intimidation can be reduced and participation promoted. Theresa and a fellow group member wrote "Community Conversations on Health Care," a brochure that describes HMOs and that is used in discussing issues surrounding selection of a primary care provider, health plans, and grievance procedures.

NEW SOLUTIONS

In addition to political response to the ever-changing health care scene, 1996 found the center addressing its own financial survival. The 3-year Rainbow Bridge Project funding was winding down, and Theresa and the volunteer staff began aggressively to seek new operations funding. They met with community hospitals in the Monongahela Valley and discussed the possibility of working with them while maintaining a community health center focus. Facing the need to merge to survive in a rapidly evolving managed care environment, these hospitals were unable to commit themselves to the Rainbow Health Center. Theresa next explored the possibility of designation as a Federally Qualified Health Center (FQHC). This designation is awarded to a health center that serves a medically underserved area and meets other standards determined by the Health Care Financing Administration and several other criteria. In July 1996, it was determined that the center met these requirements. The Rainbow Health Center merged with an existing FQHC, resulting in the addition of pediatrics, midwifery, expanded family practice, laboratory services, and reduced prescription costs for the center's clients. The volunteer professional team continued to provide care, and with the addition of the new doctors and midwife, the clinic began to operate a full-time and full-service health center.

The FQHC designation also meant that patients apply for sliding-fee eligibility based on income and family size. Initially the staff members were concerned that the patients would no longer visit the clinic, but this has not been the case; incomes of patients are so low that the majority pay only a nominal fee. The clinic staff remain committed to the goal of never denying access to the center's services despite inability to pay, but they envision a time when it may no longer be possible to meet the goal. Recently, clinic staff were instructed to deny care to an undocumented immigrant who had fled persecution in her own country. And Theresa has been told by the parent agency that the restrictions associated with Medicaid HMOs will make it impossible for the volunteers who were the mainstay of the clinic for so long to continue providing patient care. The challenges thus continue.

LESSONS LEARNED

Fifteen years have passed since Theresa began her work with the Mon Valley Unemployed Committee. During that period, Homestead has slid further into economic disaster, with increases in all the attendant social ills: teenage pregnancy, drug abuse, gangs, and violence. The health care situation has been worsened by growing numbers of employers who do not provide health insurance for their workers, and this situation has been exacerbated by the state's decision to cut medical assistance to the working poor.

The establishment of the Rainbow Health Center has taught us several lessons:

1. Knowing how to deliver high-quality care efficiently is no longer enough; one must also be knowledgeable about health care financing. One must know what public funds are available. For example, becoming an FQHC has allowed us to participate in the federally financed and state-administered "Vaccines for Children" program. It is important to remain knowledgeable about the availability of foundation funding for health care. We recently were awarded, for example, a small grant from the March of Dimes for a community health fair to be held in a local housing project during the summer.

2. We must never tire of telling our stories to policymakers. Elected officials can't get behind what they don't know about. In 1997, Theresa represented Homestead's citizens when she testified to the Pennsylvania Department of Welfare regarding changes in welfare and her support of the WIC program.

3. The community must be given the mechanisms to define its own needs. This requires leadership—not control—by health professionals. We were pleased to be able to base our programming on two surveys, one in 1989 and the second in 1996.

It was precisely because of our leadership that the founding of the clinic was both medically and politically effective. We took a risk in our role as advocates for the medically underserved population of the Mon Valley. If it were not for our risk taking, scores of residents would possibly never have access to health care services. Though we can congratulate ourselves on our work to date, it is imperative to appreciate the magnitude of the health care and economic problems and to meet their challenges both clinically and politically, as we have shown that we are capable of doing.

We, nurses, were able to show that we could choreograph the provision of services through the years by building a dedicated multidisciplinary team and by engaging in persistent networking and fund raising. The volunteer nurses and doctors have been able to contribute to the mission of the clinic's work with their individual skills, interests, and commitment. By not working in isolation, practicing extensive outreach into the neighborhoods and other health institutions, and grasping the importance of political activities, we have tried to establish the Rainbow Health Center as a 1990s nursing model of care.

References

Chalich, T. (1984). *People's health care: Problems and solutions*. Homestead, PA: Steel Valley Unemployed Committee, Homestead, Pernnsylvania.

Chalich, T. (1989). *Household health care survey: Homestead, PA*. Homestead, PA: Rainbow Kitchen.

Chalich, T., & Gula, M. J. (Eds.). (March 1996). *Bridging the gaps: A report on the Rainbow Bridge Project Community Health Care Utilization Survey*. Pittsburgh: Rainbow Health Center and the Western Pennsylvania Hospital.

Geiger, J. (1992). *Assuring access: Community health centers as a comunity-based model of coordinated care*. Paper presented at the National Primary Care Conference, Washington, DC, March 29–31, 1992.

Hall, C. G. L. (1997). *Steel phoenix: The fall and rise of a steel industry*. New York: St. Martin's Press.

Healthy people. National promotion and disease prevention objectives. (1990). Washington, DC: U.S. Department of Health and Human Services, Public Health Service. (DHHS Publication No. [PHS] 91-50213.)

Higgins, I., & Chalich, T. (Eds.). (1996). *Getting to know you: A dialogue for community health*. Pittsburgh: Community Literacy Center and Rainbow Health Center.

Lifecycles: A framework for developing a clinical strategy for primary care. (1986, September). Washington, DC: U.S. Department of Health and Human Services.

END CASE STUDY

Nurses, Consumers, Activists, and the Politics of AIDS

Karen A. Ballard and Peter J. Ungvarski

THE EARLY YEARS

The history of the human immunodeficiency virus/acquired immunodeficiency syndrome (HIV/AIDS) epidemic in the United States is a story of people, policies, and politics in conflict. It shows courage and cowardice, hope and despair, compassion and discrimination, and the struggle between scientific facts and irrational fears. It also reveals the emergence of activism and intolerance in the face of the inequities of health care in the United States.

EMERGENCE OF DISEASE IN THE UNITED STATES

The first report on the epidemic appeared on June 5, 1981, in a Centers for Disease Control (CDC) weekly publication, *Morbidity and Mortality Weekly Report.* Although the article described five previously healthy homosexual men, the title, *"Pneumocystis* Pneumonia—Los Angeles," omitted any reference to homosexuals. According to Shilts (1987), this omission was intentional in an attempt to avoid offending the gay community and inflaming homophobes. Thus politics was part of the HIV/AIDS epidemic from the beginning.

Between June 1981 and May 1982, CDC received reports of 355 cases of Kaposi's sarcoma and/or serious opportunistic infections among previously healthy persons, including homosexual and bisexual men (281 cases, or 79%), heterosexual men (41 cases, or 12%), men of unknown sexual orientation (20 cases, or 6%), and heterosexual women (13 cases, or 4%) (CDC, 1982a). Blood transfer through intravenous drug use was implicated in the majority of the affected heterosexual men and women. By July 1982, the problem was also noted in heterosexual Haitian immigrants to the United States and in recipients of blood products (CDC, 1982b, 1982c). Although the evidence was clear that this was not a disease exclusively of homosexual men, it was being referred to as the gay plague. In September 1982, CDC designated the disease as AIDS and for the first time defined its characteristics.

By 1983, there was a pervasive attitude that AIDS was a disease of a "disposable" portion of society—gay men and intravenous drug users. Walker (1991) describes it best by noting that, although the average American viewed AIDS as a sad affair, it was something that affected "them," not "us," and "they" (being undesirables) were dispensable. Baker (1983, p. 33) explains the feelings of the times by quoting Congressman Henry A. Waxman, of California, then chairman of the House Subcommittee on Health, at a Congressional hearing on AIDS in 1983: "There is no doubt in my mind that if the same disease had appeared among Americans of Norwegian descent, or among tennis players, rather than gay males, the responses of both the government and the medical community would have been different."

French and American scientists were working diligently to identify the etiologic agent of AIDS. In May 1983, Luc Montagnier, head of viral oncology at the Pasteur Institute in Paris, and colleagues published the first article describing a T-lymphotropic retrovirus as the etiologic agent of AIDS (Barre-Sinoussi et al., 1983). The French named the virus lymphadenopathy-associated virus (LAV). In September, the French scientists sent isolates of LAV to American scientists in order to validate their findings (Shilts, 1987). The following May, Robert Gallo and associates, of the National

Cancer Institute, in Bethesda, Maryland, published an article announcing the discovery of the retrovirus and named it the human T-cell lymphotropic virus type III (HTLV-III) (Popovic, Sarngadhran, Read, & Gallo, 1984). This started an international political rivalry between France and the United States over who would be recognized as the discoverer of the etiologic agent of AIDS and who would receive the most funding for continued research. The ramifications were significant and resulted in an immediate cessation in the exchange of scientific information. While French and American scientists engaged in parochial disputes, the virus was spreading around the world, and the cost to science and humanity was wasted time and death (Shilts, 1987).

Concomitantly, West Coast scientists at the University of California School of Medicine in San Francisco were studying the same virus and had named it the AIDS-associated retrovirus (ARV) (Levy et al., 1984). Attempting to search the literature became a trying endeavor because cross-referencing was necessary by looking for AIDS-related literature by the names LAV, HTLV-III, and ARV. Each author's political affiliation was evident by the viral name used in the title. Even authors who attempted to remain neutral by using all three names had to decide which to place first. Ultimately LAV, IITLV-III, and ARV were found to be variants of the same virus (Ratner, Gallo, & Wong-Staal, 1985).

The issue of what to call the virus was settled in the summer of 1986 when the International Society on the Taxonomy of Viruses arbitrated and changed the name to the human immunodeficiency virus. Not as easily settled was the dispute over who had discovered it. In 1985 the Pasteur Institute filed a multimillion dollar lawsuit against the National Cancer Institute for a share in the royalties accrued from its AIDS blood test patent. Two years later the French and Americans reached an accord recognizing Montagnier and Gallo as codiscover-

ers of HIV and agreeing to share royalties from patents of the HIV antibody blood test (Shilts, 1987). Gallo, however, came under investigation for alleged misappropriation of Montagnier's work (Hilts, 1992). At the end of 1992, the Federal Office of Research Integrity reported that Gallo was guilty of scientific misconduct in his false claim of having isolated the virus.

DISSEMINATION OF DISEASE AND DENIAL

Throughout the first decade of the HIV epidemic, the politics of downplaying the spread of this disease through heterosexual activity resulted in significant numbers of HIV-infected heterosexual persons. At the First International Conference on AIDS, held in Atlanta, Georgia, in April 1985, papers presented by Dr. Charles Rabbin, a medical epidemiologist with New York City's AIDS activity office, and Dr. Robert Redfield, of the Department of Virus Diseases at the Walter Reed Army Institute for Research, in Washington, D.C., provided evidence for, and warned against, the increasing heterosexual spread of HIV. They were labeled doomsayers (Goldsmith, 1986). CDC (1985a), concerned about public apathy regarding heterosexual spread of this virus, warned that all sexually active persons should take precautions to prevent disease transmission. Ironically, at the same time, new data indicated that homosexual men were changing their sexual behaviors in an attempt to stop the spread of HIV (CDC, 1985b). As of September 16, 1985, there were 133 heterosexual contact cases of AIDS (118 women and 15 men) in the United States (CDC, 1985b). Whereas decreases continued to occur in the 1990s among men who had sex with men, increases continued to occur among adults who acquired HIV through heterosexual activities. By 1996, cumulative totals of reported AIDS cases attributed to heterosexual contact accounted for 3% of the cases in men and 38% of the cases in women (CDC, 1996). The price paid for the denial of increasing heterosexual transmission of HIV infection is reflected in the increasing mortality rate among heterosexual Americans.

The issue of AIDS in women reveals the medical, political, and social bias against women by viewing them as mere vectors of the HIV disease rather than as a population at risk in their own right. Interest in women with HIV appears to be secondary to the potential for vertical transmission of HIV to children and horizontal transmission to men (Marte & Allen, 1992). According to Smeltzer and Whipple (1991), public policy, research, education, and treatment programs basically ignored the special needs of women infected with HIV. For example, women with HIV disease who have gynecological problems, such as chronic vulvo-vaginal candidiasis, cervical cancer, and pelvic inflammatory disease, had more trouble getting disability payments than men because the standard definitions of AIDS excluded these HIV-related problems. Studies concerning HIV transmission between women who have sex with women were nonexistent. By 1994, HIV infection had become the leading cause of death among all U.S. women aged 25 to 44 years and the leading cause of death among black women in this age group (CDC, 1995a).

Although some progress has been made in treating women with HIV infection, numerous problems remain. Some of the unresolved issues include the following: (1) gynecological examinations are not routinely performed; (2) women still have difficulty in gaining access to clinical trials; (3) women have a difficult time in gaining access to drug treatment programs (24 states have criminal prosecution laws for women who use drugs during pregnancy, and only nine of them have any treatment available for these women); (4) there are few family-focused programs of HIV/AIDS care, and (5) little attention has been paid to the issue of violence and abuse of women related to HIV disclosure to sex partners or negotiation of condom use (Cooper, 1995). When addressing the spectrum of HIV disease and women, health care professionals must be aware that they are tackling 5,000 years of sexism (Marks, 1992).

Perhaps one of the biggest failures of American society in the decade of the AIDS epidemic was its refusal to ensure that our youth, our nation's future, did not become infected. HIV continued to spread as federal, state, and local authorities, including school boards and parents, argued and moralized about matters of sex. In April 1992 the House Select Committee on Children, Youth and Families expressed alarm at the spread of HIV among adolescents and "condemned the Federal government's response as a 'national disgrace'" ("U.S. Response," 1992, p. 23). By 1996, in the United States, AIDS had been diagnosed in 18,955 individuals between the ages of 13 and 24 years, all because of sexual activity (CDC, 1995a). Kann et al. (1996) reported that substantial morbidity was occurring among school-age youth and young adults related to unintended pregnancies and to sexually transmitted diseases, including HIV infection. The study also revealed that 53.1% of all high school students had had sexual intercourse, and 45.6% of the sexually active students had not used a condom at the last sexual intercourse (Kann et al., 1996). In 1996 it was estimated that between 27 and 54 Americans younger than 20 years were becoming infected with HIV daily (Office of National AIDS Policy, 1996). Clearly we have failed our children.

THE NATION'S RESPONSE

NATIONAL INERTIA: THE REPUBLICAN YEARS

Although the HIV epidemic continued to escalate during the first half of the 1980s, there was a noticeable lack of leadership coming from the federal government. In October 1986, the surgeon general, C. Everett Koop, issued his report on AIDS. Prepared at the request of President Ronald Reagan, the report provided detailed information on AIDS and outlined preventive measures for reducing the transmission of the disease. The report, which caught everyone's attention, released for the first time statistical projections, including an anticipated 270,000 cases of AIDS by the end of 1991 (Koop, 1986).

Although the report prompted strong disagreements in Washington over the use of explicit language to describe transmission of HIV and the surgeon general's recommendation to use condoms to reduce the transmittal risk, it was well received by Congress, and members began to request large numbers of the report to mail to their constituents ("AIDS Education," 1988). The popularity of the report resulted in widespread distribution, and by July 1987 an additional printing was necessary. On July 27, however, the U.S. Department of Health and Human Services requested a delay in additional printing until a meeting could be held between the surgeon general and the White House. The White House wanted the surgeon general to amend the report by removing his recommendation that condoms be used during sexual intercourse ("AIDS Education," 1988). No changes were made, however, and the report was eventually printed and distributed in its original form. The effect of the surgeon general's report on the politicians in Washington was self-evident in the requests for hundreds of thousands of copies by members of both the House and the Senate ("AIDS Education," 1988). By 1987, it was apparent that significant involvement by the federal government in the AIDS epidemic was woefully lacking. There was, however, a distinct record of morally motivated legislation, such as the amendment sponsored by Senator Jesse Helms, of North Carolina, restricting federal funding of AIDS education programs that provided sexually explicit materials, especially concerning homosexual practices.

In June 1987, President Reagan, by executive order, created an advisory commission to investigate the spread of HIV and AIDS. The commission was charged with advising on public health dangers, including the medical, legal, ethical, social, and economic impact of the epidemic. Additionally, it was asked to recommend measures that federal, state, and local officials could take to protect the public from contracting HIV, assist in finding a cure, and care for those who already had the disease.

Kristine Gebbie, a member of the commission and a registered nurse, stated that many in Washington believed that the report would identify a few bureaucratic roadblocks and "announce that the epidemic would end by Christmas of 1990" (Gebbie, 1989, p. 869). However, the final report challenged the Reagan Administration's narrow and very political view of the epidemic. According to Gebbie (1989) the least of the problems revealed were the bureaucratic hurdles of competing cabinet secretaries, financial roadblocks, and limited staff in key agencies. Looking at health care in the United States through the eyes of AIDS "revealed gaping holes and huge problems" (Gebbie, 1989, p. 869). Some of the major issues addressed were failure to offer each child born in the United States a comprehensive health and health education program that would provide the basis for a healthy adult life, failure to construct a coherent system of delivering illness care services and of paying for those services, and failure to understand the dangers of creating a permanent underclass, a drug-linked culture that does not participate in the ordinary obligations and benefits of the social system (Gebbie, 1989). The commission concluded that if some of these problems were not addressed and resolved, the United States would not be able to contain the epidemic. Two nurse members of the commission, Colleen Conway-Welch and Kristine Gebbie, made admirable contributions to the success of the report. The commission completed its report and disbanded in the summer of 1988. The Presidential commission's recommendations were never used as the basis for a national strategy, as was originally intended. This failure on a federal level to adopt the recommendations and to mobilize the necessary resources to respond to the recommendations indicated a glaring need for a national plan to coordinate a response to the HIV epidemic in the United States (National Commission on AIDS, 1991).

In the summer of 1989, President George Bush appointed a second commission and changed the name to the National Commission on AIDS. The initial response by HIV clinicians was that the new title reflected a step backward because the first commission's report, in its summary, had pointed out that the "term 'AIDS' is obsolete. 'HIV infection' more correctly defines the problem. . . . Continual focus on AIDS rather than the entire spectrum of HIV disease has left our nation unable to deal adequately with the epidemic" (Presidential Commission on the HIV Epidemic, 1988, p. xxii). However, this soon proved to be an unfounded fear; one month after being appointed, the new commission began making formal statements on issues of funding and care for the HIV epidemic. The composition of the second commission also differed significantly from the first in that the members appointed had expertise in HIV/AIDS and included a person with AIDS. Notably, for unknown reasons, the second commission did not include nurses.

Keenly aware of the problems at hand by December 1989, the commission advised President Bush that "significant changes must be made not only in our health care system but how we think about the system and the people it serves" (National Commission on AIDS, 1989, p. 2). On April 24, 1990, the commission again wrote to the president, indicating that a national plan, with clearly delineated responsibilities and agreement on the roles of federal, state, and local governments and the private sector, was long overdue (National Commission on AIDS, 1990).

By September 1991, the commission had published eight statements of support or endorsements concerning the HIV epidemic, five interim reports, and two annual reports to the President and Congress. But after a decade of the HIV epidemic in the United States, there was still no national plan for preventing and treating HIV disease. Nevertheless, the federal government had spent $6 million between 1987 and 1992 studying the problem.

According to Greenberg (1991), the Bush Administration was undecided about what, if anything, to do about health care in the United States, although Dr. Louis W. Sullivan, Secretary of Health and Human Services, studied the problem. According to Greenberg (1991), "The Bush Administration [saw] no paydirt in attempting serious alterations in the complexities of the health care system. The poor don't vote, and they are the main victims of the system's inadequacies" (p. 935). Ironically, the major recommendations of the 1991 National Commission on AIDS report included implementing (1) a national plan to prevent and treat HIV disease, (2) universal health care coverage for all persons living in the United States, and (3) increased federal funding for all HIV-related health care activities, including prevention, education, research, and care (National Commission on AIDS, 1991).

Correcting the inadequacies of the health care system required more taxes and government involvement, which explains why the previous administration chose to continue to study the problem (Greenberg, 1991). No one could accuse the president of doing nothing as long as the problem was under study.

In June 1988, the first major national report was published by the Reagan-appointed Presidential Commission on the HIV Epidemic. The federal response was to ignore the report. In August 1989 the Bush administration commissioned another panel of AIDS experts to study the problem of HIV disease and AIDS in the United States. Their major findings were published in August 1990 (National Commission on AIDS, 1990) but with the same result as the first report: virtually no action was taken on the recommendations.

In 1989, charges of the inadequacy of federal spending were supported by comparing HIV disease funding to amounts spent on cancer or heart disease (Winkenwerder, Kessler, & Stolec, 1989). These authors noted that expenditures for HIV research were double those for education and prevention, reflecting the American tendency to devote more resources to cures than to prevention. Rogers (1989) viewed the same study as providing potent data supporting insufficient funding for the HIV epidemic by pointing out the cavalier approach to the treatment of intravenous drug use and HIV disease. New York City had an estimated 200,000 intravenous drug users and an HIV seroprevalence rate ranging from 40% to 70%, and yet facilities for treatment were available to fewer than 38,000 of them. This is precisely the point of the reports of the Presidential commissions: the United States has been unable to cope with the many problems of the epidemic.

PROGRESS: INDIVIDUAL EFFORTS

Although federal leadership was absent in the arena of AIDS care, principles of AIDS service programs were tested nationwide. In November 1986, the Robert Wood Johnson Foundation (RWJF), the country's largest health care philanthropy, granted $17.1 million to fund nine projects nationwide known as the AIDS Health Services Programs (AHSP). The RWJF trustees approved the funding as a national competitive health services demonstration, testing the efficacy of the model of AIDS care developed by the San Francisco community. The model was based on keeping persons with AIDS (PWAs) at home for as long as possible by providing case management for both support and health services and minimizing hospital lengths of stay (Weisfeld, 1991).

The AHSP demonstration project was historically unique in that it required the creation of a community consortium. The money would be given not to individual organizations or institutions providing care to PWAs but to groups that demonstrated they could work together with a common goal: to provide care for PWAs. Incredibly—although not without competition, political maneuvering, arguing, and hurt feelings—it worked. The power of the purse worked. Agencies came face to face, and, most important, the cooperation among agencies filtered down to staff involved in the care of PWAs. The experience of the RWJF demonstration in AIDS care was remarkably edifying and taught much about community action and the power of synergy (Osborn, 1991).

Individual leadership on Capitol Hill was most notably present in the work of Senator Edward M. Kennedy, of Massachusetts. In 1987, together with Senator Orrin Hatch, of Utah, he introduced the first comprehensive legislation on AIDS in an attempt to accelerate and coordinate the nation's response to the epidemic. After much debate and amending, the bill addressed education of health care workers, establishment of treatment networks, acceleration of AIDS research, and voluntary, confidential testing.

In 1989, Americans viewed the grief and anguish caused by the San Francisco earthquake and hurricane Hugo in South Carolina. The response of the American public reflected a sense of communal compassion appropriate to the tragedy and the antithesis of the American response to the AIDS epidemic (Osborn, 1991). Both the earthquake and the hurricane were immediately declared disasters by the federal government, and funds were made available. Seizing the moment, Senator Kennedy identified AIDS as a public health disaster and introduced a bill into the Senate to provide grants to improve the quality and availability of care for individuals with AIDS and HIV disease.

The bill, known as the Ryan White Comprehensive AIDS Resources Emergency (CARE) Act, was signed into law in August 1990. It was named after Ryan White, a young farm boy from Indiana with hemophilia, who had inspired the nation with his tremendous courage in fighting the discrimination he suffered while living with HIV disease. The CARE Act provided funding for the metropolitan areas hardest hit by AIDS and support to states for developing early intervention and services for people with HIV living in less affected areas where resources are limited. Although the CARE Act authorized $350.5 million, the actual amount to be distributed was reduced to $144 million (National Commission on AIDS, 1991).

PROGRESS AT LAST: BIPARTISAN EFFORTS

In June 1995, President Bill Clinton, by executive order, established the Presidential Advisory Council on HIV/AIDS. The group was charged with advising the secretary of health and human services on prevention, research, and treatment of persons living with HIV disease and AIDS (Office of the Press Secretary, 1995). One of the most notable figures appointed to the council was basketball star Earvin "Magic" Johnson. After serving less than a year, he resigned from the council because of its inability to make any changes in AIDS policy. The council's activities and powers were limited to making recommendations, many of which were contained in the work of the previous two commissions. Most of the work performed by the council was behind closed doors and received minimal media coverage. One of nursing's prominent leaders, Helen Miramontes, served on the council.

After 15 years of the HIV/AIDS epidemic in the United States, on December 17, 1996, President Clinton unveiled the first national AIDS plan endorsed by a President of the United States (Rovner, 1997). The plan, developed by the Presidential Advisory Council, produced six major goals to combat HIV disease in the United States: (1) develop a cure for

HIV infection and an HIV vaccine to prevent new infection, (2) reduce the incidence of HIV infection in the United States to zero, (3) ensure access to health care, housing, and supportive services for all HIV-infected individuals, (4) eliminate discrimination against HIV-infected individuals, (5) support international efforts to fight the HIV epidemic, and (6) ensure that advances in research are applied to improve HIV prevention programs and to better care for HIV-infected individuals. One notable aspect of the plan was the fact that most of the 40-page document restated initiatives already in place, rather than supplying any new strategies. At the press conference, the President also noted that in the first 4 years of his Administration, funding for programs related to HIV/AIDS had increased by 55% (Rovner, 1997).

Even though the Presidential Advisory Council on AIDS strongly recommended funding for needle exchange programs (NEPs), the Clinton plan to combat AIDS omitted any recommendation or mention of this topic. NEPs, also referred to as syringe exchange programs (SEPs), have been widely implemented in Australia, Canada, the Netherlands, and the United Kingdom. Studies have shown that NEPs not only reduce the spread of HIV, as well as hepatitis B and C, but do not increase or promote injection drug use (CDC, 1995b; General Accounting Office, 1993). Researchers at the University of California, San Francisco, and Montefiore Medical Center in the Bronx estimated that nearly 10,000 new HIV infections among injection drug users, their sexual partners, and their children could have been prevented between 1987 and 1995 if NEPs had been available ("Ban on Needle Swaps," 1996). However, shortly after the Clinton plan was announced, the director of the National Institutes of Health announced that $2.4 million had been approved to study the efficacy of NEPs beginning in 1997 ("NIH Director," 1996).

THE GAY COMMUNITY AND ITS POLITICAL INFLUENCE

AIDS has transformed politics and activism primarily as a result of the actions of the gay community. To understand the gay community and its political involvement in the HIV epidemic, one must go back to the summer of 1969, when, in response to increasing police harassment of the gay community in New York City, patrons of a gay bar in Greenwich Village, the Stonewall, staged a 3-day riot. This became known as the Stonewall riots and is credited with the beginning of the modern-day gay rights movement. In the United States during the 1970s, gay communities participated in the so-called sexual revolution, as did heterosexuals. However, the gay community also fought for equal rights and an end to society's oppressive attitude and condemnation of the homosexual life style.

The gay rights movement of the 1970s took root in major cities across the country, with San Francisco heralded as the most progressive city in addressing the issues. By the 1980s the gay community in San Francisco was well organized and had elected officials who were openly gay as representatives in city government. Consequently, as soon as the HIV epidemic became evident in San Francisco in 1981, the community response, both politically and economically, represented a coordinated effort. By mid-1983 the San Francisco gay community had spearheaded AIDS prevention and education programs, opened the first AIDS ward at San Francisco General Hospital, and assisted in the development of a special program of home and hospice care for PWAs. Politicians, policymakers, and clinicians throughout the nation looked to San Francisco's model AIDS program.

New York City, the city with the largest cumulative total numbers of AIDS cases since the beginning of the epidemic, attempted to replicate San Francisco's program of care for PWAs but found it as difficult as putting a square peg into a round hole. As soon as a hospital in New York opened an AIDS ward, administrators found they had insufficient beds to keep up with the escalating numbers of cases. Moreover, the composition of AIDS cases differed widely between the two cities. In San Francisco, AIDS is primarily a gay, white disease; in New York it is also a disease of the poor, racial and ethnic minorities, intravenous drug users, women, and children. Additionally, New York experienced continued political inaction, attributed by some to the fact that AIDS was increasing in intravenous drug users, minorities, and the poor (Weisfeld, 1991).

In 1982, in an attempt to address the complex problems of AIDS, two gay men, Bobbi Campbell and Dan Turner, of San Francisco, formed the first organization of, for, and by people with AIDS and AIDS-related complex (PWArc). At the same time in New York, Michael Callen and Richard Berkowitz formed Gay Men With AIDS. According to Callen and Turner (1988), "New York PWAs and PWArcs began to express growing frustrations at attending GMHC [Gay Men's Health Crisis] forums where those of us with AIDS would sit silently in the audience and hear doctors, nurses, lawyers, insurance experts and CSW's [social workers] tell what it is like to have AIDS. . . . [T]he 'real experts' [people with AIDS], we realized, weren't up there" (p. 290).

NATIONAL ASSOCIATION OF PEOPLE WITH AIDS

In 1983, the National Association of People With AIDS was formed in Denver at the Second Annual AIDS Forum, sponsored by the Gay Health Education Foundation. According to Navarre (1988), "Because AIDS is so often perceived as a moral problem instead of a health crisis, and because of the connection between AIDS and gay men, AIDS has from the beginning been a political issue, tied to the long and bitter struggle for gay and lesbian rights" (p. 20). The formation of the National Association of People With AIDS represented the beginning of self-empowerment for PWAs

(Callen & Turner, 1988). To articulate their position clearly, these PWAs adopted a statement of principles in 1983 known as the Denver Principles; the four essentials of the statement are recommendations for health care professionals, recommendations for all people, recommendations for PWAs, and the rights of PWAs (see Box).

Was this necessary? Did PWAs have to band together and state their demands? By March 1983, AIDS activist Larry Kramer noted, "Patients are now more and more being treated like lepers as hospital staffs become increasingly worried that AIDS is infectious. . . . If all of this had been happening to any other community for two long years, there would have been, long ago, such an outcry from that community and all its members that the government of this city

---

THE DENVER PRINCIPLES

Statement from the Advisory Committee of People with AIDS

We condemn attempts to label us as "victims," a term which implies defeat, and we are only occasionally "patients," a term which implies passivity, helplessness, and dependence upon the care of others. We are PEOPLE with AIDS.

Recommendations for Health Care Professionals

1. Come out, especially to their patients who have AIDS.
2. Always clearly identify and discuss the theory they favor as to the cause of AIDS, since this bias affects the treatments and advice they give.
3. Get in touch with their feelings (e.g., fears, anxieties, hopes) about AIDS and not simply deal with AIDS intellectually.
4. Take a thorough personal inventory and identify and examine their own agendas around AIDS.
5. Treat people with AIDS as a whole person, and address psychosocial issues as well as biophysical ones.
6. Address the question of sexuality in people with AIDS specifically, sensitively and with information about gay male sexuality in general, and the sexuality of people with AIDS in particular.

Recommendations for All People

1. Support us in our struggle against those who would fire us from our jobs, evict us from our homes, refuse to touch us or separate us from our loved ones, our community or our peers, since available evidence does not support the view that AIDS can be spread by casual, social contact.
2. Not scapegoat people with AIDS, blame us for the epidemic or generalize about our life-styles.

Recommendations for People With AIDS

1. Form caucuses to choose their own representatives, to deal with the media, to choose their own agenda, and to plan their own strategies.
2. Be involved at every level of decision making and specifically serve on the boards of directors of provider organizations.
3. Be included in all AIDS forums with equal credibility as other participants, to share their own experiences and knowledge.
4. Substitute low-risk sexual behaviors for those which could endanger themselves or their partners; we feel that people with AIDS have an ethical responsibility to inform their potential sexual partners of their health status.

Rights of People With AIDS

1. To as full and satisfying sexual and emotional lives as anyone else.
2. To quality medical treatment and quality social service provision without discrimination of any form including sexual orientation, gender, diagnosis, economic status, or race.
3. To full explanations of all medical procedures and risks, to choose or refuse their treatment modalities, to refuse to participate in research without jeopardizing their treatment, and to make informed decisions about their lives.
4. To privacy, to confidentiality of medical records, to human respect, and to choose who their significant others are.
5. To die—and to LIVE—with dignity.

Reprinted with permission from National Association of People with AIDS.

[New York] and this country would not know what hit them" (Kramer, 1989, p. 35). Attitudes and care continued to get worse.

In June 1985, Robert Cecchi, of the ombudsman's office of the Gay Men's Health Crisis, submitted a detailed report to the New York State Department of Health AIDS Institute. Although the report cited major problems encountered by PWAs in hospitals—among them, housekeeping, dietary, admissions, emergency departments, and medical care—the report began by addressing "the common nursing complaints of ignoring the patient" (p. 2): call bells unanswered for hours, incontinent patients lying in excreta for entire shifts, nurse-patient contact limited to medication administration, no one to bathe or feed patients, dirty linens, noticeable lack of skin care and the development of decubiti, and nursing staff refusing to identify themselves.

This report prompted the New York State Department of Health (1985) to distribute a memorandum demanding that PWAs receive humane, clinically necessary care and treatment. In fact, it mandated that PWAs (1) receive the same consideration as any other patient for admission purposes, (2) be accorded proper nursing care and treatment, and (3) be afforded a safe environment, including clean linen and nourishment.

ACTIVISM

By the mid-1980s, the gay community, as well as PWA and AIDS organizations, became increasingly alarmed at the national apathy toward the AIDS epidemic. At the First International Conference on AIDS, held in Atlanta in April 1985, scientists and clinicians heard for the first time from gay activists known as the Lavender Hill Mob. "They got more attention than anything else at that meeting. They protested, they yelled and screamed and demanded and were blissfully rude to all those arrogant epidemiologists who are ruining our lives" (Kramer, 1989, p. 135).

The sentiments and anger among the gay community swelled, and in March 1987, under the encouragement and leadership of Larry Kramer, author, playwright, and activist, the AIDS Coalition to Unleash Power (ACT-UP) was formed. Originally a community group committed to fighting for the release of experimental drugs, this nationwide group has expanded its focus to all aspects of HIV-related care and issues that affect health care delivery. ACT-UP is a powerful group of activists that is feared by politicians, scientists, clinicians, administrators, and health care organizations. The media follow them. They have become a driving force for health care policy reform as the watchdog of the HIV epidemic in North and South America, Europe, Australia, and South Africa (Carter, 1992). ACT-UP has continued to advocate access to drugs, improved treatment, and policy change throughout the HIV/AIDS pandemic.

ORGANIZED NURSING'S RESPONSE

The HIV epidemic has presented a unique challenge to organized nursing. Early in the epidemic, individual nurse advocates urged their local, state, and national nurses associations to be responsive to the epidemic by providing leadership in the many issues related to practice, education, research, and policy development.

INTERNATIONAL COUNCIL OF NURSES

In 1987 the International Council of Nurses (ICN) and the World Health Organization (WHO) released a joint declaration emphasizing that HIV/AIDS is an international health problem of extraordinary urgency and highlighting the need for international leadership, cooperation, and collaboration to control the spread of the epidemic (ICN, 1987). The ICN/WHO AIDS Project, a 30-month project, commenced in 1990 to mobilize national nurses' associations in eight African countries to prevent the spread of HIV, to improve the care of AIDS patients, and to support the families of these patients (ICN, 1990). In 1997, ICN released *On the Continuum of HIV/AIDS Care,* a publication that addresses HIV research and nursing practice, how an HIV nursing network provides support for nurses involved in AIDS care, and the professional challenges and personal experiences of nurses in the pandemic (ICN, 1997).

AMERICAN NURSES ASSOCIATION

The American Nurses Association (ANA) provided leadership for the profession by developing numerous position statements and through the work of many organizational units and the ANA House of Delegates, train-the-trainer and other HIV-focused grant-sponsored initiatives, and ongoing advocacy by its professional staff in the development of federal policy and national networking with such groups as the National Leadership Coalition on AIDS, National Organizations Responding to AIDS, and the Women and AIDS Coalition. Two early position statements addressed both the rights of all populations at risk to quality, humanistic health care and the issue of risk versus responsibility in providing nursing care (ANA, 1992).

In the summer of 1991, during a time of nationwide concern regarding the possible transmission of HIV from an infected health care professional to a patient, the ANA House of Delegates spent a considerable portion of its deliberations in discussing the nursing profession's role in the HIV epidemic. It was during this period that some nurses and other health care workers, erroneously believing that adherence to universal precautions and infection control guidelines was not adequate protection in the workplace, supported mandatory testing of potentially infected high-risk groups and the development of exposure-prone lists of procedures. Some nurses and physicians also expressed willingness to be HIV tested if they could require that all patients be HIV tested, ignoring the problems of the "window period" in the infection and how often and when

everybody would need to be tested. These attitudes, however, were not universally shared in the profession.

The 1991 ANA House of Delegates members rejected this type of thinking and supported a list of recommendations that included, among other items: (1) development and implementation of national standards governing infection control techniques for invasive procedures in all health care settings, (2) support for Occupational Safety and Health Administration (OSHA) standards requiring mandatory annual education on universal precautions and infection control for all health care personnel, (3) opposition to mandatory testing and disclosure, while supporting voluntary, anonymous, and confidential testing and voluntary disclosure of HIV status, (4) continued public education, (5) the ethical responsibilities of the nurse in regard to the epidemic, (6) the need to provide support for HIV-infected nurses, and (7) the end of discrimination within the insurance industry against HIV-infected individuals (ANA, 1991). Previous ANA conventions had endorsed resolutions ranging from support for AIDS funding, voluntary and anonymous testing, the civil and human rights of AIDS patients, and opposition to mandatory testing (ANA, 1985, 1988a).

The ANA, on the recommendation of its HIV Resource Task Force, also endorsed education and barrier use for sexually transmitted diseases and HIV infection, postexposure programs in the event of occupational exposure to HIV and hepatitis B virus, the availability of equipment and safety procedures to prevent transmission of blood-borne diseases, personnel policies on HIV in the workplace, and opposition to travel restrictions for persons with HIV/AIDS. ANA believes that antidiscrimination is the cornerstone of effective national AIDS policy (ANA, 1988b; Grimaldi, 1989). Also addressed by ANA have been such issues as access to psychological and psychosocial nursing care, condom advertising, HIV infection and teenagers, the development of AIDS-specific nursing curricula, guidelines for disclosure and confidential notification, HIV and women, HIV and correctional inmates, HIV/AIDS in socioculturally diverse populations, tuberculosis and HIV, HIV exposure from rape and other sexual assault, needle exchange programs, and the HIV-infected professional nurse.

In 1993 ANA established the Nursing and HIV/AIDS National Action Agenda, which focused on four areas (practice, education, research, and policy). Some of the major issues identified in these four areas were (1) comprehensive, holistic, humane care for persons infected with HIV/AIDS and their family members, with special emphasis on access to care for the young, the poor, and the disenfranchised, (2) ethical issues as encountered by nurses caring for PWAs, (3) the need for nursing personnel in adequate numbers to respond to the pandemic, (4) the need for model nursing curricula at all levels of nursing education, (5) the need for qualified, skilled educators and mentors, (6) the need by the profession for an HIV/AIDS nursing research agenda that specifies priorities for clinical nursing research, and (7) the need for nursing involvement in the development of legislation and policy (ANA, 1993a). New ANA publications include *Nursing and the Human Immunodeficiency Virus: A Guide for Nursing's Response to AIDS* (1993b) and, as part of its CDC-funded project, Nurses Campaign to Reduce Adolescent High Risk Behaviors, the document *Recommendations for the School Health Nurse in Addressing HIV/AIDS With Adolescents* (1997).

In January 1994 the American Academy of Nursing held an HIV/AIDS nursing care summit in Washington, D.C. The conference brought together many nursing leaders in the epidemic to discuss the myriad of HIV nursing issues. Kristine Gebbie, a nurse and then director of AIDS policy in the Clinton Administration, was the keynote speaker. It is sad to note that Dr. Gebbie had to share her significant

concerns regarding flagrant and irresponsible distortions regarding the HIV epidemic that had been published in *Revolution,* a nursing journal. Even in 1994, misinformation had an adverse impact on a responsible approach by some members of the profession to the epidemic.

ANA has consistently worked with the U.S. Senate and House leadership to address the epidemic. ANA has opposed exposure-prone lists for nursing procedures and mandatory testing and disclosure. It has provided testimony on HIV testing of health care workers (to the CDC), on the CDC recommendations and HIV-infected health care workers (to the House Energy and Commerce Subcommittee on Health and the Environment), on the reduction of occupational exposure to hepatitis B virus and HIV (to OSHA), and on health care workers and AIDS (to the House Government Operations Committee). ANA, in collaboration with the specialty nursing organizations, has pursued every opportunity to enlighten the Congress regarding the realities of the epidemic, the real problems and challenges of infected health care workers, and the role of nursing in the epidemic.

STATE NURSES ASSOCIATIONS

By the late 1980s, one fourth of the state nurses associations had addressed the HIV concerns of nurses in their states by developing specific position statements or establishing organizational units. Three state associations were providing support groups for HIV-infected nurses, and four others had pending programs. Educational offerings were of primary interest to local nurses associations, with their members expressing concerns that mirrored national interests: mandatory testing of health care workers, compensation for exposure and disease, home health care of HIV patients, safety of the blood supply, heterosexual transmission, and needle exchange programs (ANA, personal communications, 1988, 1992). By 1993, twenty-three state nurses associations had formed task forces or committees to address HIV issues. By 1995, some state governments (Florida, Minnesota, New York, Virginia, Washington) were requiring some form of HIV education in conjunction with nursing registration or licensure (ANA, 1993c).

Two state nurses associations involved in the epidemic's epicenter populations have been particularly purposeful in their activities. The New York State Nurses Association (NYSNA, 1983) and the California Nurses Association (CNA, 1985) were the first to issue statements addressing the direct-care, educational, health-counseling, advocacy, and research roles of the professional nurse in the epidemic. In 1991, NYSNA was an active leader in a statewide coalition of health care organizations that convinced the Cuomo administration to refuse to identify so-called "high risk" activities for infected health care workers and any restrictions on practice. In 1987, CNA established a unique "Train the Trainer" program, educating more than 2,000 health care workers, and was recognized by Health and Human Services Assistant Secretary Dr. James Mason for outstanding educational achievements at the 1992 federal World AIDS Day celebration.

NATIONAL LEAGUE FOR NURSING AND SCHOOLS OF NURSING

The National League for Nursing (NLN) published *AIDS Guidelines for Schools of Nursing* in 1988. These guidelines addressed institutional policy and clinical experience guidelines for faculty and students and highlighted guidelines for the prevention of HIV transmission (NLN, 1988). In 1994, in conjunction with the Association for Nurses in AIDS Care, NLN published new guidelines that called for curriculum content to include confidentiality, risk assessment, transmission, infection control/universal precautions, safer sex education, access to care issues, and attitudes and values (Corless & Nokes, 1996; NLN, 1994). In 1991,

NLN entered into a collaborative project with the AIDS Treatment Data Network, whose information is available on an interactive computer network (The Care Bank) (Fedor, 1991).

There appears to be a consensus that schools of nursing are responsible for preparing their students to meet the challenge of the HIV epidemic, but information in the literature on curriculum development or on policies regarding HIV-infected students in schools of nursing is limited. Carwein and Bowles's study (1988) identified a reluctance to develop policies addressing controversial student-related HIV issues. Chitty (1988) found that nursing education in general had responded to the epidemic but suggested that educators should use more affective and behavioral learning methods to modify the attitudes of nursing students. An article by Corless and Nokes (1996) noted that the NLN curriculum guidelines do not appear to be used in any systematic manner in nursing education.

There is an ongoing critical need for nursing programs that prepare knowledgeable nursing professionals at the master's level who can assume leadership roles in combating this epidemic. In 1990 the Hunter-Bellevue School of Nursing at Hunter College of the City University of New York received funding through the U.S. Department of Health and Human Services Division of Nursing to implement a graduate subspecialization in the care of persons with HIV-AIDS. This program, the first federally funded one of its kind, is unique with respect to students' ability to incorporate all requirements for the HIV subspecialty within one of the six specialty graduate nursing programs available at Hunter-Bellevue. Similarly funded programs can be found at Columbia University, the University of Massachusetts—Worcester, Howard University, and the Massachusetts General Hospital's Institute of Health Professions (Corless & Nokes, 1996). The University of California at San Francisco was the first in the nation to provide an opportunity for additional course-specific spe-cialization. New York University's Division of Nursing for many years provided interdisciplin-ary training programs and developed multiple curriculum guides for health care professionals.

ASSOCIATION OF NURSES IN AIDS CARE

Although the issues of nursing PWAs were being addressed through special interest groups, task forces, and other groups in nursing organizations, many of the nurses working exclusively with HIV-infected populations felt a need to join together to address the uniqueness of nursing in the wake of the HIV epidemic. In 1987, twelve nurses—Errol Chin-Loy, Jeanne Kalinowski, Joan Blanchfield, Susan Holman, Nancy Thayer, Nancy McCaslin, James Hallo-ran, Alison Moed, Michael Damon, George McKeel, Carolyn Sutton-Debarros, and Thomas O'Donnell—became the founding board mem-bers of the Association of Nurses in AIDS Care (ANAC). There was initial criticism by some nurses regarding the need for such an organiza-tion, but it quickly subsided.

ANAC has fostered the professional develop-ment of nurses involved in all aspects of AIDS and has promoted the health, welfare, and rights of all persons affected by HIV disease. ANAC publishes a peer-reviewed journal, *The Journal of the Association of Nurses in AIDS Care,* and in 1996 published *ANAC's Core Curriculum for HIV/AIDS Nursing.* ANAC also conducts a certification examination for nurses in HIV/AIDS care (AIDS-certified registered nurse [ACRN]), sponsors an annual conference and local educational programs, and has devel-oped strategic relationships with other nursing and AIDS organizations.

HYSTERIA AND POLITICS: A CASE HISTORY

Chaos and confusion have periodically sur-faced throughout the HIV epidemic in the United States. Perhaps no other report fueled the fires of hysteria as much as the case of Kimberly Bergalis, of Florida, who allegedly acquired HIV infection as a result of dental care by Dr. David Acer (CDC, 1990a). In July 1990 the news of this case sent shock waves across the country. By 1990, the CDC estimated that there were at least 1 million Americans infected with HIV and at least 40,000 new infections occurring annually among adults and adoles-cents, as well as 1,500 to 2,000 new infections among newborn infants (CDC, 1990b). Addi-tionally, an estimated 5,000 to 7,000 health care workers in the United States were infected with HIV (Altman, 1991; Physicians Association for AIDS Care, 1990). By 1989, a total of 25 cases of occupationally acquired HIV among health care workers had been reported to the CDC ("Occu-pational Exposure," 1989). Thus the issue of transmission of HIV in a health care setting had to be considered a potential risk bidirection-ally—from a patient to a health care worker, as well as from a health care worker to a patient. Hampering the investigation of the alleged dentist-to-patient transmission was the fact that the HIV-infected dentist in question died early in the investigation.

Ultimately, five of the dentist's patients were identified with HIV infection. None of the five had confirmed exposures to HIV, all had in-vasive procedures performed by the dentist, and all were infected with HIV strains that were closely related to each other and to the strain that had infected the dentist but were distinct from control patients living in the same geo-graphic area as the dental practice (CDC, 1991a, 1991b). The investigation was consid-ered inconclusive, however, because the dental records were sketchy at best (Cottone, Moli-nari, & McDonald, 1990). The CDC (1991b) found that the precise mode of transmission to these five patients could not be determined. On the basis of a hepatitis-B model and what is known about blood-borne pathogen transmis-sion from health care workers to patients, the CDC (1991b) concluded that these cases may have been the result of procedures and tech-niques used by the dentist.

The CDC (1991a) then drafted recommendations for preventing transmission of HIV and hepatitis B virus to patients during exposure-prone invasive procedures and advised that HIV-infected health care workers not perform these procedures unless they sought counsel from an expert review panel. The document did not clearly define invasive procedures. The CDC planned to consult with representative health care organizations to develop a list of those procedures and announced that the recommendations would be prepared by November 15, 1992.

Legislative backing to these recommendations was adopted on July 18, 1991, when a proposal, supported by Senator Jesse Helms, of North Carolina, won by a vote of 81 to 18 in the Senate (Tolchin, 1991). Senator Helms repeatedly cited the case of Kimberly Bergalis "as a symbol of the callousness and indifference of some health practitioners toward their professional responsibilities" (Tolchin, 1991, p. A1). The Helms amendment would set a criminal penalty of a $10,000 fine, 10 years in prison, or both for HIV-infected health care workers who had invasive physical contact with a patient, without notifying him or her of their HIV status. In a maneuver to stop the Helms amendment, Senators Edward Kennedy, of Massachusetts, Robert Dole, of Kansas, George Mitchell, of Maine, and Orrin Hatch, of Utah, submitted a proposal that would require all health care professionals engaged in invasive procedures to be tested for HIV. Those infected with HIV would be barred from performing invasive procedures unless they received permission from a panel of experts and informed their patients.

The leadership proposal was passed by an overwhelming vote of 99 to 0. This strategy backfired when Senate experts announced that passage of both bills gave them equal status (Tolchin, 1991). At that point, the House was not expected to act on the matter until after the summer recess. According to Tolchin (1991), the prospects for passage of the leadership proposal looked good because of the (assumed) lack of opposition from leading medical groups and gay rights organizations. The timing was perfect. The August congressional recess provided time for health care workers, scientists, and clinicians to respond to both bills and to the CDC proposal, and indeed they did respond.

On July 30, 1991, an emergency meeting was called by the New York City Commission on Human Rights to discuss the need to formalize a New York City and state response to both the CDC recommendations and the Senate legislation. On August 14, representatives of the major health care professions and health care organizations from New York State met in New York City to discuss the proposals and to develop an action plan. The group, known as the Coalition for Safe Health Care, was not convened by any health authority or professional organization; it was formed at the request of the leadership of ACT-UP New York. The months of August and September 1991 were filled with meetings, lobbying, letters to Congress, and public hearings.

Essentially the major opposition to both the CDC recommendations and the Senate proposal was the myopic view that the problem at hand was the practitioner instead of the practice. Review of both the case of alleged transmission during dental care and all available scientific literature pointed to an attributable risk behavior: failure on the part of a health care worker to follow established infection control guidelines.

Around the same time, John Colombotos and colleagues (1991), of the Columbia University School of Public Health, published preliminary findings from their research on physicians' and nurses' knowledge, attitudes, and practices with respect to AIDS and related issues. Their study of 1,520 nurses and 958 physicians revealed that a significant number failed to follow universal precautions and were more likely to use barrier precautions only when performing procedures on known HIV-infected patients. Swanson, Chenitz, Zalor, and Stoll (1990), in a review of nursing research on nurses' knowledge, attitudes, and practices related to the care of HIV-infected people, found identifiable gaps in nurses' knowledge regarding transmission of HIV, infection control, and how to protect themselves at work. Clearly the problems in infection control practices and the use of universal precautions needed to be addressed.

At a meeting held on August 28, 1991, in Chicago, representatives of 40 medical, nursing, and health professional organizations agreed that current data showed there was no risk of infecting patients—that is, directly from a health care worker to a patient—and refused to participate with the CDC in developing a list of invasive procedures (Altman, 1991). The meeting was sponsored by the American Medical Association (AMA). According to Dr. M. Roy Schwartz, a vice president of the AMA, "The prevailing attitude was that compiling a list implies there is a significant risk, and thus would mislead the public and capitulate to public fears" (Altman, 1991, p. A1). The former surgeon general C. Everett Koop summed up the situation: "Let me assure the American public that their chances of getting AIDS from a health care worker are essentially nil, unless they are having a sexual relationship, or shooting drugs and sharing needles with him or her" (Altman, 1991, p. A19).

At congressional hearings held in September 1991, Kimberly Bergalis, visibly debilitated from HIV disease, testified in support of mandatory testing of health care workers and restriction of HIV-infected health care workers from performing invasive procedures. According to Berke (1991), her appearance "set off a national debate that some fear threatens to reverse years of difficult progress in separating the stigma from the disease" (p. E1).

In October 1991 Governor Mario Cuomo, of New York, at the recommendation of virtually all major health care professional organizations and institutions in his state, announced that he would reject the proposed CDC guidelines, supporting the current position of voluntary, confidential HIV testing for all individuals, including health care workers, and not restrict practice (Sack, 1991). Governor Cuomo's position not only placed New York at the forefront of a national resistance movement against the CDC guidelines and federal legislation but also risked the loss of millions of dollars in federal health grants. Congress ultimately relinquished enforcement of the CDC guidelines to the individual states because professional organizations refused to cooperate with the CDC's November 15, 1991, deadline to develop lists of exposure-prone procedures (Daniels, 1992). The CDC then drafted revised guidelines recommending that local committees review the risk imposed by infected workers on a case-by-case basis (CDC, 1991c). Finally, the focus shifted from the HIV status of the practitioner to infection control procedures.

In December 1991, OSHA set standards on blood-borne pathogens that made universal precautions mandatory in all health care settings ("Occupational Exposure to Blood-borne Pathogens," 1991). In January 1992, New York State was the first to amend its state education law to include failure to follow appropriate infection control techniques as an addition to the definition of unprofessional conduct (New York State Education Department, 1992). The new rule considered it unprofessional conduct for a health professional to fail to use infection prevention techniques, appropriate to each profession, for the cleaning and sterilization of instruments, devices, materials, and work surfaces; for the use of protective garb and of covers for contamination-prone equipment; and for the handling of sharp instruments. Licensed health care workers who fail to comply with these basic standards are subject to disciplinary action for unprofessional conduct.

CONCLUSION

Sherer (1990) described the HIV-AIDS epidemic as two parallel nightmares: first, the syndromes of HIV disease and the associated suffering and death, and, second, the epidemic of fear and discrimination. History certainly attests to the reality of both. Because HIV has affected primarily the disenfranchised, it has been easy for many either to ignore the problem or to rationalize discrimination.

The gay community, although often not credited, has contributed significantly throughout the HIV-AIDS epidemic. The community's persistence and concern, as well as activism, are described as "sometimes praised, sometimes vilified, but always noticed," and as having "permanently altered American health policy" (Wachter, 1992, p. 129).

After having worked with the World Health Organization for 18 years, Dr. Michael Merson returned home to the United States in 1995 and was totally taken back by the attitudes and beliefs of the American public and politicians toward the HIV epidemic, including such facts as that (1) most believe that AIDS is still a disease of gay white men, when, in reality, 75% of all new HIV infections occur through heterosexual intercourse or intravenous drug use and are occurring predominantly among people of color, (2) there is a lack of appreciation for the global burden of AIDS, (3) school boards and chancellors are still fearful of discussing sex in the classroom, despite the fact that one in four new HIV infections now occur in people younger than 21 years, (4) many believe that condoms don't work, (5) though scientists have demonstrated that needle exchange programs work, legislators and politicians refuse to fund these programs or change existing laws, and (6) unequal access to HIV/AIDS care, including drugs, continues to be a problem (Merson, 1996). To mount the appropriate response to the problem of the HIV/AIDS epidemic, we should, as Merson suggests: (1) accept that AIDS prevention is not perfect but it works, (2) keep to a minimum the needless debates and sensationalism that detract from an appropriate response, (3) make rational policy decisions based on sound public health principles rather than on moral grounds, and (4) strengthen our research agenda, and avoid moral debates by assigning greater emphasis to cancer and cardiovascular research (Merson, 1996).

As the HIV epidemic moves into its third decade and the next millennium, the human face of AIDS is changing and the response of nurses and the profession will also need to change. Organized nursing must remain responsive. The role of individual nurses in HIV care must continue, as found in the contributions of the following nurses who have received special recognition from the assistant secretary for health: JoAnne Bennett, Mary Boland, Tracy Castelman, Barbara Fassbinder, Ronnie Leibowitz, Terry Miles, Helen Miramontes, Clifford Morrison, Carol Price, Barbara Russell, Helen Schietinger, Nancy Sears, Barbara Staton, Rose Thomas, Peter Ungvarski, and Dorothy Ward-Wimmer. In addition, there are individuals such as Linda Arnold, a nurse who, after being infected with HIV from a needlestick exposure, launched a national campaign for health care worker safety.

Recent media coverage seems to infer that AIDS is cured, but better treatment does not equal cure. The virus and the epidemic remain, and as one commentator has noted, "It will be the plaque of our professional lifetimes—and probably that of our children's lives as well" (Rogers, 1992).

Nursing will have to be responsive to the "control versus cure" stage of the epidemic; to the onset of prolonged chronicity, as opposed to a more or less predictable acute illness; and to many new faces' being seen in the epidemic—those of older individuals, increasing numbers of teenagers, women, the poor, and the homeless. Throughout the course of HIV infection in an individual, nurses play an important role in the creation and maintenance of support services for the infected person. Comprehensive HIV care, with its many shifting physical, psychosocial, socioeconomic, and spiritual needs, is basically nursing care (ANA, 1992). Nurses across the care spectrum will have to be familiar with the latest scientific findings, new pharmacological interventions and complex treatments, ethical dimensions associated with care, access-to-treatment issues, and rationing of care, while still remaining caring and compassionate in a health care industry that increasingly is unresponsive to individual human needs.

The politics of both health care and the HIV epidemic will continue to be a dominant force in the nursing profession's ability to be responsive to infected and noninfected individuals. When questions are raised regarding what care, at what cost, will be delivered to whom, nurses need to be ready to respond and to advance the needs of the infected and potentially infected marginalized members of our society. Nurses must continue to provide clear leadership in advancing the need for education, prevention, and the provision of care as both the current and future responses to this epidemic, regardless of the politics of any institution, agency, locality, or political party.

References

AIDS education: Printing and distribution of the Surgeon General's report. (1988). (Report B-230539.) Washington, DC: U.S. Government Printing Office.

Altman, L. K. (1991, August 30). Health units defy U.S. on AIDS rules. *New York Times,* pp. A1, A19.

American Nurses Association. (1985, November). *ANA urges use of CDC guidelines for care of AIDS patients.* Kansas City, MO: Author.

American Nurses Association. (1988a, August 12). *ANA urges Reagan to broaden AIDS plan.* Press release.

American Nurses Association. (1998b, September). *Personal heroism, professional activism-nursing and the battle against AIDS.* Kansas City, MO: Author.

American Nurses Association. (1991, June 30). *Nursing and the human immunodeficiency virus.* Kansas City, MO: Author.

American Nurses Association. (1992). *Compendium of HIV/AIDS—Positions, policies and documents.* Washington, DC: Author.

American Nurses Association. (1993a). *Nursing and HIV/AIDS—National action agenda.* Washington, DC: Author.

American Nurses Association. (1993b). *Nursing and the human immunodeficiency virus: A guide for nursing's response to AIDS.* Washington, DC: Author.

American Nurses Association. (1993c). Update on nursing and HIV. In *House of Delegates Report on HIV Infection and Immigration.* Washington, DC: Author.

American Nurses Association. (1997). *Recommendations for the school health nurse in addressing HIV/AIDS with adolescents.* Washington, DC: Author.

Baker, J. (1983). *AIDS: Everything you must know about acquired immune deficiency syndrome: The killer epidemic of the 80's.* Saratoga, CA: R&E Publishers.

Ban on needle swaps blamed for 10,000 U.S. infections. (1996). *AIDS Policy Law, 11*(13), 3.

Barre-Sinoussi, F., Chermann, J. C., Rey, F., Mathur-Wagh, U., Brun-Vezinet, F., Yancovitz, S. R., Rouzioux, C., Montagnier, L., & Mildvan, D. (1983). Isolation of a T-lymphotropic retrovirus from a patient at risk for acquired immune deficiency syndrome (AIDS). *Science, 220*(4599), 868–871.

Berke, R. L. (1991, October 6). AIDS battle reverting to "us against them." *New York Times,* pp. E1, E4.

California Nurses Association. (1985, September). *Resolution of mobilization of nurses for care of AIDS patients.* Resolution presented at the California Nurses Association Convention, San Francisco.

Callen, M., & Turner, D. (1988). A history of the PWA self-empowerment movement. In M. Callen, J. Rosett, & R. Dworkin (Eds.), *Surviving and thriving with AIDS: Collected wisdom* (Vol. 2, pp. 288–296). New York: People with AIDS Coalition.

Carwein, U., & Bowles, C. (1988). AIDS policy and guidelines development. *Nurse Educator, 13*(2), 14–16.

Cecchi, R. (1985). *Report to the AIDS Institute: Health care problems of people with AIDS.* New York: Gay Men's Health Crisis.

Centers for Disease Control. (1981). *Pneumocystis* pneumonia—Los Angeles. *Morbidity and Mortality Weekly Report, 30*(21), 250–252.

Centers for Disease Control. (1982a). Update on acquired immune deficiency syndrome (AIDS)—

United States. *Morbidity and Mortality Weekly Report, 31*(37), 507–514.

Centers for Disease Control. (1982b). Opportunistic infections and Kaposi's sarcoma among Haitians in the United States. *Morbidity and Mortality Weekly Report, 31*(26), 353–354, 360–361.

Centers for Disease Control. (1982c). *Pneumocystis carinii* pneumonia among persons with hemophilia A. *Morbidity and Mortality Weekly Report, 31*(27), 365–367.

Centers for Disease Control. (1985a). Heterosexual transmission of human T-lymphotropic virus type lymphadenopathy associated virus. *Morbidity and Mortality Weekly Report, 34*(37), 561–563.

Centers for Disease Control. (1985b). Self-reported behavioral changes among homosexual and bisexual men—San Francisco. *Morbidity and Mortality Weekly Report, 34*(40), 613–615.

Centers for Disease Control. (1990a). Possible transmission of human immunodeficiency virus to a patient during an invasive dental procedure. *Morbidity and Mortality Weekly Report, 39*(29), 489–493.

Centers for Disease Control. (1990b). HIV prevalence estimates and AIDS case projections for the United States: Report based upon a workshop. *Morbidity and Mortality Weekly Report, 39*(RR-16), 1–31.

Centers for Disease Control. (1991a). Update: Transmission of HIV infection during an invasive dental procedure—Florida. *Morbidity and Mortality Weekly Report, 40*(2), 22–39.

Centers for Disease Control. (1991b). Update: Transmission of HIV infection during dental procedures—Florida. *Morbidity and Mortality Weekly Report, 40*(23), 377–381.

Centers for Disease Control. (1991c, November 27). *Revised recommendations for preventing transmission of human immunodeficiency virus and hepatitis B virus to patients during invasive procedures.* Atlanta: Author.

Centers for Disease Control and Prevention. (1995a). Update: Acquired immunodeficiency syndrome—United States, 1994. *Morbidity and Mortality Weekly Report, 44*, 64–67.

Centers for Disease Control and Prevention. (1995b). Syringe exchange programs—United States, 1994–1995. *Morbidity and Mortality Weekly Report, 44*(37), 684–685, 691.

Centers for Disease Control and Prevention. (1996). *HIV/AIDS Surveillance Report, 8*(1), 3–33.

Chitty, K. (1988). *A model AIDS curriculum for schools of nursing.* University of Tennessee, Chattanooga, School of Nursing. Unpublished manuscript.

Chitty, K. (1989). Developing acquired immunodeficiency syndrome policies for schools of nursing. *Journal of Professional Nursing, 5*(6), 345–348.

Clinton offers six AIDS goals. (1996, December 18). *New York Times,* p. A22.

Colombotos, J., Macer, P., Burgunder, M., Messeri, P., & McConnell, M. B. (1991). *Physicians, nurses and AIDS: Preliminary findings from a national study Agency for Health Care Policy and Research program note.* (AHCPR publication No. 0024.) Rockville, MD: U.S. Department of Health and Human Services.

Cooper, E. B. (1995). Historical and analytical overview of policy issues affecting women living with AIDS: A blueprint for learning from our past. *Bulletin of the New York Academy of Medicine, 72*(1), 283–299.

Corless, I., & Nokes, K. (1996). Professional nursing education's response to the HIV/AIDS pandemic. *Journal of the Association of Nurses in AIDS Care, 7*(1), 15–22.

Cottone, J. A., Molinari, J., & McDonald, R. (1990). The Kimberly Bergalis case: An analysis of the data suggesting possible transmission of HIV infection from a dentist to his patient. *PAACNOTES 2*(8), 267–275, 307.

Daniels, N. (1992). HIV-infected professionals, patient rights, and the switching dilemma. *Journal of the American Medical Association, 267*(10), 1368–1371.

Fedor, M. (1991). AIDS: Advocacy and activism at work. *Nursing and Health Care, 12*(11), 458–459.

Gebbie, K. (1989). The President's Commission on AIDS: What did it do? *American Journal of Public Health, 79*(7), 868–870.

General Accounting Office. (1993). *Needle exchange programs: Research suggests promise as an AIDS prevention strategy.* Report to the chairman, Select Committee on Narcotics Abuse and Control, House of Representatives. Washington, DC: Author.

Goldsmith, M. (1986). More heterosexual spread of HTLV-III virus seen. In J. M. Cole & G D. Lundberg (Eds.), *AIDS from the beginning* (pp. 96–97). Chicago: American Medical Association.

Greenberg, D. S. (1991). Louis Sullivan is still studying the health system. *Lancet, 338*, 935–936.

Grimaldi, C. (1989). Board of directors expands policies on HIV infection. *American Nurse, 21*(6), 5.

Hilts, R. J. (1992, March 2). American co-discoverer of HIV is investigated anew. *New York Times,* p. B-9.

International Council of Nurses. (1987). *ICN/WHO Joint Declaration on AIDS.* Geneva, Switzerland: Author.

International Council of Nurses. (1990). *Spotlight: Nursing and HIV/AIDS*. Geneva, Switzerland: Author.

International Council of Nurses. (1997). *On the Continuum of HIV/AIDS Care*. Geneva, Switzerland: ICN Publications.

Kann, L., Warren, C. W., Harris, W. A., Collins, J., Williams, B., Ross, J., & Kolbe, L. (1996). Youth at risk behavior surveillance—United States, 1995. *MMWR CDC Surveillance Summary, 45*(4), 1–84.

Koop, C. E. (1986). Surgeon general's report on acquired immune deficiency syndrome. Washington, DC: U.S. Government Printing Office.

Kramer, L. (1989). *Reports from the holocaust: The making of an AIDS activist*. New York: St. Martin's Press.

Levy, J. A., Hoffman, A. D., Cramer, S. M., Landis, J. A., Shimabukuro, J. M., & Oshiro, L. S. (1984). Isolation of lymphocytopathic retroviruses from San Francisco patients with AIDS. *Science, 225*(4664), 840–842.

Marks, R. (1992). Avoiding women [Editorial]. *Focus: A Guide to Research and AIDS Counseling, 7*(1), 2.

Marte, C., & Allen, M. (1992). HIV-related gynecologic conditions: Overlooked complications. *Focus: A Guide to AIDS Research and Counseling, 7*(1), 1.

Merson, M. H. (1996). Returning home: Reflections on the USA's response to the HIV/AIDS epidemic. *Lancet, 347*, 1673–1676.

National Commission on AIDS. (1989). *Failure of the US health care system to deal with HIV epidemic*. Washington, DC: U.S. Government Printing Office.

National Commission on AIDS. (1990). *Leadership, legislation and regulation*. Washington, DC: U.S. Government Printing Office.

National Commission on AIDS. (1991). *America living with AIDS*. Washington, DC: U.S. Government Printing Office.

National League for Nursing. (1988). *AIDS guidelines for schools of nursing*. New York: Author.

National League for Nursing. (1994). *NLN-AIDS guidelines*. New York: Author.

Navarre, M. (1988). Fighting the victim label. In M. Callen, J. Rosett, & R. Dworkin (Eds.), *Surviving and thriving with AIDS: Collected wisdom* (Vol. 2, pp. 19–22). New York: People with AIDS Coalition.

New York State Department of Health. (1985). *Hospital care of acquired immune deficiency syndrome (AIDS) patients* (Series 85–83). New York: Author.

New York State Education Department. (1992, January 7). *Proposed amendment of section 29.2 of the rules of the Board of Regents pursuant to sections 207, 6504,*

6506(1), and 6506(9) of education law relating to the definition of unprofessional conduct in the professions. Albany, NY: Author.

New York State Nurses Association. (1983, September 27). *The role of the professional nurse re: Human immunodeficiency virus (HIV) infection and acquired immune deficiency syndrome (AIDS)*. Guilderland, NY: Author.

NIH director endorses needle exchange research. (1996, October 16). *The Washington Post*, p. A12.

Occupational exposure to blood-borne pathogens: Final rule. (1991). *Federal Register, 56*(235), 64175–64182.

Occupational exposure and HIV infections. (1989). *Federal Register, 54*(102), 23053–23057.

Office of National AIDS Policy. (1996, March). *Youth and HIV/AIDS: An American agenda* [Press release]. Washington, DC: The White House.

Office of the Press Secretary (1995, June 14). *Executive Order No. 12963: Presidential Advisory Council on HIV/AIDS* [Press release]. Washington, DC: The White House.

Osborn, J. (1991). Preface. In V. D. Weisfeld (Ed.), *AIDS health services at the crossroads: Lessons for community care* (pp. v–viii). Princeton, NJ: Robert Wood Johnson Foundation.

Physicians Association for AIDS Care. (1990). Ethical considerations in HIV testing of health care workers and restrictions on seropositive health care workers: A position statement. *PACCNOTES, 2*(6), 271, 272, 307.

Popovic, M., Sarngadharan, M. G., Read, E., & Gallo, R. C. (1984). Detection, isolation, and continuous production of cytopathic retrovirus (HTLV-III) from patients with AIDS and pre-AIDS. *Science, 224*(4648), 497–500.

Presidential Commission on the HIV Epidemic. (1988). *Report of the Presidential Commission on the HIV Epidemic*. Washington, DC: U.S. Government Printing Office.

Ratner, L., Gallo, R. C., & Wong-Staal, E. (1985). HTLV-III, LAV, ARV are variants of same AIDS virus. *Nature, 313*(6004), 636–637.

Rogers, D. E. (1989). Federal spending on AIDS—How much is enough? *New England Journal of Medicine, 320*(24), 1623–1624.

Rogers, D. E. (1992). Report card on our national response to the AIDS epidemic: Some A's, too many D's. *American Journal of Public Health, 82*, 522–524.

Rovner, J. (1997). President Clinton wages war against AIDS. *Lancet, 349*, 39.

Sack, K. (1991, October 9). Albany plans to allow surgery by doctors with AIDS virus. *New York Times*, pp. A1, B6.

Sherer, R. (1990). AIDS policy in the 1990s. *Journal of the American Medical Association, 263*(14), 1972–1974.

Shilts, R. (1987). *And the band played on.* New York: St. Martin's Press.

Smeltzer, S. C., & Whipple, B. (1991). Women and HIV infection. *Image, 23*(4), 249–256.

Swanson, J. M., Chenitz, C., Zalor, M., & Stoll, P. (1990). A critical review of human immunodeficiency virus infection and the acquired immunodeficiency syndrome-related research: The knowledge, attitudes and practice of nurses. *Journal of Professional Nursing, 6*(6), 341–355.

Tolchin, M. (1991, July 19). Senate adopts tough measures in health care workers with AIDS. *New York Times*, pp. A1–A14.

U.S. response to youth and AIDS is criticized. (1992, April 12). *New York Times*, p. A2

Wachter, R. M. (1992). AIDS, activism and the politics of health. *New England Journal of Medicine, 326*(2), 128–132.

Walker, R. S. (1991). *AIDS today tomorrow: An introduction to the HIV epidemic in America.* Atlantic Highlands, NJ: Humanities Press.

Weisfeld, V. D. (Ed.). (1991). *AIDS health services at the crossroads: Lessons for community care.* Princeton, NJ: Robert Wood Johnson Foundation.

Winkenwerder, W., Kessler, A. R., & Stolec, R. M. (1989). Federal spending for illness caused by the human immunodeficiency virus. *New England Journal of Medicine, 320*(24), 1598–1603.

AFTERWORD

Suzanne Gordon

I recently addressed a nursing conference about the important role nurses play in health care and how they can make their contributions visible to the public. During this session we discussed how nurses present themselves to patients and negotiate the charged, hierarchical, status-laden relationships with physicians. Whether they call physicians by their last name and title and allow physicians to call them by their first names in front of patients was a part of the conversation. As the nurses talked about their care of very sick patients in hospitals and other settings, one of them waved her hand. She proudly announced how she had solved the problem of self-presentation. "I now view my patients as my business partners," she exclaimed.

I had long been hearing nurses and many of their professional organizations refer to even the sickest patients as "consumers" or "customers." But I had not heard the caregiver–cared-for relationship recast in such stark business terms before.

This was, however, only the beginning. The following week at another conference I attended a community-health nurse raised her concerns about the invasion of market rhetoric and practice into health care. She reported that the administrators of her clinic would no longer permit their nurses to see patients on a one-to-one basis. When nurses argued for the primacy of the nurse-patient relationship, administrators—some of them nurses—accused them of being "power hungry." The administrators informed the staff that they needed to reconceptualize their mission and think of their patients not simply as "customers" but as "producers of health."

And last, but certainly not least, I talked recently with a nurse practitioner who directs a nurse-run health center. This nurse described the types of well-insured "clients" the center cares for and detailed the many managed care contracts the center had been able to secure. When I asked whether the center cared for any of the underserved populations NPs traditionally have served, the nurse retorted haughtily, "We don't have to take the *leftovers* any more. We don't have to do the typical nurse thing and take whatever they give us and smile."

These anecdotes illustrate the depth and breadth of the revolution taking place in our health care system. Whether it is in a hospital or clinic, doctor's office, community center for the homeless, or at home, the market not only is revolutionizing the financing and delivery of health care but also reshaping our cultural imagination and redefining the mission of those who provide care and the identities of those to whom that care is provided.

In discussions about health care today, clinicians and policy makers alike routinely refer to the sickest patients as "clients," "consumers," "customers," "cost centers," or "business partners and producers of health." Insurers and employers trade in "covered lives," while hospital administrators develop obstetrical, surgical, or orthopedic "product lines." People who cannot pay their own way become the "leftovers." Hands-on caregivers are metamorphosed into "providers," "case managers," "utilization reviewers," and "business partners." Dollars spent on care are considered the "medical loss ratio." Money siphoned away from the bedside and into the pockets of CEOs and shareholders is viewed as the "premium paid for cost saving" by "society," which is also conveniently redefined—as "insurers and employers."

In nursing—and in this book—there is division on the wisdom of this transformation. Some of the contributors to this book, like other market advocates, consider this an extraordinary opportunity. Many advocates of turning our health care system into another market apparently believe that market-driven health care will wring the waste out of a profligate fee-for-service system, discipline undisciplined doctors and hospitals, and standardize care. They insist this will save money, improve quality, and liberate patients from medical paternalism. Metamorphosed into "customers and consumers," patients will have more choice and, of course, like all customers, always be considered right.

As for nurses, the market promise is also alluring. Many believe the market will help them loosen the medical yoke and find great new opportunities. Inside the hospital they will become acute care nurse practitioners who take over the work of medical residents. In other types of advanced practice, nurses will have far more autonomy. In home care, they will escape the stifling hospital hierarchy and exert more control over their practice. Wherever they practice, if they are managers of care—as one consultant once put it—they will be liberated to move to a higher stage of nursing. Many believe that these changes will bring the profession the societal credibility and legitimacy that nurses have long sought and that too often has eluded them.

I wish I could share this enthusiasm. From literally hundreds of conversations with nurses, physicians, social workers, psychologists, and—most importantly, from discussions with their patients—I have come to believe market health care poses a grave challenge not only to nurses but also to the very project of caregiving in our society. While I have always believed that the fee-for-service system was extremely wasteful and that our obsessive focus on the work of physicians has blinded us to the importance of others who work in the health care system, it

has also been clear that the traditional medical system contained at least some social space for caregiving.

Although that space was radically constricted, nurses—as long as they did not get too uppity and demand too much of a voice in their institutions or in the larger system—could create, implement, and refine theories and models of care that were of great benefit to patients and professionals alike. After a long and hard fight, palliative care practitioners could take care of at least a small percentage of the dying. Home care nurses and physicians could—again with greatly reduced resources—deliver excellent quality of care in the home with a minimum of intrusion. Physicians in private practice who were content to make a living rather than a killing could do the moral thing and provide time, attention, and appropriate treatment and care to their patients. Medicare was able to give some security to the elderly.

In our employment-based, private benefit system, employers with health plans and the insurance companies have always had more say than covered employees about what health care was provided. Although they also drained far too many resources from the system and were intrusive and wasteful, they never tried to exert control over the health care delivery system in its entirety. And while the system certainly exhibited enormous confusion about its ultimate mission—whether its goal was to make a few physicians, administrators, entrepreneurs and CEOs rich or to deliver a fundamental social good—American health care was at least partially grounded in a service ethic.

Today I fear that the social space and imagination for caregiving is rapidly eroding. At the end of this valuable collection about health care, it seems appropriate to spend a moment reflecting on the moral meaning and material consequences of turning health care into a market.

When compared with health care systems in other industrialized nations, the American health care system has always been deeply influenced by profit. Physicians in this country have earned far more than those in any other. American health care has also provided a lucrative avenue for pharmaceutical and medical equipment companies, for-profit hospital chains, a nursing home industry dominated by for-profit companies, and for-profit home care agencies. But today the health care system is moving from one characterized by pockets of profits to an almost entirely profit-driven system.

We must all remember that the CEOs and boards of directors of for-profit companies have a legal responsibility to protect the interests of their shareholders, not their patients or customers. They are legally obligated to maximize the return on their shareholders investments. This focus on short-term profit maximization has produced health care companies that waste millions on CEO salaries, micromanagement of clinician practice, and advertising and marketing.

In the United States one has only to visit a physician's office or open the daily paper to see evidence of this trend. Two decades ago an American physician might have had a secretary and a nurse working for him or her. Today the average physician practice employs a veritable platoon of clerical workers who spend their days trying to figure out which health plan demands which form and information, which drugs the patient can be prescribed (depending on the managed care organization's [MCO's] drug formulary), whether the patient can go to the emergency room, whether he or she can see a specialist and which one, how many days the patient can spend in the hospital, how much home care or other clinical services the patient is permitted, and when the doctor will be paid.

Similarly, as MCOs, hospitals, and other health care institutions vie for employer dollars, the amount of money spent on advertising in the media has increased exponentially. Today it is hard to open up a newspaper without seeing several full page advertisements promising that this or that managed care company truly cares for patients. These advertisements may cost as much $75,000 for a full-page in a paper like the *New York Times* and up to hundreds of thousands for a television spot during prime time.

It is difficult to understand how spending more money on advertising, marketing, and administration will enhance patient care.

That is why any moral reflection on health care must also include a critical consideration of another of its central tenets—that sick patients are in fact consumers, customers, business partners, or producers of health and that this transformation will give them greater choice as it liberates them from medical paternalism.

Think about it for a moment. What this reconceptualization of the patient does is transforms the sick people who depend on the services of hospitals and other health care institutions into customers strolling through the shopping mall. These newly informed assertive consumers are supposed to protect themselves from harm and fight for better care when they need it.

Unfortunately this kind of market thinking is incapable of drawing distinctions between those users of the health care system who are sick and vulnerable and those who are healthy and essentially require few services and little care. It ignores the fact that many patients are too vulnerable, anxious, frightened, isolated, old, and simply too sick and exhausted to protect their own interests. Many do not have family members to help them. Those who do may find that family members are also too anxious themselves to fight for better care for a loved one. This is why, until recently at least, the ethic of health care was that first articulated by Hippocrates and then reaffirmed by Florence Nightingale—"first do no harm," not the motto of the marketplace, which is "caveat emptor," "let the buyer beware."

Placing responsibility on the consumer rather than on the caregiver also explains another contemporary phenomenon. In a market-driven system grounded in competition to cut costs rather than in the enhancement of quality, compassion, collaboration, and access, much of the burden of the care of the sick is increasingly being shifted onto the shoulders of ill-prepared family members. These informal caregivers are now asked to act as surrogates for busy nurses in the hospital. And they are forced to replace the nurse when patients are inappropriately discharged to the home.

But when it comes to both access and quality, the most significant problem of a market-driven system is the following: whatever costs are saved are not channeled back into the health care system in improvements in quality and access, research and teaching, but into the pockets of CEOs and shareholders. This is all too evident in one startling fact: the number of uninsured Americans is skyrocketing. In 1996, 42 million Americans were uninsured at any one time in the United States.

Market-driven health care is an enormously appealing ideology. Because of the successes of public health and biomedical innovation and because of the cost of technology, health costs are escalating in industrialized countries. Enter the notion of the efficient, self-regulating market that promises to "manage care" and give employers and insurers a way to get a handle on out-of-control expenditures. Market categories also provide a way for business people and politicians—who have no experience in caring for the sick and who view that entire enterprise, as one California businessman recently expressed it, as "infuriatingly unpredictable,"—to control the *experience* of health care.

Managed care offers decision makers a way of reconceptualizing health care through its pre-assigned lengths of hospital stays, its micromanagement of clinical practice through a mazelike system of prior approvals, its imposition of industrial models of care like critical pathways and clinical guidelines that promise standardization of treatment, and its redefinition of the patient as customer. The infuriatingly unpredictable world of the sick and vulnerable suddenly becomes reassuringly familiar as patients are turned into predictable units of production, health into a product, and caregivers into business people, managers, and sales or customer service staff. In an era when market ideology is on the ascendancy and private interests and political representatives are trying to turn the entire world into one interconnected

global marketplace, it is comforting to believe that one can find a final solution to the intractable realities of human infirmity, vulnerability, and mortality.

This is also what makes the ideology of market health care so appealing to ordinary citizens. In the latest version of our longstanding societal exercise in the denial of human vulnerability and mortality, patients become customers. They can thus fantasize that they will be in control even at their most vulnerable, out-of-control moments. It is hard to imagine a more reassuring myth.

Finally, for many nurses the language and ideology of managed care represent a conflict-free way out of some perennial nursing dilemmas. The promise of shifting care from the hospital to home and community suggests that nurses too will be liberated—from the yoke of medicine and its hierarchical definitions of status and importance—all of which were sheltered and reproduced in the hospital. Dramatic changes in health care have also given nurse educators an opening to promote advanced practice nursing as a way to deal with nurses' need for better education. Those nurses who have moved into consulting and some entrepreneurial roles because of hospital restructuring and the shift to managed care find lucrative new business opportunities. Others who have found employment in MCOs in utilization review now believe they have turned the tables: where once doctors controlled nurses' practice, nurses are now saying no to the doctor. To those who are now "managing" the care that others who are paid less actually deliver, it may seem that nurses have finally been elevated to a higher plane. Some believe that they have escaped negative societal stereotypes of bedpan emptiers, pillow fluffers, and physician handmaidens and finally gained social legitimacy.

But when it comes to market-driven health care the question nurses must ask is who is really in charge? Have nurses finally gotten control of their practice or have they simply exchanged one hierarchy for another? Have they discarded the role of physician handmaiden only to become HMO handmaidens?

To truly support caregiving I believe we must all think critically about and ultimately reject the attempt to turn health care into just another market and fight to preserve and expand the social space for caring. We must all struggle for the creation of comprehensive, universal health care. Some form of tax-supported universal health care is more than a practical necessity. It is a moral imperative. In the United States we can no longer tolerate a health care system that turns the rich against the poor, the young against the old, the sick against the well—and now in the age of the human genome project—the potentially sick against the potentially well. We must insist on a health care system that acknowledges our common vulnerability and mortality and that pools our social resources so that we can effectively care for each other.

To face the market assault on caregiving and to cope with the traditional devaluation of nurses' work, nurses must become more vocal about the importance of their work and more assertive in sharing their insights into the meaning of caregiving with the public. Market health care's definition of both patients and caregivers is grounded in the invisibility of nursing and the societal devaluation of caregiving and women's work. Only those who have never cared for the sick, who are determined to live in denial of human vulnerability and mortality—or who have distanced themselves from the experience and realities of illness—can perform the mental alchemy necessary to turn vulnerable people into customers strolling through a shopping mall. And only the concerted efforts of caregivers and those they care for can reverse a global process that is threatening to eliminate any social space for caregiving. By working together, I believe we can not only protect the social space for caregiving but also expand it and in the process create a genuine health care system in America.

This book will help nurses do just that. By educating nurses about the crucial issues in health care, it will give them the information essential to informed action. And by encouraging nurses to think critically about what is happening in health care it will help them clarify their own views. To care for patients, nurses have to know not only how to care for the sick patient in the bed but also how to care for a sick health care system. This important book will help to initiate the type of critical dialogue that nurses must then promote in their own workplaces, in their professional organizations, in their communities, and in the nation at large. It is only through advancing that dialogue that we will advance the practice of caregiving. Or as Florence Nightingale put it in 1887, in her book *Notes on Hospitals,* "If we were perfect, no doubt an absolute hierarchy would be the best kind of government for all institutions. But, in our imperfect state of conscience and enlightenment, publicity, and the collision from publicity, are the best guardians of the interests of the sick."

Appendix A

INTERNSHIPS IN POLICY AND POLITICS

JEFFREY P. O'DONNELL

For those interested in pursuing educational experiences in health-related public policy, presented below is a list of public policy internships and fellowships. Included is information on the type, purpose, eligibility criteria, and duration for each program. Financial data have been provided on the basis of the best available information at the time of printing. Address, telephone number, and Universal Resource Locator (URL) to access the program's Internet site have been provided wherever possible.

NAME OF PROGRAM	TYPE	PURPOSE	ELIGIBILITY	FINANCIAL DATA	DURATION	APPLICATION REQUESTS
American Fellowships	Support women doctoral candidates writing their dissertations and scholars seeking postdoctoral/research leave funds.	To offset a scholar's living expenses while she completes her dissertation. Education is the key to achieving equity for women of all ages, races, creeds, and nationalities.	One-year postdoctoral/research leave fellowships for women who will have earned a doctorate by Nov. 15. Dissertation fellowships for women who will complete their dissertations between July 1 and June 30.	One-year postdoctoral/research leave fellowship stipend $27,000; dissertation fellowship stipend $14,500	July 1 to June 30	AAUW Educational Foundation Department 60 2201 N. Dodge St. Iowa City, IA 52243-4030 (319) 337-1716, ext. 60. URL: *www.aauw. org/3000/ fdnfelgra.html*

| Brookings Institution Fellowships
—Economic Studies
—Foreign Policy Studies
—Governmental Studies | Resident fellowships for policy-oriented predoctoral research in economic, foreign policy, and governmental studies during the coming academic year. | Fellowships are designed for doctoral candidates whose dissertation topics are directly related to public policy issues and thus to the major interests of the Institution. | A graduate department must nominate candidates; sponsorship by individual faculty members cannot substitute for the formal designation of the department. | Fellowships carry a stipend of $15,000, payable on a 12-month basis. Supplementary assistance will be provided for copying and other essential research requirements in an amount not to exceed $600, reimbursement for transportation, up to $500, for research-related travel, plus some access to computer facilities. | Eleven months of research in residence at Brookings and 1 month of vacation | The Brookings Institution 1775 Massachusetts Ave., NW Washington, DC 20036-2188 (202) 797-6000 URL: *www.brook. edu/pa/int/el/ fellow.htm* |

Table continued on following page

NAME OF PROGRAM	TYPE	PURPOSE	ELIGIBILITY	FINANCIAL DATA	DURATION	APPLICATION REQUESTS
Carter Center Internship Program	Internship program designed for those who wish to combine academic study with practical application and experience. Interns participate in Center projects and conduct research under the guidance of academic fellows and project staff.	Offers unique and diverse opportunities for undergraduate, graduate, and professional students who are interested in contemporary international and domestic issues.	Offered throughout the year to students who have demonstrated superior academic ability and who have course work, professional or personal experience, and career interests related to Carter Center programs.	Financial support is not provided for internships. A summer graduate assistantship program, open to graduate and professional school students, does provide grants. Housing is not provided for interns, though information about the residential areas surrounding the Center and apartment finder service numbers are available.	Most interns commit to a minimum of 15 hours per week for at least one semester. Many interns are encouraged to extend their internship	Internship Coordinator The Carter Center One Copenhill 453 Freedom Parkway Atlanta, GA 30307 (404) 420-5151 URL: *www.emory. edu/CARTER CENTER/ intern.htm*

| Congressional Black Caucus Foundation (CBCF) Congressional Fellows Program | Provide students with financial resources; create opportunities for minority students to obtain a college education; and enhance their political education and exposure to the legislative process. | The goal of the CBCF Fellows Program is twofold: to offer talented men and women the opportunity to work on Congressional committees and learn all aspects of the legislative process; and to provide scholarly research on critical issues before Congress. | Open to individuals who are full-time graduate or law students, professionals with five or more years of experience who are pursuing part-time graduate studies, or college faculty members who have an interest in the legislative policy-making process; must be U.S. citizens. | CBCF Fellows will receive compensation in the amount of $15,000. Fellows are responsible for their own travel arrangements, expenses, and housing. | All Fellows must serve for the 9 months of the academic year. | Congressional Black Caucus Foundation 1004 Pennsylvania Ave., SE Washington, DC 20003 (202) 675-6730 |

Table continued on following page

NAME OF PROGRAM	TYPE	PURPOSE	ELIGIBILITY	FINANCIAL DATA	DURATION	APPLICATION REQUESTS
Congressional Hispanic Caucus Institute Fellowships and Edward R. Roybal Fellowship	Open to candidates pursuing careers in any field of public policy, such as economics, education, international affairs, journalism, and law. Edward Roybal Health Fellowship is offered specifically to individuals specializing in public health administration.	Through in-depth discussions of public policy, presentations by Members of Congress, policy experts, and professional and leadership skills workshops, the meetings offer participants concrete opportunities to find their own niche and strategies to accomplish their personal goals.	Recent college graduates (within 1 year of graduation) and currently enrolled graduate students interested in pursuing careers in public policy. Applicants must demonstrate active community involvement and participation through public service, excellent communication and analytical skills, an interest in pursuing a career in public policy, and a cumulative GPA of 3.0+ on a 4.0 scale.	Round-trip transportation to and from Washington, D.C., within the United States, health insurance coverage, and a monthly stipend.	Program runs from September to May.	Congressional Hispanic Caucus Institute 504 C St., NE Washington, DC 20002 (202) 543-1771 (800) EXCEL-DC (800) 392-3532 URL: *www.chci.org/ fellows2.htm*

Congressional Research Grants Program	Funds the study of research projects about Congress, particularly leadership in Congress and such public policy areas as energy, environment, trade, taxation, and regulation.	To foster study of Congress in order to enhance public understanding and appreciation of the legislative branch of the federal government.	No special requirements.	Ranges from $250 to $3,500 per award.	Program runs 1 year.	The Everett McKinley Dirksen Congressional Leadership Research Center 301 S. Fourth St. Pekin, IL 61554 (309) 347-7113 URL: *www.pekin. net/dirksen/ index.html*

Table continued on following page

Name of Program	Type	Purpose	Eligibility	Financial Data	Duration	Application Requests
Congressional Science and Engineering Fellows Program	Fellows spend 1 year working as special assistants in legislative areas requiring scientific and technical input for the staffs of Members of Congress or Congressional committees. Fellows are integrated into the staff and often must apply their science broadly. Committee assignments may provide an opportunity to focus more specifically on a scientific or technical legislative area of interest.	To provide a unique public policy learning experience, to demonstrate the value of science-government interaction, and to make practical contributions to the more effective use of scientific and technical knowledge in government.	Applicants must have a Ph.D. or equivalent doctoral-level degree at the time of application (January), but persons with a master's degree in engineering and at least 3 years of postdegree work experience may apply. All applicants must be U.S. citizens. Applications for the fellowships are invited from candidates in any physical, biological, or social science or any field of engineering. It is acceptable to apply to more than one society. Stipends, application procedures, timetable, and deadlines vary.	Provides $43,000, plus an allowance for relocation and travel expenses.	Fellowship year begins in September.	American Association for the Advancement of Science (AAAS) 1200 New York Ave. NW Washington, DC 20005 (202) 326-6600 URL: *www.aaas. org/spp/ dspp/stg/ COVER.HTM* Note: AAAS selects and funds two of its own Fellows, and runs an umbrella program for the Fellows selected and funded by other national scientific and engineering societies.

Coro Fellows Program in Public Affairs	Programs immerse participants in the many facets of society to study the intricate relationships among organizations and social systems. Participants experience at first hand the breadth, complexity, and pressures of public affairs, developing tools to become tomorrow's leaders.	To strengthen the democratic process by preparing individuals for effective and ethical leadership in the public arena.	Seeks bright, self-motivated risk takers as candidates for the Fellows Program. The strongest applicants are those who have demonstrated leadership ability, integrity and a commitment to public service. A bachelor's degree or equivalent experience is required, and postgraduate academic and/or work experience is desirable. Successful candidates have been active in civic or campus activities.	Tuition for the Fellows Program is $3500. Deferred payment plans are available. Financial stipends are available, on the basis of financial need, to assist with living expenses. Financial assistance is intended to assist with living and program-related expenses.	Program runs 9 months.	Coro Centers URL: *www.coro.org/* 44 Wall St., 21st Floor New York, NY 10005 (212) 248-2935 1730 S. 11th St., Suite 102 St. Louis, MO 63104 (314) 621-3040 811 Wilshire Blvd., Suite 1025 Los Angeles, CA 90017-2624 (213) 623-1234 690 Market St., Suite 1100 San Francisco, California 94104 (415) 986-0521

Table continued on following page

Name of Program	Type	Purpose	Eligibility	Financial Data	Duration	Application Requests
Employee Benefit Research Institute (EBRI) Fellows	Fellows program is designed to aid the institute in carrying out its mission of research and education. It allows individuals from the government, private sector, academia, and media to undertake projects on health, retirement, and other economic security issues.	To build a closer alliance between academics interested in employee benefits and economic security policy and the researchers at EBRI, its sponsors, and its wider constituency in the government, the media, and the private sector.	Must have a demonstrated knowledge and expertise in the employee benefits field based on an accomplished career in academia, government, the media, or the private sector. Applicants must be able to apply quantitative or practical skills to relevant public policy questions.	Varies according to type of Fellow	Varies according to type of Fellow	Employee Benefit Research Institute Fellows Program 2121 K St., NW Suite 600 Washington, DC 20037-1896 (202) 659-0670 URL: *www.ebri.org/ ebrifel.htm*

John Heinz Senate Fellowship Program	Fellow will be in a position to be active in developing legislative proposals, attend hearings, participate in conferences, and brief legislators for committee sessions and floor debates.	To develop the knowledge and leadership capabilities of applicants by providing professional first-hand experience in issues that affect children and/or the aging. Children's issues will be the focus in odd-numbered years, and seniors in even-numbered years.	Must already be active in the appropriate interest area and must display the potential for future contributions to that area after a year of hands-on experience as a Fellow.	Fellows will be paid annual stipends not to exceed $53,300, plus standard federal government benefits options.	Duties will commence each September and end the following August.	Heinz Family Foundation 3200 CNG Tower Pittsburgh, PA 15222 (412) 497-5775

Table continued on following page

NAME OF PROGRAM	TYPE	PURPOSE	ELIGIBILITY	FINANCIAL DATA	DURATION	APPLICATION REQUESTS
Judicial Fellows Program	One-year fellowship beginning September 1	Unique opportunity for a select group of young professionals for creative work and broad first-hand experience in judicial administration.	Candidates should have one or more postgraduate degrees and at least 2 years of professional experience.	Negotiable on the basis of education, experience, and salary history of fellow; not to exceed GS 15, step 3 level, presently $78,857.	Program runs 1 year; exact duration mutually agreed on between fellow and executive director.	Supreme Court of the United States Executive Director 1 First St., NE, Room 5 Washington, DC 20543 (202) 479-3374
Kellogg National Fellowship Program	Program designed for individuals in the early years of their professional careers. Fellows spend 25% of their time on fellowship-related activities, including a self-designed learning plan for personal and professional development.	Basically, to assist future leaders in developing skills and competencies that transcend traditional disciplinary and professional methods of addressing problems.	U.S. citizens able to take part in all program activities and able to schedule 25% release time to complete individual interdisciplinary learning activities.	Fellows may receive a stipend of up to $32,000 for the 3 years, according to the type and tax status of their employer.	Program runs 3 years.	Kellogg National Fellowship Program W. K. Kellogg Foundation PO Box 5196 Battle Creek, MI 49016 (800) 819-9997

Table continued on following page

Program	Description	Purpose	Primary criterion	Fee/Expenses	Dates	Contact
Morris K. Udall Scholarship Program	Awards scholarships to undergraduate students, and dissertation fellowships to doctoral candidates whose dissertation is in the area of environmental public policy and conflict resolution.	To preserve and protect the national heritage by the recruitment and preparation of individuals skilled in effective environmental public policy conflict resolution.	Primary criterion for fellowship awards is scholarly excellence. Dissertation fellowship applicant must be U.S. citizen or permanent resident. Fellowships are open to scholars in the area of environmental public policy and conflict resolution.	Dissertation fellowships are intended to cover both academic and living expenses. Fellowships carry a stipend of a maximum of $24,000.	Fellowship year begins July 1.	Morris K. Udall Scholarship and Excellence in National Environmental Policy Program 2201 North Dodge St. PO Box 4030 Iowa City, IA 52243 URL: *www.act.org/udall/udisser.html*
*Nurse in Washington Internship (NIWI)**	Program speakers from federal agencies, special interest groups, congressional staffs, and knowledgeable insiders will discuss their role in the development, implementation, and monitoring of health policy.	To provide information on current health policy initiatives and describe how health policy develops and how programs are funded.	Registered nurses and student nurses interested in better understanding health policy and the legislative/regulatory processes.	Registration fee $595 for NFSNO members, $695 for nonmembers. Recipient must assume responsibility for any travel, hotel, and incidental expenses.	Program runs 4 days in March.	National Federation for Specialty Nursing Organizations East Holly Ave. Box 56 Pitman, NJ 08071 (609) 256-2333 URL: *www.awhonn.org/intern.htm*

*The editors, contributors, and publisher of this book sponsor an annual NIWI "Policy and Politics Scholarship."

Name of Program	Type	Purpose	Eligibility	Financial Data	Duration	Application Requests
Open Society Institute: Individual Project Fellowships	For individuals pursuing research, writing, or other efforts to promote an open society in the United States or internationally.	To deal with criminal justice; access to the courts and legal services; drug policy; death and dying; education; immigration and civic identity; professional and ethical conduct in law, medicine, and journalism; political participation; and reproductive health and teenage pregnancy.	Ascertain the significance of the contribution that the project will make by providing new information, perspectives, or valuable public discourse on issues of importance to the promotion of an open society. The qualifications of the applicant will be relative to the project goals, and implementation requirements will relate to the soundness of the implementation plan.	Range from $15,000 to $100,000. Renewals will be in the same range.	Awarded for a term of up to 18 months and may be renewed for up to another 18 months.	Open Society Institute 400 West 59th St. New York, NY 10019 (212) 887-0187 URL: *www.soros.org*

President's Commission on White House Fellowships	White House Fellows spend a year as full-time paid assistants to senior White House staff, the Vice President, Cabinet officers, and other top-ranking government officials.	Engagement in the work of the federal government lies at the center of the White House Fellowships. Work assignments can bring broad access and ever-changing issues and challenges, but also long hours and unglamorous chores requiring as much perseverance as ability. Fellowship's education program augments and amplifies the work experience.	U.S. citizens only. Employees of the federal government are not eligible for the program, with the exception of career military personnel. No formal educational requirements or age restrictions; however, the fellowship program was created to give young men and women the experience of government service early in their careers.	Fellows receive a salary and benefits from the agency where they work. Salary is paid at the federal pay grade GS-14, step 3 (approximately $66,000).	Fellowship year runs from September 1 to August 31.	President's Commission on White House Fellowships 712 Jackson Place, NW Washington, DC 20503 (202) 395-4522 URL: *www. whitehouse. gov/WH Fellows/*

Table continued on following page

NAME OF PROGRAM	TYPE	PURPOSE	ELIGIBILITY	FINANCIAL DATA	DURATION	APPLICATION REQUESTS
Public Policy and International Affairs Fellowship Program	Programs offer the analytical, quantitative, linguistic, and communications skills needed for the twenty-first century.	To recruit and empower a new generation of culturally diverse and dedicated public servants. Targets the segment of the U.S. population that will constitute the majority of new workers hired in the new millennium—people of color.	U.S. citizens or permanent residents; people of color historically underrepresented in public policy and international affairs, including African Americans, Asian Americans, Pacific Islanders, Hispanic Americans, Alaska Natives, or Native Americans; and persons demonstrating a strong interest in public policy and/or international affairs.	Provides $15,000 in funding.	Study period of 2 years.	Public Policy and International Affairs at the Academy for Educational Development 1875 Connecticut Ave., NW Washington, DC 20009-1202 (800) 613-PPIA (7742) (202) 884-8632 URL: *www.aed.org/ppia/*

Robert Wood Johnson Health Policy Fellows	Fellows have an extensive orientation, which brings them into contact with key policy leaders in the nation's capital and prepares them for their 9-month work assignments with members of Congress or the Executive Branch.	To provide a better understanding of major issues in health policy and insight into how federal health programs are established.	Faculty member at an academic health center or a college or university with a medical school. Candidates for the fellowship program must be nominated by the chief executive officer of their home institution.	Annual stipend equal to salary before entering the program, up to $45,000.	Fellowship runs 1 year.	Robert Wood Johnson Health Policy Fellows Institute of Medicine National Academy of Sciences Marion Ein Lewin 2101 Constitution Ave. Washington, DC 20418 (202) 334-1506 URL: *www.rwjf.org/*
Women in Leadership	Provides an in-depth exposure to and an understanding of the variety and complexity of public policy. Participants gain significant insights into six major sectors of public affairs arena: business, labor, community organizations, political campaigns, government, and media.	To help participants improve on the skills necessary to compete in today's challenging public environment.	Women, salaried or volunteer, who are committed to achieving personal, career, and community involvement goals are strongly encouraged to apply. Applicants reflect a rich diversity of background and experiences.	Tuition for the program is $950.00 not including a nonrefundable application fee of $35.00. A limited number of need-based tuition scholarships are available.	Part-time program runs 6 months.	Coro Midwestern Center 1730 S. 11th St., Suite 102 St. Louis, MO 63104 (314) 621-3040 URL: *www.coro.org/stl/*

Table continued on following page

Name of Program	Type	Purpose	Eligibility	Financial Data	Duration	Application Requests
Women's Law and Public Policy Fellowship Program	Fellows are supervised by attorneys at different organizations, including women's rights groups, civil rights groups, Congressional offices, government agencies, and the Georgetown University Law Center Sex Discrimination Clinic, and they are required to work exclusively on women's rights issues.	To enable law graduates with a special interest in women's rights to work in the nation's capital on legal and policy issues affecting women.	Law graduates interested in spending 1 year working on women's rights issues in the Washington, D.C. area.	Provides $28,000 stipend and health insurance.	Program runs 1 year.	Women's Law and Public Policy Fellowship Program 600 New Jersey Ave., NW, Suite 334 Washington, DC 20001 (202) 662-9650
Women's Research & Education Institute–Congressional Fellowships on Women and Public Policy	A Fellow works 30 hours per week as a legislative aide on policy issues affecting women.	To train women to analyze and shape public policy.	Available to scholars who are currently enrolled in a graduate school or professional degree program at an accredited institution in the United States.	Carries a living stipend of $9,500, $500 for the purchase of health insurance, and up to $1,500 for tuition remission.	Fellowship runs from August to April	Congressional Fellowship Program Women's Research and Education Institute 1750 New York Ave., NW, Suite 350 Washington, DC 20006

Woodrow Wilson Dissertation Grants in Women's Studies	Fifteen awards will be made with the support of the Philip Morris Companies, Inc., and other donors. Awards will be made in mid-February.	To encourage original and significant research about women on such topics as the evolution of women's role in society, women in history, the psychology of women, and women as seen in literature and art.	Students in doctoral programs who have completed all predissertation requirements in any field of study at graduate schools in the United States. Candidates must have completed all predissertation requirements including approval of the dissertation prospectus by October 31 and must expect to complete their dissertations by the summer.	Grants of $1,500 are awarded to be used for expenses connected with the dissertation. These may include, but are not limited to, travel, books, microfilming, taping, and computer services. Special grants of $2,000 each are available for dissertations regarding women's health.	One-time grant.	The Woodrow Wilson National Fellowship CN 5281 Princeton, NJ 08543-5281 (609) 452-7007 URL: *www.woodrow. org/programs/ fellowships/*

Appendix *B*

POLITICAL ACTIVITY AND GOVERNMENT-EMPLOYED NURSES

Mary Chaffee

The U.S. Government restricts the type of political activity that government-employed nurses, as well as other employees, may participate in. This policy may appear to be a restriction of political freedom and the right to free speech, but the limits serve as a means of protecting the employee from coercion. Nearly 60,000 nurses nationwide are subject to these restrictions.

Two major regulations affect the political behavior of government-employed nurses. First, the Hatch Act limits the political activity of civilian nurses serving in a variety of government agencies, including the Veterans Administration, the Department of State, the U.S. Public Health Service, and the civil service system. Second, a Department of Defense regulation limits the political activity of nurses who serve on active duty in the army, navy, and air force.

THE HATCH ACT

The Act to Prevent Pernicious Political Activities, more commonly known as the Hatch Act, was passed in 1939. Because the original Hatch Act was extremely restrictive, multiple attempts have been made to amend the legislation and

loosen restrictions. In 1993 President Clinton signed Hatch Act reform into law. The translation of the amendment into specific regulations was published by the Office of Personnel Management (OPM) in the July 5, 1996, *Federal Register.*

Who is affected by the Hatch Act? Nurses employed by the federal government in any status (full-time, part-time, permanent, or temporary) are subject to restrictions on political activity. Nurses covered by the Hatch Act include the following:

1. Federal employees
2. District of Columbia employees
3. Employees of state or local agencies in programs funded by the federal government
4. Commissioned officers in the U.S. Public Health Service

Why are Hatch Act restrictions in place? The political activity of government employees is restricted to protect the employee from coercion by corrupt politicians and political organizations. In the 1930s a Senate panel discovered that certain federal employees had been coerced to support specific political candidates in order to keep their jobs. As a result, Senator Carl Hatch, of New Mexico, introduced legislation that was enacted in 1939 to end this practice. Senator Hatch also feared the development of a giant national political machine of federal employees following the directions of their employers. Additionally, the Hatch Act maintains the political neutrality of government offices.

The views expressed in this article are those of the author and do not reflect the official policy or position of the Department of the Navy, the Department of Defense, nor the U.S. Government.

How does the Hatch Act affect a nurse's political activity? For nurses covered by the Hatch Act, a wider range of political activities is now possible because of Hatch Act reform, with some specific restrictions.

*Nurses covered by the Hatch Act **may:***

- Register to vote, and vote as desired
- Assist in voter registration drives
- Express opinions about candidates and issues
- Contribute money to political organizations
- Attend political fund-raising functions
- Attend and be active at political rallies and meetings
- Join and be an active member of a political party or club
- Sign nominating petitions
- Campaign for or against referendum questions, constitutional amendments, or municipal ordinances
- Campaign for or against candidates in partisan (political party affiliated) elections
- Be a candidate for public office in nonpartisan elections
- Make campaign speeches for candidates in partisan elections, as long as the speech does not contain an appeal for political contributions
- Distribute campaign literature in partisan elections
- Help organize a fund-raising event, as long as the employee does not solicit or accept political contributions
- Display a partisan bumper sticker on a private automobile used occasionally for official business
- Contribute to a political action committee through a payroll deduction plan

*Nurses covered by the Hatch Act **may not:***

- Solicit, accept, or receive political contributions from the general public
- Coerce other employees to make a political contribution
- Become personally identified with a fund-raising activity
- Participate, even anonymously, in phone-bank solicitations for political contributions
- Solicit political contributions in campaign speeches
- Display partisan buttons, posters, or similar items on federal premises, on duty, or in uniform
- Participate in partisan political activity while:
  - On duty
  - Wearing an official uniform
  - Using a government vehicle
  - In a government office
- Sign a campaign letter that solicits political contributions
- Use official authority or influence to interfere with an election
- Solicit or discourage political activity of anyone with business before their agency
- Be a candidate for public office in a partisan election

Although Hatch Act reform has resulted in greater opportunity for political participation, handling political contributions remains off limits. Personally accepting, soliciting, or receiving political contributions is not permitted under current regulations.

Who enforces the Hatch Act? The U.S. Office of Special Counsel (OSC) is an independent federal agency charged with enforcing the Hatch Act and several other federal laws. Headquartered in Washington, D.C., the OSC investigates and, when warranted, prosecutes violations before the Merit Systems Protection Board.

The OSC also provides advisory opinions to anyone seeking advice about political activity and the Hatch Act. Advice may be requested in writing or by calling the OSC:

Hatch Act Unit
U.S. Office of Special Counsel
1730 M Street, NW, Suite 300
Washington, DC 20036-4505

Telephone: (800) 854-2824
(202) 653-7143

What are the penalties for violating the Hatch Act? Federal employees who violate the Hatch Act may be punished by removal or by a minimum 30-day suspension without pay. Violations of the Hatch Act applicable to state and local employees are punishable by removal or by forfeiture, by the employer, of an amount equal to up to 2 years of the charged employee's salary. In matters not sufficiently serious to warrant prosecution, the OSC will issue a warning letter to the employee.

DEPARTMENT OF DEFENSE REGULATIONS

Restrictions similar to those in the Hatch Act regulate the political behavior of the 11,520 nurses on active duty in the army, navy, and air force. The "spirit and intent" of Department of Defense Directive 1344.10 prohibits any activity that may be viewed as associating the defense department with a partisan political cause or candidate.

Nurses in the army, navy, or air force **may:**

- Register, vote, and express their personal opinions on political candidates and issues, but not as representatives of the uniformed services
- Encourage other military members to vote, without attempting to influence or interfere with the outcome of an election
- Contribute money to political organizations, parties, or committees favoring a particular candidate
- Attend partisan and nonpartisan political meetings or rallies as spectators, when not in uniform or on duty
- Join a political club and attend meetings, when not in uniform
- Serve as a nonpartisan election official, if:
  - Not in uniform
  - It does not interfere with military duties
  - Approval is provided by their commanding officer
- Sign a petition for legislative action, or to place a candidate's name on a ballot, but in the service member's personal capacity

- Make personal visits to legislators, but not in uniform or as an official representative of their branch of service
- Write a letter to the editor of a newspaper or other periodical expressing personal views on public issues or political candidates
- Display a political bumper sticker on a private vehicle
- If an officer, seek and hold nonpartisan civil office on an independent school board that is located on a military reservation

Nurses in the army, navy, or air force **may not:**

- Use their official authority to influence or interfere with an election
- Solicit votes for a particular candidate or issue
- Require or solicit political contributions from others
- Participate in partisan political management, campaigns, or conventions
- Write or publish partisan articles that solicit votes for or against a party or candidate
- Participate in partisan radio or television shows
- Distribute partisan political literature
- Participate in partisan political parades
- Display large political signs, banners, or posters on a private vehicle
- Use contemptuous words against the President; the Vice President; Congress; the secretaries of defense, transportation, or the military departments; or the governors or legislators of any state or territory where the service member is on duty
- Engage in fund-raising activities for partisan political causes on military property or in federal offices
- Attend partisan political events as an official representative of the uniformed services
- Campaign for, or hold, elective civil office in the federal government, or the government of a state, territory, the District of Columbia, or any political division in those areas

Nurses serving in the military are encouraged to obtain an official opinion from a military lawyer if they are unsure about participating in a specific political activity.

CONCLUSION

American nurses are becoming increasingly active and visible in political and policymaking arenas. Many have translated professional nursing skills into effective political skills. In remarks to the American Nurses Association on June 27, 1997, First Lady Hillary Rodham Clinton congratulated nurses on their accomplishments and told them: "You must continue speaking up and speaking out about the critical health care needs we face. We need your perspective. We need your voices." Government-employed nurses should have their voices heard and may participate actively in the political process. However, it is essential that they be aware of and abide by the laws and regulations designed to offer them a nonpartisan workplace, and protection from coercion.

REFERENCES

American Nurses Association. (1992). The political nurse: Your rights under the Hatch Act. *Capital Update, 10*(1), 4–5.

Hatch Act Reform Amendments of 1993, 5 U.S.C. §§ 7321–7326.

Maze, R. (1996, July 8). Do military officers and politics mix? *Navy Times*, p. 9.

Political activities by members of the armed forces on active duty. Department of Defense Directive 1344.10, June 15, 1990 (with Change 1, dated January 7, 1994).

Shafritz, J. M. (1993). *American government and politics*. New York: HarperCollins.

Un-Hatched for campaign '96. (1996, July 10). *The Washington Post*, p. A15.

Un-Hatched workers practice their politics. (1996, August 26). *The Washington Post*, p. A11.

U.S. Office of Special Counsel Homepage, http://www.access.gpo.gov/osc

Appendix *C*

NURSING'S AGENDA FOR HEALTH CARE REFORM

America's nurses have long supported our nation's efforts to create a health care system that assures access, quality, and services at affordable costs. This document presents nursing's agenda for immediate health care reform. We call for a basic "core" of essential health care services to be available to everyone. We call for a restructured health care system that will focus on the consumers and their health, with services to be delivered in familiar, convenient sites, such as schools, workplaces, and homes. We call for a shift from the predominant focus on illness and cure to an orientation toward wellness and care. The basic components of nursing's "core of care" include:

- A restructured health care system which:
  - Enhances consumer access to services by delivering primary health care in community-based settings.
  - Fosters consumer responsibility for personal health, self care, and informed decision making in selecting health care services.
  - Facilitates utilization of the most cost-effective providers and therapeutic options in the most appropriate settings.
- A federally defined standard package of essential health care services available to all citizens and residents of the United States, provided and financed through an integration of public and private plans and sources:
  - A public plan, based on federal guidelines and eligibility requirements, will provide coverage for the poor and create the opportunity for small businesses and individuals, particularly those at risk because of preexisting conditions and those potentially medically indigent, to buy into the plan.
  - A private plan will offer, at a minimum, the nationally standardized package of essential services. This standard package could be enriched as a benefit of employment, or individuals could purchase additional services if they so choose. If employers do not offer private coverage, they must pay into the public plan for their employees.
- A phase-in of essential services, in order to be fiscally responsible:
  - Coverage of pregnant women and children is critical. This first step represents a cost-effective investment in the future health and prosperity of the nation.
  - One early step will be to design services specifically to assist vulnerable populations who have had limited access to our nation's health care system. A "Healthstart Plan" is proposed to improve the health status of these individuals.
- Planned change to anticipate health service needs that correlate with changing national demographics.
- Steps to reduce health care costs include:
  - Required usage of managed care in the public plan and encouraged in private plans.
  - Incentives for consumers and providers to utilize managed care arrangements.
  - Controlled growth of the health care system through planning and prudent resource allocation.

- Incentives for consumers and providers to be more cost efficient in exercising health care options.
- Development of health care policies based on effectiveness and outcomes research.
- Assurance of direct access to a full range of qualified providers.
- Elimination of unnecessary bureaucratic controls and administrative procedures.
- Case management will be required for those with continuing health care needs. Case management will reduce the fragmentation of the present system, promote consumers' active participation in decisions about their health, and create an advocate on their behalf.
- Provisions for long-term care, which include:
  - Public and private funding for services of short duration to prevent personal impoverishment.
  - Public funding for extended care if consumer resources are exhausted.
  - Emphasis on the consumers' responsibility to financially plan for their long-term care needs, including new personal financial alternatives and strengthened private insurance arrangements.
- Insurance reforms to assure improved access to coverage, including affordable premiums, reinsurance pools for catastrophic coverage, and other steps to protect both insurers and individuals against excessive costs.
- Access to services assured by no payment at the point of service and elimination of balance billing in both public and private plans.
- Establishment of public/private sector review—operating under federal guidelines and including payers, providers, and consumers—to determine resource allocation, cost reduction approaches, allowable insurance premiums, and fair and consistent reimbursement levels for providers. This review would progress in a climate sensitive to ethical issues.

Additional resources will be required to accomplish this plan. While significant dollars can be obtained through restructuring and other strategies, responsibility for any new funds must be shared by individuals, employers, and government, phased in over several years to minimize the impact.

INDEX

Note: Pages in *italic* indicate illustrations; those followed by a t refer to tables.